A CORE CURRICULUM FOR DIABETES EDUCATION

Third Edition

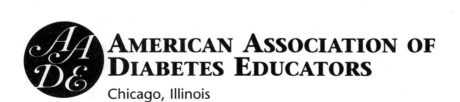

AMERICAN ASSOCIATION OF DIABETES EDUCATORS

Chicago, Illinois

A CORE CURRICULUM FOR DIABETES EDUCATION

Third Edition

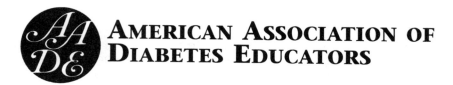

AMERICAN ASSOCIATION OF DIABETES EDUCATORS

Martha Mitchell Funnell, MS, RN, CDE
Cheryl Hunt, RN, MSEd, CDE
Karmeen Kulkarni, RD, MS, CDE
Richard R. Rubin, PhD, CDE
Peggy C. Yarborough, RPh, MS, CDE, FAPP, FASHP

Publisher: Janet Schwarz
Medical Editor: Karen Lloyd
Proofreader: Candace Kurinsky
Compositor: Montronics Corporation

A Core Curriculum for Diabetes Education, 3rd Edition
Published by the American Association of Diabetes Educators

©1998, American Association of Diabetes Educators, Chicago, Illinois.

Addendum to Second Edition
©1996, American Association of Diabetes Educators, Chicago, Illinois.

Second edition
©1993, American Association of Diabetes Educators, Chicago, Illinois.

First edition published under the title *Diabetes Education: A Core Curriculum for Health Professionals*
©1988, American Association of Diabetes Educators.

ISBN 1-881876-04-7

Printed and bound in the United States of America. Printer: Port City Press, Inc.

TABLE OF CONTENTS

Diabetes and the Life Cycle

Complications

Research

Acknowledgements

We are very pleased to present the third edition of The American Association of Diabetes Educators' *A Core Curriculum for Diabetes Education*. This project has truly been a team effort by the editorial group and staff. It would not have been possible without the willingness of many people to share their time, expertise and talents.

I would like to express my very deep appreciation for the considerable efforts and support of the Associate Editors: Cheryl Hunt, Karmeen Kulkarni, Richard Rubin, and Peggy Yarborough. Each of you worked tirelessly with multiple authors and brought a wealth of knowledge and experience to the content and presentation of this material. The publisher, Jan Schwarz and Karen Lloyd, medical editor, worked patiently with us to create a useful and attractive book. I also want to acknowledge Virginia Peragallo-Dittko, Kathryn Godley, Julie Meyer, Diana Guthrie and the other editors of the first and second editions of the Core Curriculum who created much of the design and set such a high standard for this book. I have gained new insight and appreciation for your contributions, and stand in awe of you for them.

I particularly want to thank the authors for sharing their knowledge, and for their responsiveness to deadlines, the editorial team and the reviewers. The quality of this book is a direct reflection of your expertise and your writing ability. I also want to acknowledge and thank the many experts who served as reviewers. Your questions and comments helped to ensure the accuracy and relevance of the content provided.

This book was written for you, the diabetes educator. It is intended to provide the core of information that you need as you work with, teach, and touch the lives of people with diabetes. We hope that you will find it to be a useful resource as you carry out the important and essential work that you do as a diabetes educator.

INTRODUCTION

Diabetes care has changed dramatically since the announcement of the results of the Diabetes Control and Complications Trial in 1993. The increased emphasis on the prevention, early detection, and appropriate treatment for the complications of diabetes, the development of new and more effective therapeutic options, and the focus on early diagnosis and standards of care have served to improve the quality of life for people with diabetes.

Diabetes education has also changed. The role of the person with diabetes as the primary decision maker and the role of a healthcare team to support these efforts has become increasingly recognized and emphasized. The importance of diabetes self-management education for informed choice and self-directed decision making and the emphasis on outcomes has resulted in the development and implementation of new strategies and teaching methods.

We can anticipate that the number of effective treatments and educational strategies will only increase as the attention given to diabetes care and education is reflected in research efforts. As diabetes educators, our role is not only to understand the implications of diabetes treatment and outcomes research, but to effectively interpret and translate these results for our patients until a cure is discovered. While we cannot anticipate all of the relevant findings, we can prepare ourselves by increasing our understanding of diabetes and its complications and the impact of this disease on the lives of our patients.

The choice of chapters and content included in this third edition of *A Core Curriculum for Diabetes Education* reflects the changes in both care and education across the lifespan and in the many culturally diverse groups affected by diabetes. It acknowledges both the importance of blood glucose control and the patient's role in choosing and achieving their goals, and was also designed to provide the skills you need in order to interpret and incorporate new findings into your practice.

The overall purpose of this book is to provide information for diabetes educators in such a way that they can then assist people with diabetes to become effective self-directed decision makers for their own diabetes care, health and well-being.

AUTHORS

Robert M. Anderson, EdD
University of Michigan
Ann Arbor, Michigan

James D. Anderst, BS
Medical College of Wisconsin
Milwaukee, Wisconsin

Jesse Ahroni, MSN, RN
Seattle VA Medical Center
Seattle, Washington

Marla Bernbaum, MD, MPH
St. Louis University School
of Medicine
St. Louis, Missouri

Jean E. Betschart, MSN, MN,
CPNP, CDE
Childrens Hospital of
Pittsburgh
Pittsburgh, Pennsylvania

Elaine Boswell, MSN
Vanderbilt University DRTC
Nashville, Tennessee

R. Keith Campbell,
RPh, MBA, CDE
Washington State University
Spokane, Washington

Anne S. Campbell-Daly,
MS, RD, CDE
Springfield Diabetes and
Endocrine Center
Springfield, Illinois

Belinda P. Childs
RN, MN, ARNP, CDE
Mid-America Diabetes
Associates
Wichita, Kansas

Mayer B. Davidson, MD
Cedars-Sinai Medical Center
Los Angeles, California

Kristina Ernst, RN, BSN, CDE
Grady Health Systems
Atlanta, Georgia

James A. Fain, RN, PhD,
FAAN
University of Massachusetts
Medical Center
Graduate School of Nursing
Worcester, Massachusetts

Marion J. Franz, MS,
RD, CDE
International Diabetes Center
Minneapolis, Minnesota

Martha Mitchell Funnell, MS,
RN, CDE
University of Michigan DRTC
Ann Arbor, Michigan

Linda Gonder-Frederick, PhD
University of Virginia
Behavior Science Center
Charlottesville, Virginia

Sandra J. Gillespie, MMSc,
RD, LD, CDE, FADA
Atlanta Diabetes Associates
Atlanta, Georgia

Douglas A. Greene, MD
Michigan Diabetes Research
and Training Center
University of Michigan
Medical School
Ann Arbor, Michigan

Diana W. Guthrie
RN, ARNP, FAAN, CDE
University of Kansas School
of Medicine
Wichita, Kansas

Richard A. Guthrie MD, CDE
Mid-America Diabetes
Associates
Via Christi Regional
Medical Center
University of Kansas School
of Medicine
Wichita, Kansas

Deborah Hinnen, RN, MN,
ARNP, CDE
Diabetes Treatment &
Research Center
Wichita, Kansas

Cheryl Hunt, RN, MSEd, CDE
Health and Education
Resources
Alexandria, Virginia

Donna L. Jornsay, RN, BSN,
CPNP, CDE
North Shore University
Hospital
Great Neck, New York

Joy A. Kistler, MS, CDE
Joslin Diabetes Center
Boston, Massachusetts

Karmeen Kulkarni, RD,
MS, CDE
Salt Lake City, Utah

Jane Lipps, RN, MS, CDE
Vanderbilt University DRTC
Nashville, Tennessee

Anne T. Nettles, MS, RD, CDE
Diabetes Careworks
Waysata, Minnesota

Virginia Peragallo-Dittko, RN,
MA, FADA, CDE
Winthrop-University Hospital
Levittown, New York

Michael A. Pfeifer, MD
East Carolina University
Greenville, North Carolina

James W. Pichert, PhD
Vanderbilt University School
of Medicine
Nashville, Tennessee

Robert E. Ratner, MD, CDE
Medlantic Clinical Research
Center
Washington, DC

Lynne S. Robins, PhD
Department of Medical
Education
University of Michigan
Ann Arbor, Michigan

Richard R. Rubin, PhD, CDE
Johns Hopkins Medical
Center
Baltimore, Maryland

Stephanie Schwartz,
MPH, RN, CDE
Children's Mercy Hospital
Kansas City, Missouri

Tamara Stitch,
RN, MSN, CDE
St. Louis University Health
Science Center
Division of Endocrinology
St. Louis, Missouri

Jackie Two Feathers
The University of New
Mexico
School of Medicine
Albuquerque, New Mexico

Frank Vinicor, MD, MPH
Centers for Disease Control
and Prevention
Atlanta, Georgia

John R. White, Jr., PharmD
Washington University
College of Pharmacy
Spokane, Washington

Peggy C. Yarborough, RPh,
MS, CDE, FAPP, FASH
Wilson Community Health
Center
Wilson, North Carolina

REVIEWERS

JoAnn Ahern, APRN,
MSN, CDE
Yale-New Haven Hospital
Pediatric Endocrinology
New Haven, Connecticut

Ann L. Albright, PhD, RD
University of California
California Department of
Health Services
San Francisco, California

Barbara J. Anderson, PhD
Joslin Diabetes Center
Harvard University School
of Medicine
Boston, Massachusetts

Gary M. Arsham, MD, PhD
Arsham Consultants, Inc.
San Francisco, California

Anita K. Austin, RPh, BS, CDE
Austin and Associates
Sarver, Pennsylvania

Patti Bazel Geil,
MS, RD, FADA, CDE
University of Kentucky
Medical Center
Lexington, Kentucky

David S. H. Bell, MB, BCh,
FRCI, FRCPS, FACP
University Medical School
Birmingham, Alabama

Kathy J. Berkowitz, RN, FNP,
CDE
Grady Health System
Diabetes Unit
Atlanta, Georgia

Shari A. Biggins, RN, CDE
WEDCO District Health Dept.
Cynthiana, Kentucky

Barbara H. Bodnar,
RN, MS, CDE
Pennsylvania Dept. of Health
Pittsburgh, Pennsylvania

Cecilia Casey Boyer,
RN, MS, CDE
The Ohio State University
Medical Center
Division of Endocrinology
Columbus, Ohio

Vasti Broadstone, MD
University of Louisville
Louisville, Kentucky

Ann Marie Brooks, RN, CDE
Diabetes Clinician
Diabetes Treatment Center
St. Mark's Hospital
Salt Lake City, Utah

Sharon A. Brown, PhD, RN
University of Texas at Austin
School of Nursing
Austin, Texas

Thomas A. Buchanan, MD
University of Southern
California
School of Medicine
Los Angeles, California

John B. Buse, MD, PhD
University of North Carolina
at Chapel Hill
Chapel Hill, North Carolina

Denise Charron-Prochownik,
PhD, RN, CPNP
University of Pittsburgh
School of Nursing
Pittsburgh, Pennsylvania

Belinda Childs, RN, MN,
ARNP, CDE
Mid-America Diabetes
Associates
Wichita, Kansas

Beth Ann Coonrod,
PhD, MPH, RN, CDE
The Medical Center, PA, Inc.
Beaver, Pennsylvania

Alicia Correa, BSN, MBA,
RN, CDE
University Health Systems
Texas Diabetes Institute
San Antonio, Texas

Margaret A. Cunningham,
RN, MS, CDE
Loyola University Hospital
Diabetes Care Center
Maywood, Illinois

Marjorie Cypress, RN, CDE
Lovelace Medical Center
Department of
Endocrinology
Albuquerque, New Mexico

Paul F. Dunn,
MSN, FNP, CDE
University of North Carolina
at Chapel Hill
Department of Family
Medicine
Chapel Hill, North Carolina

Mary Sullivan Ellinger,
RD, CDE
The INOVA Diabetes Center
Fairfax, Virginia

Kristina Ernst, RN, BSN, CDE
Grady Health Systems
Atlanta, Georgia

Janine Freeman, RD, LD, CDE
Columbia Dunwoody
Medical Center
Atlanta, Georgia

Russell E. Glasgow, PhD
Oregon Research Institute
Eugene, Oregon

Kathryn Godley,
MS, RN, CDE
New York State Department
of Health
Diabetes Control Program
Albany, New York

Diana W. Guthrie, BSN, MSPH, EdS, PhD, ARNP, CDE
University of Kansas School of Medicine
Department of Pediatrics
Wichita, Kansas

Richard A. Guthrie, MD, FAAP, FACE, CDE
Mid America Diabetes Associates, Inc.
Wichita, Kansas

Lee Ann Holzmeister, RD, CDE
Phoenix Childrens Hospital
Tempe, Arizona

Bonita Irvin, MS, RD, CDE
Hudson, North Carolina

Debra Haire-Joshu, PhD
Diabetes Education Center
Internal Medicine Dept.
St. Louis, Missouri

Leo E. Hendricks, PhD, LICSW, CDE
LHCA Diabetes Self-Management Training Center
Wheaton, Maryland

Rosetta T. Hendricks, MSN, RN, C, FNP, CDE
VA Medical Center
Washington, DC

Gary M. Ingersoll, PhD
Indiana University School of Education
Bloomington, Indiana

Timothy J. Ives, PharmD, MPH, CDE
University of North Carolina at Chapel Hill
Department of Family Medicine
Chapel Hill, North Carolina

Scott J. Jacober, DO, FACOI, CDE
Wayne State University School of Medicine
Detroit, Michigan

Dennis Janisse, CPed
National Pedorthic Services
Milwaukee, Wisconsin

Mark W. Johnson, MD
University of Michigan Medical School
Department of Ophthalmology
Ann Arbor, Michigan

Ginger Kanzer-Lewis, RNC, EdM, CDE
The Valley Hospital
Ridgewood, New Jersey

Wahida Karmally, MS, RD, CDE
Irving Center for Clinical Research
Columbia University
New York, New York

Julienne K. Kirk, RPh, PharmD, CDE
Bowman Gray School of Medicine
Department of Family Medicine/Endocrinology
Winston-Salem, North Carolina

David E. Klein, DPM, CDE
Gouverneur Hospital
Diabetes Management Clinic
New York, New York

Joseph C. Konan, MD, MSPH
Carolinas Medical Center
Department of Family Medicine
Charlotte, North Carolina

Davida F. Kruger, MSN, RN, C, CDE
Henry Ford Health Systems
Detroit, Michigan

Andrea J. Lasichak, MS, RD, CDE
University of Michigan
Ann Arbor, Michigan

Daniel L. Lorber, MD, FACP, CDE
Diabetes Control Foundation
Flushing, New York

David G. Marrero, PhD
Indiana University School of Medicine
Diabetes Research and Training Center
Indianapolis, Indiana

Melinda D. Maryniuk, RD, MEd, FADA, CDE
Joslin Diabetes Center
Boston, Massachusetts

Kathleen McDonald, RN, MSN, CDE
Voorhees, New Jersey

John H. Osler, III, MD, PA
Voorhees, New Jersey

Randy P. McDonough, RPh, MS
The University of Iowa College of Pharmacy
Iowa City, Iowa

Susan M. McLaughlin, BS, RD, CDE, LMNT
St. Joseph Villa Homecare and Hospice
Omaha, Nebraska

Arlene M. Monk, RD, LD, CDE
International Diabetes Center
Minneapolis, Minnesota

Arshag D. Mooradian, MD
St. Louis University
Health Science Center
St. Louis, Missouri

Kathryn Mulcahy, RN, MSN, CDE
Fairfax Hospital
INOVA Diabetes Center
Fairfax, Virginia

Charlotte Reese Nath, MSN, RN, EdD, CDE
West Virginia University
Department of Family Medicine
Morgantown, West Virginia

Janet A. Nicollerat, RN, CDE
Duke University
Cary, North Carolina

Joyce G. Pastors RD, MS,CDE
Virginia Center for Diabetes
Professional Education
Charlottesville, Virginia

Suzanne Pecoraro,
RD, MPH, CDE
Diabetes Education Society
Denver, Colorado

Martha J. Price,
DNSc, ARNP, CDE
Group Health Cooperative
Diabetes Clinical Roadmap
Seattle, Washington

Diane M. Reader RD, CDE
International Diabetes Center
Minneapolis, Minnesota

Dawn Satterfield,
RNC, MSN, CDE
Centers for Disease Control
and Prevention
Atlanta, Georgia

J. Terry Saunders, PhD
Virginia Center for Diabetes
Professional Education
University of Virginia
Charlottesville, Virginia

Deborah O. Sauve,
MSN, RN, CDE
Leesburg, Virginia

Lorraine Schafer, PhD
Marshfield Clinic
Department of Psychiatry
Marshfield, Wisconsin

Barbara Schreiner,
RN, MN, CDE
Texas Children's Hospital
Diabetes Care Center
Houston, Texas

Jeffrey T. Soukup, MSS, CSCS
Providence Hospital
Adult Wellness Program
Mobile, Alabama

Elizabeth A. Walker,
RN, DNSc, CDE
Albert Einstein College
of Medicine
Diabetes Research and
Training Center
Bronx, New York

Hope S. Warshaw,
MMSc, RD, CDE
Hope Warshaw Associates
Alexandria, Virginia

Madelyn L. Wheeler,
MS, RD, FADA, CDE
Indiana University
Medical Center
Diabetes Research and
Training Center
Indianapolis, Indiana

Neil H. White, MD, CDE
Washington University
School of Medicine
St. Louis Children's Hospital
St. Louis, Missouri

Ann Sawyer Williams,
RN, MSN, CDE
Cleveland Heights, Ohio

Donald K. Zettervall,
RPh, CDE
The Diabetes Center
Old Saybrook, Connecticut

EDUCATION

EDUCATION

Educational Principles and Strategies   **1**

Robert M. Anderson, EdD
Michigan Diabetes Research and Training Center
University of Michigan
Ann Arbor, Michigan

INTRODUCTION

1 Most of the chapters in this core curriculum are concerned with the content of diabetes patient education programs, that is, the knowledge and skills to be acquired by patients.

2 Diabetes educators need to be knowledgeable about diabetes, but they also need to be skilled teachers to be effective.

3 This chapter is concerned with the educational process relevant to diabetes patient education and focuses on the program design and educational methods used to help patients learn about diabetes.

4 How diabetes knowledge and skills are taught can have as much impact on patient outcomes as what is taught.

5 The instructional design of a diabetes patient education program can affect patients' acquisition of knowledge and skills, their attitudes about diabetes, their motivation to practice appropriate diabetes self-care, their willingness and ability to change behavior and their degree of psycho-social adjustment to diabetes.

OBJECTIVES

Upon completion of this chapter, the learner will be able to

1 Explain the similarities and differences between the compliance and empowerment approaches to diabetes patient education.
2 Describe nine issues to consider when designing a diabetes patient education program.
3 Explain the similarities and differences between formative and summative evaluation.
4 Explain the rationale for employing a multidisciplinary team in diabetes education.
5 List eight areas to consider when assessing an individual patient's needs and readiness to learn.
6 Describe four characteristics of adult learners.
7 List ten teaching and learning strategies used in diabetes patient education.

8 Describe seven techniques that can be used to enhance learning and decision making.

9 Explain the importance of follow-up diabetes patient education.

APPROACHES TO EDUCATION

1 The compliance-based approach[1,2] to diabetes patient education is intended to improve patient adherence to the treatment recommendations of healthcare professionals.

  A This approach is based on the assumption that healthcare professionals are diabetes care experts and that patients should, in most cases, comply with their recommendations regarding diabetes self-care.

  B Patient education is seen as a means of influencing patients to follow treatment recommendations to improve their glucose control and prevent the short- and long-term complications of diabetes.

2 In the empowerment approach,[3-7] the primary purpose of diabetes patient education is to prepare patients to make informed decisions about their own diabetes care.

  A This approach assumes that most patients with diabetes are responsible for making important and complex decisions while carrying out the daily treatment of their diabetes.

  B The empowerment approach also assumes that because patients are the ones who experience the consequences of having and treating diabetes, they have both the right and responsibility to be the primary decision makers regarding their own daily diabetes care.

3 Very few educators use one approach all the time to the exclusion of the other approach.

  A Most educators will use some combination of the two approaches based on their own values and understanding of the purposes and methods of patient education as well as the needs of their patients.

  B Patients will have varying needs and tolerance for autonomous decision-making in their diabetes self-care based on a number of factors. For example, a newly diagnosed patient with diabetes may wish to have the majority of decisions made by the healthcare team until he or she becomes more familiar with the cost and benefits of various options in diabetes self-care.

CONSIDERATION IN THE DESIGN OF PATIENT EDUCATION PROGRAMS

1 An education program needs to be designed to fit a particular setting and group of patients. It is important to gear program and educational materials to the disease type, age, education, experience, needs, abilities, and cultural background of patients.

2 Program philosophy is an important consideration because it shapes the design and conduct of the program.

    A The program educators need to agree on whether they believe in the compliance approach, the empowerment approach, or some other educational philosophy that expresses the values and sense of purpose shared among the program educators.

    B A written philosophy statement can be a very useful tool for developing and expressing the program philosophy.

    C The program philosophy provides the context for program goals and objectives and each patient encounter and educational session.

3 Designing a diabetes patient education program requires first selecting appropriate goals and objectives, and then determining the level(s) of comprehensiveness for the program (ie, deciding what material to include and in what depth).

    A Diabetes patient education programs need clear and realistic goals. These goals can be somewhat general in nature, such as "The program will prepare patients to make informed choices about their diabetes care goals and methods." Well-written goals will guide the formulation of the program objectives.[8]

    B The specific patient behaviors that will contribute to achieving a goal should be expressed as behavioral objectives, such as "Patients will use their own meters to demonstrate the ability to assess their own blood glucose levels with no errors." Write objectives in terms of observable and measurable behavior that contain a criterion for acceptable performance.[9]

    C Diabetes education programs need to offer courses of study with different levels of comprehensiveness. Patients cannot, and should not, learn everything there is to know about diabetes in one course of study.

- The basic course should focus on the initial skills that newly diagnosed patients must learn immediately to care for their diabetes.
- A more comprehensive course in the self-management of diabetes is needed to be available for patients who have had time to adapt to having diabetes.
- Diabetes education should be available for specific topics such as an overall review, lifestyle flexibility, and special situations (eg, instruction about insulin adjustment when traveling across time zones and the availability of visual aids if visual changes occur).

4 Other important design considerations are issues related to educational format.

   A One-to-one teaching and group teaching both have advantages and disadvantages to consider (eg, groups allow patients to share experiences while one-to-one teaching allows the focus of the entire session to be on one patient).[10,11]

   B Other issues to consider are when and where classes will be held and whether classes will be limited to just one type of patient (eg, only those patients with type 1 diabetes).

   C Flexibility and adaptability are the keys to developing appropriate educational formats.

5 The design of a patient education program needs to reflect the philosophy, needs, and values of those groups of people (stakeholders) who have an investment in the program and its outcomes.

   A Examples of program stakeholders are patients, referring physicians, hospital or clinical administrators, the patient's family, and the program educators.

   B A program benefits from having an advisory committee with representatives from each stakeholder group. Diabetes is cared for in the patient's home and community, which makes community representation on the advisory committee appropriate.

6 Availability of resources is an important design consideration.

   A The availability of financial resources has a significant impact on the design of the program. The availability of people to teach in the program is an equally important resource.

   B Another important consideration is physical resources, such as space, equipment, education materials, etc.

7 The makeup of the multidisciplinary educational team (eg, nurse, dietitian, physician, psychologist, pharmacist, exercise physiologist,) is crucial to the design of a program and should be identified early in the planning process. Team teaching provides the significant benefit of professionals with multidisciplinary expertise, although it also requires investment of time for planning and team meetings.

8 Another important issue is documentation and record keeping.

    A Diabetes education programs need to include a system that allows for documentation of educational assessment, education, and follow-up.

    B Such documentation may be required to meet standards such as the National Standards for Diabetes Self-Management Education Programs[12] and achieve certification or recognition from the American Diabetes Association (ADA).

9 A resource to help in designing diabetes patient education are the ADA National Standards for Diabetes Education Self-Management Programs.[12] These standards address important issues such as needs assessment, program planning and management, communication and coordination, patient access to teaching, content of the educational curriculum, qualifications of the instructors, the importance of follow-up education, patient and program outcomes, evaluation, record keeping, and documentation.[12]

EVALUATION OF PROGRAM OUTCOMES

1 Formative evaluation,[13-15] also called process evaluation, involves collecting information about how well the program is functioning.

    A This type of formative evaluation provides information that can be applied almost immediately to change the program and increase its effectiveness.

    B Formative evaluation data often are gathered by having patients complete questionnaires about their level of satisfaction with the course content, physical and social environment, teaching, audiovisual materials, etc.

2 Summative evaluation,[13-15] also called outcome evaluation, involves gathering and analyzing information to determine whether the program achieved the intended outcomes.

    A Summative evaluation domains include knowledge, attitudes, self-care practices, and psychosocial adaptation. Certain metabolic indices such as blood glucose control and weight are sometimes considered outcome measures by education programs.[16]

    B In general, choose to measure outcomes that occur shortly after the end of the program and outcomes that can be attributed to the program with a high degree of confidence.[17-19]

MULTIDISCIPLINARY TEAMS IN DIABETES EDUCATION[20]

1 A coordinated team approach is recommended in diabetes care because of the multidisciplinary nature of the treatment.[20] This approach is particularly appropriate for patient education where learners must acquire knowledge and skills from a variety of disciplines.

2 Additional benefits of multidisciplinary teams include improved coordination of care and education, multiple reinforcement of the same educational objectives, and consistency of approach to treatment. For example, although a physician may not spend much time teaching, he or she can reinforce the importance of diabetes patient education and transmit other core messages to the patient, such as the fact that diabetes is a serious disease.[21]

3 A program coordinator should be chosen to plan and coordinate the efforts of the educational team. This person is responsible for scheduling team meetings and preparing the agenda.

4 Team membership is crucial and should include, whenever possible, a nurse, a dietitian, and a physician as core team members. Other team members will vary depending on need and availability but could include a psychologist, social worker, pharmacist, exercise physiologist, or podiatrist.

5 Team meetings can be used for a variety of purposes:

    A To share information gained from individual patient assessments (eg, nursing, nutrition, medical)

    B To develop a plan to respond to the patient's clinical and educational priorities

    C To plan, implement, and evaluate a patient education program

    D To provide for patient referrals and follow-up care and education

ASSESSING INDIVIDUAL PATIENT EDUCATIONAL NEEDS AND READINESS TO LEARN

1 Teaching and learning are generally divided into three domains: knowledge, psychomotor skills, and affective (or attitudinal) learning. Assessment should focus on these three domains as well.

   A It is useful to assess patients' attitudes[22] and health beliefs[23] about diabetes and its care.[24,25] Patients who think they have mild diabetes or are immune from complications are not very likely to be motivated to learn.

   B It is also important to assess patients' attitudes about participating in the education program. For example, the educator could discuss patients' learning goals by asking questions about what they hope to get out of the education program and their goals related to their daily self-care.[8,26]

   C Assess the patients' metabolic goals regarding glucose control, weight, and lipids.

   D Patients' experience with diabetes and/or other health problems can shape their attitudes and affect their readiness to learn and apply diabetes self-care skills. For example, a patient who is admitted to the hospital for gallbladder surgery or a patient who is newly diagnosed with an acute illness is likely to have a diminished readiness to learn about diabetes. Acutely ill patients need to be taught only basic survival skills until they feel well enough to be more active learners.

   E Families can have a significant impact on a patients' attitudes and readiness to learn by providing or withholding support. Patients are more likely to have a positive attitude about learning when family members are supportive and enthusiastic about diabetes education.[27]

2 Current level of self-care is another important area to assess.[17,26] An educator can glean important information about patients' tolerance for complexity in the regimen and/or which self-care behaviors are most difficult to perform by assessing their current self-care practices.

3 Patients' preferred styles of learning can affect their willingness to participate in the education program and whether they actually learn.

   A Some patients prefer to read, others like to listen, and still others learn best from discussions.

   B Patients can be asked how they prefer to acquire other types of information not related to diabetes, (eg, newspapers, TV, discussion with friends). This information will provide clues about how to tailor the education to the individual's needs.

C Consider the fact that not everyone wants to be or belongs in a group program; some patients respond better to one-on-one instruction.

4 The psychological status of patients can affect their interest in learning about diabetes.

A Marked denial, depression, and anxiety can interfere with learning, while low-to-moderate anxiety about diabetes can increase readiness to learn.

B Patients will also display various degrees of alertness and ability to concentrate on educational issues.

5 Severe stress can seriously impair patients' abilities and interests in learning about diabetes.

A Stress is a reaction to factors that force persons to adapt to situations that are perceived on some level as a threat to their well-being.

B Patient education (with the possible exception of basic survival skills) should be postponed for patients experiencing severe stress (see Chapter 5, Behavior Change for more information about stress management).

6 Assess patients' social/cultural and religious milieus because of their influence on patients' interest and willingness to learn about and apply specific diabetes self-care recommendations. Tailor diabetes patient education to the specific cultural needs and perceptions of the participants.[28]

7 Literacy can be difficult to assess. Years of schooling completed provides only a clue about literacy.

A Patients' educational and literacy levels can influence how they learn (eg, reading vs listening or viewing illustrations) and the amount of complexity they can tolerate in an education program.

B Because complexity is part of diabetes self-care, the challenge lies in using this part of the assessment to direct learning and management issues (see Chapter 2, Teaching Patients With Low Literacy Skills).

8 Patients' willingness to participate in and benefit from diabetes education is most likely related to their readiness for change.

A Recent work on smoking cessation and other addictive behaviors has resulted in a stages of change model that now is being applied to diabetes education[29] (see Chapter 5, Behavior Change, for more information).

B The educational process must either create conditions that stimulate the desire for change in a patient and/or capitalize on the readiness to change if it is already present.

C The extent to which patients feel that change is necessary will indicate whether they are ready to participate in an education program.

9 Other assessment areas involve physical factors such as age, mobility, visual acuity, hearing loss, and dexterity. These factors can influence a patients' willingness and ability to learn and apply diabetes self-care skills.

CHARACTERISTICS OF ADULT LEARNERS[30]

1 Adults are usually self-directed and must feel a need to learn before they are able to participate fully in the educational process.[30]

A It is not relevant that the educator feels the patient should learn something if the patient does not also perceive this need.

B Sometimes, however, the diabetes educator will have to help patients discover what they need to know. For example, if a patient is being started on insulin for the first time, there are certain safety issues that the educator must address. In this case, the educator may have to take a leadership role in pointing out the crucial areas for diabetes education (eg, signs, symptoms, and treatment of hypoglycemia) rather than wait for the patient to discover these educational needs.

2 Adults tend to be problem-oriented learners rather than subject-oriented learners. They usually want to acquire information that will help them solve specific diabetes problems rather than complete a comprehensive study of the subject of diabetes.

3 Adults learn better when their own experience with diabetes is incorporated into diabetes education, including their past experiences and consideration of how these experiences will apply to their learning in the future (eg, Have you dealt with this problem before? What did you do to try and resolve it? What do you think might work this time?).

4 Adults usually prefer to participate actively in the learning process rather than remain passive. Education programs need to provide patients with the opportunity to ask questions, solve problems, share their own experiences, and otherwise be actively engaged in the educational process.

Teaching and Learning Strategies

1 A brief lecture is useful for presenting information. Patients participate in the learning process by listening and taking notes.

   A This kind of instruction provides a very passive learning experience for patients.

   B Sometimes this method is overused[31,32] because lectures are easier for teachers to plan and control than other more active types of instruction.

2 Discussion is a more participatory and active learning experience than a lecture; it allows patients to acquire information, ask and answer questions, and share feelings and personal experiences.

   A Discussions cannot be planned and controlled as precisely as lectures, therefore they require the educator to tolerate a certain amount of ambiguity.

   B Leading discussions effectively requires certain interpersonal skills on the part of the educator. For example, a discussion leader must know how to gracefully interrupt a nonstop talker so that other members of the group will have a chance to speak.

3 Demonstration is useful for teaching psychomotor or social skills.

   A After a skills demonstration, encourage patients to practice the skills they have seen demonstrated.[32-34]

   B Give patients the opportunity to demonstrate their skills to the educator and receive feedback. Teaching insulin injection and/or home blood glucose monitoring are the classic examples where this teaching sequence is usually employed.

4 Print materials can provide information for individual study, reinforce previously presented information, and serve as a resource for future reference and review.

   A Print materials need to employ readable type (patients with vision loss may need large type) and be written at an appropriate reading level for the learner.

B Clarity, nontechnical language, and well-designed, purposeful illustrations enhance the effectiveness of printed material (see Chapter 2, Teaching Patients With Low Literacy Skills, for more information about choosing and preparing learning materials at reading levels that are appropriate for specific patient populations).

C Printed materials do not replace interaction with the educator.

5 Audiovisual (AV) aids such as slides, films, videotapes, food models, and overhead transparencies can enhance the presentation of information.[32-34]

A Varying the presentation by using AV aids can help increase learner concentration and prevent boredom.

B Learning is reinforced when the same concepts are presented through a variety of formats.

C Homemade AV materials give the instructor flexibility. They also provide the opportunity for creativity and matching the AVs to the audience.

D The use of AV media can be very helpful for patients who do not learn well by reading.

6 Role-playing gives patients a chance to practice social skills, explore interpersonal problems (eg, family conflict), discuss alternative solutions, and share feelings in a psychologically safe environment.[35,36]

A Role-playing usually works best with a group of learners who are verbal and who know and trust each other and the instructor.

B Effective role-playing requires an instructor who has good interpersonal skills and has had training and experience in leading small groups.

7 Games can make learning more enjoyable and improve learner participation.

A Many board games (eg, Trivial Pursuit®) or television game shows (eg, Jeopardy®) can be adapted for diabetes patient education. Some games that are appropriate for diabetes education are produced commercially.

8 Computers have been used in diabetes education for the past 10 years. Computerized clinical problems and simulations can provide a useful mechanism for testing and increasing patient knowledge and improving problem-solving skills.[37,38]

9 Patient examples and problem-based case studies provide a psychologically safe and useful way for learners to explore problems related to having diabetes and to discuss solutions. Patient examples can be written to meet the needs of different types of learners and address a variety of learning domains (eg, knowledge, self-care behavior, or attitudes).[39,40]

10 Affective exercises[35,36] are techniques for helping patients express, explore, and change feelings and personal values related to having diabetes.

    A Affective exercises can include some of the previously described techniques such as discussion and role-playing, or can employ activities designed specifically to elicit an affective response.

    B Existing books on values clarification[41] and human relations training[42] provide many techniques that can be adapted for diabetes education.

TECHNIQUES THAT ENHANCE LEARNING AND DECISION-MAKING

1 Most diabetes educators want their patients to be motivated, involved, responsible and committed learners.

2 Diabetes education is much more rewarding and enjoyable for both the educator and the patient when the patient is an active and committed learner.

3 The techniques listed can enhance the involvement and learning of most patients.

    A Learning is enhanced when it is related to what the learner already knows. Match what is being taught with the patient's existing frame of reference.[39]

    B Learning is improved when patients have confidence (self-efficacy) in their ability to actually perform the behavior being taught. Continually reinforce the idea that the patient is a person who can master diabetes self-care skills. This process is enhanced when diabetes patient education is structured as a series of carefully planned, successful experiences.[43,44]

    C Practice and rehearsal increase the retention of knowledge and skills. Patients need to be given opportunities to practice both psychomotor and social skills (eg, asking family members for their support when following a meal plan).[39]

D Learning is enhanced by feedback. Provide feedback to patients about how well they are acquiring knowledge and skills. Continued learning can be encouraged by making patients aware of their incremental progress.

E Learning is reinforced and retained when it can be applied immediately and repeatedly. Patients will retain knowledge and skills longer if they have opportunities for frequent application. For example, having patients who might have to use insulin someday attend a class on insulin injection is unlikely to produce any important or lasting learning, because the information/skills cannot be used at this time.

F Educators will occasionally need to adjust the pace at which they teach to accommodate variations in patients' ability to absorb and retain information. Patients do not always learn at a constant rate. Periodic plateaus occur in learning due to the mood, stress level, and health of patients.

G Review and update core diabetes knowledge and skills on a regular basis.

FOLLOW-UP LEARNING OPPORTUNITIES

1 Learning needs to be an ongoing activity.

    A One of the most serious impediments to effective diabetes education is the notion that diabetes patient education is a one-time event. Patients change, their situations change, and their health status changes, so new learning needs arise.

    B Patient education also can provide the continuous emotional support and behavioral reinforcement that is necessary for diabetes self-care.

    C To be most effective, patient education should be thought of as an ongoing process (similar to medical care) that plays a lifelong role for people with diabetes.[45-47]

2 Look for opportunities to provide continuing education to your patients.

    A These opportunities include interactions with patients that occur during ongoing diabetes care, such as returning to the provider's office or clinic.

    B Educators can also offer courses that are promoted as diabetes updates or refresher courses for patients who have already completed basic diabetes education.

C Support groups, periodic health appraisals and screenings, and annual meetings of diabetes professional and patient organizations also provide opportunities for follow-up diabetes education.

SELF-REVIEW QUESTIONS

1 Explain the similarities and differences between the two educational philosophies, compliance and empowerment approaches.

2 If you were asked to design a patient education program, what would you do first and why?

3 When designing a patient education program, whose input would you seek and why?

4 How would you decide what to evaluate in your patient education program?

5 Describe characteristics of adult learners that appear to be most relevant for diabetes patient education.

6 Describe the teaching/learning strategies you think are most useful in diabetes patient education.

7 Describe the teaching/learning strategies you think are least useful in diabetes patient education.

8 Describe four techniques that you believe could enhance the learning of patients.

9 How would you justify the team approach in diabetes education to your supervisors?

10 What could you say to a patient to reinforce the idea that diabetes patient education needs to be ongoing?

CASE STUDY 1

JR is a nurse educator in a 200-bed hospital in a rural town in Wisconsin. For the past 2 years, the hospital has offered individual education to outpatients with diabetes on an as-needed basis. However, she and the dietitian who have been responsible for the program have become overwhelmed with the number of patients who are being referred to them for teaching. In addition, the hospital would like their services to be reimbursed. JR and the dietitian decide to revise the program to include group sessions and to seek recognition in order to receive reimbursement. Along with the other aspects of meeting national standards, choosing evaluation measures is part of the process.

QUESTIONS FOR DISCUSSION

1   How should JR begin to develop an evaluation plan?
2   What aspects of the program should be evaluated and how should they be evaluated?

DISCUSSION

1   JR begins by establishing an Advisory Committee, which is a requirement for meeting national standards. The committee is comprised of program stakeholders such as herself, her supervisor, the dietitian, a person with diabetes from the community who has received education and who is involved in several civic organizations, a referring physician, and a social worker. She decides to limit membership of the Advisory Committee at this point. However, she knows that she may choose others who also have an investment and interest in the educational program or who can offer clinical marketing, evaluation or other expertise to the program as it develops.

2   As part of the program plan, the Advisory Committee can help JR develop an evaluation plan by making recommendations about what to measure and how. In order to get the most helpful recommendations, JR asks the following questions of the committee at the first meeting:
   A   What is the purpose of the evaluation?
   B   Are both formative and summative evaluation data needed?
   C   For whom are we collecting data?
      • For example, if the major purpose is to achieve program recognition status, then the Advisory Committee should have examined the guidelines and information provided by the recognizing body to determine the requirements.
      • Evaluation should also be linked to the program staff's desire to improve the quality of the education program. The Advisory Committee should design an evaluation that will help answer meaningful questions about the program.
   D   Does the hospital know how the program is perceived by patients?
   E   Do patients find the program helpful and do they recommend it to others with diabetes?
   F   Does the program produce changes in diabetes knowledge, attitudes, or self-care behaviors?
   G   Based on the philosophy, content, and emphasis of the program, what outcomes is the program most likely to influence?

H What is the cost of the program?

I Does the program currently generate revenue or need to do so in the future?

3 The important first step in developing a program evaluation is setting priorities among the questions to be answered.

A Measures can then be either developed or selected to obtain answers to those questions. Valid and reliable measures of knowledge, attitudes, psychosocial adaptation, and self-care behavior already exist and can be employed or adapted if they represent the areas that the Advisory Committee believes would be most useful information to have.

B The most important questions that the Advisory Committee needs to answer concern the planned use of the information and the areas in which the program is expected to have its greatest impact. It is important to have reasonable answers to these questions before proceeding with choosing an evaluation measure.

4 The Advisory Committee decides to collect both formative and summative evaluation data to measure the effectiveness of the program.

A Because the program is new, collecting data about patient satisfaction is thought to be important for evaluating their efforts. The committee decides to develop a simple questionnaire using five items that can be rated using a five-point scale and two open-ended questions to evaluate satisfaction. In addition, it is believed that tracking attrition levels and referral rates will also provide data about the perceived effectiveness of the program.

B In terms of summative evaluation, the Advisory Committee decides to focus on three main areas.

- Because the target audience for the program is largely older adults with type 2 diabetes, a major emphasis of the program is the importance of foot care. The committee decides to collect pre-, immediate post-, and follow-up information about foot care practices of patients who have attended. Although HbA$_{1c}$ data are available on most patients who participate, it is decided by the committee that this is not the measure of choice at this time because the program has little influence on physician care at this stage of development. The committee does however decide to collect this information as available and use the data when making a decision about the evaluation process for the second year of the program because of this measure to reimbursement agencies.

- Based on a review of the literature, JR learns that improving self-efficacy is a major factor in behavior change for patients in this target population. Therefore, all of the sessions will include information about behavior change and strategies to increase levels of self-efficacy. Self-efficacy is therefore chosen as an additional outcome measure. Through the literature reviewed, JR is able to locate a self-efficacy instrument that has been validated. JR will obtain permission from the authors to use this instrument as part of the evaluation process.

- Behavioral goal setting is also an important area of emphasis for this target population. Each patient who participates in the program will be asked to write at least one behavioral goal at the end of the program, and report on their progress at the follow-up visit. It is decided to collect and summarize this data as part of the evaluation.

CASE STUDY 2

JL is a dietitian who has recently finished her master's degree and a 1-year internship. She has been hired to be a diabetes educator for an 800-bed urban hospital in Texas. For 6 months JL will work with the experienced dietitian who currently is teaching the nutrition component of the diabetes education program. JL is confident that she will know enough about diabetes and nutrition to teach the classes when she takes over in 6 months. However, she is concerned because the current dietitian gives the two 1-hour classes entirely as lectures. JL has been taught that lecturing to patients for 2 hours is not the best educational technique, but she is unsure about what she should substitute for the lectures.

QUESTIONS FOR DISCUSSION

1 JL has 2 hours worth of material to teach about nutrition and diabetes. Which part of the class should be lecture and which part should be changed to another educational method?

2 How can JL decide which alternative methods to use instead of a lecture?

Discussion

1 JL could begin by following a simple rule of thumb: most adults have an attention span of about 15 to 20 minutes for a lecture. Using this rough guideline she could decide that she wants to use two to three different teaching/learning activities for each hour of class.

2 Another concept that could help JL choose effective teaching methods is that patients should be able to interact with the information they have learned after 15 to 20 minutes of lecturing. For example, JL could give a 15 to 20 minute presentation about diabetes and nutrition followed by a discussion session among the patients about applying this information in their own lives. This session could be followed by an opportunity to do some problem-solving such as calculating carbohydrate content of favorite foods or practicing how to read nutrition information labels on food.

3 JL's teaching choices should be directed by the following guidelines:
A Introduce two or three new methods per hour.
B Provide an opportunity for patients to participate actively in the learning process.
C Include activities that will move the patients closer to applying the knowledge in their own lives.
D Include activities that will give patients the opportunity to share their own experiences and express and meet their own needs to ensure that the education is personally relevant.

Case Study 3

MW is a patient with type 2 diabetes who has been using meal planning alone as treatment for the past 5 years. MW's physician has referred him for patient education because his diabetes control has been worsening for the past 18 months and he is being started on oral agents. MW informs you that he doesn't see why he needs diabetes education. He said, "Do they think I'm an idiot, that I can't take a couple of pills without going to an education program? Besides, I feel fine, I don't know why I have to take these pills anyway." The physician is convinced that MW is denying the seriousness of his diabetes and expects you to change his attitude. MW seems resentful that he has been referred to the diabetes patient education program. You are not sure whether he will actually show up for classes.

QUESTION FOR DISCUSSION

1   What other approaches would you suggest in working with this patient?

DISCUSSION

1   The answer to this question involves judgment, and judgment is always debatable. It is unlikely that you can (or should) persuade MW to value and attend the education program. When trying to persuade people that their point of view is wrong, they are likely to defend that point of view with increasing vigor. It is psychologically threatening to one's self-image to be told that one's point of view is wrong or inappropriate; most people resist such threatening messages.

2   The approach that probably would be most useful with MW would be to ask him a series of questions about his diabetes: how long he has had diabetes, how he feels about having it, his concerns, what he knows about the progression of the disease, etc. Listen closely and nonjudgmentally to his responses, giving him an opportunity to express and explore his point of view and perceptions. Such exploration may give him a chance to work through some of his thoughts and feelings. It will also help you be perceived as an ally rather than as someone who is judging him.

3   If at the end of such a discussion MW is still unconvinced that he needs to attend the education program, you could acknowledge the validity of his point of view. You should also, however, suggest that he may wish to consider attending at some future time, and that you and the program are available to him if and when he should desire to use them.

4   You could suggest as another alternative that MW try at least one class or to meet for one-to-one education that will only address his concerns or answer questions.

5   Tell the referring physician that MW is not open to attending a patient education program at this time and that pushing him to do so may in fact increase rather than decrease his resistance to diabetes patient education.

6   If MW feels safe, accepted, and valued by you he is likely to return at some point and participate in the education program.

REFERENCES

1 Raymond MW. Teaching toward compliance: a patient's perspective. Diabetes Educ 1984;10:42-44

2 Resler MM. Teaching strategies that promote adherence. Nurs Clin North Am 1983;18:799-811.

3 Funnell MM, Anderson RM, Arnold MS, et al. Empowerment: an idea whose time has come in diabetes education. Diabetes Educ 1991;17:37-41.

4 Anderson RM. Patient empowerment and the traditional medical model: a case of irreconcilable differences? Diabetes Care 1995;18:412-15.

5 Arnold MS, Butler PM, Anderson RM, Funnell MM, Feste C. Guidelines for facilitating a patient empowerment program. Diabetes Educ 1995;21:308-12.

6 Anderson RM, Funnell MM, Butler P, Arnold MS, Fitzgerald JT, Feste CC. Patient empowerment: results of a randomized control trial. Diabetes Care 1995;18:943-49.

7 Feste C, Anderson RM. Empowerment: from philosophy to practice. Patient Educ Couns 1995;26:139-44.

8 American Diabetes Association: Diabetes education goals. 2nd ed. Arlington, Va; American Diabetes Association, 1995.

9 Mager RF. Preparing instructional objectives. Belmont, Calif: Fearon Publishers, 1975.

10 Rabkin SW, Boyko E, Wilson A, Streja DA. A randomized clinical trial comparing behavior modification and individual counseling in the nutritional therapy of non-insulin-independent diabetes mellitus: comparison of the effect on blood sugar, body weight, and serum lipids. Diabetes Care 1983;6:50-56.

11 Tattersall RB, McCulloch DK, Aveline M. Group therapy in the treatment of diabetes. Diabetes Care 1985;8:180-88.

12 American Diabetes Association. National standards for diabetes education programs and American Diabetes Association review criteria. Diabetes Care 1998; (Suppl 1): 595-98.

13 Haire-Joshu D. Systematic evaluation of diabetes self-management programs. In: Haire-Joshu D, ed. Management of diabetes mellitus. St. Louis: CV Mosby, 2nd ed. 1996:553-73.

14 Gronlund NE. Measurement and evaluation in teaching. 6th ed. New York: MacMillan Publishing Co, 1990.

15 Mehrens WA, Lehmann IJ. Measurement and evaluation in education and psychology. 3rd ed. New York: Holt, Rinehart, and Winston, Inc, 1984.

16 D'Eramo-Melkus GA, Wylie-Rosett J, Hagan JA. Metabolic impact of education in NIDDM. Diabetes Care 1992;15: 864-69.

17 Glasgow RE, Osteen VL. Evaluating diabetes education: are we measuring the most important outcomes? Diabetes Care 1992;15:1423-32.

18 Rubin RR, Peyrot M, Saudek CD. Effect of diabetes education on self-care, metabolic control, and emotional well-being. Diabetes Care 1989;12:673-79.

19 Rubin RR, Peyrot M, Saudek CD. Differential effect of diabetes education on self-regulation and life-style behaviors. Diabetes Care 1992:14;335-38.

20 Anderson RM. The team approach to diabetes: an idea whose time has come. Occup Health Nurs 1982;30(12):13-14.

21 Anderson RM, Funnell MM. The role of the physician in patient education. Practical Diabetol 1990;9(3):10-12.

22 Anderson RM, Donnelly MB, Dedrick RF. Measuring the attitudes of patients towards diabetes and its treatment. Patient Educ Couns 1990;16:231-45.

23 Becker MH, Janz NK. The health belief model applied to understanding diabetes regimen compliance. Diabetes Educ 1985;11:41-47.

24 Beeney LJ, Dunn SM. Knowledge improvement and metabolic control in diabetes education: approaching the limits? Patient Educ Couns 1990; 16:217-29.

25 Funnell MM, Merritt JH. Diabetes mellitus and the older adult. In: Haire-Joshu D, ed. Management of diabetes mellitus. 2nd ed. St. Louis: CV Mosby, 1996: 755-809.

26 Houston C, Haire-Joshu D. Application of health behavior models to promote behavior change. In: Haire-Joshu D, ed. Management of diabetes mellitus. 2nd ed. St. Louis: CV Mosby, 1996: 527-52.

27 Fain JA, D'Eramo-Melkus G. Diabetes mellitus in young and middle adulthood. In: Haire Joshu D, ed. Management of diabetes mellitus. 2nd ed. St. Louis: CV Mosby, 1996:729-54.

28 Murphy FG, Satterfield D, Anderson RM, Lyons AE. Diabetes educators as cultural translators. Diabetes Educ 1993;19:113-16,118.

29 Ruggiero L, Prochaska JO. Introduction: readiness for change: application of the transtheoretical model to diabetes. Diabetes Spectrum 1993;6:22-24.

30 Knowles M. Adult learner: a neglected species. Houston, Tex: Gulf Publishing Co, 1990.

31 Padgett D, Mumford E, Hynes M, Carter R. Meta-analysis of the effects of educational and psychosocial interventions in the management of diabetes mellitus. J Clin Epidemiol 1988;41:1007-30.

32 Funnell MM, Donnelly MB, Anderson RM, Johnson PD, Oh MS. Perceived effectiveness, cost and availability of patient education methods and materials. Diabetes Educ 1992;18:139-45.

33 McCulloch DK, Mitchell RD, Ambler J, Tattersall RB. Influence of imaginative teaching of diet on compliance and metabolic control in insulin dependent diabetes. Br Med J 1983;287:1858-61.

34 Clement SC, Gay N. A better method for demonstrating the relationship between factors affecting glycemic control. Diabetes Educ 1992;18:243-46.

35 Anderson RM. The personal meaning of diabetes: implications for behavior and education, or kicking the bucket theory. Diabetic Med 1986;3:85-89.

36 Anderson RM, Nowacek GW, Richards F. Influencing the personal meaning of diabetes: research and practice. Diabetes Educ 1988;14:297-302.

37 Lewis D. Computer-based patient educators: use by diabetes educators. Diabetes Educ 1996;22:140-45.

38 Noell J. Changing health-related behaviors: new directions for interactive media. Med Educ Technol 1994; 4:4-8

39 Pichert JW, Smeltzer C, Snyder GM, Gregory RP, Smeltzer R, Kinzer CK. Traditional vs anchored instruction for diabetes-related nutritional knowledge, skills, and behavior. Diabetes Educ 1994;20:45-48.

40 Cox DJ, Irvine A, Gonder-Fredrick L, Nowacek G, Butterfield J. Fear of hypoglycemia: quantification, validation, and utilization. Diabetes Care 1987;10: 617-21.

41 Simon S, Howe L, Kirschenbaum H. Values clarification. New York: Hart Publishing Co, 1972.

42 Pfeiffer JW, ed. The 1st-25th annuals: developing human resources. San Diego, Calif: University Associates Inc, 1971-1996.

43 Johnson JA Self-efficacy theory as a framework for community pharmacy-based diabetes education programs. Diabetes Educ 1996;22:237-41.

44 Hawkins RM. Self-efficacy: a cause of debate. J Behav Ther Exp Psychiatry 1995;26:235-40.

45 Falkenberg MG, Elwing BE, Goransson AM, Hellstrand BE, Riis UM. Problem oriented participatory education in the guidance of adults with non-insulin-treated type II diabetes mellitus. Scand J Primary Health Care 1986;4:157-64.

46 Scott RS, Beaven DW, Stafford JM. The effectiveness of diabetes education for non-insulin-dependent diabetic persons. Diabetes Educ 1984;10:36-39.

47 McNabb WL, Quinn MT, Rosing L. Weight-loss program for inner-city black women with non-insulin-dependent diabetes mellitus: PATHWAYS. J Am Dietetic Assn 1993;93:75-77.

SUGGESTED READINGS

Association for Supervision in Curriculum Development. Perceiving, behaving, becoming: a new focus for education. Washington, DC: National Education Association, 1962.

Bonwell C, Eison J. Active learning: creating excitement in the classroom. Washington, DC: ERIC Clearinghouse on Higher Education, George Washington University, School of Education and Human Development, 1991.

Browne M, Keeley S. Asking the right questions: a guide to critical thinking. 3rd ed. Englewood Cliffs, NJ: Prentice Hall, 1990.

Clement SC. Diabetes self-management education: a technical review. Diabetes Care 1995;18:1204-14.

Funnell MM, Arnold MS, Barr PA, eds. Life with diabetes: a series of teaching outlines. Alexandria, Va: American Diabetes Association, 1997.

Funnell MM, Haas LB. National standards for diabetes self-management education programs: a technical review. Diabetes Care 1995; 18:100-16.

Glasgow RE. A practical model of diabetes management and education. Diabetes Care 1995;18:117-26.

Kurfiss JG. Critical thinking. Washington, DC: ERIC Clearinghouse on Higher Education, George Washington University, School of Education and Human Development, 1988.

Meyers C, Jones T. Promoting active learning: strategies for the collect classroom. San Francisco: Josey Bass Publishers, 1993.

Tiberius RG. Small group teaching: a troubleshooting guide. Monograph Series/22. Toronto, Can: Ontario Institute for Studies in Education, 1990.

Vella J. Learning to listen, learning to teach: the power of dialogue in educating adults. San Francisco: Josey Bass Publishers, 1994.

Walker EA, Wylie-Rosett J, Shamoon H. Health education for diabetes self-management IN Porte Jr D, Sherwin RS eds. Ellenberg and Rifin's diabetes mellitus. 5th ed. Appleton & Lange, Stamford, Conn: 1997.

Westberg J, Hillard J. Fostering learning in small groups: a practical guide. New York: Springer Publishing Co, 1996.

Whitman NA. Peer teaching. Washington, DC: ERIC Clearinghouse on Higher Education, George Washington University, School of Education and Human Development, 1988.

Teaching Persons with Low Literacy Skills **2**

James D. Anderst, BS
Medical College of Wisconsin
Milwaukee, Wisconsin

James W. Pichert, PhD
Diabetes Research and Training Center
Vanderbilt University School of Medicine
Nashville, Tennessee

INTRODUCTION

1 One reading expert notes that literacy is like money.[1] Persons with little money find it more difficult to meet their basic needs than those with a lot of money. Similarly, persons with limited or no reading ability find it far more challenging to pursue their educational, vocational, and healthcare goals than their literate peers. Even greater challenges confront those whose reading problems are caused or compounded by language barriers, cognitive impairments, or mental handicaps. Fortunately, many low-literate persons succeed despite enormous challenges because they are remarkably resourceful and/or have significant social supports.

2 Educators help persons with diabetes by understanding the magnitude and health-related implications of the literacy problem, knowing how to assess literacy skills, and teaching in ways that maximize patients' abilities and resources. Doing these things well dramatically affects patients' abilities to achieve their healthcare goals and improve their quality of life.

OBJECTIVES

Upon completion of this chapter, the learner will be able to
1 Define *functional literacy*.
2 Explain the magnitude and health-related implications of the literacy problem in the United States.
3 Compare and contrast the strengths and weaknesses of several common strategies for assessing literacy in clinic populations.
4 Examine whether their current teaching strategies meet the needs of persons with low literacy skills.
5 Define criteria for producing patient education materials and evaluating the appropriateness of existing materials for patients with low literacy skills.

DEFINING LITERACY

1 In the National Literacy Act of 1991, literacy was defined as "an individual's ability to read, write, and speak in English and compute and solve problems at levels of proficiency necessary to function on the job and in society, to achieve one's goals, and to develop one's knowledge and potential."[1] In simpler terms, functional literacy is the ability to use

reading, writing, and computational skills at levels adequate to meet the needs of everyday situations. These or similar definitions have been used to guide recent nationwide literacy assessments.

2   Literacy levels extend across a continuum of skills. Individuals exhibit varying degrees of literacy and cannot be strictly classified as literate or illiterate. For example, a patient's literacy skills may be sufficient to function at home or work, but not in healthcare settings or in situations that require self-care and diabetes-related decision making.

3   Grade-level equivalents do not adequately define an individual's level of literacy. Many people read at levels higher or lower than the last grade they completed in school or the level determined by the most common readability formulas. Therefore, functional assessments are more useful than grade equivalents for identifying literacy skills. When their literacy skills permit them to fully function in society, people are said to be functionally competent.

4   Low literacy does not necessarily imply low intelligence or functioning. Large numbers of Americans with low literacy skills hold jobs and live productive lives, demonstrating both intelligence and motivation. Some, it seems, have learned coping systems far more complex than reading itself.

5   Defining literacy levels for persons whose first language is not English poses special challenges. Some will have high literacy levels in all their languages, some will be highly literate in one language but not another, and still others will have low literacy levels in all their languages. Literacy is best assessed not only with respect to a person's ability to understand English-language materials, but also those printed in the native languages(s). Finally, some persons with low literacy simply come from oral cultures where the spoken word is the standard medium of communication and literacy is a non-issue.

IDENTIFYING THE MAGNITUDE OF THE LITERACY PROBLEM

1   In 1992, the National Adult Literacy Survey,[1] funded by the US Department of Education, assessed the nation's literacy by testing more than 15 000 Americans.[1] Some of the results of this survey are shown in Table 2.1.

TABLE 2.1. SELECTED RESULTS AND IMPLICATIONS FROM THE NATIONAL ADULT LITERACY SURVEY[1]

Literacy Level	Number of Adult Americans Surveyed	Probable Diabetes-Related Skills*	Teaching Tips for Diabetes Educators
1	40 million	Capable of calculating total carbohydrates from a meal if number of carbohydrates for each food is provided; some may be able to use a pie graph to determine the percentage of calories that should come from each food group; can identify a sentence in a pamphlet that explains how to test blood glucose, but most likely will not understand the directions; some at Level 1 may not be able to perform any of these skills	Repeated demonstrations and oral instruction may be necessary. Use of audiotapes and videotapes may help those patients who have the necessary playback equipment in their homes. After instructing the patient, ask the patient to repeat or demonstrate what was just taught. Negotiate attainable goals each teaching session and focus on actions and behaviors rather than theories and concepts. Try to identify relatives or friends of the patient who can read and may be able to assist. Be careful not to rush these patients. Be certain fundamental prerequisites have been learned before moving on to more complex concepts.
2	50 million	Capable of underlining the meaning of a term in a diabetes brochure but may not understand the term; some may be able to interpret instructions for a blood glucose meter; may need one-on-one counseling to adequately understand material at elementary school level	Provide Level 2 patients with simple educational material and be prepared to counsel patients on the material. Audiotapes and videotapes may prove useful. These patients have the potential for improving their understanding of educational material if they are taught common diabetes-related terms such as *insulin, hypoglycemia, glucose,* etc.
3	61 million	Can use glucose log table to determine how carbohydrate intake must be modified; can explain difference between type 1 and type 2 diabetes after reading a brochure; capable of low-level inferences and integration such as understanding the connection between glucose levels, exercise, and insulin; cannot make high-level inferences such as explaining the differences between two different regimens for treating diabetes	Provide Level 3 patients with current diabetes material, but be sure they completely understand it. These patients are often high-school graduates or even college educated, and are accustomed to understanding written material. If they do not understand something, they may feel particularly reluctant to call it to your attention.
4,5	40 million	Generally capable of higher-level inferences and integration; likely capable of doing some self-education with materials written at a level too complex for the general public	Additional reading and educational materials may be suggested for these patients if they express an interest. Patients at Levels 4 and 5 should be able to progress to independent problem solving with encouragement and support.

*Skills and teaching tips are for illustration only. Assessment results and instructional needs will vary from patient to patient.
Source: Adapted from Kirsch et al.[1]

2 Based on the 5-point scale used in this literacy survey, just over 20% of study participants (approximately 40 million American adults) demonstrated skills at Level 1, the lowest level of proficiency. Another 25% (approximately 50 million adults) performed at Level 2.

    A Persons who perform at Level 1 proficiency can, at best, accomplish routine tasks that involve short, simple documents and texts (eg, locating an expiration date on a driver's license, identifying one piece of information from a brief article, or performing simple addition). Persons at Level 1 usually are not able to comprehend the instructions on a prescription label or written meal plan without assistance.

    B Persons who perform at Level 2 also have important functional literacy limitations, including great difficulty with such diabetes self-care tasks as determining algorithmic insulin adjustments, which require complex mathematical problem solving, and following written sick-day guidelines, which require higher-level reading skills.

3 The majority of subjects who performed at Levels 1 and 2 did not perceive themselves as having low literacy skills.

    A Simply asking patients if they can read does not provide an adequate assessment of literacy.

    B When offering reading materials to patients, it is important to refrain from describing the materials as simple or "easy to understand." Patients who struggle with so-called "simple" material may feel ashamed of their performance, and this negative feeling can interfere with the patient/educator relationship. Instead, inform patients that the information contained in the reading material is important and worth taking the time and effort to read and understand.

4 The findings from the 1992 National Adult Literacy Survey[1] are consistent with previous studies and suggest that the literacy problem is not improving.

    A Results from a 1986 study showed that 72 million Americans functioned at marginal or low literacy levels.

    B Results from a 1976 study indicated that 20% of American adults had reading abilities below the 5th grade level and another 30% had only marginally competent reading skills.

5 The literacy proficiencies of young adults assessed in 1992 were, on average, lower than the literacy proficiencies of young adults assessed in 1985.

6 However, more than one half of all low-literate persons in America are Caucasians. African Americans, Hispanics, Native Americans/Alaskan Natives, and Asian/Pacific Islander adults performed, on average, at lower literacy levels than Caucasian adults.

   A Appearance, race, and speech are poor indicators of literacy.

   B Research[2] shows that some poorly dressed working people tested at far higher reading levels than well-dressed, articulate workers.

ASSESSING PATIENTS' FUNCTIONAL LITERACY

1 The most straightforward way to assess patients' understanding of educational material is to give the patients something to read, then ask them to read and explain the meaning of what they have read.

   A Self-reports of education level often are poor indicators of reading ability.

   B Recent studies[2,3] indicate that the functional reading abilities of patients in medically related programs generally are four to five grade levels below their reported final education level.

   C Many low-literate patients attempt to conceal their lack of skills by making up excuses such as "I forgot my glasses." Others may carry magazines or newspapers in hopes of hiding their inability to read.

   D Patients can be asked to independently read a brief text (at home, while waiting in the clinic, or between provider visits) and circle everything in the booklet or brochure that (1) is new to them, (2) is different from what they had previously understood, and (3) raises questions. Following up on this request can provide a lot of information about patients and their literacy skills.

2 Literacy assessment tests may provide a general gauge of a patient's reading level if a reading deficiency is suspected.

   A Grade levels, despite their limitations, are a popular unit for characterizing both a patient's literacy level and the difficulty level of reading materials.

   B Once the patient's reading level is approximated, appropriate educational materials may be offered. The patient, however, is the final arbiter of the usability and comprehensibility of the materials.

   C Most general literacy assessment tests are not designed for clinical use and may be too time consuming and complex to administer. Examples of such tests are the SORT-R (Slosson Oral Reading Test), the

WRAT-R (Wide Range Achievement Test, Revised), the PIAT-R (Peabody Individual Achievement Test, Revised), and the Cloze procedure.

3 The Test of Functional Health Literacy in Adults (TOFHLA)[3] was specifically developed for use in research studies to assess the health literacy of persons in health care settings.

A The TOFHLA consists of actual materials from hospital settings, such as appointment slips, prescription vials, and informed consent documents.

B The TOFHLA is administered in two parts, reading comprehension and numeracy. Thus, both comprehension and mathematical skills are assessed.

C A Spanish version of TOFHLA, referred to as TOFHLA-S,[3] has also been developed.

D The TOFHLA is highly correlated with the WRAT-R and REALM (see below); however, because the TOFHLA can take up to 22 minutes to administer it may be too time consuming for clinical use.

4 Since 1993, two other literacy assessment tests[4,5] have been developed for routine clinical use.

A The Rapid Estimate of Adult Literacy in Medicine (REALM)[4] is a fast, efficient method for evaluating reading ability.

- REALM consists of 66 medically related words that range in difficulty from simple to complex (eg, fat and germs to colitis and impetigo). These words are set in a large print and divided into three columns across the page. The test is administered by asking patients to read the words aloud; scoring is based on their ability to correctly pronounce each word.

- The patient's raw score is then converted to an estimated grade range using a conversion chart. The conversion chart describes types of materials that might be appropriate for patients who read at each grade range.

- REALM can be administered in 2 to 3 minutes; it correlates well with more time-consuming tests such as SORT-R, WRAT-R, and PIAT-R; and it is designed for use in clinical settings.

- REALM has limitations. First, REALM assesses pronunciation rather than comprehension. However, REALM is correlated with the WRAT-R, which, in turn, is correlated with reading comprehension tests such as the Stanford Achievement Test. Therefore, REALM may provide a reasonable gauge of reading comprehension for some patients. The second limitation of REALM is that it does not assess patients' ability to understand and perform quantitative operations. Finally, since REALM is also obviously a reading test, some patients who want to hide their poor literacy skills may not want to take this test.

B The Medical Achievement Reading Test (MART)[5] is another rapid test designed for clinical use.

- MART consists of only medically-related terms that are set in small print on glossy (light reflecting) paper, similar to the label on a prescription bottle.

- The format of MART was designed purposefully to provide built-in excuses for not being able to read the words. Patients can avoid admitting that they cannot comprehend the material by blaming the glare from the glossy covering or the small print. Thus, the test is intended to be less threatening.

- MART, like REALM, correlates positively with other tests such as the WRAT-R, which is correlated to standardized reading comprehension tests.

- A limitation of MART, like REALM, is that neither comprehension nor quantitative capabilities are tested directly.

5 Readability formulas have been used increasingly to evaluate patient education materials. However, these formulas were originally designed only to rank the difficulty level of a series of written materials.[6]

A Formulas that are commonly used to evaluate word and sentence length are the SMOG, Flesch, Fry, and Dale-Chall. The National Cancer Institute (NCI) recommends the SMOG as one tool for assessing readability (The procedure for using the SMOG is available from the NCI—see the Suggested Readings).

B To use readability formulas appropriately, writers and evaluators can follow three principles:

- Use readability formulas only in concert with direct testing of materials on target audience members.

- Use formulas only when the intended audience is similar to the group that participated in validating the formula.

- Do not write a text with readability formulas in mind.

C Readability formulas will not help persons who are illiterate; text readability does not matter if the patient cannot read at all.

Teaching Approaches for Persons with Low Literacy Skills

1 Patients with low literacy skills benefit most when educators conscientiously use educational and behaviorial strategies that are known to be effective.

    A Directed questioning and active listening are essential for rapport-building and comprehensive assessment.

- Acknowledge the problem of limited reading skills by saying something like "A lot of our patients have trouble reading prescriptions and education materials. Is that a problem for you?" or "Is there anyone you usually ask to help you read your prescriptions or the booklets and pamphlets we give you?"
- Personalize all messages to patients. Instead of saying "Meal planning is the cornerstone of diabetes management," personalize the message by saying something like "Managing your diabetes begins with keeping track of what you eat."
- Invite and encourage patients to describe their strengths by saying "Ms. Jackson, tell me the ways you prefer to learn, and the strategies you've developed for doing your job/homemaking tasks."
- Assure patients that they are not alone in having reading problems and that they can succeed.

    B Tailor objectives for self-management education so that their attainment depends less on reading than on other modes of learning.

    C Limit the number of educational objectives and amount of material to be taught in a particular session to what is essential for meeting patients' needs and desires. It is better to set modest goals and teach more if a patient is able rather than set overly ambitious goals that may result in the patient feeling like a failure.

    D Repetition is a key to success. State important points at the beginning of instruction and repeat these points during the instruction process. Patients can then be asked to rehearse the important points at the end of the session.

    E Concrete illustrations, demonstrations, and hands-on experiences presented from the patient's point of view are more effective than information-telling. Emphasize actions and behaviors over theories and concepts.

- Storytelling may help some patients learn because the information is embedded in a memorable structure and may represent a more culturally appropriate way to teach.

- Analogies drawn from a patient's experience may be similarly helpful.

F Be especially sensitive to word usage.

- Most patients can learn any and all diabetes-related terms if, when the terms are introduced, they are repeatedly stated carefully and defined in context, and the patients are shown illustrations of what the words mean and how they look in print. Patients can benefit further by using the terms in return demonstrations.
- Many patients with low-to-moderate literacy skills can improve their functional ability to read patient education publications by several "grade" levels if they are taught the meaning and spelling of the 12 to 20 most common diabetes-related words (eg, *diabetes, insulin, blood glucose, hypoglycemia, hyperglycemia, nutrition, hospital*).

G Pause frequently to ask patients to repeat what has been said or to perform a return demonstration. Be sure that the prerequisites have been mastered before continuing to teach. Achieving success in one area is better than teaching five areas and discovering that the patient is bewildered.

H Being patient is essential; persons with low literacy and other learning problems do especially poorly if they feel they are being rushed.

I Recommend aids to recall, including mnemonic devices such as visualizing, categorizing, and use of associations and acronyms.

J Offer encouragement and specific feedback about patient performance.

K Provide audiotapes or videotapes to reinforce and extend patient learning for those who have the necessary playback equipment at home. Multimedia resources provide patients with the opportunity to learn in a more private, relaxed environment that helps to preserve their dignity. In many cases, homemade videotapes will be better received than professional productions, especially if the people in the video look and sound like the intended viewing audience and model effective diabetes management. If you donate one or more copies of videos to local video rental stores, they will often be happy to lend these videos free of charge.

L Identify family members, friends, or members of community agencies who can read and are willing to help. Such persons are usually the key to achieving diabetes goals when low literacy is accompanied or caused by cognitive dysfunction or mental handicaps.

M Personalize printed materials by placing the patient's name on the cover of each item. Print patient-specific information inside the materials.

N Schedule more frequent, short visits if possible and review what was taught during the previous sessions.

O Simplify patients' regimens; work up to complex goals as patients (and/or caregivers) experience success and become confident.

P Highlight one or two of the most important take-home messages. Stress their importance and ask patients or family members to repeat them.

Q Provide education materials in both English and the native language for persons whose first language is not English.

R Use small group methods to encourage storytelling and group brainstorming and problem solving. Persons with low literacy may be more comfortable learning from others' experiences.

2 Both educators and patients with low literacy skills may benefit when the curriculum includes topics not usually taught to literate patients, such as how to access ancillary services. Addressing such topics as a routine part of the content helps those persons with low literacy who feel ashamed of their lack of reading ability. Their shame can be exacerbated by health professionals who become frustrated or angry when a patient cannot find a particular location in the medical center, complete a form, or read even the most straightforward instructions.[7] Community outreach programs that assist with these needs can be very helpful. Good relationships with patients can be solidified by being sensitive to their needs for the following assistance:

A Many patients don't show up or are chronically late for appointments because they need help navigating around the medical building(s) in which they receive their care.

- Familiar words (*diabetes* rather than *endocrinology*) should be used on hallway signs.
- Color coding for hospital/clinic floors and parking levels can help identify locations.
- Strategically placed information desks staffed by persons attuned to the needs of low-literate clients should be considered in larger institutions.

B Completing forms and registering for care can be the most difficult and embarrassing tasks for persons with low literacy levels.

- Simplify forms as much as possible.

- Advise clerks, receptionists, social workers and other staff to be sensitive and alert for someone struggling to a complete a form. Support can be offered by saying something like "Many of our patients have trouble with these forms. Would it help if I read the questions to you?" Some large clinics with significant numbers of low-literate patients employ surrogate readers for this purpose.

C Medication and other self-care errors due to patients' inability to read or understand the instructions are among the most troubling and life-threatening problems for low literate persons.

- Simplify medication and self-care regimens as much as possible (eg, use combination drugs rather than separate pills, or avoid multi-drug regimens that require patients to take different drugs on different schedules).

- Include family members, friends, or agency workers identified by patients as surrogate readers when providing medication and treatment instructions.

- Ability to follow a meal plan is especially challenging for persons with low literacy. Many such persons benefit from educator-led "field trips" to neighborhood groceries. Those who cannot base food selection on nutrition labeling can, if they wish, be taught to make appropriate choices based on characteristics of food packaging, such as colors and shapes of the items.

D Many patients with low literacy skills say they have little or no difficulty understanding appointment reminders if the card or slip of paper is identified as such. Most will then keep the reminder card and obtain assistance from others if they cannot decipher the date, time, and location messages.

E Many patients with low literacy express an interest in attending adult literacy classes. Be prepared to make referrals to such courses by having and posting a list of telephone numbers of literacy classes available in your area; help patients locate these courses if necessary.

3 Review and prepare educational materials for use with patients.

A The National Cancer Institute's publication,[8] *Clear and Simple: Developing Effective Print Materials for Low Literate Readers* provides a description of five tests that can be used to create educational materials or evaluate those made by others.

- Define the target audience by identifying the segment of the population to be reached.
- Know the target audience by learning about behaviors that help or hinder prevention or self-care; knowledge and attitudes; utilization of existing services; cultural habits, preferences, and sensitivities related to the message(s) being communicated; and common barriers and motivators.
- Develop a concept for the item by defining behavioral objectives; determining a limited number of points that are key to achieving those objectives; selecting the best presentation methods (eg, audio, audiovisual, print, interactive computer); estimating the functional reading level appropriate for print materials; and organizing topics in the way they will be used by the target audience.
- Develop content and visuals using the guidelines presented in Table 2.2.
- Pretest and revise draft materials with the goal of determining whether representative members of the target audience understand the message before going to the expense of publishing and distributing the materials. Besides comprehension, other factors that can be used to in assess educational materials are audience attraction, acceptance, and personal relevance. The materials should be pilot tested with 25 to 50 persons, although results from testing with smaller groups can still provide valuable information. Be sure that the individuals who are participating in the pretest understand that it is the materials, not them, that are being evaluated.

B If the foregoing steps are used to review and prepare educational materials, the use of readability formulas will be largely unnecessary.

C Direct translations of reading materials from English into other languages are rarely successful. Other-language versions of reading materials should also be developed using the steps suggested above.

Table 2.2. Checklist for Evaluating/Developing Patient Education Materials

Content/Style	• The material is interactive and allows for audience involvement. • The material presents "how-to" information. • Peer language is used whenever appropriate to increase personal identification and improve readability. • Words are familiar to the reader. Any new words are defined clearly. • Sentences are simple, specific, direct, and written in the active voice. • Each idea is clear and logically sequenced (according to audience logic). • The number of concepts is limited per piece.
Layout	• The material uses advance organizers or headers. • Headers are simple and close to text. • Layout balances white space with words and illustrations. • Text uses uppercase and lowercase letters. • Underlining or bolding rather than all caps give emphasis. • Type style and size of print are easy-to-read; type is at least 12 point.
Visuals	• Visuals are relevant to text, meaningful to the audience, and appropriately located. • Illustrations and photographs are simple and free from clutter and distraction. • Visuals use adult rather than childlike images. • Illustrations show familiar images that reflect cultural context. • Visuals have captions. Each visual illustrates and is directly related to one message. • Different styles, such as photographs without background detail, shaded line drawings, or simple line drawings, are pretested with the audience to determine which is understood best. • Cues, such as circles or arrows, point out key information. • Colors used are appealing to the audience (as determined by pretesting).
Readability	• Readability analysis is done to suggest the approximate reading level.

Source: Reprinted with permission from the National Cancer Institute.[8]

KEY EDUCATIONAL CONSIDERATIONS

1   Nearly one half of all Americans have poor functional literacy. Understanding common diabetes educational materials and dealing with the healthcare system can be frustrating and challenging both for these people and their health professionals.

2   Literacy assessment tools such as REALM and MART may be useful for identifying and evaluating patients with low literacy skills; however, they are best used to approximate someone's ability to comprehend written materials.

3   Diabetes educators can serve low-literate clients most effectively by using teaching strategies that serve patients' specific needs. These strategies may include limiting or simplifying learning objectives, using audiovisual teaching aids, repeating main points, and assessing patient mastery before moving on to new topics.

4   Important considerations for preparing or evaluating patient education materials are knowing the target audience, having a clear concept of the audience's information needs, choosing content and visuals consistent with audience needs, and pretesting the materials with representatives from the target audience.

5   Low-literate patients may experience shame when confronted with written materials commonly found in healthcare environments (eg, forms, reading materials, and insurance papers) that they are unable to read. They may also experience problems accessing healthcare services because of their reading difficulties. Consider examining the extent to which your institution and practices help or hinder low-literate patients.

SELF-REVIEW QUESTIONS

1   Define functional literacy. Characterize the distribution of functional literacy skills in the general population of the United States.

2   What are the health-related implications of the literacy problem in the United States?

3   Name three tools you might use to assess literacy in the population of patients you serve. What are the strengths and weaknesses of each strategy?

4 Describe at least six teaching strategies that may help meet the needs of persons with low literacy skills.

5 Describe five criteria for producing patient education materials or evaluating the appropriateness of existing materials for your patients.

6 Compare and contrast the utility of different teaching approaches for helping patients with different levels of functional literacy.

CASE STUDY 1

PJ is a 45-year-old male recently diagnosed with type 2 diabetes. He is 5'8", weighs 190 lb (86.3 kg), and has a blood pressure of 135/90. PJ holds a daytime job as a housekeeper at a metropolitan hotel where he has been working since he dropped out of high school after the 10th grade. At night he tends bar at a local pub to help his sister pay for their mother's nursing home bills. His mother was placed in the nursing home about 2 years ago after having a stroke. She is 75 years old and has had uncontrolled diabetes for many years. PJ states that when his sister is not busy with her work as an accountant, the two of them often visit their mother together.

PJ was diagnosed with type 2 diabetes at a workplace screening program. He has no symptoms of diabetes, although he does complain of fatigue that he attributes to his rigorous work schedule. PJ expresses that he would like to make an effort to control his diabetes; he is concerned since his mother's physician told him that her stroke was partly due to her uncontrolled diabetes. PJ takes oral diabetes medications exactly as ordered and feels that the pills should be sufficient treatment for his diabetes. He does not understand the relationship between exercise, diet, and diabetes.

While asking PJ about his nutritional habits, you discover that he eats many of his meals at the restaurant in the hotel where he works because he gets a big employee discount. He also tells you that his favorite foods are potato chips and hot dogs, and he would really like to continue eating them on a regular basis. PJ states that he does not like exercise and feels he does not have time to cook healthy foods for himself.

You initially give PJ a diabetes education pamphlet designed for the general population. To determine PJ's understanding of the material, you select one sentence in the pamphlet and ask him what it means. You point to a sentence that says, "Reducing cholesterol and fat in your diet, in combination with a regular exercise program, will help you control your diabetes." You ask PJ to read the sentence and tell you what it means. PJ replies that the sentence tells him he should go on a diet to lose fat, and that exercise will help control his diabetes. You realize that PJ did not understand the word *cholesterol*, and that, in this context, he did not really grasp the meaning of most the words that he read, so you decide to administer the REALM literacy test. PJ scores in the 4th to 6th grade range on the REALM scoring scale, indicating that he should respond well to direct instructions, but may require some additional counseling to adequately understand material written at an elementary school level.

Questions for Discussion

1 How would you characterize PJ's literacy level?
2 What obstacles would you encounter in teaching PJ?
3 What are some strategies for teaching this patient about diabetes and health management?

Discussion

1 The characteristics displayed by PJ place him at a very low literacy level.
   A Although PJ completed the 10th grade before dropping out of school, he is an example of a person who reads at a level lower than the last grade completed.
   B PJ reads at the 4th to 6th grade level based on the REALM scoring scale and would likely fall into the Level 1 category of literacy proficiency (Table 2.1).
      • Skills common to this level are identifying a country in a short article, locating an expiration date on a driver's license, or calculating a total for a bank deposit entry.
      • Although the Level 1 tasks seem very simple, about 1 of every 5 Americans (40 million people) perform at Level 1 literacy at best, and are able to perform "simple, routine tasks involving uncomplicated texts and documents."

2 Much of the educational material designed for the general public is written at a level too complex for many patients to understand.
   A PJ, like much of the US population, reads at a level lower than the final grade he completed. His misinterpretation of the pamphlet serves as

an example of how patients with low literacy skills may skip words they do not know and use limited meanings for words they know from other contexts.

  B These patients often will not make inferences or interpret words in the context in which they are presented.

3 Many obstacles must be overcome to properly teach PJ about diabetes.

  A Because of PJ's poor literacy skills, materials such as educational audio tapes and videotapes may be useful.

  B Another possibility is to have PJ's sister assist him in reading and understanding diabetes education material.

  C Consistently repeating important information may be useful in working with PJ because many reading-impaired patients use memorization as a coping strategy.

  D Competing priorities in PJ's life must also be addressed. It is important to help PJ find a way to make controlling diabetes an important focus in his life while still allowing him to handle his difficult work schedule, his mother and her condition, and the stresses associated with both.

  E Finally, PJ may have difficulty forming new habits (eg, eating properly, exercising regularly) and affording some diabetes treatments if his insurance does not cover these expenses.

4 Strategies for teaching PJ include focusing on specific behaviors he agrees to perform and teaching only one or two essential objectives during each session.

  A After discussion with PJ, the two of you may decide that the following are some realistic goals for PJ to try to accomplish before his next appointment.

  • Substitute a low-fat variety of hot dogs for his regular brand
  • Take his mother for walks in her wheelchair for 20 minutes each time he visits her

  B You may also want to ask PJ to see if there is a worksite wellness program at the hotel where he works. If PJ can successfully accomplish his initial goals, he may want to get involved in the worksite wellness program or, if one is not available, to enroll in a diabetes management class. He is more likely to attend if he receives assistance in working these into his schedule.

Case Study 2

LM is a 59-year-old female who lost her job as a light machinery operator at a local paper plant due to company downsizing 3 months ago. Her blood pressure is 160/94, she is 5'3" and she weighs 160 lb (72.6 kg).

LM arrived 45 minutes late for her appointment today, and you notice in her chart that she has a history of missing appointments. She states that her family responsibilities often cause her to be late or miss appointments. At her last visit 5 weeks ago, LM started two medications in addition to her oral diabetes medication. The two medications were an antihypertensive and a drug that inhibits cholesterol formation so as to prevent atherosclerosis. LM has been instructed to take the antihypertensive 2 times per day, the anticholesterol drug once a day, and the oral diabetes medication 3 times per day. LM reports that she has not been feeling well lately. She complains of headaches, sleeplessness, and frequent urination, although the vaginal itching she complained of at the last appointment has since been resolved. You also note that she has not yet been accepted to Medicaid, even though she was given application forms immediately after she lost her job and company insurance.

LM's laboratory test results indicate that her blood glucose is 230 mg/dL (12.78 mmol/L) after a 12-hour fast and her cholesterol level is 160, which is down from 240 the last time she visited. When you ask LM if she has been taking her medications, she responds that she has taken them exactly as ordered. LM then takes her bag of medications out of her purse so you can look at the bottles. You notice that she has a bottle of antibiotics with her husband's name on it instead of the blood pressure medication that was prescribed. Sensing that LM may not be able to read prescription labels, you decide to give her the REALM reading test. She refuses, stating that she forgot to bring her glasses today.

Questions for Discussion

1 What are LM's physical problems? Why might she be feeling so poorly?
2 What characteristics of poor literacy is LM displaying?
3 What are some strategies for helping LM?

DISCUSSION

1 LM has confused her medications. She appears to be taking her husband's antibiotics instead of her blood pressure pills. In addition, her high blood glucose and very sharp reduction in blood cholesterol since her last visit suggest that she may have switched the dosing for the diabetes pills with the dosing for the cholesterol pills (ie, LM is taking the diabetes pills once a day and the cholesterol pills 3 times per day).

2 Patients with low literacy skills commonly cope by memorizing information about their medications. When confronted with several different medications with different dose directions, some persons may become confused about what they have memorized and take pills in the wrong doses and/or at the wrong times.

3 Patients with low literacy also commonly forget appointments or arrive late. They must often rely on their memories to recall the correct date and time of appointments. Some patients may even get lost on their way to the appointment because they cannot read the road signs or the signs within the hospital/clinic. One reason LM may not have been accepted to Medicaid is that she did not properly complete the forms (or fill them out at all). Accessing health care, from getting to the clinic to taking medications to filling out forms and becoming properly educated about one's diagnoses, requires a fairly high level of literacy. Living with low literacy skills can make navigating the healthcare system a nightmare for some patients.

4 A very important aspect of LM's coping style is the schemes she has created to attempt to hide her poor literacy skills. Claiming she forgot her glasses and that her family is the reason for her poor or late appointment attendance are simple mechanisms to hide the fact that she cannot read very well.

5 All of these characteristics point to the tremendous amount of shame that many people feel about having poor reading skills. Many illiterate people are able to hold jobs for years and function quite well in society even though they cannot read. It is important to not confuse poor reading and writing skills with lack of intelligence; a high degree of intelligence may be necessary to function in society without being able to read.

6 A variety of strategies can be used to help LM cope with her reading problems.

   A Provide telephone reminders of her appointments to improve her attendance.

   B If she is interested, tell her where to obtain and then demonstrate how to use a pill organizer with different containers for her pills each day (some pharmacies provide these free to customers, but, if not, an egg carton may be used if LM cannot afford a pill organizer).

   C Enlist the help of family members, friends, or social services to assist her with the aspects of her life that require literacy, such as filling out Medicaid forms and properly taking her medications.

   D Simplify LM's medications by requesting that her provider prescribe pills that are different colors or sizes to make them easy to identify and distinguish from one another.

   E Assist her in enrolling in an adult literacy class if she wishes to learn to read and can make the time to attend class.

   F Perhaps most importantly, end each teaching session with LM repeating/demonstrating to you what you have taught her that day.

7 When dealing with functionally illiterate patients, be sensitive to the shame they may feel because they cannot read.

   A When you suspect a patient is illiterate, take steps to reduce their embarrassment. For instance, when giving them a piece of literature to read to see if they understand the meaning, a helpful comment might be "many of our patients cannot understand this pamphlet, tell me if you have trouble with it," or "the glossy covering on this prescription bottle makes it hard to read for some patients; tell me if it bothers you." These statements and others like them provide excuses for the patients. They do not have to admit directly that they cannot read the material; but you can still find out if they are functionally illiterate.

   B Reduce potential for shame associated with LM having taken the wrong medications: "When two or more family members take several medicines it's pretty easy to get them mixed up, and it looks like that might have happened in your home. It's good that we caught the mix-up early. This time I want to be sure I've been clear about your medications so you can go home and get the medicine you need and your husband gets what he needs..."

REFERENCES

1   Kirsch L, Jungeblut A, Jenkins L, Kolstad A. Adult literacy in America: a first look at the results of the National Adult Literacy Survey. Washington, DC: National Center for Education Statistics, Department of Education, 1993.

2   Doak C, Doak L, Root J. Teaching patients with low literacy skills. 2nd ed. Philadelphia: Lippincott-Raven Publishers, 1996.

3   Parikh NS, Parker RM, Nurss JR, Baker DW, Williams MV. Shame and health literacy: the unspoken connection. Patient Educ Couns 1996;27:33-39.

4   Davis TC, Long SW, Jackson RH, Mayeaux EJ, George RB, Murphy PW, Crouch MA. Rapid estimate of adult literacy in medicine: a shortened screening instrument. Family Medicine, 1993;25:391-5.

5   Hanson-Divers EC. Developing a medical achievement reading test to evaluate patient literacy skills: a preliminary study. J Health Care for the Poor and Underserved 1997;8:56-69.

6   Pichert JW, Elam P. Readability formulas may mislead you. Patient Educ Couns 1985;7:181-91.

7   Baker DW, Parker RM, Williams MV, et al. The health care experience of patients with low literacy. Arch Fam Med 1996;5:329-34.

8   National Cancer Institute, National Institutes of Health. Clear and simple: developing effective print materials for low literate readers. Bethesda, Md: National Institutes of Health, undated.

Suggested Readings

Combined health information database. At Web site http://chid.nih.gov.

Diabetes educational materials for people with limited reading skills. Searches-on-file, topics in diabetes. Bethesda, Md: National Diabetes Information Clearinghouse, Mar 1997. Contact the NDIC at 1 Information Way, Bethesda, MD 20892-3560. Telephone 301-654-3327.

Patient education materials (many described as low literacy, only a few directly related to diabetes). At Web site http://lib-sh.lsumc.edu

Mettger W. Communicating nutrition information to low-literate individuals: an assessment of methods. Bethesda, Md: National Cancer Institute, National Institutes of Health, 1989. To order, contact: Office of Cancer Communications, NCI, Building 31, Room 10A03 9000 Rockville Pike, Bethesda, MD 20892. Telephone 1-800-4-CANCER.

National Cancer Institute, National Institutes of Health. Detailed guidelines for writers who wish to communicate effectively with low literate audiences. "Clear and Simple" and "Making Health Communications Work," and "Theory At A Glance" may be downloaded free at Web site http://www.nci.nih.gov or by calling 1-800-4-CANCER. If you use the internet, go to the NCI website and search the alternatives under "Information for Patients, Public and the Mass Media" in order to find these program planning publications.

Bernoff RA. Teaching clients with low literacy skills. Better teaching skills for the diabetes educator. Issue 3. Elkins Park, NJ: Educational Programs Inc, 1995.

Beyond the Brochure: Alternative Approaches to Effective Health communications (PDF-821K). Free from the Centers for Disease Control and Prevention. May be downloaded from the "cancer" publications section of the CDC website at www.cdc.gov/

Resources for teaching may be obtained from the Office of Minority Health Resource Center. Telephone: 1-800-444-6472. Web site http://www.omhrc.gov. OMH lists many Spanish language health materials.

Cultural Appropriateness in Diabetes Education and Care

3

Lynne S. Robins, PhD
University of Michigan
Department of Medical Education
Ann Arbor, Michigan

Jackie Two Feathers
The University of New Mexico
School of Medicine
Albuquerque, New Mexico

INTRODUCTION

1 Cultural appropriateness is an important consideration in providing diabetes education and care:

   A The incidence of diabetes is increasing disproportionately among various ethnic populations in the United States.

   B The cultural distance between patients and healthcare professionals is increasing as the patient population diversifies.

2 There are benefits to providing culturally appropriate diabetes education and care:

   A Improved treatment outcomes

   B Increased patient satisfaction

3 The theory behind culturally appropriate diabetes education and care involves key anthropological concepts:

   A Everyone has a culture of origin and cultures of affiliation.

   B Healthcare professionals are influenced by their own personal cultures and the culture of biomedicine.

   C Cultural competence provides a means of bridging cultural differences.

4 Designing culturally appropriate diabetes education and care programs requires engaging both the individual and the community.

OBJECTIVES

Upon completion of this chapter, the learner will be able to

1 Define culturally appropriate diabetes education and care.

2 Describe the influence of culture on the beliefs and practices of patients and diabetes educators.

3 Explain strategies for providing culturally appropriate diabetes education and care.

4 Describe the prevalence of diabetes among people from underserved cultural groups.

5 Explain the principles of providing culturally appropriate diabetes education and care.

6 Describe specific applications of the principles for providing culturally appropriate diabetes education and care.

THE IMPORTANCE OF BEING CULTURALLY COMPETENT

1   The premise of this chapter is that diabetes educators can offer more compassionate and effective care to their patients by becoming culturally competent. Adopting the understandings and conceptual tools of anthropology can foster fuller understanding and appreciation of patients' cultural beliefs, behaviors, and perspectives (worldviews) and their influence on diabetes self-care behaviors.

2   Diabetes educators, more so than many other health professionals, need to understand the cultural contexts in which patients conduct their self-care routines. Daily blood glucose measurement, use of a meal plan, use of medications, and physical activity impinge on such culturally defined phenomena as family relationships, food preferences and preparation rituals, and beliefs about health and illness.

3   Helping patients navigate through cultural barriers to self-care requires a recognition of these barriers, an appreciation of their power to impede patients' progress toward health, and an understanding of how these barriers might be negotiated. It is also important to recognize and support strengths that patients derive from their cultural and religious beliefs.

DEFINING CULTURALLY APPROPRIATE HEALTH CARE

1   *Culturally appropriate* health care and education acknowledges and strives to accommodate patients' understandings about health and sickness. Questions and concerns, beliefs about death and bereavement, personal hygiene practices, dietary preferences, religious behaviors, modesty norms, family involvement, and language preferences are taken into account in a nonjudgmental fashion.[1]

2   Other terms used to describe this type of care include culturally relevant, culturally sensitive, and culturally competent health care.

3   Achieving the cultural competence necessary to provide culturally appropriate patient education and health care and is a developmental learning process that requires time, effort, active awareness, practice, and introspection. Bennett,[2] a noted researcher on the development of cultural sensitivity, observed that intercultural sensitivity is not natural and has little

historical precedent. It is neither part of our primate past nor has it characterized most of human history. Rather, cross-cultural contact has historically been accompanied by bloodshed, oppression, or genocide.

A *Anthropology.* The social scientific discipline that seeks to understand the particulars and universals of human behavior by studying people in their cultural contexts.

B *Culture.* A set of beliefs and behaviors that are learned and shared by members of a group. Culture serves as a guide for acting and for interpreting experience.

C *Ethnicity.* A shared cultural identity or cultural heritage that forms a part of the lifestyle and shared sense of identity of the members of a group. Ethnicity is a cultural, not a biological, characteristic and is changeable.

D *Enculturation.* The process of learning or acquiring one's culture of origin.

E *Acculturation.* The process of adapting to a culture other than one's culture of origin or first learned culture.

F *Conventional Medicine.* The officially sanctioned medical system of the United States; also called Western, academic, or scientific medicine, or biomedicine.

G *Worldview.* The metaphorical lens through which human beings view and interpret experience. Worldviews determine the character of what is real or true and how it is reliably to be known.

H *Ethnocentric.* The belief that one's own culture is superior to others. The conscious or unconscious practice of interpreting other cultures or the actions of their members in terms of the values and norms of one's own culture.

I *Ethnographer.* A social science researcher, typically an anthropologist, who collaborates with his/her subjects, respondents, or informants to attempt to understand them and the cultural groups to which they belong by gaining an "insider's" perspective.

UNDERSTANDING CULTURALLY APPROPRIATE HEALTH CARE

1 Many of the concepts used to describe and provide a theoretical basis for culturally appropriate diabetes education and care are borrowed from the discipline of anthropology.

2 Everyone has a culture.

A   *Culture* is defined as a set of beliefs and behaviors that are learned and shared by members of a group. Culture shapes the way group members view and experience the world.

B   As children, all human beings learn a particular cultural tradition through a process called enculturation.

C   All people are additionally influenced by the many group cultures to which they belong, in addition to their cultures of origin and rearing.
  • These cultures include religious groups; ethnic, gender, and sexual orientation/identity groups; social classes; and voluntary and professional organizations.
  • The process of learning, borrowing, and then assimilating values and behaviors from these additional cultural groups into a person's cognitive and behavioral repertoires is called acculturation.

D   Providing *culturally appropriate health care* requires a willingness to
  • Learn from patients about their health beliefs.
  • Incorporate patients' concerns and perspectives into structuring and delivering education and health care.
  • Modify personal thinking and behaviors to facilitate mutual respect and rapport.
  • Develop treatment and prevention plans to meet the patients' needs and goals.
  • Establish a true working partnership with patients.[3]

3   All diabetes education and care is essentially cross-cultural.
  A   Culture is not a factor of significance only for underserved groups or patients. Cultural differences require at least two reference points.[3]
    • Anthropologist Robert Hahn[4] observed that patients and professionals may appear to understand one another and communicate effectively because they use a common language and share concepts and behavioral patterns. But he warned that these appearances may be deceptive.
    • At least two very different reference points are represented in every professional/patient encounter, and the potential for miscommunication is great unless they are explicitly discussed.
  B   Healthcare providers can be thought of as a cultural group with a worldview and language that distinguishes them from their patients.
  C   The intensive training of all healthcare professionals has been likened to the process of acculturation.[5]

- Through the process of education, healthcare professionals acquire a worldview that influences the way they interpret sickness, explain its causes and progression, understand its symptoms, and orchestrate methods of treatment.

- Conventionally trained healthcare professionals, for example, learn a biomedical model of health and illness. In this model, disease is characterized as a biochemical or physiological abnormality. The therapeutic goal of disease treatment is to restore the patient to health by addressing the underlying physiological disorder.[6]

- In the same vein, diabetes educators may judge each other on patient outcomes, such as "All my patients have HbA$_{1c}$ levels in the near-normal range" or "I brought that patient's hemoglobin down into the normal range."

- In contrast, a more holistic model of health and illness focuses on the patient's experience of his or her illness and attempts to respond to that experience. This approach entails understanding hidden aspects of illness reality and working to transform that reality.

D Attitudes about how sick people and professionals are expected to interact are also learned in the context of health professional education.

- The traditional medical model of health professional/patient relationships is derived from the acute care model of disease treatment. According to this model, health professionals are characteristically active, in charge of, and responsible for treatment of the patient's illness, while the patient is passive, accepting, compliant, and dependent on the provider's knowledge and good will.[7]

- Perhaps most noticeable is that healthcare professionals acquire a style of speaking that differs in form and content from that of the general public, and a knowledge base and set of skills that are rarely shared by those who have not gone through this acculturation process.

BENEFITS OF PROVIDING CULTURALLY APPROPRIATE DIABETES EDUCATION AND CARE

1 Many health professionals believe that their approaches to health and illness are superior to all others.

A This belief is a form of *ethnocentrism,* which is defined as a view that one's own culture does things the right (or natural) way and that all other ways are inferior. Adopting such a view about patients' beliefs is unproductive.

B Research[8] has suggested that a failure to acknowledge and accommodate patients' health beliefs and behaviors can result in patient dissatisfaction and poor treatment outcomes.

2 Awareness of one's own professional cultural values and worldview is a prerequisite for becoming culturally competent, or able to provide culturally appropriate health care.[9]

3 Like all individuals, diabetes educators belong to many cultural groups. Organizations like the American Association of Diabetes Educators (AADE) provide opportunities for socialization and affiliation through which professional values and behaviors specific to diabetes education and treatment are transmitted.

   A The perspective that diabetes is largely self-managed is a predominant belief among diabetes educators, and one that is reinforced through professional meetings, publications, and recommendations.

   B Patients may have a different perspective, as many have been acculturated to the roles and responsibilities associated with the traditional medical model. Some patients expect to turn over their care to their health professionals, preferring to play a more passive role in their treatment. Others may believe it is the responsibility of their spouse, adult children, or other family members. These differences in perspective can lead to problems if not recognized, explored, and addressed.

4 *Cultural relativism* is defined as the attitude that other ways of doing things are different but equally valid and that behavior needs to be understood in its cultural context. Adopting this attitude is a necessary first step toward culturally appropriate and more effective care and education.

THE PREVALENCE OF DIABETES

1 When comparing people with diabetes with people in the US without diabetes, the following tends to be true:

   A People with diabetes are older. In 1989, the median age for the population with diabetes was 63 years as compared with the median age of 40 years for all adults.[10]

B A higher proportion of adults with type 2 diabetes are women (58.4%) than men (41.6%). These higher proportions of women are found for non-Hispanic Caucasians, African Americans, and Mexican Americans. The difference is greatest for African Americans with type 2 diabetes.[10]

C People with diabetes are often members of traditionally underserved cultural groups. All of these groups, except natives of Alaska, have a prevalence of type 2 diabetes that is 2 to 6 times greater than that of Caucasian persons. Diabetes-related mortality is higher for non-whites, and both prevalence and mortality rates are rapidly increasing.[11]

- African Americans:[12] In 1993, 1.3 million African Americans were known to have diabetes. On average, African Americans are 1.6 times more likely to have diabetes than Caucasians of similar age. African Americans with diabetes are more likely to develop diabetes complications and experience greater disability from the complications than Caucasian Americans with diabetes. African Americans have a higher incidence of and greater disability from diabetes complications such as kidney failure, visual impairment, and amputations.

- Native Americans:[11] Native Americans comprise more than 500 tribal organizations. High prevalences of diabetes among most Native American tribes have been reported; Indian Health Service data indicate that the overall prevalence is 2.8 times the overall US rate. The Pima tribe in Arizona has one of the highest rates in the world.

- Hispanic Americans:[13] On average, Hispanic/Latino Americans are almost twice as likely to have diabetes as non-Hispanic Caucasians of similar age. More than 1 in 10 Hispanic American adults (1.8 million) have type 2 diabetes. Among Hispanic persons living in the US, the prevalence of type 2 diabetes is greatest for Puerto Ricans and Hispanic persons living in the southwest and is lowest for Cubans.

- Asian Americans and Pacific Islander Americans:[11] The Seattle Japanese-American Community Diabetes Study found the prevalence of diabetes to be higher than that reported for the US Caucasian population. Filipinos had the highest prevalence of diabetes among the four largest ethnic Asian groups in Hawaii (Chinese, Filipino, Japanese, and Korean); all groups had higher prevalences than those of Caucasians.

D People with diabetes are less educated.[10] Even after accounting for age, persons with type 2 diabetes have less education than persons without diabetes.

E People with diabetes are poorer. According to a Gallup Organization survey,[14] households in the lowest economic group had the highest prevalence of diabetes. At all ages and for both men and women, a greater percent of persons with type 2 diabetes were at lower income levels than persons without diabetes.[10]

2 The reason these social and cultural characteristics are important is because they are likely to distance patients from the Caucasian, middle-class educators and professionals with whom they often interact unless these professionals make an attempt to bridge the barriers.

CULTURE AND DIABETES EDUCATION AND SELF-MANAGEMENT

1 Understanding patients' cultures is especially relevant for managing a chronic illness such as diabetes because of its lifelong course and influence on culturally embedded behaviors. Diabetes and its self-management affect virtually every aspect of a patient's life, and patients are often asked to substantially reshape the ways in which they live.[15]

2 The cultural distance between professionals and patients becomes an issue when either fails to live up to the expectations of the other. Diabetes educators can acquire the skills in understanding, communicating, and intervening that will help them mediate between the mainly Caucasian, middle-class, healthcare system and the many historically underserved populations with diabetes.[14]

A Diabetes educators often express frustration when patients fail to live up to their expectations to follow nutritional recommendations.
- A fact often overlooked is that patients may view their educators' expectations about meal planning as unrealistic or culturally insensitive. One assumption that educators often make is that individuals have control over their own food preparation and consumption.

B Focus group discussions with patients have revealed that this assumption is ethnocentric. In a focus group with Latino patients, Anderson et al[16] learned that for Latino women, barriers to following dietary guidelines included their culturally defined roles as food preparers within the family, and family members' desires to have traditional foods of their culture prepared for them. Latino women explained that their own health was a lower priority than meeting their family's expectations related to food as revealed in the following comments:

- "I cook for my daughter and son and take care of all my grandchildren and cook for them, too. It is too difficult to make time to prepare something different and sometimes I don't have time to eat."
- "What I prepare for my family I also eat because I work a lot and I'm too tired to cook something separate for myself."
- The behaviors of the women quoted might have been interpreted as noncompliant or difficult. Viewing these behaviors in a cultural context reveals that they were responding to cultural constraints on their behavior related to food preparation. Asking these women about the meaning of food in their lives would have brought into focus the constraints on their ability to control their meals and may also have reduced frustrations on both sides.

3 Listening to others of all traditions is the hallmark of the anthropological perspective and practice. A central goal is to understand how things look from the other person's point of view.

   A Listening serves multiple purposes in the process of education, including establishing rapport with the patient, understanding the patient's condition, recognizing the patient's goals, and assessing effective modes of therapy.[4]

   B Healthcare providers also can strive to understand the context of their patients' healthcare needs and concerns.

4 Avoid making assumptions about patients' beliefs based on ethnic identification.

   A An individual's identification with an ethnic group does not determine his or her beliefs, values, or behavior in line with the norms of that group.

- Factors that lead to variation among people of the same ethnic group include the length of time they have spent in the US, the age at which they came here, their desire to assimilate, whether they live in ethnic enclaves, whether they are from rural or urban areas, and their level of education.
- Social and economic class cross-cut ethnic boundaries and may sometimes be more important than ethnic background.[17]

   B It is important to recognize that there is variation within cultural traditions.

- Knowledge of a pattern of health beliefs common to a given identity-group may provide a useful frame of reference when working with these patients, but it is not predictive.[9]

- Behaviors, values, or worldviews cannot be categorized by culture. This process fosters the stereotyping and falsely implies that the dominant culture, against which all others are compared, is somehow standard.
- Avoid making assumptions about patients' behaviors based on cultural background or ethnicity. As examples, not all Hispanic American patients incorporate ethnic foods and not all Muslim patients with diabetes fast during Ramadan.

C Rather than make assumptions about cultural beliefs and practices, educators need to take time to ask questions about them.

D It is important to assess these areas, even when the educator and patient share a cultural or ethnic identity.

5 Asking questions of patients is the best way to find out what is important to them, what explanatory model of diabetes they hold, what goals and expectations they have for treatment, and what personal beliefs and values might affect their responses. It is also critical to elicit information about cultural and religious practices that might affect the patient's diabetes self-management.

A Most people view health professionals as persons in positions of authority, and often as persons with very fixed ideas about what is right or important.[3]

- Patients become very cautious about revealing anything they feel might jeopardize their access to medical services, having their deeply felt concerns dismissed as trivial, or being made to feel foolish by provoking irritable reactions.
- Patients manage degrees of disclosure in their encounters according to their own assessments of the situation; they are the ones who make the final decisions about how they will respond to recommendations.
- As an example, professionals working in African-American communities report that older African Americans may not give their healthcare professionals much information about their diabetes. They believe it is the health professional's job to discern their problems and that it would be insulting to the health professional to offer such information. A diabetes educator who is aware of this belief can ask appropriate questions to bring this view out into the open.
- It is important to elicit from patients in a compassionate and nonjudgmental way their important concerns, beliefs, and values that

may have implications for their health and health care. Several relevant pieces of information usually can be learned with just a few well-put questions and an accepting manner. This is especially important for brief encounters and when time to spend with a patient is limited. Findings can be used to jointly develop a treatment plan that will be more likely to succeed.

B Key questions for exploring patients' specific values, beliefs, and practices relevant to health and illness include

- What concerns you most about (caring for) your diabetes?
- What is most difficult for you in (caring for) your diabetes?
- How does your culture affect how you care for your diabetes?
- How do your religious practices and beliefs affect how you care for your diabetes?
- What kinds of home remedies do you use for your diabetes or other health conditions? Are there herbs, medicines, or other treatments you use to care for your diabetes or other health concerns?
- Do you see other health practitioners or healers to help you with your diabetes?
- Tell me a little bit about who you consider family and kin.
- What does your family do to help you take care of your diabetes?
- Who helps you when the going gets tough?
- What is your real passion for living?
- What do you want from your doctor or other providers?
- What can I do to be most helpful to you?

CULTURALLY APPROPRIATE DIABETES EDUCATION PROGRAMS

1 To be effective, diabetes education programs must be relevant, acceptable, and understandable to intended learners. There must also be a consonance or agreement of purpose between professional and client for each to take and sustain action.[18] Educational programs that are not meaningful to their intended audiences risk failing to attract, retain, or aid the people for whom they are designed.

2 The notion of cultural relevancy is based on the understanding that cultural subgroups differ from one another on the basis of their worldviews, value systems, behavioral styles, and often languages. Consequently, what may be real and relevant to members of one group may not have the same salience and value in another.[18]

A For example, there is often a strong sense of the present within African American communities. Orientation toward the future and the necessity of preventive health measures such as annual eye examinations are not consistent with this cultural pattern.[19]

B The problem is compounded by the fact that type 2 diabetes is often a silent disease until complications are quite advanced. Therefore, a program focused solely on blood glucose control to prevent future complications might not be as effective among patients who are focused on the present as a program that also includes immediate benefits.

3 A key to designing culturally appropriate educational programs is the commitment to doing the work of discovering what learners believe about the world and what they think they need to learn.

A This approach requires educators to enter the community unencumbered by preconceived notions about what communities need or how they need to go about achieving healthcare goals.

B Healthcare professionals may need to put aside the ethnocentric belief that patients should sacrifice now for better health tomorrow. There are cultures in which this idea does not resonate. For these cultures, it would be more beneficial to highlight the immediate benefits of glucose control (eg, not having to get up at night to use the bathroom) than to focus on future or long-term health benefits.

CULTURALLY APPROPRIATE COMMUNITY OUTREACH

1 A set of four tenets has been developed[20] for conducting diabetes community outreach programs specifically designed to address the needs of African Americans.

2 These tenets provide a valuable set of planning principles for designing culturally appropriate community programs and education for *all* cultural groups.

A Involve community members and community leaders. Involve community members in each stage of the planning and implementation of health education and care programs intended to be used by them. Such input will help ensure that diabetes programs will be relevant and credible.

B Empower people. *Empowerment* is defined as the process of increasing personal, interpersonal, and political control so that individuals can take action to improve their life situations. Personal empowerment enables individuals in problem situations to use their own skills and abilities to change their own behavior and to influence the behavior of individuals and organizations that affect their quality of life (see Chapter 1, Educational Principles and Strategies, for educational strategies based on an empowerment philosophy). As patients gain a sense of control over their diabetes, they are often better able to become empowered in other aspects of their lives.

C Respect the cultural diversity of the community. Individuals belonging to the same cultural or ethnic group may be bound together by similar experiences, but they are not monolithic in their attitudes or behaviors.

- Social and economic class cross-cut ethnic boundaries and may sometimes be more important than ethnic background.
- Diabetes education programs must seek to optimize the quality of life for cultural group members while respecting their diverse cultural beliefs, traditions, and lifestyles.

D Provide a service. Research institutions should avoid studying patient populations without providing an appropriate and adequate service to them. It is unrealistic to expect any group to participate actively in a program whose only goal is to generate new knowledge for the sponsoring institution.

KEY EDUCATIONAL CONSIDERATIONS

1 Culture influences the way that people think about and behave in relation to health and illness. Due to cultural differences, professionals and patients may have very different perspectives on how to interpret diabetes, explain its causes and progression, understand its symptoms, and orchestrate methods of treatment.

2 Awareness of one's own professional cultural values and worldview is a prerequisite for becoming culturally competent or able to provide culturally appropriate diabetes care.

3 Cultural values influence both the choices patients make each day as they care for their diabetes and the ways that diabetes educators interpret and react to their choices. It is helpful to examine how your values influence the decisions you make so that you can better understand your patients' decisions and work with them to achieve their goals.

4 Understanding patients' cultures is especially relevant for a chronic illness such as diabetes because of the lifelong course of the disease and its influence on culturally embedded behaviors.

5 Critical areas to explore as part of the cultural assessment are beliefs about diabetes; role of the patient in self-care; health and healing; values and priorities; communication styles and preferences; and common family, cultural, and religious rituals and practices.

6 While a complete cultural assessment may not be possible in all situations (eg, brief encounter in a busy clinic), treating patients with courtesy, focusing attention on the patient rather than acting in a hurry, sitting at the patient's level, and asking at least one culturally related question (eg, "Do you have any religious, family or cultural practices that influence how you care for your diabetes") conveys concern and sensitivity.

7 Educators can do a great deal to decrease cultural barriers during any encounter by manifesting a caring, concerned and understanding manner. Respect for patients and their culture can be demonstrated through honoring appointment times, not making assumptions about educational level or profession, asking patients how they would like to be addressed, and being sensitive to historical and current cultural differences.

8 Effective communication is essential for an accurate diagnosis, meaningful discussion of treatment options and patient education. Determine the patient's primary or preferred language and any secondary languages. Use interpreters as needed and ask patients in what language they would prefer written materials, because some people are better able to read English than the language they typically speak (see Chapter 2, Teaching Patients with Low Literacy Skills, for more information).

CASE STUDY 1

TM is an Hispanic-American woman with type 2 diabetes. She sees a traditional healer and takes an herbal home remedy to decrease her blood glucose levels. For years she had been seeing her physician about her diabetes, and all that time he had recommended that she begin insulin therapy. TM refused, explaining that she just didn't want to go "on the needle." Interpreting her fear as an aversion to the discomfort of insulin shots, her physician never questioned TM further to determine why she would not follow his recommendation. TM is beginning to experience neuropathy and microalbuminuria as a result of her ongoing elevated blood glucose levels.

QUESTIONS FOR DISCUSSION

1 How can the diabetes educator find out what is influencing TM's behavior?

2 What strategies could you use when working with her that demonstrate cultural appropriateness?

DISCUSSION

1 Asking TM directly about her concerns regarding insulin can open the way for discovering why she has been unwilling to begin this therapy. In response to your question, she tells you that her mother and others she has known have died once they started on insulin, so she has decided to use herbs and other alternative medicines instead.

2 TM needs to understand that the insulin taken by injection is very similar to that produced by the body and is therefore safe. It is unlikely, however, that this information will change her deeply held beliefs. Other strategies for helping TM understand the safety of using insulin include

  A Introduce TM to others Hispanic American women who have diabetes and take insulin as well as alternative medicines.

  B Offer referral to a support group.

  C Offer referral for promotores or other community health resources.

  D Provide tailored written and video materials that reflect her language, culture, and literacy level.

3 TM may not have spoken with her physician about her insulin concerns for a number of reasons.

    A She holds physicians in general in high esteem.

    B She feels intimidated by him.

    C She distrusts Western medicines.

    D She received advice from her healer telling her not to talk with her physician.

    E She may have difficulty completely expressing herself in English.

4 It would be helpful to find out what is in the herbal medicines that TM is taking to be sure that she is not experiencing any adverse effects.

CASE STUDY 2

LC is a 60-year-old European-American man with diagnosed type 2 diabetes who has difficulty using his meal plan. LC is an engineer by profession and is employed in the auto industry. He explains that he knows he needs to limit his food intake but just can't seem to help himself when he is around food. He says that he knows very little about food and leaves that up to his wife. However, he resents his wife telling him what or how much he should eat and reacts by eating even more. LC has expressed a reticence to begin taking pills for fear that he would feel like he had license to eat everything. Furthermore, he tells you that he hasn't been testing his blood sugar levels because his diabetes wasn't that bad.

QUESTIONS FOR DISCUSSION

1 What cultural influences are affecting LC's behavior?

2 What strategies could you use when working with him that demonstrate cultural appropriateness?

DISCUSSION

1 LC's behavior is typical of many European American men of his generation. Preparing food and caring for the family's health are perceived as a woman's responsibilities; being in charge and in control of situations is viewed as the man's role. One way that this value is expressed is by minimizing the seriousness of illnesses.

2 To address LC's need to be in charge, you might begin each visit by asking about his concerns and asking what he would like to learn about or discuss.

A Asking LC about his thoughts or concerns about his diabetes will likely be more successful than asking about his feelings.

B Discuss treatment options, blood glucose monitoring and use of the results in terms of how they will help him be in control of his diabetes.

3 The process of blood glucose monitoring should be discussed in terms of data collection and conducting experiments with foods to test their effect on blood glucose levels. This approach may appeal to someone with an engineering background and may be more acceptable than trying to teach him about foods and their ingredients. Learning through his own explorations may also help decrease the tensions between he and his wife regarding food issues.

CASE STUDY 3

AK is a 53-year-old Asian American man of Japanese descent who was recently diagnosed with type 2 diabetes. He eats a traditional diet that is high in carbohydrates (eg, rice and starchy vegetables), high in sodium, and low in proteins. AK understood that being on "a diabetic diet" meant eating fewer foods, especially fried foods and desserts. Therefore, he eats two large meals that are very high in carbohydrates and low in fat. He was referred to you by his doctor because his glycosylated hemoglobin remains elevated. He comes to you very frustrated because he does not understand why he is always hungry and why his blood glucose levels are high all the time despite the changes he has made.

QUESTIONS FOR DISCUSSION

1 What cultural influences are affecting AK's behavior?

2 What strategies could you use when working with him that demonstrate cultural appropriateness?

DISCUSSION

1 AK's eating pattern is based on traditional Asian foods and his understanding of his meal plan is based on traditional Western foods.

2 Offer AK nutritional information that is compatible with his preferred food choices.

   A Let him know that he will feel less hungry and be able to lower his blood glucose levels by decreasing the portion sizes of some of the carbohydrate foods he eats and filling in with lean meat or other protein foods.

   B Explain that spreading his food consumption over three or more meals per day helps prevent overloading his pancreas and thus promotes more even blood glucose levels throughout the day. He may also notice that he is less hungry and more energetic.

CASE STUDY 4

CD is a middle-aged Asian Indian man with diabetes. He eats a vegetarian diet of traditional foods including chapatis, rice, and high-starch vegetables, and he eats relatively infrequently. CD's food habits are working against his desire to lower his blood sugar and avoid taking insulin.

QUESTIONS FOR DISCUSSION

1 What cultural influences are affecting CD's behavior?

2 What strategies could you use when working with him that demonstrate cultural appropriateness?

DISCUSSION

1 CD's vegetarianism is influenced both by religion and culture. All aspects of his treatment program need to be adjusted to accommodate these culturally influenced eating preferences.

2 Offer suggestions such as adding heart-healthy oils to increase satiety and eating small meals throughout the day. Nonmeat protein alternatives such as limited amounts of nuts and seeds can be used to increase the protein content of his diet.

3 Offer referral to a registered dietitian with expertise in this area.

CASE STUDY 4

LS is a 64-year-old African-American female who lives in an urban high-rise with her daughter and two grandchildren. She has had diabetes for 15 years and is now hospitalized with a severe foot infection. She was referred to you for inpatient diabetes education for weight loss and foot care. During the assessment she tells you that her grandchildren are the most important thing in the world to her and she likes to bake for them because she can't afford to buy them toys and other things. She is concerned that they are not being fed right while she is in the hospital. She tells you she has tried to follow a diabetes meal plan but she cannot afford it. She cooks many foods in the traditional way because that is how her mother taught her. She tells you that she copes by "turning it over to the Lord - He takes care of me and my sugar." The guild nurse at her church recently started a support group for women with diabetes. LS explains that she attends when she can but transportation is a frequent problem.

QUESTIONS FOR DISCUSSION

1 What cultural influences are affecting LS's behavior?

2 What strategies could you use when working with her that demonstrate cultural appropriateness?

DISCUSSION

1 LS eats traditional foods that are a valued part of her cultural identity. Eating these foods is often viewed as a way of showing respect for the culture; not eating them may be viewed as rejection or being "too good". Cooking and preparing food are viewed as expressions of love and family continuity. Her religious beliefs are a source of comfort, and she seems to be somewhat fatalistic about her future health.

2 Acknowledge her many efforts to care for her grandchildren and her diabetes in spite of the many obstacles she faces. Ask if she can identify benefits for lowering her blood glucose level and caring for her feet that are more oriented toward the present (eg, more energy for her grandchildren, avoiding hospitalizations so she can be with her family).

3   An appropriate starting point might be using meal planning for blood glucose control. Assess her willingness to modify traditional recipes to lower the fat or sugar content of her meals (eg, using turkey neck bones instead of fat back in vegetables).

4   Assess her level of interest in weight loss, and explain how focusing on meal planning for better blood glucose control may have a side benefit of weight loss.

5   With LS's permission, contact the guild nurse about providing follow-up support for her. You could consider offering your services to the support group for consultation, diabetes education or cooking demonstrations.

Case Study 6

ML is a 58-year-old Navajo woman whose first language is Navajo. She lives with her son, his wife, and their four children on a Navajo reservation. She was diagnosed with type 2 diabetes during a free screening at the mall one year ago. She states that the screening people told her that she needed to see her doctor right away because if she did not she might go blind or lose a foot. They also told her that she should go on a diet, exercise, and get some medicine from her doctor. She is in today with symptoms of fatigue, blurred vision, increased thirst, frequent urination, and weight loss. Her HbA$_{1c}$ is 10.8% (normal=4.0% to 6.0%), cholesterol level is 276 mg/dL, triglyceride level is 240 mg/dL. Current weight is 200 lb (91 kg) and height is 5'4" tall (160 cm). She states that she did not visit the doctor a year ago as she thought that the diagnosis was wrong because she did not feel sick then.

Questions for Discussion

1   What cultural influences are affecting ML's behavior?
2   Considering ML's culture, how would you explain diabetes to her?
3   What strategies could you use when working with her that demonstrate cultural appropriateness?

DISCUSSION

1   Diabetes, which may be asymptomatic in the early phases, is a condition that can be difficult to explain because in many Native American cultures people do not feel they are ill unless they have visible symptoms or pain.

2   In ML's case, a Navajo interpreter who is knowledgeable about diabetes will be needed for the explanation and visits. The interpreter should be from the same culture as the client (and preferably the same community) since culture and health cannot be separated. The diabetes educator should remain aware of his/her communication style and body language even though an interpreter is being used.

3   ML will need the support and understanding of her family in order to make any needed lifestyle changes to lower her blood glucose levels, so it will help if they participate in the education process. If ML chooses to include a method of healing in addition to Western medicines, the diabetes educator should respect and acknowledge her choice.

4   Along with other aspects of self-care, ML needs to be taught how she can prevent the complications of diabetes, described to her in the third person.

5   In addition the educator can
   A   Explain the importance of regular visits to the clinic even when she feels well.
   B   Describe to ML what she can expect during the clinical encounter.
   C   Schedule ML for more than one appointment per visit, especially if transportation is limited.
   D   Offer information to ML and her family about available diabetes resources and sponsored activities such as community diabetes education classes, cooking classes, grocery store tours led by a dietitian, and community-wide walking/fitness programs if they are available.
   E   Ongoing support and information from a community health worker may be helpful to ML.

References

1 Barclay J. Shaping the care of the future...meeting the needs of all individuals. Nursing: J Clin Prac Educ Manag 1991;4(31):20-22.

2 Bennett M. Towards ethnorelativism: a developmental model for intercultural sensitivity. In: Paige R, ed. Education for the intercultural experience. 2nd ed. Yarmouth, Maine: Intercultural Press, 1993:21-71.

3 O'Connor BB. Healing traditions. Alternative medicine and the health professions. Philadelphia: University of Pennsylvania Press, 1995.

4 Hahn R. Sickness and healing, an anthropological perspective. New Haven, Conn: Yale University Press, 1995:265.

5 Pachter LM. Culture and clinical care. Folk illness beliefs and behaviors and their implications for healthcare delivery. JAMA 1994;271:690-94.

6 Good BJ, Good MJ. The meaning of symptoms: a cultural hermeneutic model for clinical practice. In: Eisenberg L, Kleinman A, eds. The relevance of social science for medicine. Dordrecht, Holland: D. Reidel Publishing Co, 1992;165-96.

7 Anderson RM, Funnell MM, Arnold MS. Beyond compliance and glucose control: educating for patient empowerment. In: Rifkin H, Colwell JA, Taylor SI, eds. Diabetes. Amsterdam, Netherlands: Elsevier Science Publishers, 1991;1285-89.

8 Penn NE, Kar S, Kramer J, Skinner J, Zambrana RE. Ethnic minorities, health care systems, and behavior. Health Psychol 1995;14:641-46.

9 Galanti GA. Caring for patients from different cultures. Philadelphia: University of Pennsylvania Press, 1991.

10 Cowie CC, Eberhard MS. Sociodemographic characteristics of persons with diabetes. In: Diabetes in America. 2nd ed. National Diabetes Data Group, eds. Bethesda, Md: National Institute of Diabetes and Digestive and Kidney Diseases, 1995; NIH Publication No. 95-1468:85-116.

11 Carter JS, Pugh JA, Monterrosa A. Non-insulin-dependent diabetes mellitus in minorities in the United States. Ann Intern Med 1996;125:221-32.

12 National Institutes of Health. Diabetes in African Americans. Bethesda, Md: National Institute of Diabetes, Digestive and Kidney Diseases, 1997; NIH Publication No. 97-3266.

13 National Institutes of Health. Diabetes in Hispanic Americans. Bethesda, Md: National Institute of Diabetes and Digestive and Kidney Diseases, 1997; NIH Publication No. 98-3926.

14 Murphy FG, Satterfield D, Anderson RM, Lyons AE. Diabetes educators as cultural translators. Diabetes Educ 1993;19:113-16,118.

15 Anderson RM. Patient empowerment and the traditional medical model: a case of irreconcilable differences? Diabetes Care 1995;18:412-15.

16 Anderson RM, Goddard C, Vasquez F, Garcia R, Guzman R. Using focus groups to identify diabetes care and education issues for Latino people with diabetes. Diabetes 1998;47(Suppl 1):128.

17 Harwood A. Ethnicity and medical care. Cambridge, Mass: Harvard University Press, 1981.

18 Gilbert MJ. Cultural relevance in the delivery of human services. In: Keefe SE, ed. Negotiating ethnicity: the impact of anthropological theory and practice. NAPA Bull 1989;32:706-16.

19 VanSon AR. Crossing cultural and economic boundaries. In: VanSon AR, ed. Diabetes and patient education: a daily nursing challenge. New York: Appleton-Century-Crofts, 1984;160-77.

20 Anderson RM, Herman WH, Davis JM, Freedman RP, Funnell MM, Neighbors HW. Barriers to improving diabetes care for blacks. Diabetes Care 1991;14:605-9.

SUGGESTED READINGS

Anderson LA, Janes GR, Ziemer DC, Phillips LS. Diabetes in urban African Americans. Body image, satisfaction with size, and weight change attempts. Diabetes Educ 1997;23:301-8.

Anderson RM. Patient empowerment and the traditional medical model. Diabetes Care 1995;18:412-15.

Anderson RM, Goddard C, Vasquez F, Garcia R, Guzman R. Using focus groups to identify diabetes care and education issues for Latino people with diabetes. Diabetes 1998;47(suppl 1):128.

Bennett PH, Calles-Escandon J: Diabetes in Hispanic Americans. Diabetes Care 1991;14:615-705.

Bolderman KM, Mersey JH. Faithful fasting. Diabetes Forecast 1996;49(9): 48-50.

Bradley E. Spiritualicise mind-body exercise program. Diabetes Educ 1996;22:117-18.

Brown SA, Hanis CL. A community-based, culturally sensitive education and group-support intervention for Mexican Americans with NIDDM: a pilot study of efficacy. Diabetes Educ 1995;21:203-210.

Burden ML, Burden AC. Management of diabetes mellitus during the holy month of Ramadan. Practical Diabetes Internation 1998;15(suppl 1):S1-S23.

Carter C. Soul food buffet. Diabetes Forecast 1991;44(2):29-31.

Carter JS, Gilliland SS, Percy GE, Levin S, et al. Native American Diabetes Project: designing culturally relevant education materials. Diabetes Educ 1997;23:133-39.

Carter JS, Pugh JA, Monterrosa A. Non-insulin-dependent diabetes mellitus in minorities in the United States. Ann Intern Med 1996;125:221-32.

Corkery E, Palmer C, Foley ME, Schechter CB, Frisher L, Roman SH. Effect of a bicultural community health worker on completion of diabetes education in a Hispanic population. Diabetes Care 1997;20:254-57.

Cowie CC, Eberhard MS. Sociodemographic characteristics of persons with diabetes. In: Diabetes in America. 2nd ed. National Diabetes Data Group, eds. Bethesda, Md: National Institute of Diabetes and Digestive and Kidney Diseases, 1995; NIH Publication No. 95-1468:85-116.

Cravener P. Establishing therapeutic alliance across cultural barriers. J of Psychosocial Nursing 1992;30(12):10-14.

Cross cultural counseling: A guide for nutrition and health counselors. US Dept of Agriculture FNS 150; United States Department of Health and Human Services. 1990:1-26.

Delamater AM, Albrecht DR, Postellon DC, Gutai JP. Racial differences in metabolic control of children and adolescents with type I diabetes mellitus. Diabetes Care 1991:14:20-25.

Edwards GJ, Coleman-Burns P. A culturally sensitive approach to patient care. Caring for African American patients. Practical Diabetology 1996;15(3):4-9.

Fitzgerald JT, Anderson RM, Funnell MM, Arnold MS, Davis WK, Aman LC, Jacober SJ, Grunberger G. Differences in the impact of dietary restrictions on African Americans and Caucasians with NIDDM. Diabetes Educ 1997;23:41-47.

Friedman MM. Transcultural family nursing: application to Latino and Black families. Pediatric Nursing 1990;5:214-22.

Gaillard TR, Schuster DP, Bossetti BM, Green PA, Osei K. Do sociodemographics and economic status predict risks for Type II diabetes in African Americans? Diabetes Educ 1997;23:294-300.

Gilbert MJ. Cultural relevance in the delivery of human services. In: Keefe SE, ed. Negotiating ethnicity: the impact of anthropological theory and practice. NAPA Bull 1989;32:706-16.

Gohdes D, Kaufman S, Valway S. Diabetes in American Indians: an overview. Diabetes Care 1993;16(suppl 1):214-382.

Harwood A. Ethnicity and medical care. Cambridge, Mass: Harvard University Press, 1981.

Hosey GM, Freeman WL, Stracqualursi F, Gohdes D. Designing and evaluating diabetes education material for American Indians. Diabetes Educ 1990;16: 407-14.

Jaber LA, Slaughter RL, Grunberger G. Diabetes and related metabolic risk factors among Arab Americans. Annals of Pharmacotherapy 1995;29:573-77.

Keenan DP. In the face of diversity: modifying nutrition education delivery to meet the needs of an increasingly multicultural consumer base. J Nutr Ed 1996;28:86-91.

Kulkarni K. Nutrition counseling for Indian and Pakistani patients. Practical Diabetology 1996;1S(2):19-20.

Ledda MA, Walker EA, Basch CE. Development and formative evaluation of a foot self-care program for African Americans with diabetes. Diabetes Educ 1997;23:48-51.

Magnus MH: What's your IQ on cross-cultural nutrition counseling? Diabetes Educ 1996;22:57-60, 62.

McCarren M. The in-between diabetes. Diabetes Forecast 1994;48(4):20-24.

McNabb, WL. Delivering more effective weight-loss programs for black American women. Diabetes Spectrum 1994;7:332-333.

Murphy FG, Satterfield D, Anderson RM, Lyons AE. Diabetes educators as cultural translators. Diabetes Educ 1993;19:113-18.

National Institutes of Health. Diabetes in African Americans. Bethesda, Md: National Institute of Diabetes and Digestive and Kidney Disease 1997; NIH Publication No. 97-3266.

National Institutes of Health. Diabetes in Hispanic Americans. Bethesda, Md: National Institute of Diabetes and Digestive and Kidney Disease 1997; NIH Publication No. 98-3926.

Pichert JW, Briscoe VJ. A questionnaire for assessing barriers to healthcare utilization, part I. Diabetes Educ 1997;23:181-191.

Pichert JW, Briscoe VJ. Strategies for overcoming barriers to healthcare utilization, part II. Diabetes Educ 1997;23:251-56.

Rankin SH, Galbraith ME, Huang P. Quality of life and social environment as reported by Chinese immigrants with non-insulin-dependent diabetes mellitus. Diabetes Educ 1997;23:171-77.

Raymond NR, D'Eramo-Melkus G. Non-insulin-dependent diabetes and obesity in the black and Hispanic population: culturally sensitive management. Diabetes Educ 1993;19:313-17.

Reid BV. It's like you're down on a bed of affliction: Aging and diabetes among black Americans. Soc Sci Med 1992;34(12):1317-23.

Rempusheski VF. The role of ethnicity in elder care. Nursing Clinics of North America 1989;24:717-24.

Skelly AH, Marshall JR, Haughey BP, Davis PJ, Dunford RG. Self-efficacy and confidence in outcomes as determinants of self-care practices in inner-city, African-American women with non-insulin-dependent diabetes. Diabetes Educ 1995;21:38-46.

Tripp-Reimer T, Afifi LA. Cross-cultural perspectives on patient teaching. Nursing Clinics of North America 1989;24:613-19.

VanSon AR. Crossing cultural and economic boundaries. In: VanSon AR, ed. Diabetes and patient education: a daily nursing challenge. New York: Appleton-Century-Crofts, 1982;160-77.

Westberg J. Patient education for Hispanic Americans. Patient Education and Counseling 1989;13:143-60.

Wing RR, Anglin K. Effectiveness of a behavioral weight control program for blacks and whites with NIDDM. Diabetes Care 1996;19:409-12.

National Diabetes Education Program; NIDDK; NIH: 1-800-438-5383.

National Diabetes Information Clearinghouse; NIDDK; NIH: 301-654-3327; www.niddk.nih.gov.

Combined Health Information Database (CHID); http://chid.nih.gov

Psychosocial Issues

Psychosocial Issues

Psychosocial Assessment

4

Richard R. Rubin, PhD, CDE
The Johns Hopkins University School of Medicine
Departments of Medicine and Pediatrics
Baltimore, Maryland

INTRODUCTION

1 Diabetes is a demanding disease for those who have it as evidenced by the fact that at least 99% of diabetes care is self-care. Given this considerable demand on the person with diabetes, personal, family, and other resources are critical to a person's success in day-to-day diabetes management.

2 The first step in helping individuals make informed choices concerning their diabetes is to conduct a comprehensive educational assessment that includes psychosocial aspects of diabetes.

3 The purpose of incorporating psychosocial assessment is to systematically identify an individual's strengths and vulnerabilities when it comes to the resources available for diabetes self-care.

4 The issues involved in such an assessment include: social support; health beliefs, attitudes, and intentions; psychosocial adjustment; readiness to change; and contextual factors such as individual barriers to learning, cultural and religious influences, and socioeconomic factors.

5 A complete assessment needs to be performed when the person with diabetes is seen for the first time, and on a regular basis thereafter. Informal reassessment is done at every visit and formal reassessment is done as indicated by changes in the patient's life or therapy, or by crises such as the onset of complications.

6 Once an assessment is done, an individual education and treatment plan can be developed with the patient (For more on using information from the psychosocial assessment to facilitate behavior change, see Chapter 5, Behavior Change. For more on using information from the psychosocial assessment to help manage psychological disorders, see Chapter 6, Psychological Disorders).

7 Most educators do not have the time to do a complete psychosocial assessment. This chapter will suggest expedient approaches to identifying critical psychosocial issues for individual patients. More detailed assessment may then be done in areas that seem to be problems for the patient.

OBJECTIVES

Upon completion of this chapter, the learner will be able to

1   State the goals of psychosocial assessment for patients with diabetes.

2   Identify psychosocial factors that may affect an individual's capacity for diabetes self-care.

3   Explain the role that each psychosocial factor may play in influencing self-care behavior.

4   Describe practical, effective approaches for assessing relevant psychosocial factors.

5   Select and use tools and techniques for assessing relevant psychosocial factors.

GOALS OF PSYCHOSOCIAL ASSESSMENT

1   Certain factors are assessed to determine an individual's capacity to effectively manage diabetes on a day-to-day basis.

   A   Health beliefs, attitudes, and self-care intentions

   B   Current level of self-care skill

   C   Psychosocial adjustment, including coping skills and emotional well being

   D   Health status

   E   Social support

   F   Contextual factors

- Regimen complexity and aversiveness
- Barriers to learning
- Cultural and religious influences
- Socioeconomic and organizational factors related to healthcare delivery

   G   Readiness to change

2   The results of the psychosocial assessment are used to create an individual plan for diabetes education and treatment with the patient.

DETERMINANTS OF DIABETES-RELATED BEHAVIOR

1   Health beliefs

2   Locus-of-control

3   Self-efficacy

4   Self-care/self-management intentions and skills

5 Coping skills

6 Emotional well-being

7 Health status

8 Social support

9 Cognitive maturity

10 Regimen complexity

11 Organizational factors related to healthcare delivery

12 Readiness to change

IMPORTANCE OF HEALTH BELIEFS

1 According to the Health Belief Model,[1] behavior reflects a person's subjective interpretation of a situation. In the context of diabetes self-care, the behavior of patients is influenced by four perceptions:

   A Susceptibility, or how vulnerable the person feels to the negative consequences of the illness:

     • People with type 2 diabetes may feel less susceptible if they think they have a "milder" form of diabetes. Conversely, people who have type 1 diabetes, or people who are suffering from complications of diabetes may feel more susceptible to negative consequences. According to this theory, the more susceptible a person feels, the more likely that person is to practice self-care.

   B Severity of diabetes and its complications:

     • Perceptions of issues such as impairment, disability, and job loss are relevant. The more severe the perceived consequences of having diabetes, the more likely a person is to care for his or her diabetes.

   C Benefits of self-care:

     • Patients who feel that active diabetes self-management will yield benefits are more likely to devote themselves to self-care than patients who are pessimistic that self-management will make a difference.

   D Cost of self-care:

     • Financial costs, personal costs such as extra time involved in efforts to actively manage diabetes, and other costs of active management such as increased incidence of hypoglycemia and weight gain all influence self-care behavior. To be open to active self-care, a person must believe that the benefits outweigh the costs.

Table 4.1. Statements for Assessing Health Beliefs People With Diabetes

Benefit	• I'll be healthier in later life if I control my diabetes.
	• I believe that exercise can help me control my diabetes.
	• Controlling my blood sugar will help me avoid heart disease.
	• Changing my eating habits would help me control my diabetes.
	• Even if I took my medicine as I should, I wouldn't be able to control my diabetes.
	• I can control my diabetes if I follow my regimen closely.
Cost	• It will take a lot of effort to control my diabetes.
	• I would have to change too many habits to use a meal plan.
	• Taking my medication interferes with my daily activities.
	• I'm always hungry when I stick to my meal plan.
	• It takes a lot of effort to exercise.
Severity	• Diabetes is a serious disease if you don't control it.
Susceptibility	• My diabetes would be worse day-to-day if I did nothing about it.
	• I'm more likely to have eye problems if my control is poor.
	• If my diabetes isn't controlled, I'm likely to die sooner.

2 Research yields some support for the predictions of the Health Belief Model. In particular, perceived susceptibility and severity seem to predict self-care. These relationships may be curvilinear. For example, those experiencing the lowest and highest levels of susceptibility may have the lowest levels of self-care. Those who feel extremely susceptible may not be able to change their behavior because they feel overwhelmed or fatalistic.

Assessing Health Beliefs

1 Health beliefs may be assessed by asking patients to complete a brief questionnaire rating how strongly they agree or disagree with a series of statements that reflect elements of the Health Belief Model as it applies to diabetes and its management, or by incorporating a few questions into the complete educational assessment.

2 Statements that might be included in an assessment of diabetes-related health beliefs are shown in Table 4.1. These statements represent beliefs related to benefit, cost, severity, and susceptibility. Self-care can be facilitated by identifying and discussing beliefs that support and undermine active self-management. Special attention needs to be given to helping patients recognize the behavioral and health effects of beliefs concerning benefits and costs of diabetes care (See Chapter 5, Behavior Change for more on this topic).

3 Health beliefs may be expediently assessed by asking the patients how much he or she agrees (on a scale of 1 to 10) with any single statement from the benefit and cost categories of Table 4.1.

IMPORTANCE OF LOCUS OF CONTROL

1 Beliefs concerning who or what controls health-related outcomes also influence self-care behavior. The Locus-of-Control Theory[2] suggests three such beliefs (often called orientations): internal orientation, powerful other orientation, and chance orientation.

   A *Internal orientation*: people who have an internal orientation tend to believe that diabetes-related health outcomes are controlled primarily by their own efforts.

   B *Powerful other orientation*: people who have a powerful other orientation tend to believe that outcomes are controlled primarily by other people, generally by healthcare providers, but often by family members and others as well.

   C *Chance orientation*: people who have a chance orientation believe that outcomes are determined primarily by chance or fate.

2 Recent research by Peyrot and Rubin[2] supports some important elements of the Locus-of-Control Model.

   A Internal orientation actually consists of two components, autonomy and self-blame. Autonomy was associated with a range of positive outcomes including fewer high blood glucose levels and better emotional adjustment. Self-blame was associated with a range of negative outcomes including less frequent SMBG and insulin dose adjustment.

   B Powerful other orientation also consists of two components, healthcare provider, and nonmedical other family and friends, each of which was associated with different aspects of self-care. High healthcare provider locus-of-control orientation was associated with less insulin dose adjustment, and high nonmedical other locus-of-control orientation was associated with less insulin doses adjustment, fewer late shots, and less binge eating.

C Chance orientation was associated with a variety of outcomes that reflect a pattern of dysfunction, including more frequent hyperglycemia, less exercise, lower self-esteem, and more depression and anxiety.

Assessing Diabetes Locus of Control

1 Diabetes-specific locus of control can be assessed comprehensively by means of standardized questionnaires.[2,3]

2 The patient's beliefs about who or what controls diabetes-related health outcomes can provide critical information concerning approaches that are likely to be meaningful for that individual. Patients with predominantly a chance orientation are at special risk for negative outcomes; they need a great deal of support and assistance to shift from this orientation.

3 Locus-of-control orientation can be assessed by asking patients to complete a brief questionnaire rating how strongly they agree or disagree with a series of statements that reflect locus of control orientation as it applies to diabetes and its management or by incorporating a few questions into the complete educational assessment.

4 The statements in Table 4.2[2] might be included in an assessment of diabetes-related locus-of-control. Self-care can be facilitated by identifying and discussing locus-of-control orientations that support and undermine active self-management. Special attention needs to be devoted to helping patients recognize the potential effects of a high chance of locus-of-control orientation.

5 Diabetes locus-of-control orientation may be expediently assessed by asking patients how much (on a scale of 1 to 10) they agree with any single item from each of the categories in Table 4.2.

TABLE 4.2. STATEMENTS FOR ASSESSING LOCUS OF CONTROL IN PEOPLE WITH DIABETES

Internal locus of control - autonomy	• I can avoid complications. • What I do is the main influence on my health. • I am responsible for my health.
Internal locus of control - blame	• When my sugar is high, it's because of something I've done. • When my blood sugar is high it's because I made a mistake. • Complications are the result of carelessness.
Chance locus of control	• Good health is a matter of good fortune. • If it's meant to be I'll avoid complications. • My blood sugars will be whatever they will be. • Blood sugars are controlled by accident. • I never know why I'm out of control. • Good control is a matter of luck.
Powerful other locus of control - health professional	• Regular doctor's visits avoid problems. • I should call my doctor whenever I feel bad. • I can only do what my doctor tells me. • Health professionals keep me healthy.
Powerful other locus of control - nonmedical	• My family is a big help in controlling my diabetes. • Other people have a big responsibility for my diabetes.

IMPORTANCE OF SELF-EFFICACY

1   According to Self-Efficacy Theory,[4] a person's sense of self-efficacy or confidence affects self-care behavior. The more confident a person feels about performing a set of behaviors, the more likely a person is to actually engage in those behaviors.

2   Some studies[5] suggest that people with diabetes who have a high degree of self-efficacy are more active in the care of their diabetes, and have better emotional well-being and glycemic control than people who have a low degree of self-efficacy.

Assessing Diabetes Self-Efficacy

1 A 30-item questionnaire,[6] originally developed for use with adolescents, is an effective way to measure a patient's perceptions of diabetes self-efficacy, or the confidence a person feels about performing diabetes self-care behaviors. These perceptions provide useful data about the patient's overall confidence and specific behaviors that might need special attention during the education process.

2 Diabetes self-efficacy can be assessed by asking patients to complete a brief questionnaire rating how strongly they agree or disagree with a series of statements that reflect how confident they feel about managing a variety of daily diabetes-related activities or by incorporating a few questions into the complete educational assessment.

3 The statements in Table 4.3 might be included in an assessment of diabetes-related self-efficacy. This questionnaire, based on the work of Grossman and associates[6] has been used by Rubin and Peyrot in their ongoing research.[7-9] Respondents are asked how sure they are that they can do what is stated.

4 Diabetes self-efficacy may be expediently assessed by asking patients how confident they feel (on a scale of 1 to 10) about their ability to manage their diabetes on a daily basis.

Importance of Behavioral Intentions

1 Behavioral intentions, in addition to health beliefs, locus-of-control orientation, and self-efficacy, may predict actual self-care behavior.

2 Work by Peyrot and Rubin[10] suggests that a person's intention to make changes in diabetes self-care behavior powerfully predicts actual behavior change 6 and 12 months later. This relationship is stronger for self-regulation behaviors such as SMBG and insulin adjustment than it is for lifestyle behaviors such as diet and exercise. Self-regulation behaviors appear to be more amenable to change, whereas lifestyle changes are more difficult for most people to maintain.

TABLE 4.3. STATEMENTS FOR ASSESSING SELF-EFFICACY IN PEOPLE WITH DIABETES[9]

I feel sure I can:

1   Take insulin or other medication
2   Figure out meals and snacks at home
3   Figure out foods to eat when away from home
4   Keep track of blood sugar levels
5   Test for ketones
6   Adjust insulin timing or dosage for a lot of extra exercise
7   Figure out how much to eat before activities
8   Figure out how much insulin to take when sick
9   Prevent low blood sugar reactions
10 Talk to my doctor and get the things I need
11 Sleep away from home in a place where no one knows I have diabetes
12 Keep myself free of high blood sugars
13 Avoid having ketones
14 Change my doctor if I don't like him/her
15 Stop a reaction when I'm having one
16 Ask for help when I'm sick
17 Tell a friend or people at work that I have diabetes
18 Argue with my doctor if I feel he/she is not being fair
19 Prevent blindness and other complications from my diabetes
20 Get as much attention from people when my diabetes is under control as I get when it isn't
21 Regularly wear a medical alert tag or bracelet which says I have diabetes
22 Sneak food without anyone but me knowing
23 Follow my doctor's orders for taking care of my diabetes
24 Run my life the same as if I didn't have diabetes

ASSESSING BEHAVIORAL INTENTIONS

1   Peyrot and Rubin[10] developed an approach for assessing self-care behavioral intentions in people with diabetes. A questionnaire was used to measure self-reported, self-care behavior in patients entering a 5-day intensive outpatient diabetes education program. At the end of the program participants were asked to complete a questionnaire to determine what they *intended* to do regarding each of the same self-care behaviors. Six months later, participants completed a third questionnaire identical to the preprogram instrument, which assessed actual self-care behavior.

2 The specific behaviors that might be included in an assessment of diabetes-related self-care behaviors and intentions are shown in Table 4.4. Respondents are asked how often they do (or intend to do) what is stated.

3 The results of an assessment of behavioral intentions can be formalized in a behavioral contract with the patient that can be used as a guide and reminder for ongoing self-care. At the next visit to the educator, actual behavior can be compared with earlier behavioral intentions, allowing the patient to adjust intentions and plan for future changes (For more on contracting as a means to facilitate behavior change, see Chapter 5, Behavior Change).

TABLE 4.4. SPECIFIC BEHAVIORS FOR ASSESSING OF DIABETES SELF-CARE BEHAVIORS AND INTENTIONS

How often do you plan to:
1 Monitor blood glucose levels
2 Adjust insulin doses
3 Take medications on time
4 Use your meal plan
5 Walk or do other exercise

IMPORTANCE OF CURRENT LEVEL OF SELF-CARE

1 Behavior may also be influenced by the degree of actual self-care and self-management skills that a person has achieved.

2 Skill may be defined as knowledge in action because it is achieved through the acquisition of knowledge and through guided practice.

3 Self-care skill involves specific abilities, including the ability to accomplish specific tasks (eg, accurately self-monitor blood glucose levels (SMBG), correctly administer insulin, and use a meal plan). The ability to coordinate a variety of specific tasks to promote physical and emotional well-being (eg, coordinate the amount and timing of food, medication, and exercise when attending a party).

4   The foundation of self-care skill is the ability to solve problems by coordinating activities and using information and experience to make decisions. The ability to solve problems and set goals may be thought of as self-management skills.

ASSESSING CURRENT LEVEL OF SELF-CARE

1   The patient's ability to carry out critical day-to-day self-care tasks, which reflects the level of self-care skills, guides the planning of individual treatment or education.

2   The level of these skills is best assessed by observation when possible (eg, procedure of insulin administration or SMBG), or by having the patient describe in detail how the activity is performed (eg, meal planning or sick-day management).

3   The patient's ability to coordinate activities to maintain physical well-being and quality of life can also be assessed by asking patients how they deal with typical potentially problematic diabetes-related situations. The level of these problem-solving skills seems to be a powerful predictor of health outcomes.

4   Techniques for helping patients reach self-care goals are addressed in Chapter 5, Behavior Change.

IMPORTANCE OF COPING SKILLS

1   Self-care behavior can be affected by a person's skill in coping with the emotional stresses of day-to-day life with diabetes. Clinical experience reveals that the major barriers to self-care are often emotional (eg, denial and feeling overwhelmed).

2   Improved coping skills can lead to improved metabolic control indirectly by facilitating self-care, and directly, by reducing the acute effects of stress on glycemia.[11]

3   Some evidence suggests that improved diabetes-specific coping skills may be associated with better self-care and glycemic control.[9]

ASSESSING COPING SKILLS

1 Coping style can be evaluated using structured instruments.[12]

2 Coping skills may be expediently assessed by asking patients how they would respond to typical day-to-day diabetes-related problems.

3 Examples of specific questions to include are: "Is your diabetes and its care causing you stress? If so, how?" "What are you currently doing to try to cope with the stress? "What could help you cope better?"

IMPORTANCE OF PSYCHOSOCIAL ADJUSTMENT: QUALITY OF LIFE, EMOTIONAL WELL-BEING

1 Active diabetes self-care is demanding and pervasive.
   A Requires attention 24 hours a day, 365 days a year
   B Affects every aspect of a person's life
   C Frequently involves tasks that are unpleasant, such as finger sticks, food restrictions, and, for some people, insulin injections
   D Presents substantial risks
      • Efforts to optimize blood glucose levels may increase the likelihood of hypoglycemia without a guarantee of reduced risk of complications.
      • Some factors that affect glycemia and risks for complications are not under the patient's control.

2 Issues of psychosocial adjustment are critical to self-care. Those who have adjusted to diabetes and its demands are much more likely to take effective day-to-day control of their diabetes than those who have not.

ASSESSING QUALITY OF LIFE

1 Health-related quality of life (HRQL) refers to an individual's subjective perception of well-being as it relates to health status.

2 HRQL assessment is multidimensional and typically includes several domains: physical functioning, role functioning, pain, emotional well-being, and satisfaction with treatment.

3 Two broad approaches to assessing HRQL are generic and illness-specific measurement.

4   Some popular generic measures of HRQL are the Medical Outcomes Survey (SF-36),[13] the Quality of Well-Being Instrument,[14] and the Sickness Impact Profile.[15]

5   Illness-specific measures focus on specific problems posed by an individual illness. For example, a diabetes-specific quality-of-life assessment could evaluate the impact of experiences such as hypoglycemia, insulin injections, blood glucose monitoring, and dietary restrictions.

6   Illness-specific measures and situation-specific questions are probably the most effective way of assessing HRQL in people with diabetes.

7   The Diabetes Quality of Life Measure (DQOL) is the most widely used diabetes-specific assessment of quality of life.[16] The DQOL was originally developed by the Diabetes Control and Complications Trial (DCCT) Research Group to evaluate the relative burden of different diabetes treatment approaches.

8   The DQOL consists of 46 items and assesses quality of life in four areas: satisfaction with treatment, impact of treatment, worry about the future effects of diabetes, and worry about social and vocational issues.

9   Other measures that may be useful for assessing HRQL in people with diabetes are the 8-item Diabetes Treatment Satisfaction Questionnaire[17] and the 24-item Problem Areas in Diabetes Scale (PAID).[18]

10   The presence of potential problems with diabetes-related quality of life may be expediently identified by asking the patient, "How is diabetes affecting your quality of life?"

ASSESSING EMOTIONAL WELL-BEING

1   Emotional well-being is positively correlated with patient self-care behavior. The causal relationships between emotional status and self-care are probably reciprocal (ie, high levels of emotional well-being tend to facilitate self-care and high levels of self-care tend to facilitate emotional well-being).

2 Specifically, self-esteem is positively related to self-care, and depression and anxiety are negatively related to self-care.[2,5]

3 Major depression affects approximately one of every five patients with diabetes and severely impairs quality of life and all aspects of functioning, including sleep patterns, sexual functioning, self-care behavior and metabolic control.[19,20]

    A Several standardized tests are available to help the healthcare provider screen for common psychiatric disorders, including depression, that can have a significant impact on the management of diabetes. One of the most frequently used measures is the SF-36 scale.[13]

    B Patients can complete the SF-36 in less than 10 minutes and the measure can be scored by hand.

    C The educator can screen patients for depression by asking a series of simple questions concerning symptoms. A person who has five or more specific symptoms for a period of at least 2 weeks is probably clinically depressed. The symptoms of clinical depression are listed in Table 4.5. Ask patients if they have each symptom; if yes, ask for how long and how often.

TABLE 4.5. SYMPTOMS OF CLINICAL DEPRESSION

1 Depressed mood (feeling sad or empty) most of the day, nearly every day

2 Significant weight loss when not dieting or weight gain (eg, a change of more than 5% of body weight in a month), or decrease or increase in appetite nearly every day

3 Trouble sleeping or sleeping too much nearly every day

4 Feeling very agitated or physically sluggish nearly every day

5 Fatigue or loss of energy nearly every day

6 Markedly diminished interest or pleasure in all or almost all activities most of day, nearly every day

7 Feeling worthless or excessively or inappropriately guilty nearly every day

8 Diminished ability to think or concentrate, or indecisiveness, nearly every day

9 Recurrent thoughts of death (not just fear of dying), recurrent thoughts of suicide, a suicide attempt or a specific plan to commit suicide

D Because some of the symptoms of clinical depression (specifically items two through six in Table 4.5) are similar or identical to symptoms of hyperglycemia, it may be difficult to ascertain whether a patient with these symptoms is depressed, hyperglycemic, or both. Thus, it is important to pay especially close attention to the other symptoms listed in the table when a possibly depressed patient is chronically hyperglycemic.

E While most educators are not mental health professionals, an understanding of current treatment options may be useful. Approaches to treating depressed patients who have diabetes are addressed in Chapter 6, Psychological Disorders.

4 Clinical anxiety disorder is another problem common among people with diabetes.[20] This disorder often interferes with a person's ability to effectively manage diabetes and with other aspects of life as well.

A An educator can screen patients for anxiety by asking a series of simple questions concerning symptoms. A person that has been uncontrollably anxious for at least 6 months about a number of events and activities, and during that period has had five or more specific symptoms for more days than not is probably suffering from a clinical anxiety disorder. The symptoms of clinical anxiety disorder are listed on Table 4.6.

TABLE 4.6. SYMPTOMS OF CLINICAL ANXIETY DISORDER

1 Restlessness or feeling keyed-up or on-edge
2 Being easily fatigued
3 Difficulty concentrating or mind going blank
4 Irritability
5 Muscle tension
6 Sleep disturbance (difficulty falling or staying asleep, or restless, unsatisfying sleep)

B Some of the symptoms of clinical anxiety disorder overlap with those of clinical depression because certain psychological problems share similar symptoms and people can suffer from more than one clinical psychological disorder.

C Approaches to treating patients who have diabetes and suffer from anxiety disorder are addressed in Chapter 6, Psychological Disorders.

5 The problem of eating disorders in people with diabetes has received increased attention in the past few years. There are two types of eating disorders.

A Anorexia nervosa is characterized by a severe, self-imposed restriction in caloric intake, often combined with extreme levels of exercise.

B Bulimia nervosa is characterized by binge eating followed by purging, usually in the form of vomiting or the use of diuretic medications or laxatives.

C Either type of eating disorder enormously complicates diabetes management, often leading to acute emergencies and contributing to chronic complications.

D Even subclinical eating disorders (ie, disordered eating that does not meet the criteria for either anorexia or bulimia) can seriously compromise metabolic control and long-term health.

E Although some young men suffer from clinical eating disorders, anorexia and bulimia are about ten times more common among young women, probably because of the far more intense pressure that our society places on young women to be thin. Subclinical eating disorders are common in all persons with diabetes, including those with type 2 diabetes.

F The healthcare provider can screen patients for clinical and subclinical eating disorders by asking a series of simple questions concerning symptoms. Keep in mind that it may be difficult for a patient to acknowledge an eating disorder especially anorexia or bulimia. Sometimes it may also be difficult to distinguish between a normal (and even) positive focus on food and body image, which are part of living with diabetes, and the abnormal concerns and behavior that reflect an eating disorder. The educator can ask the patient if he or she has any of the signs and symptoms in Table 4.7. A person who has any of these signs and symptoms is probably suffering from a clinical eating disorder.

G Insulin manipulation is an especially troubling manifestation of eating-disordered behavior that is unique to people with diabetes. Researchers estimate that between one third and one half of all young women with diabetes frequently take less insulin than required for blood sugar control in order to control their weight.[21]

H Approaches for treating patients who have diabetes and suffer from clinical or subclinical eating disorders are addressed in Chapter 6, Psychological Disorders.

TABLE 4.7. SIGNS AND SYMPTOMS OF CLINICAL EATING DISORDERS

1 Weighs less than 85% of normal weight for height, bodyframe, and age
2 Has intense fear of gaining weight or becoming fat, even though underweight
3 Sees self as fat when others say too thin
4 Exercises far more than is necessary to stay fit
5 Misses at least three consecutive menstrual cycles
6 Denies the seriousness of low body weight
7 Binge eats (eats very large amounts of food at a single sitting) at least twice a week for 3 months
8 Feels unable to stop eating or control what or how much is eaten

IMPORTANCE OF HEALTH STATUS

1 A patient's health status influences self-care behavior. Acute and chronic complications of diabetes may either hamper or facilitate behavior change in the direction of active self-care.

2 Acute complications may adversely affect self-care behavior. For example, hypoglycemic episodes may discourage efforts to achieve tight control, and hyperglycemia may lead to exhaustion which, in turn, may sap energy required for self-care.

3 Acute complications may also encourage self-care. For example, blurry vision caused by hyperglycemia may be so frightening that the patient is motivated to more actively manage his or her diabetes.

4 Chronic complications can also have an adverse effect on self-care. For example, neuropathy or cardiovascular complications may interfere with exercise, and poor vision may interfere with the patient's ability to self-monitor blood glucose levels.

5 Chronic complications may also encourage better self-care. Patients often report that they were "scared straight" by the onset of complications.

Assessing Health Status

1 A complete history of the patient's health status, including acute and chronic complications of diabetes and other health issues and problems, is essential for effective educational or treatment planning.

2 These issues may critically influence a patient's ability and motivation for self-care.

Importance of Social Support

1 Self-care behavior may be powerfully affected by amount and type of social support provided by family, friends, and others, and even by the healthcare provider.[22] Much of diabetes self-care takes place in a social context, so assessing and understanding social influences is often critical to facilitating effective self-care. The major social influences on diabetes in patients throughout the lifespan is shown in Table 4.8.

2 Social support may help patients mobilize positive coping strategies for dealing with the demands of daily life with diabetes, or it may help by buffering the effects of stress on these patients.

3 Patients are often more able to engage in self-care when their social networks provide practical and emotional support for diabetes self-management efforts.

4 Patients whose social networks are unsupportive, either practically or emotionally, are often less motivated to take care of their diabetes.

Table 4.8. Major Social Influences on Diabetes Self-Care Through the Life Span

Patient	Major Influence
Children	Parents
Adolescents	Peers
Adults	Spouses, other family members, friends, coworkers

ASSESSING SOCIAL SUPPORT

1 To clarify the strengths and weaknesses of a patient's social support networks, the educator may ask all or some of the questions in Table 4.9 to determine the following information:

   A What practical and emotional help patients receive from those around them

   B What barriers to self-care other people represent

   C What changes the patient wants in the area of support

2 The educator may find it useful to involve important members of the patient's social network in assessment, education, and treatment plans. Some comprehensive education programs use this approach as do many support groups (see Chapter 5, Behavior Change, for more information on these and other interventions).

TABLE 4.9. CRITICAL QUESTIONS FOR ASSESSING SOCIAL SUPPORT AVAILABLE TO PEOPLE WITH DIABETES

1 Who helps you the most when it comes to day-to-day diabetes management?

2 What does that person do that you find helpful? Please be as specific as possible.

3 Would you say this support is more practical or emotional?

4 Does anyone provide you with practical/emotional support (whichever was not mentioned in response to prior question) for managing your diabetes? If someone does, tell me about it, being as specific as possible.

5 Does anyone important to you make it harder for you to manage your diabetes? If so, who is this person? What does this person do that makes it harder for you to manage your diabetes? Please be as specific as possible.

6 What would you like in the way of support for day-to-day diabetes management that you are not getting now?

7 What one thing could you do to make it more likely you will get the support you want?

8 What can I do to help you get the support you want? (Suggest options such as joint meeting with family, materials for family to read, educational or support group programs to attend, etc.)

Importance of Contextual Influences: Barriers to Learning, Substance Abuse, Economic Factors, and Cultural and Religious Influences

1 Self-care behavior reflects the level of cognitive maturity a person has achieved.

A Some young people (up to age 15) are not cognitively ready to assume responsibility for independent self-care.[23]

B To be considered cognitively mature, a young person must be able to reason about abstract concepts that are inherent in diabetes management (eg, balancing multiple unknowns).

C Parents, motivated by frustration or the advice of health professionals, often withdraw from responsibility for their child's diabetes care. When young children aren't ready to assume the responsibility divested by their parents, gaps in care may develop.[24] These gaps can go unrecognized and lead to critical health-related difficulties.

D Some adults may also be cognitively immature or have other learning difficulties that pose problems for independent diabetes self-care (see Chapter 2, Teaching Patients With Low Literacy Skills for more information about this issue).

2 Substance abuse, in the form of smoking, excessive consumption of alcohol, or abuse of prescription or so-called recreational drugs, can cause serious problems for diabetes-self care and metabolic control. These types of abuses may also dramatically increase the risk for developing long-term complications of diabetes.

3 Paying for essential health services is a problem for many people who have diabetes, even for those with medical insurance coverage. Out-of-pocket medical expenses for people with diabetes are three times greater than for people who don't have diabetes. In addition, there are patients who are not able to pay for basic necessities such as food and shelter. Effective self-care and good health are hard to attain for those who lack the resources to pay for food, housing, and basic medical care.

3 Cultural influences on diabetes care must be recognized as well. We are all influenced by our cultural background and religious beliefs. Some cultural values (ie, the view that being overweight is desirable) and practices (ie, considering it impolite to refuse food that is offered when visiting another person's home) may be inconsistent with standard

approaches to diabetes self-management. In some cultures fasting is a religious practice, and in others, having diabetes may be seen as a sign of imperfection or contamination. On the other hand, some cultural and religious beliefs and practices can be sources of support in coping (see Chapter 3, Culturally Appropriateness in Diabetes Education and Care, for more information about these issues).

4 Once rapport has been established, the educator can quickly screen for the possibility that religious or cultural beliefs may affect a person's diabetes care by asking about this directly.

Assessing Cultural Influences

1 Recognizing, assessing, respecting, and working with cultural influences can be a challenge for many educators.

2 To communicate effectively with some patients, the educator may need to work with an appropriate interpreter.

Assessing Barriers to Learning

1 Cognitive immaturity may preclude children and young adolescents from assuming substantial responsibility for their self-care. Although the educator may choose to not assess cognitive maturity directly, this issue should be considered when working with young patients (see Chapter 17, Childhood and Adolescence for more information about these issues).

2 Assessing literacy skills in patients presents a challenge to many educators (see Chapter 2, Teaching Patients With Low Literacy Skills for information about assessment and education of persons with low literacy skills).

Assessing Substance Abuse

1 Symptoms of excessive alcohol intake may appear similar to ketoacidosis, including fruity-smelling breath, flushed face, irritability, staggering gait, drowsiness, and coma.

   A Excessive alcohol intake may also trigger or mimic hypoglycemia.

    B Ask patients directly about their alcohol consumption, including questions about how much alcohol is consumed each week, how much is the most consumed in 1 day over the past 3 months, and how much it takes to make the person intoxicated.

2 Signs of drug abuse vary as widely as a function of the substance abused.

    A Some typical signs of drug abuse include bloodshot eyes, constricted or dilated pupils, confusion, inappropriate behavior with emotional mood swings, anorexia or overeating, dramatically pressured or slowed speech, needle marks, and poor physical condition.

    B Stimulants such as amphetamines and cocaine, and depressants such as barbiturates and heroin affect memory and appetite, and in turn, diabetes self-care and metabolic control.

    C Hallucinogens such as lysergic acid diethylamide (LSD) phencyclidine (PCP), and marijuana can increase appetite, leading to extra caloric intake and often, higher blood glucose levels.

    D Ask patients who may be abusing drugs directly about their use even though most people will be wary about revealing that they are engaged in this activity.

3 Ask patients directly about whether and how much they smoke, and about their use of smokeless tobacco products.

    A Because smoking is a risk factor for many disease states, all of which are complicated by diabetes, smoking behavior is important to assess.

    B Ask patients who smoke if they are interested in information on or help with smoking cessation, and provide any requested resources.

    C The diabetes healthcare team needs to vigorously support patients' efforts to stop smoking.

Assessing Economic Factors

1 Because financial resources are required to pay for food, shelter, and medical care, the diabetes educator should ask patients directly about any concerns they have in this area.

2 Become familiar with community resources that may be available to help patients who cannot pay for basic necessities.

    A Medical assistance may be available through Medicaid or Medicare.

B Some organizations such as the American Diabetes Association (ADA), the Juvenile Diabetes Foundation International (JDFI), and the American Association of Diabetes Educators (AADE) offer information about services for those with limited financial resources.

C Community food banks have appropriate choices of foods for people with diabetes and may assist in providing staples on a monthly basis.

D State vocational rehabilitation agencies may provide vocational counseling, job placement, and financial assistance for job training and education.

E The Salvation Army and the American Red Cross often can help with emergency financial assistance.

Importance of Readiness to Change

1 The *transtheoretical model* postulates that the cessation of high-risk behaviors such as smoking and the acquisition of health-enhancing behaviors such as exercise, involve progression through five stages of change:

A Precontemplation—not thinking about change

B Contemplation—considering change in the foreseeable future

C Preparation—seriously considering change in the near future

D Action—in the process of behavior change

E Maintenance—continued change for an extended period

2 Assess the patient's stage of change for each diabetes-related health behavior (eg, SBGM, insulin use, meal planning) as it will likely vary for different behaviors. Approaches to facilitate or maintain each of the behaviors the individual desires will also need to vary.

Assessing Readiness to Change

1 Readiness to change any specific diabetes-related behavior may be assessed by asking the patient whether he or she is already engaged in that behavior, and if so, for more than 6 months (maintenance stage) or less than 6 months (action stage). If the patient is not engaged in the behavior, is he or she planning to do so in the next month (preparation stage), the next 6 months (contemplation stage), or not at all (precontemplation stage).

2   The results of the readiness to change assessment may be used to guide subsequent educational interventions (see Chapter 5, Behavior Change, for more information).

Key Educational Considerations

Helping patients make informed decisions concerning their diabetes is a primary responsibility of the diabetes educator. The first step in addressing this responsibility is to conduct a thorough assessment, including an assessment of psychosocial factors that may influence a person's capacity for self-care. In planning and conducting psychosocial assessments, apply the following key considerations:

1   Psychosocial factors powerfully influence not only a person's overall capacity for self-care, but also the unique details of that person's approach to day-to-day management.

2   Assess the entire range of psychosocial influences: social support; health beliefs and attitudes; quality of life, emotional well-being, and coping skills; and, contextual factors such as barriers to learning, economic considerations, religious and cultural influences; and readiness to change.

3   Assess psychosocial influences on self-care during the first meeting with a patient and on a regular basis thereafter.

4   Psychosocial assessment is useful for both the educator and the patient because it establishes at the outset that education and care are cooperative endeavors based on the unique facts of the individual patient's life.

5   Each potential psychosocial influence on behavior may be assessed using either published instruments, sample items from published instruments, or open-ended questions.

6   This chapter has identified specific questions in each psychosocial domain which may be used to expediently screen for possible problems in that domain. If such problems are identified, the educator may choose to do a fuller assessment of that domain.

7 In some cases, psychosocial assessment will reveal problems that can only be resolved using skills outside of the educator's area of expertise. Developing a network of specialists, including mental health professionals, social workers, and others, to provide expert evaluation, treatment, and case management services on an as-needed basis can greatly facilitate patient access. An important role for the educator in this network is to provide information about diabetes to these professionals.

SELF-REVIEW QUESTIONS

1 Define the educator's goals in doing a psychosocial assessment.

2 Describe how health beliefs and attitudes influence a person's self-care behavior.

3 List simple, practical instruments or questions can you use to assess various aspects of a person's diabetes-related health beliefs and attitudes.

4 Define behavioral intentions and why they are important to assess.

5 When assessing overall quality of life in a person with diabetes, should you use a diabetes-specific measure? Why?

6 List the three clinical psychological disorders that seem to be more common among people with diabetes.

7 Describe how social support influence a person's day-to-day diabetes self-care.

8 List questions you could ask a person with diabetes to assess available social support.

9 State why it is important to assess readiness to change.

10 List contextual influences to assess in patients with diabetes.

CASE STUDY 1

LB is a 44-year-old African-American female who was diagnosed with type 2 diabetes 2 years ago. She lives in the home she shared with her husband before they divorced 6 years ago. Two of her four adult children and one of her grandchildren also live with her. LB's glucose readings are generally very high, and she has problems with many aspects of diabetes self-care, especially SMBG, which she does only a few times a week, meal planning, and exercise, which she does rarely. LB is already reporting some symptoms of neuropathy, and her most recent lab work revealed albumin in her urine. Insulin treatment has been recommended to LB, but she is very upset at the prospect of taking shots. When questioned, she responds, "I just can't take it! I'm already stretched to the limit. I have lots of stress at home, I'm the only one bringing in any money, and I feel rotten all the time. No way could I deal with insulin on top of all that. Everyone else in my family died young from diabetes and I guess the same thing will happen to me."

Questions for Discussion

1 What psychosocial factors might be contributing to LB's resistance to initiating insulin therapy?
2 Which of these factors would you assess first?
3 What questions would you ask to assess these issues?

Discussion

1 LB's presentation suggests that she is feeling overwhelmed by a variety of psychosocial issues. Her family situation seems to make her life and her diabetes management more difficult rather than easier.

2 LB's diabetes-related beliefs and attitudes, based in part on the experience of other family members who had diabetes, reinforces her pessimism concerning the possibility of living well with diabetes.
   A There is a high prevalence of type 2 diabetes among African Americans.
   B Her quality of life is clearly poor.

3 LB may be depressed, her economic situation appears to be precarious, and her coping skills are not adequate for helping her take effective control of her diabetes in the face of other pressures.

4 The diabetes educator must protect herself from feeling as overwhelmed as LB feels. This will be difficult given the severity of LB's problems.

5 Under these circumstances a step-by-step triage approach is essential. A useful first step might be to simply acknowledge the frustration and pessimism LB so obviously feels.

6 Next, the educator could clarify the fact that while change may be slow, it is possible if LB and the educator work together to identify LB's most pressing problem and address that.

    A Prioritizing in this way may help both LB and the educator feel less over-whelmed and help them both focus on problem-solving.

    B Keep in mind that this approach has the best chance of success if the priorities are set by LB herself.

7 If this approach works, LB will feel more confident in her working relationship with the educator and in her own ability to deal with her diabetes-related difficulties.

8 If LB is unable to engage in setting priorities, it is probably because she is feeling unworkably overwhelmed by the stress—including the non-diabetes-related stress—in her life.

    A Consider referring LB to a social worker or mental health professional. The services of these specialists may improve LB's capacity to work with the educator and make informed choices for her life with diabetes.

CASE STUDY 2

ZM is a 62-year-old man who was diagnosed with type 2 diabetes at the age of 41 years. He takes insulin by injection three times a day, performs SMBG four times a day, and walks five times a week for at least 30 minutes. Despite ZM's efforts in these aspects of his diabetes self-care, he has hypertension and hyperlipidemia, neither of which is well controlled. ZM has also been steadily gaining weight the last 4 to 5 years and now weighs 35 pounds more than he did 5 years ago. His wife always comes to clinic visits with him.

When ZM is asked about his situation, says, "I know I have a problem. I live to eat. That's a major source of stress between my wife and me. On the one hand she's often hassling me to eat healthier, but on the other hand, she keeps bringing the cake and candy and ice cream into the house and stuffing her face with it. Now that I think about it, we hassle about a lot of things, especially when it comes to my diabetes. She's the reason I take my shots and test my blood and walk as regularly as I do. She's always reminding me, and even nagging me if she has to. She is so into my diabetes it's almost like it's her disease and not mine. Now don't get me wrong, there are times I really appreciate the help. But other times it drives me crazy. The latest thing between us is smoking. She quit 6 months ago and now she's trying to get me to do the same."

Questions for Discussion

1 What three psychosocial factors need to be addressed by ZM and the educator?

2 How important is ZM's wife to his self-care? What questions might you ask to help ZM identify what he wants from his wife in terms of diabetes care?

3 What strategies might you use to include ZM's wife in the assessment and educational process?

Discussion

1 ZM's presentation suggests 3 psychosocial issues that need to be addressed.
   A Most obvious among these issues is how ZM and his wife interact concerning his diabetes care.
   B A second related issue is ZM's attitudes about his diabetes and its management.
   C Finally, given ZM's medical history, his smoking is also a concern.

2 It appears that ZM's wife both helps and hinders his diabetes management efforts. It also seems that ZM is ambivalent about his wife's involvement, sometimes welcoming it and other times not.
   A The educator might ask ZM and his wife to say as specifically as possible what determines whether her involvement is helpful. Questions like, "When is it helpful? When is it not? What makes the difference? How do you know when it is helpful? What make the difference? How do you know when it is helpful? What happens when it is not helpful?", may be useful in identifying the determinants of true helpfulnesss in their relationship.
   B Based on this information, the educator might ask ZM if it would be helpful for he and his wife draft a "contract" specifying when and in what ways she will participate in his diabetes care.

3 The educator might also discuss with the couple the difference between support and pushing. Support is almost always helpful; pushing is generally not.
   A Support is helping someone do what he says he wants to do.
   B Pushing is trying to get someone do what you have believe he should do.

4 Assess ZM's readiness to stop smoking, and offer appropriate resources, including support from his wife.

REFERENCES

1   Becker MH, Janz NK. The health belief model applied to understanding diabetes regimen compliance. Diabetes Educ 1985;11(1):41-47.

2   Peyrot M, Rubin RR. Structure and correlates of diabetes-specific locus of control. Diabetes Care 1994;17:994-1001.

3   Ferraro LA, Price JH, Desmond SM, Roberts SM. Development of a diabetes locus of control scale. Psychol Rep 1987;61:763-70.

4   Bandura A. Social foundations of thought and action: a social cognitive theory. Englewood Cliffs, NJ: Prentice-Hall, 1986.

5   Rubin RR, Peyrot M. Psychosocial problems and interventions in diabetes: a review of the literature. Diabetes Care 1992;15:1640-57.

6   Grossman HY, Brink S, Hauser S. Self-efficacy in adolescent girls and boys with insulin-dependent diabetes mellitus. Diabetes Care 1987;10:324-29.

7   Rubin RR, Peyrot M, Saudek CD. Effect of diabetes education on self-care, metabolic control, and emotional well-being. Diabetes Care 1989;12:673-79.

8   Rubin RR, Peyrot M, Saudek CD. Differential effect of diabetes education on self-regulation and life-style behaviors. Diabetes Care 1991;14:335-38.

9   Rubin RR, Peyrot M, Saudek CD. The effect of a diabetes education program incorporating coping skills training on emotional well-being and diabetes self-efficacy. Diabetes Educ 1993;19:210-14.

10 Peyrot M, Rubin RR. The effect of self-efficacy and behavioral intentions on self-care improvement following diabetes education. Diabetes 1995; 44(Suppl 1):96A.

11 Bradley C, Lewis KS, Jennings AM, Ward, JD. Scales to measure perceived control developed specifically for people with tablet-treated diabetes. Diabetic Med 1990;7:685-94.

12 Kurtz SMS. Adherence to diabetes regimens: empirical status and clinical applications. Diabetes Educ 1990;16:50-59.

13 Ware JE Jr, Shelbourne CD. The MOS 36-item short-form health survey (SF-36). I: conceptual framework and item selection. Med Care 1992;30:473-83.

14 Bush JM, Kaplan RM. Health-related quality of life measurement. Health Psychol 1982;1:61-80.

15 Bergner M, Bobbitt RA, Carter WB, et al. The sickness impact profile: development and revision of a health status measure. Med Care 1981;19:787-805.

16 Jacobson A. Quality of life in patients with diabetes mellitus. Semin Clin Neuropsychiatry 1997;2:82-93.

17 Bradley C, Lewis KS. Measures of psychological well-being and treatment satisfaction developed from the responses of people with tablet-treated diabetes. Diabetic Med 1990;7:445-51.

18 Polonsky W, Anderson BJ, Lohrer PA, Welch G, et al. Assessment of diabetes-related distress. Diabetes Care 1995;18: 754-60.

19 Gavard JA, Lustman PJ, Clouse RE. Prevalence of depression in adults with diabetes: an epidemiological evaluation. Diabetes Care 1993;16:1167-78.

20 Peyrot M, Rubin RR. Levels and risks of depression and anxiety symptomatology among diabetic adults. Diabetes Care 1997;20:585-90.

21 Rydall AC, Rodin GM, Olmsted MP, et al. Disordered eating behavior and microvascular complications in young women with insulin-dependent diabetes mellitus. N Engl J Med 1997;336:1849-54.

22 Peyrot M, McMurry JF, Jr. Psychosocial factors in diabetes control: adjustment of insulin-dependent adults. Psychosom Med 1985;47:542-57.

23 Ingersoll GM, Orr DP, Herrold AJ, Golden MP. Cognitive maturity and self-management among adolescents with insulin-dependent diabetes mellitus. J Pediatr 1986;108:620-23.

24 Brackenridge BP, Rubin RR. Sweet kids: how to balance diabetes control and good nutrition with family peace. Alexandria, Va: American Diabetes Association, 1996.

25 Ruggiero L, Prochaska JO, eds. From research to practice: readiness for change. Diabetes Spectrum 1993; 6:21-60.

SUGGESTED READINGS

Anderson B, Rubin RR, eds. Practical psychology for diabetes clinicians: how to deal with the key behavioral issues faced by patients and health care teams. Alexandria, Va: American Diabetes Association, 1996.

Bradley C. Handbook of psychology and diabetes. Chur, Switzerland: Harwood Academic Publishers, 1994.

Cox D, Gonder-Frederick L. Major developments in behavioral diabetes research. J Consulting Clin Psychol 1992;60:628-38.

Feste C. The physician within, 2nd edition. Alexandria, Va; American Diabetes Association, 1992.

Peyrot M, Rubin RR. Living with diabetes: the patient-centered perspective. Diabetes Spectrum 1994;7:204-205.

Peyrot M, Rubin RR, Psychosocial aspects of diabetes care. In: Leslie D, Robbins D, eds. Diabetes: clinical science in practice. Cambridge: Cambridge University Press, 1995:465-77.

Rubin RR, Biermann J, Toohey B. Psyching out diabetes: a positive approach to your negative emotions. Los Angeles, Calif: Lowell House, 1992.

Saudek CD, Rubin RR, Shump C. The Johns Hopkins guide to diabetes: for today and tomorrow. Baltimore, Md: The Johns Hopkins University Press, 1997.

PSYCHOSOCIAL ISSUES

Behavior Change

5

Richard R. Rubin, PhD, CDE
The Johns Hopkins University School of Medicine
Departments of Medicine and Pediatrics
Baltimore, Maryland

INTRODUCTION

1 Self-care behavior is critical for maintaining physical and emotional health for people who have diabetes. Although technological advances in recent years have offered the promise of better health, the trade-off of additional self-care demands has been considerable.

2 The key to helping patients with diabetes achieve their desired level of self-care is understanding the factors that determine diabetes-related behavior. These factors include health beliefs, self-efficacy, social support, self-care skills, coping skills, locus-of-control orientation, emotional well-being, cognitive maturity, health status, patient-provider communication, regimen complexity and aversiveness, and organizational factors related to health-care delivery. Assessing these factors in individual patients is addressed in detail in Chapter 4, Psychosocial Assessment.

3 The patient and educator need to work together to develop an individualized treatment or education plan designed to foster and maintain patterns of self-management that the patient has chosen to follow.

4 One rationale for supporting efforts by patients to make behavioral changes is the knowledge that these have the potential to improve physiologic outcomes including glycemia, weight, and lipid levels, which, in turn, reduce the risk of long-term complications and resulting costs.

5 Recent years have seen a growing awareness that behavior change and improved glycemic control may also contribute to improved quality of life.

6 The assessment of psychosocial and behavioral factors which may influence self-care and a person's capacity and resources for change are addressed in Chapter 4, Psychosocial Assessment.

OBJECTIVES

Upon completion of this chapter, the learner will be able to

1 Explain the role of behavior in diabetes.
2 Identify two perspectives on behavior change in diabetes.
3 Apply the results of a comprehensive psychosocial assessment to help patients develop an effective self-care plan.

THE ROLE OF BEHAVIOR IN DIABETES

1 Self-care is a multidimensional construct.

   A Levels of self-care vary across areas of the regimen, being highest for medical aspects such as taking medications, with lifestyle aspects such as diet and exercise causing the greatest difficulty.[1]

   B Levels of self-care in different areas of diabetes management are often uncorrelated.[2] Consequently, it has been difficult to formally establish relationships between specific self-care behaviors and physiologic outcomes until recently.

2 While the relationships of self-care behavior, quality of life, and metabolic control and complications is complex, evidence supporting the existence of relationships among these variables has been increasing in recent years.

   A The results of the Diabetes Control and Complications Trial (DCCT)[3] confirm the benefits of intensive treatment, including active self-management.

   B Other research reinforces some of the findings of the DCCT.[4,5] For example, in one study,[6] people who increased the frequency of their self monitoring of blood glucose (SMBG) or exercise lowered their glycosylated hemoglobin levels by an average of 1.3%. Those who improved the frequency of both exercise and SMBG or improved their insulin administration (skipping fewer shots or adjusting doses more often) lowered their glycosylated hemoglobin levels by an average of 2.9%.

3 Burgeoning technology and therapeutic advances affect diabetes self-care behavior.

   A Examples of such advances include SMBG, intensive conventional therapy (ICT) involving multiple daily insulin injections, and continuous subcutaneous insulin infusion (CSII).

   B The impact of this progress is greatest for patients who take insulin, although the availability of new classes of oral antidiabetes medications may increase the impact of technology on people who do not take insulin.

   C The impact of technology on diabetes education and care is increasing, with developments such as electronic patient records, telemedicine, and the use of computers for assessment and education.

    D These advances are like a two-edged sword: they offer hope for better health, but often involve greater self-care demands.

4 Diabetes self-care requires substantial effort.

    A People who develop diabetes are often asked to make major lifestyle changes:

- Practice SMBG
- Follow an often-complex medication regimen
- Engage in ongoing physical activity
- Plan and manage nutritional composition and timing
- Manage hypo- and hyperglycemia and associated mood swings
- Engage in regular foot care and other preventive practices
- Stop smoking
- Maintain reasonable body weight
- Manage common illnesses

    B Research and clinical experience suggest that the behavior change required to maintain diabetes self-care is difficult for most people.[7,8]

    C Others[9,10] have discussed the reasons why diabetes self-management is difficult for many people.

PERSPECTIVES ON BEHAVIOR CHANGE IN DIABETES

1 The *compliance perspective*[11] is a traditional medical view of the relationship between health professionals and their patients.

    A The compliance perspective assumes that the healthcare professional is responsible for the diagnosis, treatment, and outcome of diabetes care, while the patient is a recipient of this care.

    B The compliance perspective assumes that change occurs as a result of the professional's efforts to get the patient to follow or comply with the prescribed treatment regimen.

2 The *empowerment perspective*[11] assumes that most of the responsibility for diabetes care rests with the person who has the disease. Therefore, final decisions regarding diabetes-related behavior are the right and responsibility of the individual.

    A The empowerment perspective holds that the costs and benefits of diabetes care must be seen in the broader personal and social context of a person's life, and that patients must be seen as experts in their own lives, while professionals are experts in the clinical aspects of diabetes. Self-care requires an effective coalition that incorporates each party's expertise.

B The empowerment perspective incorporates the fact that more than 99% of diabetes care is self-care. The vast majority of diabetes care takes place not two to four times a year in the provider's office, but literally countless times every day in the places where people with diabetes live, work, eat, and play.

C According to the empowerment perspective, behavior change takes place as healthcare professionals help patients make informed decisions about self-care. Efforts to understand the patient's perspective, acknowledge the patient's feelings, and offer relevant information to help the patient make decisions are the cornerstone of the diabetes educator's role in facilitating empowerment.[12]

D People with diabetes have always chosen what to do with recommendations they receive from healthcare professionals. Accordingly, the empowerment perspective seeks to clarify the patient's role as an informed, equal, active partner in formulating and maintaining the treatment program. This approach avoids the dilemma in which patients exercise their power to choose by vetoing recommendations made by healthcare providers and educators without effectively using their expertise to develop a more workable plan.

E Not all patients seek to be the primary decision maker in their care. Professionals must respect different styles. Some people are more comfortable in a less active role, some of the time preferring to follow the recommendations of the providers. Sometimes self-directed care may be achieved in steps.[6] For example, patients who present in very poor control or limited knowledge may first use a set treatment plan. Once they have experienced self-care, they may choose to take a more active role in self-management.

FACILITATING SELF-CARE

To care for diabetes, patients need self-management and coping skills. Developing and maintaining healthy patterns of self-care requires three basic skills: specific self-care skills, self-management skills, and coping skills, including the ability to enlist appropriate support for self-care efforts. Educational interventions need to facilitate the development of each set of skills (the assessment of these skills is discussed in Chapter 4, Psychosocial Assessment).

1 Specific self-care skills training:

    A Meta-analyses, a method of statistically combining the results of many different studies, reveal that active diabetes education that involves demonstration of skills, practice, and direct practical feedback for efforts is the most effective approach for improving self-care skills and metabolic control.[13-15]

    B More didactic approaches are less effective because they tend to increase knowledge without increasing skill or improving glycemia.

    C The key approach for facilitating behavior change is clear: don't talk; teach behavior. Although these findings may seem obvious, their implications for the design of educational interventions are profound and often not adequately taken into account.

    D To make the inherently difficult process of behavior change as manageable as possible, educators can help patients learn to make the best use of their coping skills and resources. If the goal is improved glycemic control, some studies show that performing just one new behavior (eg, situational adjustment of insulin) can lead to significantly improved glycosylated hemoglobin levels even in the absence of changes in such basic aspects of lifestyle as meal planning and exercise.[16]

2 Self-management skills training:

    A One fundamental skill is setting realistic self-care goals, goals which fit with other life goals.

    B Rigid adherence to a regimen may be less effective than juggling components of treatment in response to daily events and SMBG results.[6,17]

    C Given the demands of life with diabetes, the patient's physical and emotional well-being is most enhanced by flexibility or skill in problem solving.[18]

    D To be effective, diabetes education must incorporate interventions to foster the development of these skills. One productive approach involves discussing potential options for handling situations in which the patient finds diabetes to be problematic. The goal of this approach is to develop, practice, and refine strategies for handling these situations in ways that promote physical and emotional well-being.

3 Coping skills training:

    A The goal of diabetes coping skills training is to help patients overcome attitudinal and emotional barriers to the successful application of new knowledge and skills. A diabetes-specific cognitive behavioral model, which has been described in detail elsewhere,[9,10] provides effective coping skills training that is active and individualized.

B   In this training, patients learn that certain thoughts or attitudes trigger constructive behavior in difficult situations, while other thoughts and attitudes trigger unconstructive behavior.

C   Patients are then taught how to implement a procedure for achieving a positive approach to the troublesome diabetes-related situations, and practice this approach.

D   A final component of coping skills training is relapse prevention, which offers protection against the possibility that the inevitable slips in self-care may trigger a full-blown relapse.[19]

THE EFFECTS OF THE ORGANIZATION AND STRUCTURE OF EDUCATIONAL AND TREATMENT PROGRAMS

1   The way in which educational and treatment programs are organized or structured can facilitate or hinder patient participation rates as well as their ability to make changes.

2   Educators can incorporate specific structural issues into the interventions they design.

A   Interdisciplinary staff:
   • Given the complexity of life with diabetes, patients will generally benefit from educational and treatment interventions that allow them to consult with an interdisciplinary staff that includes physicians, nurses, nutritionists, mental health specialists, exercise specialists, and pharmacists.
   • Because few clinics can support such a staff, a viable alternative is a referral network of experienced specialists in each field. Access to specialists tends to facilitate self-care, so developing an effective and coordinated referral network is helpful to educators and their patients.

B   Educators can consider helping patients to prepare before visits with their physicians. Studies[20] show that a brief intervention focused on training patients to be more active and assertive during interviews with a physician leads to improvement in glucose control and quality of life.

C   On-call availability and follow-up contact:

- Most changes involved in maintaining healthy patterns of self-care require continuing support, yet patients typically go for months without consulting healthcare providers.
- Two options for encouraging more frequent contact (and potentially facilitating behavior change) are on-call availability and follow-up telephone contact.
- Follow-up telephone contact initiated by the patient at set times or as circumstances require or by the educator may also support the patient's self-care efforts.
- These contacts can help patients maintain their motivation to change by addressing specific problems that might lead to relapse, and by facilitating a pattern of open communication that makes it easier for the patient to call if problems arise.

D Group support:
- Whenever possible, provide opportunities for group experiences with others who have diabetes. Such opportunities can take the form of group education, or formal or informal diabetes support groups or referral to these groups.
- Groups encourage efforts to improve self-care through mutual sharing and encouragement, modeling, positive reinforcement, and personal goal setting.
- Other options for support include walking groups, diabetes-related support or educational groups, other support groups, and computer-based resources.

THE EMPOWERMENT APPROACH FOR FACILITATING BEHAVIOR CHANGE

1 Empowering patients for self-directed behavior change is gaining increased support in diabetes education.[21] Given the fact that patients make many important and often complex self-care decisions every day, the goal is to enable people to make informed decisions (see Table 5.1).

2 Several key concepts are basic to an empowerment-based practice.
A Emphasizing the whole person.
- People are more than patients. They are physical, emotional, social, and spiritual beings.
- The different aspects of a person's life are interrelated and must be taken into account in making diabetes self-care decisions.

TABLE 5.1. FOUR-STEP PATIENT EMPOWERMENT COUNSELING MODEL[21]

1 *Help patient identify diabetes-related problems and issues on which they want to work.*
"I believe that exercise can help me control my diabetes."

2 *Help patient identify thoughts and feelings associated with the issue.*
"What are you thinking and feeling when you are struggling with the problem?"

3 *Help patient identify health-related attitudes and beliefs underlying the problem and establish diabetes self-care goals.*
"What deeper attitudes and beliefs lead you to think and feel as you do when you are struggling with the problem?" "What is your ultimate goal for dealing with the problem?"

4 *Help patient develop and commit to a plan for achieving the goal.*
"What would be the steps, one by one, that would lead to reaching your ultimate goal?"

- Recognizing , respecting, and supporting this holistic dynamic helps the educator play a constructive part in the process of change.

B Acknowledging the patient's role in decision-making.

- Recognize that it is impossible to solve problems for the patient or to impose a solution.
- The effective educator assumes the role of an advisor to the patient on subjects related to the treatment of diabetes. Offering options and supporting the generation of potentially useful approaches to a given problem increase the educator's effectiveness.
- It is the patient's right and responsibility to make decisions.

C Educating for informed choice about treatment options. Two types of education are crucial to empowerment:

- The first type of education involves providing information about diabetes and its treatment to allow the patient to make wise decisions about diabetes self-care options.[21] This type of education might be called self-management training.
- The second type of education is designed to facilitate patients' self-awareness and skills for dealing with the emotional, social, intellectual, and spiritual components of their lives as they relate to the daily

decisions patients must make about their diabetes. This type of education has been called coping skills training.

D Taking into account readiness to change.

- Different approaches to facilitating behavior change are appropriate depending on the patient's stage of readiness to change.[22] The educator should keep in mind that patients may be at different stages of readiness to change regarding different aspects of self-management. (See Chapter 4, Psychosocial Assessment, for guidelines for assessing readiness to change.)

- For patients in the precontemplation stage (ie, not planning to change behavior in the foreseeable future), approaches which emphasize providing patients with personalized information and allowing them to express feelings about diabetes may be most effective.

- For patients in the contemplation stage (ie, seriously thinking about changing behavior in the next 6 months), approaches which encourage patients to develop support networks, provide positive feedback for patients' capacity to make changes, and help patients clarify ambivalent feelings concerning behavior change while emphasizing expected benefits, may be most effective.

- For patients in the preparation stage (ie, intending to change behavior in the next month), approaches which encourage the patient to set specific, achievable goals (eg, walking briskly for at least 15 minutes 3 or more times a week), and reinforce small changes already made, may be most effective.

- For patients in the action stage (ie, already modifying behavior), approaches that include referral to a diabetes self-management program and providing relevant self-help materials may be most effective.

- For patients in the maintenance stage (ie, continued in action stage for a least 6 months), approaches which encourage patients to anticipate and plan for potential difficulties (eg, maintaining dietary changes while on vacation) and providing information on community resources such as support groups, may be most effective.

E Viewing treatment plans as ongoing experiments.

- Treatment plans need to be refined periodically to reflect changes in a person's life and state of diabetes. It is critically important that both the educator and patient recognize this fact and use it to their advantage.

- The beauty of an experiment is that it produces information, not success or failure. This information is used to refine the treatment plan and produce more information, which is then used to support further refinement, and so on.
- Because this process mirrors life with a chronic disease, it is an excellent model for positive coping with diabetes.

TWELVE SPECIFIC STEPS FOR FACILITATING PATIENT EMPOWERMENT

1 Ask questions.

  A The educator can use specific concrete techniques such as asking questions using other approaches listed in Table 5.2 to facilitate patient empowerment. History-taking questions such as "Have you been having any low blood sugars lately?" or "How often are you testing your blood sugar these days?" are not particularly effective in facilitating empowerment and self-management.

  B Questions like "What's the hardest thing for you right now about dealing with your diabetes?" are more likely to generate the kind of information the patient and educator need to generate self-care strategies that will actually work for a given patient.

TABLE 5.2. TWELVE STEPS FOR FACILITATING PATIENT EMPOWERMENT

1 Ask questions.
2 Start with the patient's agenda.
3 Work with the patient to individualize the treatment plan.
4 Define the problems as specifically as possible.
5 Take a step-by-step approach.
6 Focus on behaviors, not outcomes.
7 Use contracts.
8 Involve the family and other people who are important to the patient.
9 Maintain contact between visits.
10 Facilitate problem-solving skills.
11 Nourish emotional coping skills.
12 Get help from colleagues and refer to specialists as needed.

C   Asking questions can actually save time for healthcare professionals and patients. It is a waste of valuable time when the educator attempts, visit after visit, to offer recommendations without knowing what is actually bothering the patient most. The educator often ends up making suggestions that have little meaning for the patient, so that both the professional and patient become frustrated.

2   Start with the patient's agenda.

A   Educators often feel they know what their patients need to do to improve their health, as well as the order in which these things need to be done.

B   Unfortunately, operating as if patients will follow the agenda an educator sets almost never works. Patients simply veto any suggestions that don't make sense to them.

C   Veto power is rarely expressed directly in words. More often patients express this veto power by simply not doing what the educator has recommended.

D   Starting with the patient's agenda increases the likelihood that patients will reach critical self-care goals. A more positive relationship is established, and patients are likely to become more open when they see that their needs are the educator's primary concern.

3   Individualize the treatment plan.

A   Everyone is different, so there is no single plan that works for every person with diabetes.

B   The key to successful individualization is a fundamental tool: good questions. If the patient's goal is weight loss, for example, the educator might ask how much weight the person wants to lose, what success the patient has had losing weight in the past, what facts of life will facilitate or hinder weight-loss efforts, and what the patient would like the healthcare professional to do when it comes to facilitating the weight-loss process.

4   Define the problem as specifically as possible.

A   The more specifically patient and the educator define a problem, the more likely they are to solve the problem.

B   Questions, again, are the key to success. If a patient complains of difficulties with her meal plan, for example, the educator should help the patient define the problem more specifically. Most patients have specific "sticking points" and are aware of them. In this situation, the sticking point might turn out to be a problem resisting late night snacks.

C Two benefits result from identifying specific sticking points.
- First, both patient and educator can see that the problem they face is more manageable than they originally believed (eg, snacking after dinner is less overwhelming than overall dietary failure). Thus the patient's ability and motivation is greater to make changes.
- Second, problem-solving for specific problems is usually much easier than problem-solving for general problems.

5 Take a step-by-step approach:

A Problems that seem insurmountable as a whole can often be solved one step at a time.

B Most diabetes-related problems are daunting. Educators can help their patients simplify a problem by taking a step-by-step approach. Consider the task of establishing an exercise program. The educator knows that a healthy exercise plan for most people would involve a minimum activity level equivalent to three brisk 30-minute walks per week, or more frequent activity of shorter duration. Yet many patients who want to start exercising would feel overwhelmed starting at this level.

C The patient needs to identify a first step in reaching his or her goal, such as initiating an exercise program by walking for 15 minutes twice a week. The role of the educator is to help the patient generate a list of possible strategies, assist in using the list to create a meaningful plan, and provide emotional encouragement and practical support for the patient's efforts to change behavior.

D This process provides four benefits:
- It establishes a cooperative working relationship between the educator and patient in dealing with a goal the patient has chosen.
- The first step the patient has suggested regarding exercise is a meaningful one. If the strategy is meaningful, the patient is more likely to implement it.
- A patient who succeeds in taking a first step is likely to have the confidence to take a second step, and a third.
- If the plan doesn't work, the educator can ask what the patient learned from the experience.

6 Focus on behaviors, not outcomes:

   A When an educator helps a patient work on behaviors, desired outcomes are likely to follow.

   B It's easier for patients to achieve their chosen goals such as improved blood sugar control or reduced weight, when they focus on the behaviors required to reach these goals (eg, switching from regular ice cream to fat-free or starting a walking program).

   C Behavior is something the patient can work on and ultimately control directly, while outcomes such as blood sugar levels are often influenced by factors outside the patient's control.

   D Focusing only on physiologic outcomes can lead to feelings of frustration and even helplessness. Although focusing on behavior is not a panacea, it increases the patient's sense of control.

7 Use contracts:

   A Helping patients formally specify what they will do to reach goals can facilitate self-management.

   B A useful behavioral contract might include the following elements:

      • Statement of goal in specific, measurable, behavioral terms. A goal that is both ambitious and realistic is more meaningful to patients.

      • Rewards for achieving the goal. These rewards may be anything the patient chooses, ranging from sleeping through the night (less need to awaken and urinate, improved blood sugar control) to being alive to see a grandchild graduate from high school, to feeling good about oneself for improved self-care.

      • Who the patient will turn to at the first sign of slipping in efforts to achieve the goal. The patient could choose the educator or any other appropriate person for this role.

8 Involve the family and others who are important to the patient:

   A Diabetes is a family disease powerful enough to affect the lives of everyone who loves, lives with, or cares for a person with diabetes.

   B Family members and other important people in the patient's life can significantly affect the way a person with diabetes lives with the disease.

   C Involving the family and significant others may take several forms.

      • Include important family members and significant others in office visits if at all possible, and with the patient's permission. Getting the perspective of family members can be helpful to the the patient and the educator.

- When it is not possible to include family members in education, ask questions about how the family members are involved in diabetes care. These questions include queries concerning what family members do to facilitate and hinder self-care, and what the patient needs from family members and others to make life with diabetes easier (see Chapter 4, Psychosocial Assessment).

9 Maintain contact between visits:

A Research and clinical experience show that even brief, occasional contact with a healthcare professional (between regularly scheduled visits) can powerfully affect people struggling with a chronic disease.

B Some potentially effective approaches for maintaining patient contact are through phone calls, postcards, newsletters, e-mail messages, and office-based support groups.

C Maintaining contact helps patients feel cared for, enhances motivation, and provides the educator with an invaluable early-warning system for problems that might otherwise get worse before the patient called about them.

10 Facilitate problem-solving skills:

A Living well with diabetes requires a high level of problem-solving skills. Diabetes makes life more complicated, so people with diabetes have more decisions to make and problems to solve on a day-to-day basis than people who don't have diabetes.[18]

B Patients develop diabetes-related problem-solving skills through trial and error and continuous practice. As one young man said, "I hate having diabetes, but it's forced me to be a really good problem-solver, and I wouldn't give that up for anything in the world."

11 Nourish emotional coping skills:

A One of the things that people with diabetes need most is a strong emotional foundation. Educators need to be prepared to help their patients deal with emotional issues.

B Books are available to help healthcare professionals[23] and people with diabetes[10] cope with the emotional side of diabetes.

12 Get help:

A Educators also need help and support because caring for people with diabetes can be as hard as living with it, though in different ways.

    B Getting help may mean consulting with a colleague to get suggestions for dealing with a difficult issue. Sometimes just talking things out or getting someone else's perspective can help.

    C Getting help may also mean referring a patient for specialized services for which the educator is not trained or does not have the time to provide.

REEVALUATING TRADITIONAL TEACHING METHODS TO INCORPORATE THE EMPOWERMENT APPROACH

1 Empowering patients requires diabetes educators to evaluate their teaching methods and approaches to patient care.

2 Recognize that patients are in control of their own self-care. This realization often happens indirectly. Every day educators work with patients who refuse to follow the educator's good advice about caring for their diabetes. The first and strongest response to this refusal might be frustration or perhaps disappointment. However, further thought might lead the educator to see that these patients are telling the educator in no uncertain terms that they will decide what they will and will not do.

    A Because patients truly have veto power, creating a coalition for care that helps the patient assume an initiating role rather than a defensive one decreases frustration for both patients educators.

    B The role of the educator in such a coalition is not to give advice about the "right" or "best" way to accomplish a particular goal, but rather to help patients explore the range of self-care options available and the consequences of implementing each of these options.

    C This type of exploration can be frustrating for the educator when the patient is resistant or in denial. In such a case, educators need to recognize the limits of their ability to affect change.

3 Many educators have difficulty dealing with the emotional content of patients' problems. This limitation makes it difficult for educators to encourage patients to identify, express, and explore negative emotions that are an inevitable part of living with diabetes. Diabetes educators need to therefore refocus their professional tendency to be problem solvers and support their patients' explorations of emotional issues. Emotions are not problems to be solved, but rather, feelings to be recognized, identified, expressed, and accepted.

A The educator's role is that of a thoughtful, compassionate, active, well-informed listener.

B Educators are not responsible for fixing their patients' negative emotions. Recognizing this aspect of their role may help educators feel more comfortable in helping their patients recognize and work with uncomfortable feelings.

Potential Benefits to Educators for Facilitating Patient Empowerment

1 Accepting that the educator's role is limited to education and counseling can relieve any guilt the educator might feel when patients don't follow their suggested healthy, self-care programs. The educator can feel a great relief to be able to say, "I did my job (educating and counseling) as well as I could; getting the patient to change is not part of my responsibilities."

2 Recognizing that changing patients' behavior is not part of the job description may help educators feel less frustrated with patients who choose to manage their diabetes in ways that the educator considers unhealthy.

3 When educators spend less energy trying to change patients, they relieve themselves of a self-imposed burden and free energy for other, more attainable tasks.

Key Educational Considerations

1 Supporting patients in their efforts to decide upon, initiate and maintain healthy patterns of self-care is a critical responsibility of the diabetes educator.

2 The role of the educator is to facilitate change; the role of the patient is to make change. Every encounter with the patient can be directed toward empowerment. The key is to ask questions and offer options rather than to issue directives.

3 The patient's personal model of diabetes, including health beliefs, locus-of-control orientation, and diabetes self-efficacy, powerfully influences motivation for change. Both the patient and educator need to learn to

identify and understand the effects of these attitudes and, when necessary, how they can be shifted. The power of attitudes can be demonstrated through discussions that reveal how diabetes-related behaviors flow directly from personal beliefs.

4 The support a patient receives from family, friends, co-workers, and medical staff also affects patterns of self-care. The educator can assess and make efforts to influence these factors as well. Assist patients to identify gaps in currently available support and creating plans to fill these gaps.

5 Behavior-based education is far more effective than knowledge-based education in changing patterns of self-care. Therefore, all interventions need to be presented in a practical, experience-based context. Specific self-care skills and more complex problem-solving or self-management skills can be demonstrated, practiced, observed, and refined in face-to-face interactions.

6 Coping skills training can be an invaluable component of efforts to improve self-care patterns. All too often attitudinal and emotional barriers prevent patients from making needed changes in diabetes-related behavior. Teaching patients can be taught a basic approach for managing the emotional side of living with diabetes that may help them cope more effectively with the many common self-care crises.

CASE STUDY

RT is a 57-year-old man who was diagnosed with type 2 diabetes 3 years ago. At the time of diagnosis RT was hypertensive, weighed approximately 30 lb (14 kg) above his ideal body weight, did not exercise regularly, and smoked about two packs of cigarettes a day. An oral antidiabetes agent was prescribed and RT was given a handout of a calorie-restricted diet, asked to monitor his fasting blood glucose level 3 times a week, offered a smoking cessation program, and advised to begin some form of regular exercise.

Since his diagnosis RT has canceled most of his appointments for medical follow-up of his diabetes, keeping only four appointments in 3 years. Last week he called to complain of increased fatigue, blurred vision, and frequent urination. At his appointment today his blood glucose is 220 mg/dL (12.2 mmol/L), his blood pressure is 160/95, his weight is 20 lb (4.5 kg) more than it was on diagnosis, and he acknowledges that he is not monitoring his blood glucose levels at home nor is he exercising or eating as he was told. He is still smoking two packs of cigarettes per day.

When questioned about his diabetes-related behavior, RT offers the following explanations: "Other than the little problems I had last week, I feel I'm doing fine. After all, I have the milder type of diabetes." "At my job I'm always on the go. There's no way I could eat the way you say I'm supposed to." "The cigarettes are my way of relaxing, and they haven't killed me yet." "My mother died from diabetes when she was 62 years old. I figure it's fate, and it will get me, too, sooner or later. There's nothing I can do about it." "The exercise, the diet, the blood sugar testing - the whole routine is just more than I can manage. I'm just not a structured sort of person."

"You tell me what to do, like the blood sugar testing, for instance, and I go home thinking I might be able to do it, but when I get home I realize I can't. I can't get the drop on the strip or whatever, so I get frustrated and give up." "Even when I feel like I'm really going to just do it, like start exercising, right away I flop, because it all gets so complicated, with the timing and making sure I don't go low, and all that. It's just too much to think about." "I get so mad. It's just unfair. I ask "Why me?" When the answer is 'There is no reason', I just say to forget it all. I know that's crazy, but that's just the way my mind works."

QUESTIONS FOR DISCUSSION
1 What factors seem to be creating RT's resistance to self-care?
2 What other factors might you want to assess before beginning to work with RT?
3 What empowerment-based strategies can you use with RT?
4 How would you decide which aspect of self-care to address first?

DISCUSSION
1 RT offers a classic, if all too common, example of resistance to change. His attitudes and his lack of skills interact to create a vicious cycle that leaves him stuck.

2 His motivation to change is limited by the fact that he sees his disease as relatively mild and the consequences of better self-care (coordinating diet and work, giving up cigarettes) as too costly. He also believes that diabetes-related health outcomes are controlled by chance or fate, so there's no reason to try to affect these outcomes because 'what will be, will be.'

3 RT has no confidence that he can manage the self-care, and it's clear that his education to date leaves him without sufficient skill to truly take care of himself. His skills are limited in the realms of specific diabetes self-care skills, problem-solving skills, and coping skills.

4 An effective approach for solving these problems begins by creating a coalition between the diabetes educator and RT. The educator can help RT identify some of his diabetes-related emotions and then acknowledge these feelings (if he is ready to do so). Work may then proceed at both attitudinal and behavioral levels.

5 Using an empowerment approach, the educator can ask RT questions about his fatalistic attitude toward diabetes-related health outcomes, and what gets in the way when he tries to care for his diabetes.

6 Asking questions rather than making statements is crucial to this approach.

7 Feelings of inadequacy must be recognized and acknowledged. The practical difficulty of living with diabetes also need to be acknowledged to keep the issue in perspective and create a therapeutic relationship with RT.

8 To address the behavior directly, the educator might ask RT what aspect of self-care he feels he is handling best right now. This question will usually lead to the acknowledgment that everything isn't totally hopeless. It may then be possible for RT to identify sources of strength that facilitate his handling of this issue.

9 RT should be asked if he is ready to identify an issue on which he'd like to work. It's important for the choice to be his, and he should be encouraged to be both ambitious and realistic in making his choice and setting his goals. Reaching a goal that is insufficiently ambitious provides little satisfaction, while an overly ambitious goal is generally unsuccessful and discouraging.

10 RT, like so many patients, needs intensive, behavior-based skills training. He could benefit from watching the educator demonstrate important skills, practicing the skills while being observed, using the skills at home and then demonstrating the skills later to the educator. RT also needs some basic diabetes education including nutritional counseling, so referring him to a diabetes education program may be helpful.

11 RT also needs follow-up. He seems willing to try things, but then seems to run into problems and gives up. An intervention as simple as a follow-up phone call one week after a face-to-face meeting might be helpful.

References

1 Kurtz SMS. Adherence to diabetes regimens: empirical status and clinical applications. Diabetes Educ 1990;16:50-59.

2 Ary DV, Toobert D, Wilson W, Glasgow RE. Patient perspective on factors contributing to nonadherence to diabetes regimen. Diabetes Care 1986;9:168-72.

3 The Diabetes Control and Complications Trial Research Group. The effect of intensive treatment of diabetes on the development and progression of long-term complications in insulin-dependent diabetes mellitus. N Engl J Med 1993; 329:977-86.

4 Lorenz RA, Bubb J, Davis D, et al. Changing behavior: practical lessons from the Diabetes Control and Complications Trial. Diabetes Care 1996;19:648-52.

5 Clement S. Diabetes self-management education: a technical review. Diabetes Care 1995;18:1204-14.

6 Peyrot M, Rubin RR. Modeling the effect of diabetes education on glycemic control. Diabetes Educ 1994;20:143-48.

7 Robiner W, Keel PK. Self-care behaviors and adherence in diabetes mellitus. Semin Clin Neuropsychiatry 1997;2:40-56.

8 Ruggiero L, Glasgow RE, Dryfoos JM, et al. Diabetes self-management: self-reported recommendations and patterns in a large population. Diabetes Care 1997;30:568-76.

9 Rubin RR, Walen SR, Ellis A. Living with diabetes. J Rational-Emotive Cognitive/ Behavioral Ther 1990;8:21-39.

10 Rubin RR, Biermann J, Toohey B. Psyching out diabetes: a positive approach to your negative emotions. Los Angeles: Lowell House, 1992.

11 Arnold MS, Butler PM, Anderson RM, Funnell MM, Feste C. Guidelines for facilitating a patient empowerment program. Diabetes Educ 1995;21:308-12.

12 Hampson SE, Glasgow RE, Foster, LE. Personal model of diabetes among older adults: relationship to self-management and other variables. Diabetes Educ 1995;21:300-07.

13 Padgett D, Mumford E, Hynes M, Carter R. Meta-analysis of the effects of educational and psychosocial interventions on management of diabetes mellitus. J Clin Epidemiol 1988;41:1007-30.

14 Brown SA. Effects of educational interventions in diabetes care: a meta-analysis of findings. Nurs Res 1988;37:223-230.

15 Brown SA. Studies of educational interventions and outcomes in diabetic adults: a meta-analysis revisited. Patient Educ Couns 1990;16:189-215.

16 Rubin RR, Peyrot M, Saudek CD. Differential effect of diabetes education on self-regulation and lifestyle behaviors. Diabetes Care 1991;14:335-38.

17 Sims D, Sims E. From research to practice: motivation, adherence, and the therapeutic alliance. Diabetes Spectrum 1989;2:49-51.

18 Toobert DJ, Glasgow RE. Problem-solving and diabetes self-care. J Behav Med 1991;14:71-86.

19 Marlatt GA. Situational determinants of relapse and skill-training interventions. In: Marlatt GA, Gordon JR, eds. Relapse prevention. New York: Guilford Press, 1985.

20 Greenfield S, Kaplan SH, Ware JE Jr, et al. Patients' participation in medical care: effects on blood sugar control and quality of life in diabetes. J Gen Intern Med 1988;3:448-57.

21 Anderson RM, Funnell MM, Barr PA, et al. Learning to empower patients: results of professional education program for diabetes educators. Diabetes Care 1991;14:584-90.

22 Curry SJ. Commentary on Prochaska JO, DiClemente CC, Norcross JC. In search of how people change: application to addictive behaviors. Diabetes Spectrum 1993;6:34-35.

23 Anderson B, Rubin RR, eds. Practical psychology for diabetes clinicians: how to deal with the key behavioral issues faced by patients and healthcare teams. Alexandria, Va: American Diabetes Association, 1996.

PSYCHOSOCIAL ISSUES

Psychological Disorders

6

Richard R. Rubin, PhD, CDE
The Johns Hopkins University School of Medicine
Departments of Medicine and Pediatrics
Baltimore, Maryland

INTRODUCTION

1   The relationship between diabetes and psychological disorders has received growing attention over the past 15 years.

2   Patients with diabetes may suffer disproportionately from psychological problems and certain psychiatric disorders, and the course and consequences of some of these disorders may be more severe in patients with diabetes.

3   Psychological disorders are distinct diagnoses that can be distinguished from the subclinical emotional strain associated with the predictable crises of diabetes (eg, diagnosis, onset of complications) and the daily stresses of living with diabetes.

4   The distinction between clinical psychological disorders and subclinical emotional strain is generally one of severity. Most people with diabetes experience symptoms of depression, anxiety disorder, and eating disorder, at least occasionally. Some of these people suffer from a sufficiently large number of these symptoms for a long enough period of time to warrant a diagnosis of clinical depression, anxiety disorder, or eating disorder.

5   The goal of the psychosocial assessment described in Chapter 4 is to identify patients who may suffer from either clinical or subclinical emotional problems, since both clinical and subclinical difficulties affect diabetes self-management, physiologic outcomes, and quality of life.

6   Effective approaches for working with patients who have subclinical problems include goal-setting, behavioral contracting and self-monitoring. These and other techniques are described in Chapter 5. When these approaches are successful, they reduce the likelihood that subclinical emotional strain will worsen and become a full-blown clinical disorder.

7   This chapter focuses on the treatment of clinical psychological disorders. Although the diagnosis and treatment of these disorders is outside the scope of practice of all but a few educators, screening patients for possible psychological disorders and referral to a mental specialist for formal diagnosis and treatment is critically important. This chapter is designed to acquaint the educator with effective treatments for these disorders.

Additionally, educators may find information on the side-effects of some commonly prescribed psychotropic medications useful in their work with patients.

Objectives

Upon completion of this chapter, the learner will be able to

1 Explain the relationship between diabetes and common psychological disorders

2 Identify current psychotherapeutic treatments for the psychological disorders that are common among people with diabetes

3 List current pharmacologic treatments for the psychological disorders that are common among people with diabetes

4 Describe indications for referring a patient to a mental health specialist for consultation or treatment.

Depression

1 Signs and symptoms of depression are described in Chapter 4, Psychosocial Assessment.

2 Depression appears to be more common among people with diabetes than in the general population.

    A Although estimates of the prevalence of depression vary, at least one of every five people with diabetes is likely to be affected by depression.[1] Some studies suggest that approximately 40% of people with diabetes have significantly elevated levels of depressive symptomatology;[2] not all are diagnosably clinically depressed.

    B Levels of diagnosable depression among people with diabetes are about three times the estimated prevalence in the population at large.[3]

3 Depression may be more severe in people with diabetes.

    A Depression is a recurring condition for many people who have diabetes. Only about 20% of people with diabetes who recover from an episode of depression remain asymptomatic more than 5 years.[4]

    B Individual depressive episodes may be more severe as well as more common among people with diabetes.

    C The symptoms of depression and diabetes may exacerbate one another at a neuroendocrine level. For example, hormonal disregulation associated with depression may contribute to glycemic disregulation (and vice versa).[5]

4 Depression has especially adverse effects for people with diabetes.

    A Clinical depression can severely hamper the management of diabetes. Feelings of helplessness and hopelessness that often are associated with depression can contribute to a disastrous cycle of poor self-care, worsened glycemia, and deepened depression.[6]

    B Clinical depression has been associated with poor glycemic control and an increased risk of micro- and macrovascular complications in part because of its effect on self-care and other health behaviors.[7]

    C Even subclinical depression (ie, persistent depressive symptoms that fall short of the criteria for diagnosing clinical depression) appears to be associated with diminished functioning and increased medical morbidity.[8]

5 Depression remains unrecognized and untreated in a majority of cases despite its specific relevance to diabetes.[3]

    A Reasons for underdiagnosis of depression in people with diabetes include the perception that depression in the medically ill is secondary to the medical condition and thus not of independent importance, labeling depressed patients as "noncompliant," and, concerns about the accuracy of the diagnosis of depression in this patient population.

    B Some of the symptoms of depression such as fatigue or changes in libido, appetite, and weight are also symptoms of hyperglycemia.[7]

    C Current diagnostic approaches are relatively sensitive for detecting depression in a person with diabetes. The use of tools described in Chapter 4, Psychosocial Assessment, can help the educator screen patients who may be depressed.

6 Depression in diabetes is responsive to psychotherapy.

    A Diabetes educators may refer depressed patients for psychotherapy, a treatment that is as effective as medication but without the risk of physical side effects.

    B Interpersonal therapy[9] and cognitive-behavioral therapy[10] are both proven treatments for depression in people who have no other medical conditions; the use of these psychotherapeutic approaches for people with diabetes has not been studied extensively.

C According to the model from which interpersonal therapy (IPT) is derived, stressful and conflicted relationships cause, maintain, and exacerbate depression. IPT helps patients develop and refine specific skills in communication and social interaction that help to relieve depression.

D Cognitive-behavioral therapy (CBT) is based on the observation that depressed people tend to think in negative, stereotypical ways ("Nobody likes me, I'm a failure").

- CBT involves a structured program of cognitive modification or reframing, and behavioral activation.
- Negative, self-defeating thoughts and actions are identified and efforts are made to replace them with more accurate and constructive thoughts and behaviors.
- Preliminary findings from a controlled study suggest that CBT is effective in the treatment of depression in diabetes.[11]

E Both IPT and CBT help patients build skills for coping with stressful life circumstances, which may provide more lasting relief from depression than antidepressant medications. This benefit is significant given the recurrent nature of depression in diabetes and the need for ongoing coping skills.[3]

7 Depression in diabetes is probably responsive to treatment with psycho-pharmacological agents based on studies of people who do not have diabetes. Unfortunately, very little information is available on the use of these drugs in people with diabetes.

A The effectiveness of antidepressant medications may be influenced by a different etiology and more severe course of depression in people with diabetes than those without diabetes.

B Lustman and colleagues[12] recently demonstrated that depression in diabetes could be treated successfully with antidepressant medication.

- In the first placebo-controlled trial with diabetes patients, 60% of those treated for 8 weeks with nortriptyline (a member of the tricyclic class of antidepressants) had a complete remission of their depression, while only 35% of those treated with a placebo were free of depression at the end of the study.
- Another important finding from this study was that a complete remission of depression among study participants was associated with a 0.8% to 1.2% reduction in glycohemoglobin (GHb) levels over the 8-week study period.

- Sustained reductions in GHb of this magnitude could provide the additional benefit of slowing the progression of microvascular complications such as retinopathy by as much as one third.

8 Newer classes of antidepressants are being studied that do not have some of the anticholinergic, central nervous system, cardiovascular, and weight-gain side-effects typical of the tricyclics. Many of the side effects are especially problematic for people who have diabetes.

  A Tricyclic antidepressants (amitriptyline [Elavil], desipramine [Norpramin], imipramine [Tofranil], and nortriptyline [Pamelor]) have some bothersome side effects, including dry mouth, sedation, increased appetite, and weight gain. Among the tricyclics, nortriptyline has the most benign side-effect profile.

  B A newer class of antidepressants called selective serotonin reuptake inhibitors (SSRIs) seem to be less sedating and do not lead to weight gain in most people. In fact, there is some evidence that SSRIs may actually decrease appetite in some people. Drugs in this class include fluoxetine (Prozac), paroxetine (Paxil), and sertraline (Zoloft). Unfortunately, SSRIs are more likely to cause agitation; sexual problems such as anorgasmia, decreased libido, and delayed ejaculation; and gastrointestinal distress than tricyclic antidepressants.

  C Venlafaxine (Effexor) and nefazodone done (Serzone) are members of a new class of antidepressants which came out after the SSRIs. The medications may be appropriate for some patients who do not respond to SSRIs or who have difficulty tolerating some side effects of the SSRIs such as agitation.

9 Choosing and using an antidepressant medication requires experience with these medications and close monitoring of the individual patient.

  A All the medications described have similar antidepressant effects when used in their therapeutic dosage range.

  - Depression is relieved in 50% to 60% of patients who complete 8 to 16 weeks of treatment.
  - Another 30% of those who do not respond to the initial medication will improve when they change to a second antidepressant.

  B Some improvement in mood is often seen within the first 2 to 3 weeks of treatment. Medication dosage changes are not made for 4 to 6 weeks because many patients respond to these agents slowly and incrementally.

C Unfortunately, many patients experience the side effects of antidepressant agents before they experience any beneficial effects. Side effects tend to diminish over time.

D Potential drug interactions must also be considered when choosing antidepressant medications.

E The effectiveness of all psychotropic (eg, antidepressant, antianxiety) medications is an individual matter. Different medications, even those closely related chemically, affect people differently.

F Selection of an antidepressant agent for a given patient is based on such factors as presenting symptoms, coexisting medical conditions, drug interactions, side effects, and cost. SSRIs are generally much more expensive than tricyclic antidepressants.

G Maintenance treatment with antidepressants, which is an increasingly common practice among psychiatrists caring for the depressed population at large, may also improve the prognosis for patients with diabetes. The only indications for stopping an antidepressant medication within the first 6 months of treatment are the absence of a therapeutic effect or severe side-effects.

10 To maximize the likelihood of selecting an effective depression treatment for a given patient, the patient's specific problems including initial presentation of symptoms and other medical conditions need to be matched to the known benefits of the treatments under consideration. The potential benefits of effective depression management for people with diabetes are shown in Table 6.1.

11 Many patients report flu-like symptoms including headache and fever when they discontinue treatment with any of the SSRIs or venlafaxine or nefazodone. Tapering medications especially those with the shortest half-life, such as paroxetine and venlafaxine, may help to reduce these symptoms.

ANXIETY DISORDER

1 Signs and symptoms of anxiety disorder are described in Chapter 4, Psychosocial Assessment.

Table 6.1. Potential Benefits of Effective Depression Management in Diabetes

1 Improved mood
2 Improved diabetes self-care
3 Improved functioning in work, social, and family realms
4 Improved glycemic control
5 Restoration of normal sleep and eating patterns
6 Decreased somatic preoccupation
7 Pain relief and increased pain tolerance
8 Enhanced sexual functioning

2 Anxiety disorder appears to be more prevalent among people with diabetes than in the general population.

  A Little is known about the rate of anxiety disorder among people with diabetes. However, the results from one study[2] suggest that people who have diabetes may suffer from anxiety disorder as frequently as from depression and at much higher rates than people who do not have diabetes.

  B Prevalence studies[13,14] using structured diagnostic interviews have reported an increased incidence of anxiety disorder, especially Generalized Anxiety Disorder and Simple Phobia, in people with diabetes.

3 Anxiety disorder may be more prevalent among people with diabetes because of the additional stresses of living with and managing diabetes.

  A Anxiety disorder is an exaggerated emotional response to the normal fears most people have.

  • People with diabetes often live with sources and levels of fear greater than those most people experience.

  • Fear of hypoglycemia, complications, and the effects of diabetes on day-to-day life are some of the more common fears reported by people who have diabetes.

  B In one study,[2] the only diabetes-related factor found to be associated with increased risk for symptoms of anxiety disorder was the presence of two or more complications. Type of diabetes, duration of diabetes, and glycohemoglobin level were not associated with an increased risk for anxiety symptomatology.

4 Little is known about the effects of anxiety on metabolic control in people with diabetes.

    A Severe anxiety affects quality of life and may affect metabolic control indirectly by interfering with diabetes self-care. However, no research has been conducted to test this hypothesis.

    B The direct effects of anxiety (often perceived as stress) on glycemia in people with diabetes has been the subject of numerous studies.[15]

- The results of research have been contradictory, with some studies reporting hypoglycemic responses and others reporting hyperglycemic responses to stress.[16]
- Significant evidence of the influence of stress on metabolic control in patients with type 2 diabetes, but not in those with type 1 diabetes was noted by Surwit et al.[16]
- Alterations in sympathetic nervous system activity unique to type 2 diabetes may explain this difference.

5 Anxiety disorder, like depression remains largely undiagnosed and untreated in patients with diabetes.

6 Anxiety disorder and subclinical anxiety in some people with diabetes may be responsive to psychotherapy and related treatments such as relaxation training and stress management.

    A Improved glucose tolerance and reduced long-term hyperglycemia were reported in studies[17] of people with type 2 diabetes after biofeedback-assisted relaxation training (BART).

    B The effectiveness of BART for those with type 1 diabetes is less clear-cut, although some studies[18] have reported positive findings.

    C The potential benefits of effective stress management for people with diabetes include: improved glycemic control, both directly, and indirectly as a result of improved self-care, improved emotional well-being, and improved quality of life.

7 Anxiety disorder in people with diabetes is probably responsive to treatment with psychopharmacological agents based on studies of people who do not have diabetes. Unfortunately, very little information is available on the use of these drugs in people with diabetes.

    A Lustman[19] reported improved glycemic control in patients treated with alprazolam (Xanax), a benzodiazepine regardless of whether they had a formal diagnosis of anxiety disorder.

B Treatment with fludiazepam (Erispan), a benzodiazepine, resulted in decreased anxiety ratings as well as an increase in high-density lipoproteins in a small group of patients with type 2 diabetes.[20]

8 Commonly prescribed anxiolytics (antianxiety agents) include benzodiazepines such as alprazolam (Xanax), fludiazepam (Erispan), lorazepam (Ativan), oxazepam (Serax), and clorazepate (Tranxene). Buspirone (BuSpar) which is not a benzodiazepine, is also sometimes prescribed for the treatment of anxiety.

9 There is little research to indicate which anxiolytic agent is best for people with diabetes.

A The possibility of oversedation, its effects on self-care, and potential for addiction need to be considered when prescribing any benzodiazepine. Buspirone is associated with minimal sedative and cognitive effects. Its potential for addiction is unknown.[21]

B Medications with short half-lives such as alprazolam and lorazepam may be the best choices for patients who have renal impairment.

10 The potential benefits of effective anxiety management for people with diabetes are similar to the benefits noted the effective management of depression.

EATING DISORDERS

1 Signs and symptoms of eating disorders and tools for identifying patients who may be suffering from eating disorders are described in Chapter 4, Psychosocial Assessment.

2 Eating disorders appear to be more common in people who have diabetes than in the general population.

A The problem of eating disorders in people with diabetes has received increased attention in the past few years.

B There are two types of eating disorders: anorexia nervosa and bulimia nervosa. Anorexia nervosa involves a severe, self-imposed restriction of caloric intake often combined with extremely high levels of exercise. Bulimia nervosa involves binge eating followed by a purging usually by means of vomiting or the use of diuretic medications or laxatives.

C It is difficult to estimate the actual prevalence of eating disorders in people with diabetes due to the problem of distinguishing between a normal (and even positive) focus on food and the body which is necessary for diabetes management and the abnormal concerns and behavior associated with an eating disorder. Some researchers[22] have suggested viewing this problem as an eating continuum with normal at one end, clinical eating disorders at the other end, and subclinical aspects at points in-between.

D Research in the field offers widely varying estimates of the prevalence of eating disorders in people with diabetes. Some studies[23,24] suggest that adolescents and young women with diabetes have an increased risk for eating disorders, especially bulimia nervosa; other studies[25] have not noted the same susceptibilities.

E A meta-analysis of existing data suggests a prevalence of eating disorders in those with diabetes of 1 to 1.5 times that found in the general population given the same gender and similar age and educational level.[26]

F Women who have type 1 diabetes are about ten times more likely to have an eating disorder than men with the same diagnosis.

3 There are indications that eating disorders in patients with type 1 diabetes are in some ways similar to and in other ways different from these same disorders in those without diabetes.

A Hillard and Hillard[27] note many similarities in the eating disordered behaviors and etiology of people with type 1 diabetes and people who do not have diabetes. These similarities include the type and symptoms of their eating disorder, underlying personality structure, family history of an eating disorder, and other psychiatric diseases.

B A unique and particularly troubling feature of eating disordered behavior common to many young people with diabetes is insulin purging.[27] Recent research[28] suggests that between one third and one half of all young women with type 1 diabetes frequently take less insulin than they need for glycemic control as a means of controlling their weight.[29]

4 Eating disorders have especially devastating consequences for people with diabetes.

A Eating disordered behavior, including manipulation of insulin dosage to control weight, can severely compromise diabetes self-care, glycemic control, and medical management.

B A relationship has been reported between eating problems (especially bulimia) and poor adherence to the nondiet aspects of the diabetes regimen,[30,31] poor glycemic control,[23,29] and complications.[24,32]

C Even subclinical eating disorders can interfere with glycemic control.[33]

D Insulin manipulation per se is associated with an increased risk for poor metabolic control[34] and microvascular complications.[28,32,35,36]

5 Eating disorders in people with diabetes are often unrecognized and untreated.

A Differentiating between normal concerns with food and body image and pathological concerns can be difficult in people with diabetes.

B Those suffering from eating disorders are often resistant to acknowledging the problem. Controlling eating feels crucially important for many of these patients. They are terrified at the prospect of giving up this control, which they feel they will be pressured to do if they acknowledge their eating disorder.

C It is important for educators to be alert to signs (see Table 6.2) that a patient may be suffering from an eating disorder, especially when the patient is a young woman.

TABLE 6.2. SIGNS OF AN EATING DISORDER IN PATIENTS WITH DIABETES

1 Frequent diabetic ketoacidosis (DKA)
2 Excessive exercise
3 Use of diet pills or laxatives to control weight
4 Anxiety about or avoidance of being weighed
5 Frequent and severe hypoglycemia
6 Binging with alcohol
7 Severe stress in the family

---

6 Most patients with diabetes do not eat in a manner that maximizes their chances for normoglycemia. It can sometimes be difficult to draw clear lines between normal struggles to establish and maintain patterns of healthy eating, subclinical eating disorders such as binge eating and "food addiction," and clinical eating disorders such as anorexia and bulimia.

7   The techniques for facilitating behavior change described in Chapter 5 are appropriate for working with patients who appear to have normal problems controlling their eating. These techniques may also be helpful for some people who have subclinical eating disorders.

8   Diabetes educators need to be familiar with strategies for primary prevention of eating disorders in your female patients who have diabetes (See Table 6.3). These strategies may be effective in preventing clinical eating disorders, and may also be helpful in identifying patients who require the services of a mental health specialist experienced in treating eating disorders.

TABLE 6.3. STRATEGIES FOR PREVENTION OF EATING DISORDERS IN YOUNG WOMEN WITH DIABETES[22]

1   Addressing the drive for thinness and associated body dissatisfaction
2   De-emphasizing dieting
3   Counseling patients about the need to express negative feelings about diabetes management
4   Helping the patient who is experiencing conflict over normal developmental struggles
5   Addressing metabolic reactivity during adolescence
6   Involving the family

---

9   Ongoing consultation with a mental health professional familiar with eating disorders may help prevent subclinical eating disorders from becoming full-blown clinical disorders. Such a consultation relationship should be established whenever possible. When the mental health specialist is a part of the diabetes team, patients are more likely to accept referral for treatment of emotional problems before they become more severe.

10 Eating disorders may be responsive to psychotherapy and pharmacotherapy.

   A Recent literature[37] suggests that psychoeducation directed toward specific, culturally-based cognitive distortions may be effective for individuals with mild to moderate eating disorders in the early stages.

     • Psychoeducational therapy is a highly structured treatment program in which a therapeutic setting and didactic instruction are used to help patients understand the nature, etiology, and complications of disordered eating behaviors.

- The purpose of this intervention is to foster attitudinal and behavioral change in the patient.[38]

B Because many patients suffering from eating disorders are also depressed, treatment with any of the antidepressants discussed earlier in this chapter may be considered. Some antidepressants in the SSRI class may positively affect compulsive behavior, including eating disordered behavior, as well as depression. Fluoxetine (Prozac) has been used successfully for this purpose; other agents in the same class may provide similar benefits.

PSYCHOPATHOLOGY THAT PRESENTS AS A MEDICAL CRISIS

1 In many cases a medical crisis may be the first sign that a patient is suffering from a psychiatric disorder. Examples of such medical crises are recurrent diabetic ketoacidosis; frequent, severe hypoglycemic and hyperglycemic episodes (sometimes called brittle diabetes); and severe disruption of self-care activities, especially insulin administration.

2 These destructive behaviors frequently coincide with severe psychological disturbance, including individual psychopathology,[39] family dysfunction,[40] or both.[41]

3 These psychological disturbances have been effectively treated by intensive individual therapy[42] and family therapy, often conducted at least partly in residential or inpatient settings.[43]

PSYCHOLOGICAL DISORDERS AS SEQUELAE OF LONG-TERM DIABETES COMPLICATIONS

1 Developing any of the chronic complications of diabetes could be considered an emotional crisis. However, there is little research to clarify the degree to which any of these complications contribute to psychological distress.

2 Only two diabetes-related complications have been studied in terms of their association with psychological distress: sexual dysfunction and visual impairment.

A The sexual dysfunction most often associated with diabetes is erectile impotence.

 - Impotence in a man with diabetes is almost invariably the result of psychological and organic factors.[44]
 - Sexual dysfunction is generally developed and maintained by a reciprocal process in which organic problems lead to psychological distress, and the distress in turn heightens the organic problems.

B The study of sexual problems in women with diabetes is a recent undertaking.

 - In one of the few substantial investigations in this area, Schreiner-Engel et al[45] found that women with type 2 diabetes reported significantly more sexual problems and less sexual satisfaction than nondiabetic control subjects. The authors speculate that late-onset diabetes may distort a woman's sexual body image, signalling the end of her sexual attractiveness and intensifying concerns about earlier aging.
 - Women with type 1 diabetes in the same study did not differ from controls in terms of sexual problems and satisfaction.

C Only a few reports describe psychological interventions for men with diabetes who have sexual problems, and none are available for women.

D There is some evidence that psychological distress increases dramatically during the first 2 years after diagnosis with proliferative diabetic retinopathy,[46] regardless of the severity of the visual impairment.

 - Bernbaum et al[47] reported that those with fluctuating visual impairment actually reported lower levels of psychological well-being than people with more severe yet stable impairment.
 - In another study,[48] visually impaired people with diabetes participated in a 36-session self-care training program conducted over a 12-week period. The program staff included a psychologist, and psychosocial support groups and individual counseling were available to participants. At the end of the program participants were in better glycemic control and less depressed.

3 Many people may suffer psychological distress following the onset of a diabetes-related complication and the cumulative impact of several complications may be especially severe. One study[2] revealed that both depression and anxiety symptomatology were dramatically elevated in those with more than two diabetes-related complications.

KEY EDUCATIONAL CONSIDERATIONS

1 Understanding the relationship between psychological disorders and diabetes is critical for the diabetes educator, because of the profound impact of these disorders on the education and treatment process and on a person's capacity to live well with diabetes.

2 To effectively address psychological disorders, apply the following key considerations:

A People with diabetes may suffer disproportionately from certain psychological disorders, and the course and consequences of these disorders may also be more severe.

B It is important for educators to know the signs and symptoms of depression, anxiety disorders, and eating disorders, and be able to recognize markers for these disorders in their patients. If the educator feels the patient may be suffering from a psychological disorder, referral to a mental health specialist for a definitive diagnosis and treatment is appropriate.

C It is also important for educators to recognize subclinical disorders including mild symptoms of depression or anxiety or behaviors such as uncontrolled or binge eating because they may also have adverse effects on self-care, metabolic control, and quality of life for people with diabetes.

D Subclinical disorders can often be effectively dealt with by educators, using some of the techniques described in Chapter 5, Behavior Change.

E Mental health professionals are invaluable resources for consultation concerning patients with subclinical disorders and for comprehensive assessment and treatment of patients who may be suffering from clinical disorders.

F Effective psychotherapeutic, psychoeducational, and pharmacological approaches have been identified for depression, anxiety disorders, and eating disorders. Educators need to be familiar with these approaches and have resources available for the provision of these treatments.

SELF-REVIEW QUESTIONS

1 What is the difference between clinical and subclinical disorder?

2 What are some effective approaches for helping people with subclinical psychological disorders?

3 Approximately what percentage of people with diabetes suffer from clinical depression?

4 Why is the course of depression more severe for a person with diabetes?

5 Why are the effects of depression especially devastating for a person with diabetes?

6 What forms of psychotherapy are good choices for treating depression in a person with diabetes?

7 What are some advantages of SSRI antidepressants as compared with tricyclic antidepressants for people with diabetes?

8 What are the benefits of biofeedback-assisted relaxation training?

9 Why are eating disorders in people with diabetes often unrecognized and untreated?

10 What approaches may be effective for primary prevention of eating disorders in a person with diabetes?

11 What medical crises may indicate an underlying psychological disorder?

12 What is the role of the mental health specialist in caring for patients with diabetes?

Case Study 1

SF is a 64-year-old man whose type 2 diabetes was diagnosed 12 years ago. He had signs of background retinopathy at that time. SF did well taking oral medication for his diabetes and handling self-care tasks for the first 9 years after diagnosis. His glycemic control during that period was good, and his retinopathy was stable. Three years ago SF's wife died suddenly of a heart attack, and within the last 18 months SF began to experience painful symptoms of neuropathy. In the past year microalbumin has begun to appear in his urine and he has shown signs of proliferative retinopathy. SF's glycemic control has steadily worsened, as well, to the point that an appointment was scheduled with him to discuss the possibility of initiating insulin therapy.

During this appointment SF appears very sad and questions directed to him reveal that he has been sleeping poorly and that he feels fatigued "all the time." SF says that he has lost touch with most of his former friends because he "doesn't get the pleasure from their company that he used to," and adds that he "is no fun to be around." When asked specifically about the prospect of taking insulin, SF says that while he hates the idea of shots, he feels he's "getting what he deserves," for failing to effectively control his diabetes. He adds, "I'm not much good to anyone these days, including myself."

QUESTIONS FOR DISCUSSION

1 What psychological disorder is likely affecting SF?

2 Why is it hard to be sure SF is suffering from this disorder?

3 What further information would be helpful in assessing SF's condition?

4 What treatments might be appropriate for SF?

5 What do you think about SF beginning to take insulin at this time?

DISCUSSION

1 SF appears to be depressed. He is sad and complains of sleep disturbance and fatigue. In addition, he says he has lost interest in activities he used to enjoy, and he is feeling worthless and guilty.

   A He seems to meet the diagnostic criteria for clinical depression. He has also experienced the loss of his wife and the onset of several diabetes-related complications.

   B Research shows that developing multiple complications dramatically increases a person's risk for depression.

2 While the diagnosis of depression seems reasonable in this case, SF's chronic hyperglycemia is another possible explanation for some of his symptoms.

3 To clarify what is actually going on, SF can be asked about any changes in appetite, problems in concentration, and thoughts of death or suicide.

4 If the diagnosis of depression is not clear-cut, a referral to a mental health professional for a comprehensive assessment and definitive diagnosis is appropriate.

   A Treatment options for depression include interpersonal or cognitive-behavioral psychotherapy or pharmacotherapy.

5 Initiating insulin therapy is probably not indicated for SF at this time, as major treatment changes are generally not advisable for a depressed patient because such patients often feel overwhelmed by the prospect of making changes.

CASE STUDY 2

QT is a young woman, 15 years old. Her type 1 diabetes was diagnosed when she was 6. Her family has always been actively involved in her diabetes management, and QT herself is knowledgeable and open. She maintained excellent glycemic control until about a year ago. Since then her glyco-hemoglobin levels have risen dramatically, and she has had to go to the emergency room twice for DKA.

During her last two appointments with the diabetes educator QT has been much less communicative, offering little explanation for her worsened glycemic control and associated medical crises. She says she "doesn't really know what's going on," adding, "I guess it's just harder now for me to do everything right with all my activities and such." When asked specifically about the fact that her weight has decreased by 18 lb (8.2 kg) over the past year, placing her weight at 85% of normal for her height, body frame and age, QT responds, "Don't tell me I need to gain that weight back! Last year I was too fat to make the cheerleading squad, and now I feel like I have a real chance."

QUESTIONS FOR DISCUSSION

1   What psychological disorder is likely affecting QT?
2   Why is it hard to be sure QT is suffering from this disorder?
3   What further information would be helpful in assessing QT's condition?
4   What treatments might be appropriate for QT?

DISCUSSION

1   QT appears to be suffering from an eating disorder. She is a young woman whose glycemic control has worsened dramatically, leading to episodes of DKA and significant weight loss.
    A   Her weight is now 85% of normal for her height, body frame, and age, and she is adamantly opposed to regaining the weight she has lost.
    B   QT seems to meet some of the criteria for a clinical eating disorder.

2   There are a couple of reasons why it is difficult to be sure whether QT has an eating disorder.
    A   First, she is 15 years old, so the insulin resistance of puberty might account for some of her worsened glycemic control.

B Second, she is not forthcoming about her situation, so essential information is not immediately available. Although most young women who have eating disorders actively resist acknowledging their problem, the educator needs to ask QT about her exercise, missed menstrual periods, and eating behavior, especially any episodes of binge eating.

3 Ask QT about any occasions when she did not give herself a scheduled insulin injection or reduced the dose of insulin she administered. Keep in mind that even subclinical eating disorders may have devastating consequences.

4 An ideal treatment for QT would be participating in a structured program of psychoeducation to resolve eating disordered behavior. Unfortunately, this option is not widely available.

A One possible alternative would be education and counseling that incorporates some elements of a structured psychoeducation program.

B Another alternative would be using pharmacotherapy to treat compulsive eating disordered behavior and any associated underlying depression.

5 It's important to recognize that patients with established eating disorders are not likely to change their disorder behavior on an outpatient basis. They generally require hospitalization in an eating disorders program. However, if dramatic deterioration in glycemic control is identified by the educator before a full-blown eating disorder has developed, outpatient treatment may be effective.

REFERENCES

1 Gavard JA, Lustman PJ, Clouse RE. Prevalence of depression in adults with diabetes: an epidemiological evaluation. Diabetes Care 1993;16:1167-78.

2 Peyrot M, Rubin RR. Levels and risks of depression and anxiety symptomatology among diabetic adults. Diabetes Care 1997;20:585-90.

3 Lustman PJ, Clouse RE, Alrakawi A, et al. Treatment of major depression in adults with diabetes: a primary care perspective. Clinical Diabetes 1997;15:122-26.

4 Lustman PJ, Griffith LS, Clouse RE. Recognizing and managing depression in patients with diabetes. In: Anderson BJ, Rubin RR, eds. Practical psychology for diabetes clinicians: how to deal with the key behavioral issues faced by patients and health-care teams. Alexandria, Va: American Diabetes Association, 1996:143-54.

5 Lustman PJ, Griffith LS, Clouse RE. Depression in adults with diabetes: results of a 5-year follow-up study. Diabetes Care 1988;11:605-12.

6 Rubin RR, Peyrot M. Psychosocial problems in diabetes treatment: impediments to intensive self-care. Practical Diabetol 1994;13(2):8-10,12-14

7 Lustman PJ, Griffith LS, Clouse RE. Depression in adults with diabetes. Semin in Clin Neuropsychology 1997;2:15-23.

8 Frasure-Smith N, Lesperance F, Talajic M. Depression and 18-month prognosis after myocardial infarction. Circulation 1995;91:999-1005.

9 Frank E, Kupfer DJ, Wagner EF, et al. Efficacy of interpersonal psychotherapy as a maintenance treatment of recurrent depression. Arch Gen Psychiatry 1991;48:1053-59.

10 Rush AJ, Beck AT, Kovacs M, et al. Comparative efficacy of cognitive therapy and pharmacotherapy in the treatment of depressed outpatients. Cogn Ther Res 1977;1:17-37.

11 Lustman PJ, Griffith LS, Clouse RE, Cryer PE. Efficacy of cognitive therapy for depression in NIDDM: results of a controlled clinical trial. Diabetes 1997;46(suppl 1):13A.

12 Depression Guideline Panel. Depression in primary care, vol 5: detection, diagnosis and treatment. Rockville, Md: Department of Health and Human Services, 1993;AHCPR, publication no. 93-0550 edn.

13 Lustman PJ, Griffith LS, Clouse RE, Cryer PE. Psychiatric illness in diabetes mellitus: relationship to symptoms and glucose control. J Nerv Ment Dis 1986;174: 736-42.

14 Popkin MK, Callies AL, Lentz RD, et al. Prevalence of major depression, simple phobia, and other psychiatric disorders in patients with long-standing type I diabetes meillitus. Arch Gen Psychiatry 1988;45:64-68.

15 Barglow P, Hatcher R, Edidin DV, Sloan-Rossiter D. Stress and metabolic control in diabetes: psychosomatic evidence and evaluation of methods. Psychosom Med 1984;46:127-44.

16 Surwit RS, Schneider MS, Feinglos MN. Stress and diabetes mellitus. Diabetes Care 1992;15:1413-22.

17 Surwit RS, Ross SL, McCaskill CC, et al. Does relaxation therapy add to conventional treatment of diabetes mellitus? Diabetes 1989;38(suppl 1):9A.

18 McGrady A, Bailey BK, Good MP. Controlled study of biofeedback-assisted relaxation in type I diabetes. Diabetes Care 1991;14:360-65.

19 Lustman PJ, Griffith LS, Clouse RE, et al. Effects of alprazolam on glucose regulation in diabetes. Results of double-blind, placebo-controlled trial. Diabetes Care 1995;18:1133-39.

20 Okada S, Ichiki K, Tanokuchi S, et al. Effects of an anxiolytic on lipid profile in non-insulin-dependent diabetes mellitus. J Int Med Res 1994;22:338-42.

21 Pecknold JC, Matas M, Howarth BG, et al. Evaluation of buspirone as an anti-anxiety agent: buspirone and diazepam versus placebo. Can J Psychiatry 1989;34:766-71.

22 Rapaport WS, LaGreca AM, Levine P. Preventing eating disorders in young women with type I diabetes. In: Anderson BJ, Rubin RR, eds. Practical psychology for diabetes clinicians: how to deal with the key behavioral issues faced by patients and health-care teams. Alexandria, Va: American Diabetes Association, 1996:133-42.

23 Stancin T, Link DL, Reuter JM. Binge eating and purging in young women with IDDM. Diabetes Care 1989;12:601-3.

24 Steel JM, Young RJ, Lloyd GG, Macintyre CC. Abnormal eating attitudes in young insulin-dependent diabetics. Br J Psychiatry 1989;155:515-21.

25 Fairburn CG, Peveler RC, Davies B, et al. Eating disorders in young adults with insulin-dependent diabetes mellitus: a controlled study. Br Med J 1991;303: 17-20.

26 Hall RCW. Bulimia nervosa and diabetes mellitus. Semin in Clin Neuropsychiatry 1997;2:24-30.

27 Hillard JR, Hillard PJ. Bulimia, anorexia, and diabetes: deadly combinations. Psychiat Clin North Am 1984;7:367-79.

28 Rydall AC, Rodin GM, Olmsted MP, et al. Disordered eating behavior and microvascular complications in young women with insulin-dependent diabetes mellitus. N Engl J Med 1997;336:1849-54.

29 Polonsky WH, Anderson BJ, Lohrer PA. Aponte JE, Jacobson AM, Cole CF. Insulin omission in women with IDDM. Diabetes Care 1994;17:1178-85.

30 LaGreca A, Schwartz L, Satin W, et al. Binge eating among women with IDDM: associations with weight dissatisfaction, adherence, and metabolic control. Diabetes 1990;39(suppl 1):164A.

31 Pollock M, Kovacs M, Charron-Prochownik D. Eating disorders and maladaptive dietary/insulin management among youths with childhood-onset insulin-dependent diabetes mellitus. J Am Acad Child Adolesc Psychiatry 1995;34: 291-96.

32 Rodin G, Rydall A, Olmsted M, et al. A four-year follow-up study of eating disorders and medical complications in young women with insulin dependent diabetes mellitus. Psychosomatic Med 1994; 56:179.

33 Wing RR, Norwalk MP, Marcus MD, et al. Subclinical eating disorders and glycemic control in adolescents with type I diabetes. Diabetes Care 1986;9: 162-67.

34 LaGreca AM, Schwartz LT, Satin W. Eating patterns in young women with IDDM: another look (Letter). Diabetes Care 1987;10:659-60.

35 Biggs MM, Basco MR, Patterson G, Raskin P. Insulin withholding for weight control in women with diabetes. Diabetes Care 1994;17:1186-89.

36 Olmsted MP, Davis R, Garner DM, et al. Efficacy of a brief group psychoeducational intervention for bulimia nervosa. Behav Res Ther 1991;29:71-83.

37 Davis R, Dearing S, Faulkner J, et al. The road to recovery: a manual for participants in the psychoeducation group for bulimia nervosa. In: Harper-Giuffre H, MacKenzie KR, eds. Washington, DC: American Psychiatric Press, 1992: 281-341.

38 Gill G, Robinson M, Marrow J. Hypoglycaemic brittle diabetes successfully managed by social worker intervention. Diabetic Med 1989;6:448-50.

39 Boehnert CE, Popkin MK. Psychological issues in treatment of severely noncompliant diabetics. Psychosomatics 1986; 27:11-20.

40 Coyne JC, Anderson BJ. The "psychosomatic family" reconsidered: II. Recalling a defective model and looking ahead. J Marital Fam Ther 1989;15:139-48.

41 Follansbee DJ, LaGreca AM, Citrin WS. Coping skills training for adolescents with diabetes. Diabetes 1983;32(suppl 1):37A.

42 Moran G, Fonagy P, Kurtz A, et al. A controlled study of psychoanalytic treatment of brittle diabetes. J Am Acad Child Adolesc Psychiatry 1991;30:926-35.

43 Schiavi PC, Hogan B. Sexual problems in diabetes mellitus: psychological aspects. Diabetes Care 1979;2:9-17.

44 Schreiner-Engel P, Schiavi RC, Vietorisz D, et al. The differential impact of diabetes type on female sexuality. J Psychosom Res 1987;31:23-33.

45 Wulsin LR, Jacobson AM, Rand LI. Psychosocial adjustment to advanced proliferative diabetic retinopathy. Diabetes Care 1993;16:1061-66.

46 Bernbaum M, Albert SG, Duckro PN. Psychosocial profiles in patients with visual impairment due to diabetic retinopathy. Diabetes Care 1988;11: 551-57.

47 Bernbaum M, Albert SG, Brusca SR, et al. A model clinical program for patients with diabetes and vision impairment. Diabetes Educ 1989;15:325-30.

SUGGESTED READINGS

Brackenridge BP, Rubin RR. Sweet kids: how to balance diabetes control and good nutrition with family peace. Alexandria, Va: American Diabetes Association, 1996.

Peyrot M, Rubin RR. Psychosocial aspects of diabetes care. In: Leslie D, Robbins D, eds. Diabetes: clinical science in practice. Cambridge Mass: Cambridge University Press, 1995:465-77.

Rubin RR. Working with diabetic adolescents. In: Anderson BJ, Rubin RR, eds. Practical psychology for diabetes clinicians: how to deal with the key behavioral issues faced by patients and health care teams. Alexandria, Va: American Diabetes Association, 1996:13-22.

Rubin RR, Peyrot M. Emotional responses to diagnosis. In: Anderson BJ, Rubin RR, eds. Practical psychology for diabetes clinicians: how to deal with the key behavioral issues faced by patients and health care teams. Alexandria, Va: American Diabetes Association, 1996:155-62.

Rubin RR. Psychotherapy in diabetes mellitus. Semin in Clin Neuropsychiatry 1997;2:72-81.

Rubin RR, Peyrot M. Psychosocial problems and interventions in diabetes: a review of the literature. Diabetes Care 1992;15:1640-57.

Rubin RR, Peyrot M. Psychosocial problems. In: Levin ME, Pfeifer MA, eds. Diabetes complications. Alexandria, Va: American Diabetes Association, 1998.

Saudek CD, Rubin RR, Shump C. The Johns Hopkins guide to diabetes: for today and tomorrow. Baltimore, Md: The Johns Hopkins University Press, 1997.

PATHOPHYSIOLOGY

DIABETES DISEASE STATE

Pathophysiology

7

Robert E. Ratner, MD, CDE
Medlantic Clinical Research Center
Washington, DC

INTRODUCTION

1   Diabetes mellitus is sometimes described by both patients and health professionals as "a little bit of sugar" or "high sugar." In reality, "sugar" is only one component of the pathology and clinical manifestations of the multifaceted syndrome of diabetes mellitus.

2   Diabetes mellitus may be broadly described as a chronic, systemic disease characterized by
   A   Abnormalities in the metabolism of carbohydrates, proteins, fats, and insulin.
   B   Abnormalities in the structure and function of blood vessels and nerves.

3   The pathophysiology leading to the development of the metabolic aspects of diabetes are described in this chapter. A clear understanding of these processes is helpful for diabetes educators in order to:
   A   Provide in-depth information to patients about diabetes, the symptoms and metabolic effects.
   B   Understand the actions of the nonpharmacologic and pharmacologic therapies for diabetes in order to provide both information and clinically appropriate care.
   C   Better understand the interactions between food, activity, medications, and blood glucose levels for decision-making and to prepare patients for self-management.
   D   Understand the pathogenisis of the complications of diabetes and teach patients about modifiable risk factors and symptom recognition for early treatment.

4   Although hyperglycemia plays a role in the complications of diabetes (abnormalities in the structure and function of blood vessels and nerves), other pathological processes and additional risk factors are major, and sometimes independent, etiologies (see Chapter 20, Chronic Complications of Diabetes, for more information).

5   The reader is encouraged to consider the pathophysiology of diabetes not as a discrete problem of carbohydrate-insulin abnormality, but as a dynamic interplay of etiologies.

OBJECTIVES

Upon completion of this chapter, the learner will be able to

1   Describe fuel metabolism and its hormonal control.

2   Identify the groups at risk for diabetes.

3   State the diagnostic criteria for diabetes mellitus.

4   Identify the differences among the various forms of diabetes mellitus.

5   Explain the stages of development of type 1 diabetes and the implications for early intervention and prevention.

6   Explain the mechanisms by which type 2 diabetes occurs, the risk factors for its development, and mechanisms for potential prevention.

KEY DEFINITIONS

1   *Adipocyte.* A fat cell that serves as the primary storage for excess calories.

2   *Genotype.* The specific description of a defined region of a chromosome.

3   *Glucagon.* A hormone produced by the alpha cells of the pancreatic Islets of Langerhans, and the counterregulatory hormone to insulin. Glucagon release results in an increase in the circulating glucose level by stimulating gluconeogenesis.

4   *Gluconeogenesis.* The process of glucose production in the liver from precursors such as lactate and amino acids.

5   *Glycogen.* A complex carbohydrate that serves as the primary storage form of glucose in the liver and muscle.

6   *Glycogenolysis.* The metabolic conversion of glycogen into glucose.

7   *Lactate.* An incomplete breakdown product in the anaerobic metabolism of glucose; can serve as a precursor for subsequent glucose synthesis in the process of gluconeogenesis.

8   *Substrate.* A material that may be acted upon by enzymes in a metabolic process (ie, lactate is a substrate for gluconeogenesis).

Normal Fuel Metabolism

1 Five phases of fuel homeostasis have been described by Chipkin et al.[1]

    A Phase I is the fed state (0 to 3.9 hours after meal consumption) in which blood glucose originates from an exogenous source.

- The brain and other organs use some of the glucose that has been absorbed from the gastrointestinal tract.
- The remaining glucose is added to hepatic, muscle, adipose, and other tissue reservoirs.
- Plasma insulin levels are high, glucagon levels are low, and triglyceride is synthesized in adipose tissue. Insulin inhibits breakdown of glycogen and triglyceride reservoirs.

    B Phase II is the postabsorptive state (4 to 15.9 hours after meal consumption) in which blood glucose originates from glycogen and hepatic gluconeogenesis.

- Plasma insulin levels decrease and glucagon levels increase.
- Energy storage ends in this phase and energy production begins.
- Carbohydrate and lipid stores are mobilized. Hepatic glycogen provides glucose to the brain and other tissues. Blood glucose levels are maintained.
- Adipocyte triglyceride begins to break down and free fatty acids (FFA) are released into the circulation and utilized by the liver and skeletal muscle as a primary energy source.
- The brain continues to use glucose, provided mainly by gluconeogenesis (35% to 60%) because of its inability to use FFA as fuel.

    C Phase III is the early starvation state (16 to 47.9 hours after meal consumption) in which blood glucose originates from hepatic gluconeogenesis and glycogenolysis.

- Gluconeogenesis continues to produce most of the hepatic glucose.
- In this phase of starvation, lactate makes up half of the gluconeogenetic substrate.
- Amino acids, specifically alanine, and glycerol are other major substrates.
- Insulin secretion is markedly suppressed and counterregulatory hormone (eg, glucagon, cortisol, growth hormone, and epinephrine) secretion is stimulated.

    D Phase IV is the preliminary prolonged starvation state (48 hours to 23.9 days after meal consumption) in which blood glucose originates from hepatic and renal gluconeogenesis.

- By 60 hours of starvation, gluconeogenesis provides more than 97% of hepatic glucose output. The need for gluconeogenesis is limited to conserve body protein by increased reliance of muscle and other tissues on FFA and ketone bodies, and a change from glucose to ketone bodies as fuel for the brain.
- Insulin secretion is markedly suppressed and counterregulatory hormone (eg, glucagon, cortisol, growth hormone, and epinephrine) secretion is stimulated.

E   Phase V is the secondary prolonged starvation state (24 to 40 days after meal consumption) in which blood glucose originates from hepatic and renal gluconeogenesis, the same source as in Phase IV. In Phase V, the rate of glucose being used by the brain diminishes as does the rate of hepatic gluconeogenesis.

Definition of Diabetes Mellitus

1   Diabetes mellitus consists of a group of metabolic diseases characterized by hyperglycemia resulting from defects in insulin secretion, insulin action, or both.

2   The pathogenic processes in the development of diabetes involve ß-cell dysfunction leading to impaired insulin synthesis and/or release, and peripheral insulin resistance. The ß-cell dysfunction may be due to immune-mediated insulitis, genetically determined ß-cell dysfunction, or acquired ß-cell dysfunction (including glucose toxicity).

3   Symptoms of hyperglycemia include polyuria, polydipsia, polyphagia, weight loss, blurred vision, fatigue, headache, occasional muscle cramps, and poor wound healing.

4   Signs and symptoms of chronic hyperglycemia include growth impairment, susceptibility to certain infections, and renal, retinal, peripheral vascular, and neuropathic syndromes.

5   Acute life-threatening consequences of diabetes include hyperglycemia with ketoacidosis (DKA), hyperglycemic hyperosmolar nonketotic syndrome (HHNS), and therapy-induced hypoglycemia.

Diagnostic Criteria for Diabetes Mellitus and Other Categories of Impaired Glucose Homeostasis

1 In 1997, the Expert Committee on the Diagnosis and Classification of Diabetes Mellitus[2] updated the classification and diagnostic criteria for diabetes. Diabetes mellitus is diagnosed using any one of the three following methods and must be confirmed on a subsequent day.

A Acute symptoms of diabetes plus casual plasma glucose concentration is ≥200 mg/dL (11.1 mmol/L).

- Casual implies any time of day without regard to time since last meal.

- The classic symptoms of diabetes include polyuria, polydipsia, polyphagia, and unexplained weight loss.

B Fasting plasma glucose is ≥126 mg/dL (7.0 mmol/L). Fasting is defined as no caloric intake for at least 8 hours.

C Two-hour plasma glucose is ≥200mg/dL during an oral glucose tolerance test (OGTT).

- The test should be performed as prescribed by the World Health Organization[3] (World Health Organization 1985) using a glucose load containing the equivalent of 75 gm anhydrous glucose dissolved in water.

2 Impaired Fasting Glucose (IFG) is diagnosed when fasting glucose levels are >110 mg/dL but less than 126 mg/dL. IFG represents a metabolic stage of impaired glucose homeostasis intermediate between normal and diabetes mellitus. IFG is not a category of diabetes mellitus.

3 Impaired Glucose Tolerance (IGT) is diagnosed when 2-hour OGTT values are ≥140 mg/dL (7.0 mmol/L) but less than 200 mg/dl (11.1 mmol/L). IGT represents a metabolic stage of impaired glucose homeostasis intermediate between normal and diabetes mellitus. IGT is not a category of diabetes mellitus.

4 The 1997 classifications focus on the etiology of this heterogeneous disease rather than the treatment. The terminology has been revised in the following ways:

A The terms insulin-dependent diabetes mellitus (IDDM) and non-insulin-dependent diabetes mellitus (NIDDM) are eliminated.

B Arabic numerals replace the Roman numerals; thus Type I diabetes becomes type 1 diabetes, and Type II diabetes becomes type 2 diabetes.

CLASSIFICATION OF DIABETES MELLITUS

1 The following characteristics define type 1 diabetes:

    A Develops at any age, but most cases are diagnosed before the age of 30 years.

    B Affected individuals experience significant weight loss, polyuria, and polydipsia characterized by the abrupt signs and symptoms associated with marked hyperglycemia and the strong propensity for the development of ketoacidosis.

    C Dependent on exogenous insulin to prevent ketoacidosis and sustain life.

    D Coma and death can result from a delayed diagnosis and/or treatment.

2 The following characteristics define type 2 diabetes:

    A Approximately 90% of patients in the United States with diabetes have type 2 diabetes, with disproportionate representation among the elderly and certain ethnic populations.

    B Usually diagnosed after the age of 30 years, but can occur at any age.

    C Frequently asymptomatic at the time of diagnosis, but as many as 20% may present with end-organ complications (eg, retinopathy, neuropathy, and nephropathy).

    D Endogenous insulin levels may be normal, increased, or decreased; the need for exogenous insulin is variable.

    E Insulin resistance is typically present with impaired glucose tolerance in the initial stages.

    F Not prone to ketosis.

    G Approximately 80% of patients are obese at the time of diagnosis.

3 Secondary diabetes is diagnosed when diabetes occurs as a result of other disorders or treatments. Treatment of these other disorders or discontinuation of diabetogenic agents may result in amelioration of the diabetes. However, frequently it is impossible to reverse the underlying disorder or stop the offending agent, in which case the therapy is similar to diabetes therapy in general using the modalities of medical nutrition therapy, exercise, and medications. The following disorders are classified as secondary diabetes:

A Known genetic defects associated with Maturity Onset Diabetes of the Young (MODY), glycogen synthase deficiency, and mitochondrial DNA markers.

B Pancreatic disorders such as hemochromatosis, chronic pancreatitis, and pancreatectomy.

C Hormonal disorders such as Cushing's syndrome (excess amounts of corticosteroids), thyrotoxicosis (excess thyroid hormone), and acromegaly (excess growth hormone).

D Other disorders such as cystic fibrosis, congenital rubella syndrome, and Down's syndrome.

E Concomitant diabetogenic drug therapy.

4 Gestational diabetes is a diagnosis of diabetes mellitus that applies only to women in whom glucose intolerance develops or is first discovered during pregnancy.

A After pregnancy, the diagnostic classification may be changed to previous abnormality of glucose tolerance, type 1 or type 2 diabetes or impaired glucose tolerance.

B Women whose diabetes predated the pregnancy should not be included in the gestational diabetes classification.

C The occurrence of gestational diabetes increases the future risk for progression to type 2 diabetes, or, rarely, type 1 diabetes.

NATURAL HISTORY AND PATHOPHYSIOLOGY OF TYPE 1 DIABETES

1 Type 1 diabetes results from an autoimmune attack on the ß-cell.[4]

A Type 1 diabetes is characterized by the abrupt onset of clinical signs and symptoms associated with marked hyperglycemia and the strong propensity for the development of ketoacidosis.

B The disease begins to develop long before the clinical signs become evident.

2 Pathologic and biochemical changes may occur as long as 9 years before the clinical onset of type 1 diabetes. The five stages of development are shown in Table 7.1.

A There is a genetic propensity for type 1 diabetes.

TABLE 7.1. PATHOPHYSIOLOGIC STATES IN THE DEVELOPMENT OF TYPE 1 DIABETES

Stage 1	Genetic predisposition
Stage 2	Environmental trigger
Stage 3	Active autoimmunity
Stage 4	Progressive ß-cell dysfunction
Stage 5	Overt diabetes mellitus

- The risk of type 1 diabetes in the general population ranges from 1 in 400 to 1 in 1000.[5] That risk is substantially increased (from approximately 1 in 20 to 1 in 50) in the offspring of individuals with diabetes.
- The genetic predisposition to type 1 diabetes is the result of the combination of HLA DQ coded genes for disease susceptibility offset by genes that are related to disease resistance. Genes that produce resistance are frequently dominant over those that produce disease susceptibility.
- HLA DR-3 and/or DR-4 appear to be present in greater than 90% of Caucasians with type 1 diabetes. However, 95% of these individuals are found to have DQ A-1 *0301, DQ B-1 *0302. This HLA genotype is strongly associated with the occurrence of type 1 diabetes among African American, Caucasian, and Japanese populations.
- Dominant protection from developing diabetes results from the presence of the genotype DQ B-1 *0602 or DQ W-1.2.
- Not all individuals at genetic risk for type 1 diabetes ultimately develop the disease.
- Although 40% of Caucasian individuals express the DR-3 or DR-4 haplotype, fewer than 1% ultimately develop diabetes.[4]
- A 50% discordance rate of type 1 diabetes exists between identical twins suggesting that specific genes are necessary but not sufficient conditions for its development.

B A trigger is necessary for the expression of the genetic propensity for type 1 diabetes; environmental triggers have long been suspected.

- Viral triggers are suggested by the association of type 1 diabetes with congenital rubella syndrome and Coxsackie B4 infection.

- Bovine serum albumin (BSA) is thought to be an environmental trigger by many investigators.
- BSA-specific antibodies are found in the majority of children with newly diagnosed diabetes. Thus, early exposure to cow's milk may be an important determinant of subsequent type 1 diabetes, increasing disease risk by as much as 1.5 times.[6]
- Structural similarities exist between BSA and an islet cell-surface antigen referred to as ICA-69. The cross reactivity of circulating anti-BSA antibodies with ICA-69 would provide a link between the environmental trigger and the subsequent development of auto-immunity, causing type 1 diabetes.
- Additional environmental factors that have been suggested as triggers for type 1 diabetes include sex steroids as seen in puberty and during pregnancy, environmental toxins (including N-nitroso derivatives and the rodenticide, vacor), or possibly insulin itself.[7]

C Regardless of the trigger, early type 1 diabetes is first identified by the appearance of active autoimmunity directed against pancreatic ß-cells and their products.

- Fifty percent of relatives with high titer ICAs have diabetes within 5 years of follow up. ICA negativity has a 99.9% probability of freedom from the development of type 1 diabetes.
- ICAs are composed of a variety of specific islet cell antibodies that may interact with diabetic serum. Many measurements of titers are currently available from commercial laboratories.
- Glutamic acid decarboxylase (GAD), a 64000 M_R protein appears to be the best immunologic predictor for the future development of type 1 diabetes.[8]
- Additional islet cell autobodies that may play a permissive or pathologic role in the causation of type 1 diabetes are shown in Table 7.2.
- There is also an immunologic attack on insulin, the product of the ß-cell.
- Seventy-eight percent of future cases of type 1 diabetes found in ICA-positive individuals arose from the subset with multiple autoantibodies; thus, the combination of positive antibody titers provides both increased sensitivity and specificity for disease progression.[9]

Table 7.2. Islet Cell Antibodies (ICAs) Observed in Type 1 Diabetes

Autoantigen	T-Cell Reactivity	Description
GM2-1	?	Nonspecific; in all islet cells
Glutamic acid decarboxylase (GAD)	Positive	Present as GAD-65, GAD-67, and 64 000 M_r antibodies
Insulin	Positive	Insulin autoantibodies (IAAs)
ICA-69 (IPM-1)	?	Homologous with bovine serum albumin (BSA)
38 000 M_2	Positive	Secretory granule related
52 000 M_r	?	Rubella associated
Carboxypeptidase H	?	Secretory granule related
GLUT	?	Inhibition of glucose-stimulated insulin secretion

D The combination of autoimmune attack on ß-cells and on insulin by insulin autoantibodies (IAAs) progressively diminishes the effective circulating insulin level.

- Before the clinical onset of diabetes mellitus, intravenous (IV) glucose tolerance testing demonstrates a progressive decline in first-phase insulin secretion (the insulin released within the first 5 minutes following an IV glucose stimulus) in individuals with positive immunologic markers. More than 50% of individuals with positive ICAs, but normal glucose tolerance tests, have first-phase insulin secretion that falls within the 10th percentile of the normal population.[10]

- Hyperglycemia and symptoms consistent with the diagnosis of diabetes mellitus develop only after >90% of the secretory capacity of the ß-cell mass has been destroyed.

E The clinical onset of diabetes may be abrupt, but the pathophysiologic insult is a slow, progressive phenomenon.

- At any time during the progressive decline in ß-cell function, overt diabetes may be precipitated by either acute illness or stress, thus increasing the insulin demand beyond the reserve of the damaged islet cell mass.

- Hyperglycemia will ensue until such time as the acute illness or stress is resolved; then the individual may revert to a compensated state for a variable time period in which the ß-cell mass is sufficient to maintain normal glycemia. This "honeymoon period" is a variable period of non-insulin dependency following acute decompensation.
- Continued ß-cell destruction occurs and ultimately the individual will require insulin within 3 to 12 months, after which the person will have permanent diabetes.

F Identifying these multiple stages of development of type 1 diabetes provides a provocative framework for potential interventions that focus on prevention and cure.

- Identifying HLA markers may allow recognition of populations at risk at the time of birth.
- Developing specific vaccines against identified environmental triggers, or the simple avoidance of environmental toxins such as bovine serum albumin, may prevent triggering of autoimmunity.
- Identifying active autoimmunity by measuring islet cell antibodies may serve as a marker for individuals who are destined to develop diabetes.
- The National Institutes of Health has embarked upon the Diabetes Prevention Trial–Type 1 (DPT-1) to include screening first-degree relatives of probands with type 1 diabetes via ICA measurement, including anti-GAD, and performing IV glucose tolerance testing with measurement of first-phase insulin release. Individuals are stratified according to risks and interventions with either oral insulin or subcutaneous insulin in an effort to prevent the ultimate development of type 1 diabetes.

NATURAL HISTORY AND PATHOPHYSIOLOGY OF TYPE 2 DIABETES

1 Ascertainment of type 2 diabetes remains extremely poor, with almost 30% of those affected being undiagnosed.[11] This apparent failure to identify individuals with type 2 diabetes results in progressive morbidity and mortality.

A Type 2 diabetes may be present, on average, for about 6.5 years prior to its clinical identification and treatment.[12]

B The prevalence of coronary artery disease in those with type 2 diabetes is twice that of the nondiabetic population, and cardiovascular and total mortality are two- to three-fold greater than in nondiabetic individuals.

2 Heredity plays a major role in the expression of type 2 diabetes.

A Although there is no recognized HLA linkage, offspring of individuals with type 2 diabetes have a 15% chance of developing the disease and a 30% risk of developing impaired glucose tolerance.[5]

B A greater than 90% concordance rate exists between monozygotic twins if one has type 2 diabetes, suggesting the primacy of the genetic defect in this form of the disease.

3 Identification of specific gene defects in certain groups with exceptionally high prevalence of type 2 diabetes has resulted in their designation as secondary forms of diabetes.

A The Pima Indians have a 50% prevalence of type 2 diabetes, with insulin resistance and hyperinsulinemia inherited as an autosomal trait.[13]

B In the familial form of type 2 diabetes known as MODY, diabetes is associated with alterations of chromosome 7 in close proximity to the glucokinase gene.[14]

4 Type 2 diabetes is a heterogeneous disorder characterized by variable plasma insulin levels with associated hyperglycemia and peripheral insulin resistance. This disorder has been described as the Insulin Resistance Syndrome.

5 Type 2 diabetes may be divided into several specific defects:

A Primary beta cell dysfunction

B Insulin receptor abnormalities (rare)

C Specific postreceptor defects, including altered glucose transporter function and specific enzymatic defects that modulate intracellular insulin activity.

6 Limitation in ß-cell response to hyperglycemia appears to be the cornerstone of the pathophysiology of type 2 diabetes.[15]

A A 50% reduction in ß-cell mass is seen in individuals with type 2 diabetes compared with controls, particularly when the degree of obesity is also taken into account. No evidence of autoimmune insulitis is found within these ß-cells, but the expected degree of hypertrophy and hyperfunction caused by chronic hyperglycemia is distinctly absent.

B Abnormal ß-cell recognition of glucose and its subsequent linkage to insulin synthesis and secretion are specific mechanisms by which the ß-cell plays a critical role in type 2 diabetes.

C Intrinsic abnormalities in patterns of insulin secretion are noted in most individuals with type 2 diabetes. The packaging and secretion of insulin appear to be progressive abnormalities in the transition from normal to impaired glucose tolerance and subsequently to type 2 diabetes.

D Abnormal secretion of the insulin precursor, proinsulin, has been noted in multiple populations.

E Acquired defects in ß-cell activity have been noted in response to hyperglycemia and referred to as glucose toxicity.

- ß-cells chronically exposed to hyperglycemia become progressively less efficient in responding to subsequent glucose challenges.[16]

- Thus, ß-cell dysfunction may be either primary or acquired in the pathogenesis of type 2 diabetes; however, it remains a necessary component of carbohydrate intolerance in any event.

7 A second essential trait of type 2 diabetes is the presence of resistance to the biologic activity of insulin noted in both liver and peripheral tissues.[17] Severe insulin resistance exists years before the onset of hyperglycemia.

A Resistance to the biologic activity of insulin may result in hyperglycemia with progressively increasing requirements for insulin secretion resulting in expression of either glucose toxicity or some genetic limitation in ß-cell activity.

B The relative roles of insulin resistance and insulin deficiency remain highly controversial and are frequently presented in the literature.[18]

8 In the fasting state, circulating blood glucose is maintained by hepatic glucose production via glycogenolysis and gluconeogenesis. Insulin suppresses these processes in a marked dose-response fashion.

A Those with type 2 diabetes have a substantial shift to the right of the dose-response curves, with a decrease in both the sensitivity and response of the system.

B Thus, regardless of circulating insulin levels, type 2 diabetes is associated with a persistent hepatic glucose production that increases fasting glucose levels.

9 Studies[15] using a euglycemic hyperinsulinemic clamp show both decreased sensitivity and response in peripheral glucose disposal in individuals with type 2 diabetes compared with nondiabetic controls.

10 Early suggestions of impaired insulin receptor function have not been demonstrated. Rare individuals have been identified as having altered insulin receptor structure or function. However, in the vast majority of individuals with type 2 diabetes, insulin binding to its receptor, insulin receptor number, and insulin receptor activity appear to be entirely normal.[17]

11 These premises, along with the public health demands of recognizing an insidious disorder associated with substantial morbidity and mortality, have led the National Institutes of Health to propose a prevention trial for type 2 diabetes.
  A The Diabetes Prevention Program (DPP) intends to screen high-risk populations for the presence of impaired glucose tolerance.
  B Subsequent intervention with intensive lifestyle modifications (diet, exercise, and subsequent weight loss) versus pharmacologic interventions to improve endogenous insulin action are aimed to ameliorating the specific defects prior to decompensation to a hyperglycemic state.

KEY EDUCATIONAL CONSIDERATIONS

1 Diabetes mellitus is a syndrome of metabolic diseases characterized by inappropriate hyperglycemia resulting from defects in insulin secretion, insulin action, or both, and associated with chronic microvascular and macrovascular complications.

2 Newly revised diagnostic criteria and classification of disease have been adopted.

3 Type 1 diabetes is an autoimmune disorder resulting in destruction of pancreatic ß-cells, requiring insulin therapy to prevent ketoacidosis and death.

4 Type 2 diabetes is a heterogeneous disorder in which specific secondary genetic causes of the metabolic syndrome are being rapidly identified.

5 Type 2 diabetes is characterized by variable ß-cell function and peripheral insulin resistance.

SELF-REVIEW QUESTIONS

1 Describe normal metabolism in each of the 5 phases of full homeostasis.

2 Define diabetes mellitus based on the three methods used in its diagnosis.

3 Describe three differences between type 1 diabetes and type 2 diabetes.

4 Describe the natural history of type 1 diabetes and type 2 diabetes.

REFERENCES

1 Chipken SR, Kelly KL, Ruderman NB. Hormone-fuel interrelationships: fed state, starvation, and diabetes mellitus. In: Kahn CR, Weir GS, eds. Joslin's diabetes mellitus. 13th ed. Philadelphia: Lea & Febiger, 1994:97-115.

2 Expert Committee on the Diagnosis and Classification of Diabetes Mellitus. Report of the expert committee on the diagnosis and classification of diabetes mellitus. Diabetes Care 1997;20:1183-97.

3 World Health Organization. Diabetes mellitus: report of a WHO Study Group. Geneva: World Health Organization 1985. Technical Report Series No. 727.

4 Thai A-C, Eisenbarth GS. Natural history of IDDM. Diabetes Rev 1993;1:1-14.

5 Raffel LJ, Rotter JI. The genetics of diabetes. Clin Diabetes 1985;3:49-54.

6 Gerstein HC. Cow's milk exposure and type 1 diabetes mellitus. Diabetes Care 1994;17:13-19.

7 Leslie RD, Elliott RB. Early environmental events as a cause of IDDM. Evidence and implications. Diabetes 1994;43:843-50.

8 Atkinson MA, MacLaren NK, Scharp DW, Lacy PE, Riley WJ. 64,000 Mr autoantibodies as predictors of insulin-dependent diabetes. Lancet 1990;35:1357-60.

9 Bingley PJ, Christie MR, Bonifacio E, et al. Combined analysis of autoantibodies improves prediction of IDDM in islet antibody positive relatives. Diabetes 1994;43:1304-10.

10 Maclaren NK. How, when and why to predict IDDM. Diabetes 1988;37:1591-4.

11 Centers for Disease Control and Prevention. National diabetes fact sheet. U.S. Department of Health and Human Services, Centers for Disease Control and Prevention, Division of Diabetes Translation. Atlanta;1997.

12 Harris MI, Klein RE, Welborn TA, Knuiman MW. Onset of NIDDM occurs at least 4-7 yr before clinical diagnosis. Diabetes Care 1992;15:815-19.

13 Bogardus C, Lillioja S, Nyonba BL, et al. Distribution of in vivo insulin action in Pima Indians as a mixture of three normal distributions. Diabetes 1989;38:1423-32.

14 Froguel PH, Vaxilliaire M, Sun F, et al. Close linkage of glucokinase locus on chromosome 7p. to early onset non-insulin-dependent diabetes. Nature 1992;356:162-64.

15 Leahy JL. Natural history of beta-cell dysfunction in NIDDM. Diabetes Care 1990;13:992-1010.

16 DeFronzo RA, Bonadonna RC, Ferrannini E. Pathogenesis of IDDM. A balanced overview. Diabetes Care 1992;15:318-68.

17 Reaven GM. Role of insulin resistance in human disease. Diabetes 1988;37:1595-1607.

18 Taylor SI, Accili D, Imai Y. Insulin resistance or insulin deficiency. Which is the primary cause of NIDDM? Diabetes 1994;43:735-40.

Suggested Readings

Elbein SC, Hoffman MD, Bragg KL, Mayorga RA. The genetics of NIDDM. An update. Diabetes Care 1994;17:1523-33.

Jacober S. Prediction and prevention of insulin-dependent diabetes mellitus. Diabetes Spectrum 1994;7:298-322.

Kahn CR. Insulin action, diabetogenes, and the cause of type II diabetes. Diabetes 1994;43:1066-84.

THERAPIES

THERAPIES

Nutrition 8

Marion J. Franz, MS, RD, CDE
International Diabetes Center
Institute for Research and Education
Minneapolis, Minnesota

Carbohydrate Counting Section:
Karmeen Kulkarni, RD, MS, CDE
Salt Lake City, Utah

Anne S. Daly, MS, RD, CDE
Springfield Diabetes and Endocrine Center
Springfield, Illinois

Sandra J. Gillespie, MMSc, RD, LD, CDE, FADA
Atlanta Diabetes Associates
Atlanta, Georgia

INTRODUCTION

1   Diabetes is a chronic disease that often requires lifestyle changes, especially in the areas of nutrition and exercise. The goal of medical nutrition therapy is to assist persons with diabetes in making self-directed behavior changes that will improve their overall diabetes management and/or nutritional status.

2   Medical nutrition therapy is an essential component of successful diabetes management.[1,2]

   A   Every individual with diabetes needs
   - Education related to diabetes and nutrition therapy
   - An individualized meal plan appropriate for his/her lifestyle and diabetes management goals[3]

   B   The meal plan, management goals, and self-management education need to be reviewed regularly and modified, as necessary, during the course of ongoing treatment and care.

3   Achieving nutritional goals requires a coordinated team effort by the registered dietitian (RD), registered nurse (RN), physician, exercise specialist, and behavioral specialist, with the person with diabetes being the center of the team. Family members and significant others need to be an integral part of the education and treatment program. Family members can also benefit from the same lifestyle recommendations as the person with diabetes to improve overall health through optimal nutrition.

4   For the person with diabetes, however, there are additional concerns.[4-6] A primary goal of medical nutrition therapy is to assist the patient in attaining blood glucose level goals by balancing food with insulin and activity.

5   Diabetes and dyslipidemia are each major risk factors for morbidity and mortality due to macrovascular disease. Nutrition therapy plays a preventive and therapeutic role in achieving recommended lipid levels.

6   Insulin therapy should be integrated into the usual eating and activity patterns.[4] For persons with type 2 diabetes, the goal of medical nutrition therapy is to normalize blood glucose and lipid levels. This goal can be achieved through improved eating habits, caloric restriction, proper spacing of meals, moderate weight loss, decreasing fat intake, increasing physical activity levels, and adopting new behaviors and attitudes.[4]

Objectives

Upon completion of this chapter, the learner will be able to

1 Identify medical nutrition therapy goals for diabetes management.

2 State the primary nutrition-related strategy for persons with type 1 diabetes to achieve glucose goals.

3 List five nutrition-related strategies for persons with type 2 diabetes to achieve glucose goals.

4 Explain the role of body mass index (BMI), waist-hip ratio, and reasonable body weight in defining and treating obesity.

5 Describe the role of insulin in the metabolism of carbohydrate, protein, and fat.

6 State guidelines for the role of protein in meal planning for persons with diabetes.

7 Describe the role of carbohydrate in meal planning for persons with diabetes.

8 State guidelines for the use of sucrose and fiber.

9 Explain how the term *acceptable daily intake* (ADI) relates to the use of nonnutritive sweeteners.

10 List nutrition recommendations for the amount and type of fat that is appropriate in the meal plan for persons with diabetes.

11 List recommendations for the amount of sodium in the meal plan for persons with and without hypertension.

12 List guidelines for the use of alcohol.

13 Describe four steps that are used to individualize a meal plan.

14 Describe four meal planning tools that are available for teaching food and meal planning.

15 Explain the concept of exchange lists, including the nutritive values for each group.

16 Describe the rationale of carbohydrate counting and at least four methods that are used for this meal planning approach.

17 Explain the three levels of carbohydrate counting, including the purpose, intended audience, content areas, resources and tools available, the necessary skills, and how to evaluate a client's understanding of and ability to use carbohydrate counting.

18 Explain how carbohydrate counting is useful for pattern management.

GOALS OF MEDICAL NUTRITION THERAPY

1 Restore and maintain as near-normal blood glucose levels as feasible by balancing food with insulin and activity levels.

2 Provide assistance in attaining optimal lipid levels (cholesterol, low-density lipoprotein [LDL], triglycerides, and high-density lipoprotein [HDL]). Recommended[3,6,7] values are shown in Tables 8.1, 8.2, and 8.3.

TABLE 8.1. RECOMMENDED LIPID VALUES FOR ADULTS[3,7]

	Cholesterol Levels Levels	LDL-Cholesterol Levels	HDL-Cholesterol Levels
Acceptable	≤200 mg/dL (5.17 mmol/L)	<100 mg/dL (2.59 mmol/L)	≥45 mg/dL (1.17 mmol/L)
Borderline	200-239 mg/dL (5.17-6.18 mmol/L)	100-129 mg/dL (2.59-3.34 mmol/L)	35-45 mg/dL (0.9-1.17 mmol/L)
High	≥240 mg/dL (6.20 mmol/L)	≥130 mg/dL (3.36 mmol/L)	<35 mg/dL (0.9 mmol/L)
Adults with preexisting cardiovascular disease (CVD)	≤100 mg/dL (2.59 mmol/L)		

TABLE 8.2. RECOMMENDED LIPID VALUES FOR CHILDREN AND ADOLESCENTS[3,7]

	Cholesterol Levels	LDL-Cholesterol Levels
Desirable	≤170 mg/dL (4.40 mmol/L)	≤110 mg/dL (2.85 mmol/L)
Borderline	170-199 mg/dL (4.40-5.15 mmol/L)	110-129 mg/dL (2.85-3.34 mmol/L)
High	≥200 mg/dL (5.17 mmol/L)	≥130 mg/dL (3.36 mmol/L)

TABLE 8.3. RECOMMENDED TRIGLYCERIDE LEVELS

	Adult Triglyceride Levels[3]	Child Triglyceride Levels[5]
Acceptable	<200 mg/dL (2.20 mmol/L)	Child, first decade ≤100 mg/dL (1.13 mmol/L)
		Child, second decade ≤120 mg/dL (1.35 mmol/L)
Borderline	200-399 mg/dL (2.20-4.39 mmol/L)	
High	400 mg/dL (4.40 mmol/L)	
Adults with history of CVD	<150 mg/dL (1.70 mmol/L)	

3 Provide appropriate calories for maintaining or attaining reasonable weights for adults, normal growth and development rates for children and adolescents, and adequate calories and nutrients during catabolic stress, pregnancy, and lactation.

4 Prevent and treat the acute and chronic complications of diabetes.

5 Improve overall health through optimal nutrition.

NUTRITION-RELATED STRATEGIES FOR ACHIEVING BLOOD GLUCOSE GOALS FOR TYPE 1 DIABETES[5,6]

1 The ideal management plan for persons who require exogenous insulin integrates insulin therapy into usual eating habits. Using this strategy, meals and snacks do not have to be separated into unnatural divisions or fractions. Individuals using conventional insulin therapy need to eat similar amounts with types of food at consistent times that are synchronized with the time actions of the insulin they take. They also need to monitor blood glucose levels and adjust insulin doses for the amount of food usually eaten based on blood glucose patterns.

2 Individuals can learn to make appropriate insulin adjustments by evaluating their blood glucose pattern (see Chapter 11, Monitoring, and Chapter 12, Pattern Management). After mastering pattern management, individuals can learn a more intensified style of insulin adjustment and can make compensatory and anticipatory changes in regular (short-acting) or lispro (rapid-acting) insulin based on pre- and/or postprandial blood glucose levels.

3 Individuals using intensified insulin regimens (eg, multiple daily injections [MDI] or continuous subcutaneous insulin infusion [CSII] using an infusion pump) can have more flexibility in the timing and amounts of food eaten, and still attain blood glucose gaols by determining the amount of bolus insulin needed to cover the carbohydrate content of their meals/snacks.

NUTRITION-RELATED STRATEGIES FOR ACHIEVING BLOOD GLUCOSE GOALS FOR TYPE 2 DIABETES[5,6]

1 The primary goal of nutrition therapy for persons with type 2 diabetes is to achieve and maintain normal blood glucose and lipid levels.

2 Several strategies are available to assist individuals in accomplishing this goal.

    A As research[8,9] continues to clarify why weight loss is difficult for many persons, the emphasis for persons with type 2 diabetes needs to shift from weight loss to achieving and maintaining blood glucose goals.

        • Moderate calorie restriction (250 to 500 calories less per day than the average daily intake as calculated from diet history) and a nutritionally adequate meal plan accompanied by an increase in physical activity will produce a gradual and sustained weight loss.[4]

        • A hypocaloric diet (independent of weight loss) is associated with increased sensitivity to insulin; significant improvements in blood glucose levels generally occur before much weight is actually lost.[10,11]

    A Moderate weight loss 10 to 20 lb (5 to 9 kg), irrespective of starting weight, has been shown to reduce hyperglycemia, dyslipidemia, and hypertension.[8,12,13] However, if blood glucose levels have not improved after moderate weight loss, oral antidiabetes agents or insulin (alone or in combination) may be needed.

        • The type of obesity associated with metabolic diseases (glucose intolerance, hypertension, and lipid abnormalities) is the android or abdominal distribution of adipose tissue. Upper body obesity (abdominal) is associated with hyperinsulinemia and insulin resistance, which are both risk factors for metabolic disease.[14,15] Waist-to-hip ratio (>0.95 for men, >0.8 for women) indicates risk for metabolic diseases.

- *Obesity* is the excessive accumulation of adipose tissue. Obesity and body weight can be described in several ways[16] (see Table 8.4).
- Target weights for persons with diabetes are based on a reasonable body weight, which usually is not the same as the traditionally defined desirable or ideal body weight.

C   Spreading food intake throughout the day to include five to six small meals and snacks instead of only two or three meals can help to even out blood glucose patterns.[17,18] Spacing of meals is based on the patient's schedule, blood glucose goals, monitoring results, and ability to reduce or control food intake.

D   Assist the patient to focus on behaviors and attitudes that assist with long-term lifestyle changes.[19]

E   Increase physical activity levels (see Chapter 9, Exercise).[20,21]

F   Monitor blood glucose levels to determine if the patient's goals have been met. If the person with diabetes has made all the lifestyle changes they are able or willing to make and target goals have not been achieved, a change in therapy (additions or changes in medication doses) is needed.[2,22]

3   The need to add or change medications is not as diet failure. Rather, it reflects the usual progression of therapy from nutrition/exercise therapy alone to combined nutrition, exercise, and medication therapies.

NUTRIENTS AND FOOD SOURCES

1   Carbohydrate provides 4 kcal per gram.

A   Carbohydrate is the body's major source of energy.

B   Dietary sources of carbohydrate are sugars (fruit, milk, added sugars), starches (breads, cereals, grains), and fiber, which does not supply calories.

C   After eating, carbohydrate in foods is the major predictor of postprandial blood glucose levels.

TABLE 8.4. DESCRIPTIONS OF BODY WEIGHT AND OBESITY[17]

Indicator	Definitions
Body mass index (BMI) = body weight (in kg) divided by height (in m)^2	Overweight: BMI >27; obesity: BMI >30 Based on the Koop report: the cutoff point for the BMI is 22 as being at risk, if one has comorbid diseases
Percent body fat—measured by skinfold measurement	Obesity: >25% for men and >30% for women
Morbid obesity	Weight twice the desirable weight or 100 lb (45 kg) overweight
Reasonable body weight	Weight an individual and healthcare provider acknowledge as achievable and maintainable, both short- and long-term[4]

2 Protein contributes 4 kcal per gram.

  A Protein is necessary for growth and tissue maintenance, and is a secondary source of energy.

  B Dietary sources of protein are both animal (meat, milk, and other dairy products) and vegetable (legumes, starches, nuts, seeds, and vegetables).

  • Animal proteins are called complete proteins because they contain all of the essential amino acids.

  • Vegetable proteins are deficient in one or more of the essential amino acids and must be combined to be complete. Foods that are deficient in one amino acid can be combined with other foods to result in complete proteins (eg, rice and beans, wheat [bread] and nuts [peanut butter], cereal and milk).

3 Fat contributes 9 kcal per gram.

  A Fat is used as an energy source in the form of free fatty acids (FFA).

  B Dietary sources of fat are animal sources (meat, egg yolk, dairy-fat-containing foods) and vegetables sources (margarine, oils, nuts, seeds, certain fruits [coconut, avocado], and many snack foods).

  C Fats in foods are broken down into triglycerides (three fatty acids attached to glycerol). Triglycerides are the form in which fat travels through the bloodstream and are stored in adipose tissue.

4 Vitamins and minerals are involved in a wide range of vital body functions (eg, vitamins are involved in the processing of other nutrients: carbohydrate, protein, fat, and minerals; minerals are components of many enzyme systems). They do not contribute calories or require insulin to be metabolized, although many micronutrients are intimately involved in carbohydrate and/or glucose metabolism as well as with insulin release and sensitivity.

5 Water is also considered an essential nutrient and is an important component of body tissue, accounting for between one half to three fourths of body weight.

   A Water is important in regulating body temperature and carrying nutrients to and waste products away from the cells.

   B Water is involved in all of the chemical reactions in metabolism.

   C Daily water losses need to be replaced from dietary sources such as water, beverages, and water in food.

Insulin and Metabolism

1 The therapeutic goals of diabetes care include not only striving toward euglycemia, but also the accompanying return of normal carbohydrate, protein, and fat metabolism.

2 Insulin is a hormone essential for the use and storage of these nutrients. The action of insulin is both anticatabolic (prevents breakdown) and anabolic (promotes storage), and it facilitates cellular transport. Insulin suppresses hepatic glycogenolysis and gluconeogenesis, and inhibits lipolysis and proteolysis. Insulin stimulates glycogen synthesis and facilitates the transport of glucose into muscle cells and adipocytes.

   A In the metabolism of carbohydrate, insulin facilitates entry of glucose into cells, stimulates glycogen synthesis in liver and muscle cells, and increases triglyceride stores by facilitating the entry of glucose into adipose tissue and its conversion to triglycerides. Without insulin, glucose production (gluconeogenesis) by the liver is accelerated and liver and muscle glycogenolysis occurs.

   B In the metabolism of protein, insulin lowers blood amino acids while reducing blood glucose levels, facilitates incorporation of amino acids into tissue protein, and decreases gluconeogenesis. Without insulin, gluconeogenesis increases, and proteolysis and amino acid release occurs in muscle.

   C In the metabolism of fat, insulin promotes lipogenesis by activating lipoprotein lipase, the enzyme that facilitates transport of triglycerides into adipose tissue for storage. Insulin also inhibits lipolysis and stimulates hepatic lipogenesis. Without adequate insulin, ketogenesis occurs in the liver and lipolysis and fatty acid release occur rapidly in adipose tissue, leading to excessive production of ketones and eventually ketoacidosis. Triglyceride levels also increase due to a decrease in cellular uptake of triglycerides.

3 The effects of insulin are balanced by the effects of the *counterregulatory hormones*: glucagon, growth hormone, cortisol, epinephrine, and norepinephrine.

PROTEIN IN THE DIABETES MEAL PLAN

1 The average protein intake for most Americans is approximately 12% to 20% or more of daily calories.

   A No evidence is available suggesting that persons with uncomplicated diabetes have protein requirements that are greater or less than those of the general public.[23]

   B At the present time, scientific evidence does not support either a higher or lower protein intake for those with diabetes. Protein intake in the range of 10% to 20% of daily calories is recommended.[24,25] Although 20% of the calories from protein is approximately double the adult recommended daily allowance (RDA) for protein, there is limited evidence that protein intake correlates with the development of nephropathy.[23]

   C One gram of protein per kilogram of body weight will meet the protein needs of most adults, and 1.2 g/kg will meet the protein needs for most children, adolescents, and athletes.

2 The rate of protein degradation and conversion of protein to glucose in individuals with diabetes depends on the state of insulinization and degree of glycemic control.

   A In individuals with poorly controlled diabetes, gluconeogenesis can occur rapidly and can adversely effect glycemic control.[23]

   B In contrast, the independent influence of dietary protein on blood glucose levels in individuals with well-controlled type 1 and type 2 diabetes appears to be minimal.[26,27] Even if approximately 50% of protein is converted to glucose, it appears to not have much influence on overall blood glucose levels.

C   It is speculated that although amino acids provide substrate for gluconeogenesis, they do not increase the rate of hepatic glucose release.[28]

3   Although patients have traditionally been taught to have a food source of protein before bedtime (or with other snacks), it is not clear that this protein has much clinical effect. Furthermore, under controlled conditions, treatment of hypoglycemia with a snack containing both protein and carbohydrate or carbohydrate alone was compared in six patients with type 1 diabetes; the rate of redevelopment of hypoglycemia did not differ, leading the researchers to conclude that inclusion of a protein adds calories rather than protects against subsequent hypoglycemia.[28]

4   Experimental and clinical studies have shown that protein restriction as an adjunct to blood glucose and blood pressure control slows the progression of renal disease by reducing albuminuria and preserving renal function. However, the optimal intake remains to be determined.[29]

A   With the onset of overt nephropathy, a protein intake of not less than 0.8 g/kg/day or approximately 10% of kcal is recommended.[4,5] With a lower intake of 0.6 g/kg/day, there is evidence of protein malnutrition.[30]

B   The differing effects of animal and vegetable protein on renal function are currently under investigation. Several studies suggest that animal rather than vegetable protein may be an important determinant in the progression of renal disease.[23]

CARBOHYDRATE IN THE DIABETES MEAL PLAN

1   If protein intake is between 10% and 20% of the calories, the remaining 80% to 90% of daily calories are left to be divided between carbohydrate and fat.

A   Exactly how these calories are divided depends on goals for glucose and lipid levels, weight management goals, and an assessment of changes the person is willing and able to make.[4,5]

B   An individual with a food history of 40% of kcal from fat may only be able to reduce this to 35%, resulting in approximately 45% to 50% of the calories from carbohydrate. In contrast, a vegetarian diet may contain 55% to 60% of kcal from carbohydrate.

2   It is a commonly held belief that sugars, both added and naturally occurring, are rapidly absorbed and lead to hyperglycemia and increased need for insulin.

   A   Recent studies[31-34] indicate that sucrose and other sugars do not have more of a deleterious effect on blood glucose levels and are not absorbed more rapidly than starches.

   B   The American Diabetes Association[4,5] has recommended that sucrose can be used as part of the total carbohydrate in the meal plan, not additive carbohydrate, in the context of an otherwise healthful eating plan.

   C   Research has consistently shown that sucrose and other sugars do not have a greater impact on blood glucose levels than other carbohydrates when consumed separately or as part of a meal or snack.

   • Starches, which are polymers of glucose, rapidly break down to 100% glucose due to the presence of enzymes in the intestinal tract, whereas sucrose is metabolized to 50% glucose and 50% fructose.

   • Fructose has a lower glycemic response that has been attributed to its slower rate of absorption and its rapid removal and metabolism in the liver.[35]

   D   The total amount of carbohydrate, as well as the total amount of food eaten, will have more of an effect on blood glucose levels than the source of the carbohydrate (glycemic index). Patients need to be made aware, however, that foods containing significant amounts of added sugars, (eg, regular soft drinks, syrups, desserts), not only contribute carbohydrate to the diet but may be high in calories and/or fat as well.

3   Although selected soluble fibers (eg, fiber from legumes, oats, fruits, and some vegetables) are capable of inhibiting absorption of glucose from the small intestine, the clinical significance of this effect on blood glucose levels is probably insignificant.[4,5] In contrast, insoluble fiber (eg, fiber from wheat and corn bran, whole grains, and some vegetables) is useful for increasing stool bulk and decreasing transient time of the stool, and thus may be helpful in preventing and treating constipation. Both types of fiber provide satiety value to the diet.

A The average dietary fiber intake for adults is 10 to 30 grams per day, with men averaging 19 grams and women averaging 13 grams.[5]

B The recommendation of the American Diabetes Association (ADA) is to follow the fiber recommendations for the general public concerning fiber consumption and a healthful diet. Approximately 20 to 35 grams per day of dietary fiber are from both soluble and insoluble fibers.[4]

4 Sweeteners are also included as part of the diabetes meal plan and are classified as carbohydrates.

A Nutritive (caloric) sweeteners include fructose, honey, corn syrup, molasses, hydrogenated starch hydrolysates, fruit juice or fruit juice concentrates, dextrose, maltose, and sugar alcohols such as sorbitol, mannitol, or xylitol. No evidence exists that these sweeteners have advantages or disadvantages over sucrose in decreasing amounts of carbohydrate in the diet or in improving overall diabetes control.[4,5]

- Calories from nutritive sweeteners must be accounted for in the meal plan and have the potential to affect blood glucose levels.
- Fructose provides 4 kcal per gram.
- The exact caloric value of sugar alcohols varies, and only limited evidence is available to suggest that total caloric savings can be expected by consuming foods containing sugar alcohols.[5] Sugar alcohols provide approximately 2 kcal per gram compared with the 4 kcal per gram from other carbohydrates.

B Nonnutritive sweeteners currently available include saccharin, aspartame, and acesulfame K. Other sweeteners pending approval from the Food and Drug Administration (FDA) include cyclamates, sucralose, and alitame. All FDA-approved nonnutritive sweeteners can be used by individuals with diabetes, including pregnant women. Because saccharin can cross the placenta, other sweeteners are better choices during pregnancy.[4]

- The *acceptable daily intake* (ADI) is defined as the amount of a food additive that can be safely consumed on a daily basis over a person's lifetime without any adverse effects. This determination includes a 100-fold safety factor and is determined by the FDA.
- The ADI for aspartame is 50 mg/kg/body weight. Aspartame consumption (14-day average) in persons with diabetes has been found to be 2 to 4 mg/kg/day.[36] The amount of aspartame in some common foods is (1) approximately 225 mg per 12 oz diet soft drink, (2) 80 mg per 8 oz fruited yogurt or 4 oz gelatin dessert, (3) approxi-

mately 32 mg per 3/4 cup sweetened cereal, (4) approximately 47 mg per frozen dessert, and (5) 37 mg per packet of tabletop sweetener.

- The ADI for acesulfame K is 15 mg/kg/body weight, which is the equivalent of a 132 lb (60 kg) person eating 150 grams (36 tsp) of sugar daily (or four 12 oz cans of soda containing 9 tsp sugar per can).
- When saccharin received Generally Recognized as Safe (GRAS) status in 1955, recommended consumption limits were 500 mg/day for children and 1000 mg/day for adults. However, even when saccharin was the only nonnutritive sweetener available, actual intake for persons with diabetes ranged from 54 to 173 mg/day.

FAT IN THE DIABETES MEAL PLAN

1 The recommended percentage of calories from fat is based on identified lipid problems and glucose, lipid, and weight goals. It is recommended that saturated fat intake be less than 10% of daily calories, and dietary cholesterol intake be 300 mg or less daily.[4,5]

   A People who are at a reasonable body weight and have normal lipid levels are encouraged to follow the recommendations of the National Cholesterol Education Program (NCEP)[7] in order to reduce their risk for cardiovascular disease.

   - In individuals over age 2 years, limiting fat intake to less than 30% of kcal, with saturated fat restricted to less than 10% of total kcal is recommended.
   - Polyunsaturated fat intake should be less than 10% of kcal, with monounsaturated fat in the range of 10% to 15% of kcal.

   B If LDL-cholesterol is the primary concern or if levels are elevated, further restriction of saturated fat to 7% of total kcal and dietary cholesterol to less than 200 mg/day (NCEP Step II diet) is recommended.

   C If obesity and weight loss are the primary concerns, a reduction in dietary fat can be considered.

   D If triglycerides and very-low-density lipoprotein (VLDL) cholesterol are the primary concerns, one approach that may be tried is a moderate increase in monounsaturated fat intake, with less than 10% of the kcal from saturated fats and a more moderate carbohydrate intake.

2 Several diabetes-related diet factors influence the risk of developing macrovascular disease (see Chapter 24, Macrovascular Disease).

  A Saturated fats raise blood cholesterol levels. Food sources of saturated fats are animal fats (meat, butterfat, lard, bacon, etc); coconut, palm, and palm kernel oils; dairy-fat-containing foods; and hydrogenated vegetable oils.

  B Polyunsaturated fats (omega-6) have been shown to lower cholesterol levels but have a heterogeneous effect on HDL-cholesterol levels. Food sources of polyunsaturated fats are vegetable oils (corn, safflower, soybean, sunflower, and cottonseed) and walnuts.

  C Monounsaturated fats lower total cholesterol but do not lower HDL-cholesterol levels. Food sources of monounsaturated fats are canola, olive, and peanut oil; olives; and nuts (except walnuts).

  D Omega 3 (fish oils) have an antiplatelet clotting effect and lower serum triglycerides and cholesterol levels. Food sources of omega 3 fish oils are fish from cold, deep water and (fatty) fish such as salmon, herring, albacore tuna, mackerel, and sardines. In capsule form, these oils have been shown to elevate blood glucose levels; this effect is under investigation.[37]

  E Dietary cholesterol affects LDL-cholesterol concentration by competing for cell receptors for LDL-cholesterol. Dietary cholesterol is found only in animal foods. Some individuals appear to be more sensitive to the blood-cholesterol-raising effects of dietary cholesterol than others. Food sources high in cholesterol are egg yolks, organ meats (especially liver), and dairy-fat-containing food products.

  F A diet high in total fat can increase chylomicron levels leading to atherogenic remnant particles. (Chylomicrons carry food cholesterol and triglycerides from the intestinal mucosa to the liver.)

3 Over 20 fat replacements are currently being used in food products. These replacements are generally classified according to the nutrients from which they are made.

  A Carbohydrate sources of fat replacements are dextrins, maltodextrins, modified food starches, polydextrose, cellulose, and gums.

  B Protein sources of fat substitutes are microparticulated proteins from egg whites or milk, and texturized proteins.

  C Several sources of fat replacements from fat (eg, caprenin, salatrim, and olestra) are currently are available in foods that are on the market, and others are under development.[38,39]

6 Alcohol raises triglycerides.

7 Alcohol also may potentiate or interfere with the action of other medications.

TRANSLATING DIABETES NUTRITION RECOMMENDATIONS FOR USE IN NUTRITION SELF-MANAGEMENT EDUCATION

1 The process of providing medical nutrition therapy for diabetes has shifted from nutrition prescriptions based on formulas for caloric requirements and percentage of calories from macronutrients to individualization based on assessment, goal setting, implementation of education, evaluation of outcomes, documentation, and follow-up.[46] A system for providing ongoing nutrition care is also essential.[22,47]

2 Certain assessments are needed to develop a medical nutrition therapy plan.[22,47]

    A The following minimum referral data are needed before beginning an assessment:
- Diabetes treatment program
- Laboratory data (glycosylated hemoglobin levels, fasting/nonfasting plasma glucose, cholesterol and fractionations, fasting triglycerides, and microalbumin [when appropriate])
- Blood pressure
- Medical history
- Medications that affect nutrition therapy
- Medical clearance and/or limitations for exercise

    B The following patient parameters need to be assessed:
- Anthropometric measures
- Biochemical indices and laboratory data
- Clinical signs
- Food/nutrition history
- Learning style, cultural heritage, religious practices, food-related beliefs, attitudes and concerns, and socioeconomic status

    C A complete food/nutrition history is needed. Two methods that can be used to assess eating patterns and food choices are a food history taken by the dietitian or food records (1- to 3-day) kept by the individual.

D A preliminary meal plan can be designed using the food history and the food/nutrition assessment information. The nutrition history form shown in Figure 8.1 can be used to record and modify usual food intake; calculations for the meal plan can then be done based on these data (Figure 8.2).

- A registered dietitian has the major responsibility for working with the patient to develop an appropriate meal plan. Although the nutrition history form in Figure 8.2 is based on the exchange system, it does not limit the dietitian to the use of exchanges as the meal planning approach. The advantage of this form is that it allows the meal plan to be based on the modification of usual eating habits instead of beginning with a predetermined calorie level (that may or may not be appropriate) and then calculating the percentages of calories for macronutrients.

- Nutrient values from the exchange lists (Table 8.5) are a useful tool for evaluating the nutrition assessment and calculating the meal plan.[48] However, after completing an assessment the registered dietitian may determine that the blood glucose goals and meal planning can be best achieved by employing the use of basic nutrition or diabetes nutrition guidelines.

- With increasing use of more flexible insulin regimens, it is not necessary to divide the meal (or carbohydrate) content into various fractions; insulin therapy can be adjusted to match the patient's customary food intake. However, meals and snacks still need to be synchronized with the time actions of the insulins that the patient is injecting to prevent increases or decreases in blood glucose levels.[4]

- For persons with type 2 diabetes, having smaller meals and snacks spaced throughout the day may assist in controlling postmeal hyperglycemia.

E The preliminary meal plan can be evaluated by asking the following questions:

- Are the calories appropriate?
- Is the meal plan appropriate to reach blood glucose and other diabetes goals?
- Does the meal plan encourage healthful eating?
- Does the meal plan take into account personal preferences, cultural background, and religious practices?

USING FOOD DIARIES

1 Food diaries can be helpful for all phases of self-management and education. Food diaries have been shown to be an effective strategy for helping patients make positive changes in their eating patterns as well as reach and maintain weight goals. Patients write down everything they eat with approximate amounts and the circumstances under which the food was eaten over a period of time. Food diaries can be kept for one day each week, a few days each month, or for longer periods of time.

2 Patients who might benefit from keeping a food diary are
   A Those starting a new meal plan
   B Those who want to lose weight
   C Those who are having problems with blood glucose control

3 Food diaries can be beneficial by helping patients and educators to see
   A Unconscious eating or nibbling patterns
   B Portion sizes
   C Eating from boredom, being tired, being under stress, etc.
   D Skipping planned meals and/or snacks
   E Eating food in places other than at the table
   F Food choices, such as foods high in fat, foods with hidden fats, excessive sweets, etc.
   G Level of exercise

4 The patient and diabetes educator can review the patient's food diary to determine
   A What, where, and how much food was eaten
   B Improvements that can be made
   C Progress made toward short-term goals
   D Effect of food intake and activity on blood glucose levels (correlations can be made between foods eaten and blood glucose records)

FIGURE 8.1. SAMPLE NUTRITION HISTORY FORM

Food Group	Meal/Snack/Time						Total servings/day	CHO (g)	Protein (g)	Fat* (g)	Calories
	Breakfast	Snack	Lunch	Snack	Dinner	Snack					
Starch								15	3	1	80
Fruit								15			60
Milk, Skim								12	8	1	90
Vegetables								5	2		25
Meats/Substitutes									7	(8)(5)(3)(1)	(100)(75)(55)(35)
Fats										5	45
Carbohydrate Choices											

	TOTAL				
Calories		x 4 =	x 4 =	x 9 =	Total =
Percent Calories					

To foster flexibility in meal planning, the number of servings per food group may vary at a meal but the aggregate should not exceed the total servings allotted for the day.
*Calculations are based on medium-fat meats and skim/very-low-fat milk. If diet consists predominantly of lean meats, use the factor 3 g fat instead of 5 g fat; if predominantly very-lean meats, use 1 g fat; if predominantly high-fat meats, use 8 g fat. If low-fat (2%) milk is used, use 5 g fat; if whole milk is used, use 8 g fat.
Source: Adapted from Franz M. *A new era in nutrition therapy for diabetes.* On the Cutting Edge [Newsletter] 1995; 16(2):6.

FIGURE 8.2. EXAMPLE OF COMPLETED NUTRITION HISTORY FORM

Food Group	MEAL/SNACK/TIME Breakfast 7:30	Snack 10:00	Lunch 12:00	Snack 3:00	Dinner 6:30	Snack 10:00	Total servings/day	CHO (g)	Protein (g)	Fat* (g)	Calories
Starch	2	1	2-3	1	2-3	1-2	10	15 / 150	3 / 30	1 / 10	80
Fruit	1	1	1				3	15 / 45			60
Milk, Skim	1				1		2	12 / 24	8 / 16	1	90
Vegetables			0-1		1-2		2	5 / 10	2 / 4		25
Meats/Substitutes			2		3		5		7 / 35	(8)(5)(3)(1) / 25	(100)(75)(55)(35)
Fats			1	0-1	1-2	0-1	5			5 / 25	45
Carbohydrate Choices	4	2	3-4	1	3-4	1-2					
TOTAL								230	85	60	
Calories								x 4 = 920	x 4 = 340	x 9 = 540	Total = 1800
Percent Calories								51	19	30	

To foster flexibility in meal planning, the number of servings per food group may vary at a meal but the aggregate should not exceed the total servings allotted for the day.

*Calculations are based on medium-fat meats and skim/very-low-fat milk. If diet consists predominantly of lean meats, use the factor 3 g fat instead of 5 g fat; if predominantly very-lean meats, use 1 g fat; if predominantly high-fat meats, use 8 g fat. If low-fat (2%) milk is used, use 5 g fat; if whole milk is used, use 8 g fat.

Source: Adapted from Franz M. *A new era in nutrition therapy for diabetes.* On the Cutting Edge [Newsletter] 1995; 16(2):6.

TABLE 8.5. MACRONUTRIENT AND CALORIC VALUES PER SERVING FOR 1995 EXCHANGE LIST[48]

Groups/Lists	Carbohydrate (g)	Protein (g)	Fat (g)	Calories
Carbohydrates				
Starch	15	3	1 or less	80
Fruit	15	—	—	60
Milk				
Skim	12	8	0-3	90
Low-fat	12	8	5	120
Whole	12	8	8	150
Other Carbohydrates	15	Varies	Varies	Varies
Vegetables	5	2	—	25
Meat and substitutes				
Very lean	—	7	0-1	35
Lean	—	7	3	55
Medium-fat	—	7	5	75
High-fat	—	7	8	100
Fat	—	—	5	45

5 The food diary provides information that the patient can use when setting short- and long-term goals.

  A There are two phases of nutrition self-management and education:[49]

- Initial education is the information needed at the time of diagnosis, when the patient's treatment program or lifestyle changes, or at the time of initial contact with a patient. Initial skill topics provide information about basic nutrition, diabetes nutrition guidelines, and beginning strategies for altering eating patterns, and are considered basic nutrition therapy survival skills for all persons with diabetes. Basic educational tools are used to discuss initial changes in food habits (eg, making better food choices, spreading carbohydrate-containing foods throughout the day, or eating less fat).

- Continuing/in-depth self-management education is the comprehensive level of education that includes both management skills and lifestyle changes (Table 8.6). Continuing education provides essential education for ongoing nutrition self-management. Topics emphasized or chosen are based on the patient's choice, lifestyle, level of nutrition knowledge, and experience in planning, purchasing,

TABLE 8.6. TOPICS FOR CONTINUING/IN-DEPTH EDUCATION

Management Skills
(Information required to make decisions to achieve management goals)
- Food sources of carbohydrate, protein, fat
- How to use nutrition facts on food labels
- Meal planning and insulin adjustments for
    Illness
    Delay or changes in meal times
    Drinking alcoholic beverages
    Eating sugar-containing foods
    Exercise
    Travel
    Competitive athletics
    Holidays
- Treatment and prevention of hypoglycemia
- Nutritional management during short-term illness
- How to use blood glucose monitoring for problem solving and identification of blood glucose patterns
- Behavior change strategies
- Working rotating shifts, if needed

Improvement of Lifestyle *(Problem-solving skills)*
- Eating away from home
- Eating lunch in school cafeterias
- Brown bag lunches
- Special occasions, birthdays, holidays
- Grocery shopping
- New ideas for snacks
- Recipe modifications, menu ideas, cookbooks
- Reducing and modifying fat intake
- Reducing salt intake
- Vegetarian food choices
- Ethnic foods
- Use of convenience food
- How to fit foods with fat replacers and sugar substitutes into the meal plan
- Canning and freezing

and preparing food and meals. During this second phase, which is ongoing, individuals are taught to make adjustments in meal planning for a number of situations. Flexibility in meal planning is also addressed.

6 Identify and monitor outcomes after the second or third visit (approximately 6 weeks after the initial nutrition consult) to determine whether the individual is making progress toward personal goals.

    A If no progress is evident, the individual and educator need to reassess and consider possible revisions to the nutrition plan.

    B If the patient has done all he/she can do or is willing to do and blood glucose levels are not in the target range, notify the provider that medications need to be added or adjusted.[22]

7 Appropriate documentation of nutrition self-management and education includes short- and long-term goals, meal plan, educational topics addressed, assessment of patient acceptance and understanding, behavior changes, additional skills or information needed, additional recommendations, and plans for ongoing care.[22] Effectiveness (outcomes) of nutrition interventions also need to be documented.

8 Follow-up and ongoing/continuing education and care are essential part of medical nutrition therapy.

    A Patients and team members need to understand that persons with diabetes need follow-up and ongoing, long-term nutrition care.

    B It is recommended that persons with diabetes be seen periodically by a diabetes educator for continuing education, updating of the meal plan, and support.

        • The American Diabetes Association Standards of Care indicate that adults should be seen every 6 months to 1 year or if there is any major change in work schedule, activity level, type of diabetes medication (especially insulin), blood glucose control, or medical status (development of complications). Weight management may require more frequent visits.[22]

        • Children should be seen at a minimum of every 6 months, preferably every 3 months. Calories need to be adjusted to accommodate growth and development requirements.[47]

Evaluating Caloric Needs

1 Caloric needs are based on a reasonable body weight.

    A Adult calorie needs vary depending on level of activity, age, and desired weight change.

B The most accurate method for estimating caloric needs is a detailed diet history of usual food intake to be completed by a registered dietitian.

C General guidelines for estimating adult calorie requirements are shown in Tables 8.7 and 8.8.

D Short- and long-term weight goals should be based on the individual's determination of a reasonable weight rather than an ideal or desirable body weight.

2 Calories should be prescribed to provide for normal growth and development in children and adolescents. To determine normal growth and weight profiles, growth of children and adolescents should be monitored on a weight-height growth grid at a minimum of every 3 to 6 months.

A Children's calorie requirements should be based on a diet history. The meal plan is not intended to restrict calories but is to ensure a reasonably consistent food intake and a nutritionally balanced diet. Several methods can be used to evaluate adequacy of caloric intake (see Table 8.9).[49]

B Parents of young children and adolescents need to learn to adjust insulin rather than restrict food to control blood glucose levels.

METHODS FOR TEACHING MEAL PLANNING

1 No single meal planning approach works for every patient. For each phase of education, different educational resources may be needed; basic nutrition interventions are needed for beginning education and more complex tools may be needed as the counseling process continues. Preplanned printed diet sheets are ineffective and should not be used.

TABLE 8.7. ESTIMATING MAINTENANCE CALORIES FOR ADULTS

Approximate caloric requirements for adults based on actual weight

10 kcal/lb (20 kcal/kg) = kcal for obese or very inactive persons and chronic dieters

13 cal/lb (25 kcal/kg) = kcal for persons over age 55 years, active women, and sedentary men

15 kcal/lb (30 kcal/kg) = kcal for active men or very active women

20 kcal/lb (40 kcal/kg) = kcal for very active men or athletes

TABLE 8.8. HARRIS-BENEDICT EQUATION FOR ADULT CALORIE REQUIREMENTS[49]

	BEE* wt for obese = [(actual wt - IBW†) x .25] + IBW
Females	BEE = 655 + (9.6 x W‡[kg]) + (1.8 x H§[cm]) - (4.7 x A¶[y])
Males	BEE = 66 + (13.7 x W[kg]) + (5 x H[cm]) - 6.8 x A[y])
Activity factors	Restricted 1.1 Sedentary 1.2 Aerobic 3x/wk 1.3, 5x/wk 1.5, 7x/wk 1.6; True athlete 1.7

*BEE = measure of resting energy expenditure.
†IBW = ideal body weight.
‡W = weight.
§H = height.
¶A = age.

TABLE 8.9. ESTIMATING CALORIE REQUIREMENTS FOR YOUTH[49]

- Base calories on nutrition assessment.
  - Validate calorie needs using one of the following formulas:

Method 1
- 1000 kcal for 1st year
- Add 100 kcal/y up to age 10 years
- Girls 11 to 15 years old: add 100 kcal or less per year after age 10 years
- Girls >15 years old: calculate as an adult
- Boys 11 to 15 age years old: add 200 kcal/y after age 10 years
- Boys >15 years old: 23 kcal/lb (50 kcal/kg) very active; 18 kcal/lb (40 kcal/kg) usual; 15 to 16 kcal/lb (30 to 35 kcal/kg) sedentary

Method 2
- 1000 kcal for 1st year
- Add 125 kcal x age for boys, 100 kcal x age for girls, up to 20% more kcal for activity
- For toddlers 1 to 3 years old: 40 kcal per inch length

2 Several meal planning approaches are available to teach basic nutrition and diabetes nutrition guidelines, as well as more in-depth nutrition interventions.[50] The patient and educator may begin with one meal planning approach and try other resources as the counseling process continues.

3 Many of the more in-depth educational resources are based on some system of grouping foods. *Exchange Lists for Meal Planning*, developed and published by the American Dietetic Association and the American Diabetes Association,[48,51] groups foods into lists based on calorie and macronutrient composition. Exchange lists are perhaps best used by the registered dietitian to evaluate food and nutrient intake; values for the exchange lists can be used to simplify the assessment process.

4 Any of the many meal-planning approaches can be selected to implement nutrition education and the meal plan. Each of the diabetes meal-planning systems emphasizes different aspects of nutrition therapy; selecting an appropriate educational tool is based on what the individual with diabetes will best be able to understand and use.

5 Nutrition education topics are divided into two categories: basic or initial education and continuing, in-depth education.

6 Basic nutrition education focuses primarily on providing information about general nutrition and diabetes nutrition guidelines; goal setting is included in this educational process. The following resources can be used for teaching about general and diabetes-specific nutrition:

A *Dietary Guidelines for Americans,*[52] *Guide to Good Eating,*[53] and *The Food Guide Pyramid:*[54] all can be used as an introduction to basic nutrition and to begin the process of changing eating behaviors; these resources do not address issues specific to diabetes.

B *The First Step in Diabetes Meal Planning*[55] is a basic, self-contained nutrition pamphlet based on the Food Guide Pyramid. It is designed to be given to patients to use until an individualized meal plan can be developed by a dietitian but can also be used in individualizing the meal plan.

C *Healthy Food Choices*[56] is a pamphlet designed to promote healthy eating. It is divided into two sections: guidelines for making healthy food choices (eating less fat, salt, and sugar) and simplified exchange lists that provide a general idea of what to eat and when.

D *Healthy Eating for People with Diabetes*[57] is a low-literacy booklet in which drawings are used to visually present nutrition concepts. The "plate method" for determining portion sizes is introduced.

E *Single-Topic Diabetes Resources*[58] is a set of 21 single-topic handouts that contain basic information about popular diabetes education topics as diverse as to how to treat hypoglycemia, nutrition and diabetes complications, and counseling parents of toddlers about food and diabetes. Each reproducible handout begins with a self-assessment and learning objectives, provides topic-specific content, and ends with information on problem-solving and goal-setting to help patients apply what has been learned.

7 In-depth nutrition information provides more structure to the process of meal planning and/or information about specific nutrient (eg, carbohydrate or fat) or calorie content (see Table 8.6).

A *Month of Meals 1, Month of Meals 2, Month of Meals 3, Month of Meals 4, and Month of Meals 5*[59] are five separate booklets that were developed in response to frequent requests by patients for menus. Each Month of Meals (MOM) booklet contains 28 days of complete menus for breakfast, lunch, dinner, and snacks. Menus are written for a basic meal plan of 1500 kcal daily with instructions for adjusting the calorie level up or down. Although certain elements are consistent, each volume has unique features: MOM 1 includes a special occasion section, MOM 2 has more ethnic foods, MOM 3 emphasizes time-saving meals, MOM 4 features family favorites, and MOM 5 is about vegetarian cooking.

B *Exchange Lists for Meal Planning*[48] lists groups of measured foods of approximately the same nutritional value; foods in each list can be substituted or exchanged for other foods in the same list. The exchange lists are used with an individualized meal plan that specifies when and how many exchanges from each group are to be eaten for meals and/or snacks. The exchange lists were revised in 1995 to include the following:

• Foods are grouped into three categories: carbohydrate, meat and meat substitutes, and fat. Carbohydrate-containing foods include the starch, fruit, milk, and "other" carbohydrate lists (the "other" carbohydrate list was expanded from the "occasional use" food list of past editions). Vegetables are free unless three or more servings are eaten at one meal.

• A very-lean meat list has been added to the meat and meat substitute lists.

- Fats are divided into saturated, monounsaturated, and polyunsaturated lists.
- About one third more foods were added to the lists, including newer food products such as low- or nonfat foods, vegetarian, and ethnic foods.
- The database was updated and, as a result, some portion sizes were changed.

C *Carbohydrate Counting: Adding Flexibility to Your Food Choices*[60] is a booklet that explains carbohydrate counting and how it can be added to the exchange system to increase flexibility in food choices. One choice from the starch, fruit, or milk list supplies ~15 g of carbohydrate, and each choice is a 1 carbohydrate choice. A meal plan outlines the number of carbohydrate choices each person can select for meals and snacks.

D *Carbohydrate Counting: Getting Started*[61] is a booklet that introduces carbohydrate counting. It focuses on what foods contain carbohydrate, how to count carbohydrate, keeping simple food records, and how to eat consistent amounts of carbohydrate at meals and snacks.

E *Carbohydrate Counting: Moving On*[62] is a booklet that focuses on identifying patterns in blood glucose levels related to food intake, diabetes medication (if used), and physical activity. It includes how to interpret records and take action based on blood glucose patterns.

F *Carbohydrate Counting: Using Carbohydrate/Insulin Ratios*[63] is a booklet designed for people who take insulin and have chosen intensive diabetes management using multiple daily insulin injections or an insulin pump. Food and blood glucose records are used to fine-tune diabetes management by adjusting rapid- or short-acting insulin according to anticipated carbohydrate intake and physical activity. The relationship between food eaten and insulin injected is shown as a carbohydrate-to-insulin ratio. Before a carbohydrate-to-insulin ratio can be established, blood glucose levels need to be in the target range and the usual dose of both the basal insulin and bolus insulin established. This approach requires that an experienced team of professionals, including a registered dietitian, be available to provide individualized instruction and follow-up care.

G *My Food Plan*[64] is a booklet that provides a simplified approach to carbohydrate counting and meal planning. Common foods are grouped by approximate portion sizes. A personalized food plan provides for individualization. General guidelines for making healthful food choices are included. The booklet is also available in Spanish, *Mi Plan de Comidas*.

8 *Facilitating Lifestyle Change: A Resource Manual*[65] is designed to aid educators in working with patients who want to make changes in eating habits for blood glucose and/or weight control. This publication provides an overview of the education process; monitoring forms with camera-ready originals to be used for assessment, goal-setting, intervention, and evaluation; case studies; and additional resources.

TRANSLATING DIABETES NUTRITION RECOMMENDATIONS FOR USE IN HEALTHCARE FACILITIES

1 Standardized calorie-level meal patterns based on exchange lists have traditionally been used to plan meals for hospitalized patients.

    A The nutrition prescription was usually physician-determined and ordered as an "ADA diet" with a specified calorie level and percentage of carbohydrate, protein, and fat.

    B The term *ADA diet* is no longer appropriate since the American Diabetes Association does not endorse any single meal plan or specified percentages of macronutrients.[66,67]

2 A number of alternative meal planning systems are available, each has various advantages and disadvantages. A preferred method is to implement a consistent-carbohydrate diabetes meal plan. This method uses meal plans that incorporate consistent carbohydrate intake at meals and snacks, appropriate fat modifications, and consistent timing of meals and snacks instead of specific calorie levels.

3 Meal plans labeled "no concentrated sweets," "no sugar added," "low sugar," and "liberal diabetic diets" are no longer appropriate. These diets do not reflect the current diabetes nutrition recommendations and unnecessarily restrict sucrose.

4 Patients requiring clear- or full-liquid diets should receive approximately 200 grams of carbohydrate per day spread evenly throughout the day at meal and snack times to prevent "starvation ketosis." Liquids included are not be sugar-free.

5 Providing adequate nutrition is the primary concern for residents of long-term care facilities. It is appropriate to provide residents with a regular menu that has fairly consistent amounts of carbohydrate at meals and snacks.[68] Low calorie meal plans are not generally needed.

ESSENTIAL FOOD LABEL INFORMATION FOR FOOD AND MEAL PLANNING[69,70]

1 The Nutrition Labeling and Education Act (NLEA) mandated implementation of the 1995 National Food Labeling Regulations by the Food and Drug Administration and the US Department of Agriculture Food Safety and Inspection Service (FSAS). The food label regulations expand mandatory nutrition labeling to almost all food products and provide a standard format for food labels.

2 The Nutrition Facts label includes the following required information:

A Serving size and servings per container (similar food products have similar serving sizes)

B Total calories per serving and calories from fat per serving

C Total fat (g), saturated fat (g), cholesterol (mg), sodium (mg), total carbohydrate (g), dietary fiber (g), sugars (g), protein (g), and % Daily Value (for a 2000 calorie diet) for fat, saturated fat, cholesterol, total carbohydrate, and dietary fiber

D Percentage of Recommended Dietary Allowances (RDA) for vitamin A, vitamin C, calcium, and iron

E Percent Daily Values for total fat, saturated fat, cholesterol, sodium, total carbohydrate, and dietary fiber based on a 2000 calorie diet

F Calories per gram of fat, carbohydrate, and protein

3 Nutrient content claims describe the amount of nutrient in a food.

A The following words are used as absolute descriptors for nutrient claims: *free, low, good source, high, lean,* and *extra lean.*

• Claims with descriptors such as free and low indicate to consumers that a food is modified in a dietary component such as calories, fat, saturated fat, cholesterol, or sodium.

• Claims with descriptors such as *good source* and *high* can help consumers identify foods that are more important sources of vitamins, minerals, and fiber.

- Descriptors such as *lean* and *extra lean* can be used to characterize the fat and cholesterol content for meat, poultry, seafood, and game products.

    B Comparative claims are allowed between a regular food product and a nutritionally altered product (eg, *reduced, light, less,* and *more*).

4 Label information can be helpful in various meal planning methods. For example, one carbohydrate serving is based on the amount of food (eg, a starch, a fruit, a milk, or other carbohydrates) that contains ~15 g of carbohydrate. One fat serving is based on the amount of food that contains ~5 g of fat.

ETHNIC AND CULTURAL APPROPRIATENESS

1 Sensitivity to cultural communication styles and ethnic food is essential for successful nutrition counseling.

2 Cross-cultural counseling can be improved by health professionals using a four-step process. Educators need to:

   A Become familiar with their own cultural heritage.

   B Become acquainted with the cultural background of each client.

   C Use an in-depth, cross-cultural interview to establish the client's cultural background, food habit adaptations made in the US, and personal preferences.

   D Make recommendations based on a nonjudgmental analysis of the dietary data (see Chapter 3, Cultural Appropriateness in Diabetes Education and Care).[71]

TRAVEL ADAPTATIONS

1 When traveling where the time change is only 1, 2, or 3 hours, each morning insulin injection time can be moved one-half hour ahead or behind (depending on the direction the person is traveling) until the person is back on schedule. Insulin adjustments will need to be made when traveling overseas.

   A When travel is eastbound, there may be a 6- to 8-hour difference resulting in a shorter day. Background insulins such as intermediate-acting insulins or ultralente need to be reduced. Some centers use the guideline of decreasing the dose by whatever percentage of 24 hours is lost. Regular or lispro insulins are given before meals.

B When travel is westbound, days will be longer. Injections of regular or lispro insulin can be added for every 4 to 6 hours (before meals) to cover the additional time. Different centers use different guidelines. Teach patients using insulin to talk with their healthcare team about how to adjust insulin before traveling.

2 Remind patients to carry their medications, blood glucose monitoring equipment, and urine ketone testing materials when traveling. They also need to wear medical identification that shows that they have diabetes. Teach patients how to protect strips and insulin from extremes in temperature.

3 Patients need to be prepared for delays, cancelled flights or changes in travel plans. Many flights offer only beverages and peanuts or pretzels. Teach patients to carry extra snacks with them to help prevent hypoglycemia.

4 Airplane travel is not the only time that an eating schedule may be disrupted. In many countries, it is customary to eat very late evening meals. With planning and flexible insulin regimens, travel and mealtime changes can be handled safely.

5 Other precautions include carrying carbohydrate for extra activity and for treating hypoglycemia, teaching travel companions how to give glucagon, carrying guidelines on how to handle acute illnesses, and carrying spare prescriptions for medications.

RATIONALE OF CARBOHYDRATE COUNTING

1 Carbohydrate counting is becoming a more widely used meal planning approach for persons with diabetes.

    A It has been used in the US since insulin was discovered[24,72] and was one of the four meal planning approaches that was used successfully in the Diabetes Control and Complications Trial (DCCT).[25]

    B Scientific evidence and clinical observations have shown that carbohydrate is the main factor affecting postprandial blood glucose excursion and, thus, insulin requirements.[73-76]

    C Carbohydrate counting offers patients benefits such as greater flexibility in food choices and improved glucose control.

D Carbohydrate counting also requires more self-monitoring of blood glucose and decision making by the patient.

2 Emphasis should be placed on the total amount of carbohydrate rather than the type. Sucrose and other sweeteners may be substituted for other carbohydrate in the diet as part of a meal plan. Healthy eating remains the bottom line.[77]

3 When using carbohydrate counting, other nutrients, fat, and protein also must be considered because of the potential for weight gain even though, in usual amounts, they have minimal effect on blood glucose.

4 Patients with all types of diabetes—newly diagnosed as well as those with diabetes of long-standing duration—are appropriate candidates for carbohydrate counting.

5 Many variations of carbohydrate counting are used:
  A Counting carbohydrate servings or choices
  B Counting exchanges
  C Counting carbohydrate grams
  D Counting carbohydrate plus protein
  E Counting total available glucose (TAG), which incorporates carbohydrate, protein, and fat

6 Carbohydrate counting may be used as a follow-up to a basic guidelines approach such as the Food Guide Pyramid. Patients who are familiar with and skilled in using the exchange system will find it easier to use carbohydrate counting. In addition, carbohydrate counting may be a welcome alternative for patients who are frustrated with other meal planning systems.

7 Carbohydrate counting may be combined in various ways with other meal planning approaches and educational tools (eg, *Single Topic Diabetes Resources*[58] handouts and lifestyle change monitoring forms from *Facilitating Lifestyle Change*[65]).

8 Three levels of carbohydrate counting[78-80] have been identified based on the increasing levels of complexity and skills required.

A In Level 1 (basic), the concept of carbohydrate counting is introduced emphasizing consistent amounts of carbohydrate at meals and snacks (Table 8.10).

B In Level 2 (intermediate), the relationships among food, medication, activity, and blood glucose are presented and the concept of pattern management is introduced (Table 8.10).

C In Level 3 (advanced), the concept of matching insulin to carbohydrate intake using carbohydrate-to-insulin ratios is taught to patients using multiple daily injections or continuous subcutaneous insulin infusions (Table 8.10).

LEVEL 1 CARBOHYDRATE COUNTING

1 There are several factors to consider when offering carbohydrate counting as an option:

   A Blood glucose goal attainment

   B Desire for flexibility of food choices

   C Dissatisfaction with current meal planning approach

   D Lack of understanding of current plan

   E Desire for a new meal planning approach

2 Education for Level 1 carbohydrate counting covers the following concepts:

   A Why carbohydrate intake is important in relation to blood glucose levels

   B Which foods contain carbohydrate

   C What portion sizes are equal to one carbohydrate choice or one serving of carbohydrate

   D How to find and use carbohydrate information

   E What portion tools are needed

   F Food exchange information about carbohydrate intake

      • One carbohydrate choice = 15 grams carbohydrate

      • One carbohydrate choice = 1 starch exchange, 1 fruit exchange, or 1 milk exchange

      • One carbohydrate choice = 1½ cups vegetables

      • A *free food* is defined as any food or drink that contains less than 20 calories and 5 grams or less of carbohydrate per serving

Table 8.10. Carbohydrate Counting Checklist

Activities		Level 1	Level 2	Level 3
Patient contact	Pre	1 to 3	1 to 3	1 to 3
Contact intervals		1 to 4 weeks	1 to 2 weeks	1 to 2 weeks
Length of visit		30 to 90 minutes	30 to 60 minutes	30 to 60 minutes
Nutrition/ diabetes history	X			
Why count carbohydrate		X		
Starch vs sugar		X		
Effects of carbohydrate		X	X	X
Effects of protein, fat		X	X	X
Good nutrition		X	X	X
Intro to carb choices		X		
Portion control		X	X	X
Food labels		X	X	X
Carbohydrate resources			X	X
Set goals for carb*		X	X	X
Set goals for BG*		X	X	X
Keep food, BG, and medication records			X	X
Assess readiness for next level*	X	X	X	
Review BG records*			X	X
Evaluate BG patterns*			X	X
Adjust plan*			X	X
Restaurant meals			X	X
Combination foods			X	X
Fiber			X	X
Choices vs grams		X	X	X
Estimate carb/ insulin ratio				X
Use carb/insulin ratios				X
Snacking		X	X	X
Alcohol		X	X	X
Avoid weight gain		X	X	X

*Contact/activities can be done at visit, by phone, or by fax.
Source: Reprinted with permission from the American Dietetic Association. *Diabetes medical nutrition therapy.* Chicago: American Dietetic Association, 1997.
©1997, The American Dietetic Association. *Diabetes Medical Nutrition Therapy.* Used with permission.

3 A variety of activities are used to help patients become familiar with carbohydrate counting.

    A Practice exercises to assess previous knowledge and skills regarding carbohydrate counting.

        • Food labs provide an opportunity for hands-on demonstrations with carbohydrate foods. Patients "guesstimate" portion size and carbohydrate content before they actually measure, and then compare their guess with the actual answer.

        • Written quizzes can also be used.

    B Identify usual food intake and portion sizes through the use of food records or food recall, which enables patients to determine usual carbohydrate intake at meals and snacks. Resources typically used for information about the carbohydrate content of foods include the nutrition facts panel on a food label, carbohydrate food lists, and other reference books or materials (see Suggested Readings).

    C Plan sample meals to demonstrate what patients have learned about carbohydrate counting.

4 Carbohydrate target ranges for meals and snacks are determined by the patient and registered dietitian based on usual carbohydrate intake and distribution, nutrition goals set by the patient and the dietitian, medication, and level of physical activity.

TABLE 8.11. FIGURING CARBOHYDRATE FOR YOUR MEAL PLAN

Meal/Snack	Time	Usual Carbohydrate Intake (from Step 1)	Time	Agreed-Upon Carbohydrate Goals (Step 3)
		___ carbohydrate choices or ___ g carbohydrate		___ carbohydrate choices or ___ g carbohydrate
		___ carbohydrate choices or ___ g carbohydrate		___ carbohydrate choices or ___ g carbohydrate
		___ carbohydrate choices or ___ g carbohydrate		___ carbohydrate choices or ___ g carbohydrate
		___ carbohydrate choices or ___ g carbohydrate		___ carbohydrate choices or ___ g carbohydrate
		___ carbohydrate choices or ___ g carbohydrate		___ carbohydrate choices or ___ g carbohydrate
		___ carbohydrate choices or ___ g carbohydrate		___ carbohydrate choices or ___ g carbohydrate

Source: Reprinted with permission from The American Dietetic Association. Diabetes medical nutrition therapy. 1997[55]

5 Self-monitoring of blood glucose provides the information needed by patients using Level 1 carbohydrate counting and their healthcare team to determine the plan's effectiveness in reaching the target blood glucose levels.

6 In most cases, consistency of carbohydrate intake is appropriate to reduce fluctuations in postprandial glucose levels. When variation in carbohydrate intake is desired, patients can be taught to adjust medication and activity in order to maintain target blood glucose levels.

LEVEL 2 CARBOHYDRATE COUNTING

1 Level 2 carbohydrate counting is designed to teach patients about the relationship between nutrition, activity, and blood glucose so that they can effectively manage their diabetes.

2 During the initial phase, patients continue to use the target carbohydrate ranges that were established in Level 1 and keep a diabetes diary.

3 The information record includes (see Figure 8.3)
    A Medication/insulin: type, dose
    B Blood glucose levels: premeal, postmeal
    C Food intake: time of day, type, amount
    D Carbohydrate intake: choice or gram method
    E Level of physical activity: type, amount

4 Patients continue to weigh and measure food portions and learn to identify portions more accurately.

5 As patients gain more experience with weighing and measuring food, they become more skilled at estimating and recording carbohydrate intake using either the choice or the gram method.

FIGURE 8.3. EXAMPLE OF DIABETES DAILY RECORD

Name: JD
BG Goal: 80 to 150 mg/dL

Day/Date	Time	Med/Insulin Type/Dose	BG, mg/dL Premeal	Postmeal	Food Intake Amt.	Type (food/drink)	Carbohydrate Info Choices	Grams	Exercise Type/Amount
Tues. 4/15	5:30 PM	Glucotrol/2.5 mg	160		4 oz	Ground beef		0	Watch TV
					8 oz	Baked potato		43 g	
					1 c	Corn		30 g	
								73 g Total	
	9:00 PM			212					
Wed. 4/16	5:30 PM	Glucotrol/2.5 mg	141		2 c	Macaroni and cheese		60 g	Shop, walk in mall 1 hour
					1 c	Green peas		30 g	
					1 pc	Bread		12 g	
								102 g Total	
	9:00 PM			183					
Thurs. 4/17	5:45 PM	Glucotrol/2.5 mg	170		3 pc	Fried chicken		27 g	Walk 15 minutes
					1 c	Mashed potatoes		30 g	
					1/2 c	Gravy		6 g	
					3 oz	Biscuit		34 g	
								97 g Total	

6 Patients need certain skills to be able to use and benefit from Level 2 carbohydrate counting.

   A How to perform addition, subtraction, multiplication, and division (a calculator can be used if necessary)

   B How to use a variety of resources such as reference books, carbohydrate lists, and nutrition labels to calculate the carbohydrate content of more complex foods (eg, combination food items, restaurant foods)

   C How to determine the role of protein, fat, and fiber in the carbohydrate counting system

   D How to identify patterns related to blood glucose, food, medication, and activity

   E How to perform pattern management. The diabetes daily record (see Figure 8.3) demonstrates an example of pattern management (developed through practice exercises and evaluating self-care daily records for a 2-week period). Practice exercises for pattern management also include making adjustments to food, medication, and activity.

7 If patients plan to begin intensive insulin therapy, they can use what they have learned at Level 2 carbohydrate counting or Level 3.

LEVEL 3 CARBOHYDRATE COUNTING: CARBOHYDRATE-TO-INSULIN RATIOS

1 There are three principles of using carbohydrate-to-insulin ratios:

   A Accurately estimating the anticipated carbohydrate intake at meals and snacks

   B Determining the carbohydrate intake based on grams of carbohydrate or carbohydrate choices (15 gram equivalents or carbohydrate exchanges), or a combination of grams and choices

   C Administering a rapid- or short-acting premeal insulin dose based on a predetermined carbohydrate-to-insulin ratio

2 Certain prerequisites are necessary for moving to Level 3 carbohydrate counting and using carbohydrate-to-insulin ratios:

   A Mastery of Levels 1 and 2 carbohydrate counting

   B Intensive insulin therapy (eg, multiple daily injections [MDI] or use of a continuous subcutaneous insulin infusion [CSII] insulin pump)

   C Proficiency in self-adjustment and supplementation of insulin

   D Insulin doses adjusted to meet blood glucose goals while patient consistently uses Level 2 CHO guidelines

E   Food, blood glucose, and insulin records for at least 1 to 2 weeks to use for determining carbohydrate-to-insulin ratio

F   Carbohydrate-to-insulin ratio (C:I) is based on matching fast-acting food (CHO) to fast-acting insulin. C:I can be different for different people. For example, weight, physical activity, etc influence the calculation of C:I. There is variation from meal to meal, and different ratios are used based on insulin requirements; the C:I is always individualized.

3   Figure 8.4 outlines a possible protocol to determine carbohydrate-to-insulin ratios using carbohydrate grams.

A   The grams-per-unit ratio is obtained by dividing the grams of carbohydrate consistently consumed at a given meal by the number of units of rapid- or short-acting insulin needed to meet blood glucose goals.

B   To adjust insulin for more or less than the usual carbohydrate intake, the total grams of carbohydrate to be consumed are divided by the carbohydrate-to-insulin ratio. For example, a patient who consistently has 60 grams of carbohydrate at a meal and requires 6 units of regular insulin to achieve target blood glucose levels would have a ratio of 10 grams carbohydrate per 1 unit insulin. To adjust insulin for intake of 80 grams of carbohydrate, the 80 grams would be divided by 10 to obtain the appropriate insulin requirement of 8 units.

4   The following procedure can be used to determine carbohydrate-to-insulin ratios using carbohydrate choices (or exchanges) (see Figure 8.5):

A   The units-per-carbohydrate-choice ratio is obtained by dividing the number of units of rapid- or short-acting insulin needed to meet blood glucose goals by the number of carbohydrate choices consistently consumed at a given meal.

B   To adjust insulin for more or less than the usual carbohydrate choices, multiply the number of carbohydrate choices by the units-per-carbohydrate-choice ratio. For example, a patient who consistently consumes 6 carbohydrate choices at a meal and requires 9 units of regular insulin to achieve target blood glucose levels would have a ratio of 1.5 units per carbohydrate choice. To adjust insulin for an intake of 8 carbohydrate choices, the 8 carbohydrate choices would be multiplied by 1.5 to obtain the appropriate insulin requirement of 12 units.

Figure 8.4. Procedure for Determining Carbohydrate-to-Insulin Ratios Using Carbohydrate Grams

Case Example

RO has kept food, activity, and blood glucose records for 2 weeks. Based on a consistent intake of carbohydrate (CHO) and appropriate insulin adjustments to meet target blood glucose levels, you observe the following:

    Breakfast: 8 units regular insulin for 65 grams CHO
    Lunch: 6 units regular insulin for 65 grams CHO (50 grams for lunch, 15 grams for
        midafternoon snack)
    Dinner: 7 units regular insulin for 75 grams CHO
    Use this information and follow the steps below to calculate RO's
    carbohydrate-to-insulin ratio.

1   Record the grams (g) carbohydrate that are consistently eaten at each meal based on blood glucose and food records.
    Breakfast _____ g   Lunch _____ g   Dinner _____ g

2   Record meal doses of regular (R) insulin that consistently meet target blood glucose levels.
    Breakfast _____units   Lunch _____units   Dinner _____units

3   For each meal, determine the carbohydrate grams per unit of insulin by dividing total carbohydrate grams for each meal by the number of units of regular insulin.
    Breakfast = B   Lunch = L   Dinner = D
    CHO g   =_____   B____ = ____   L____ = ____   D____ = ____
    units R insulin g/unit   g/unit   g/unit g/unit

4   If the answers to step 3 vary from each other by no more than one gram of carbohydrate, add together the three answers and divide by 3 to get the average grams carbohydrate per unit of insulin.
    B_____ + L_____ + D_____ = _____ total g/unit÷ 3 = _____
                                                      average g/unit
    The appropriate carbohydrate-to-insulin ratio is _____ g/unit.

5   If the answers to step 3 vary from each other by more than one gram of carbohydrate, and you and the rest of the diabetes healthcare team agree that your basal insulin doses are well adjusted, use the answers to step 3 as carbohydrate-to-insulin ratios for each meal.
    The appropriate carbohydrate-to-insulin ratios are
    B _____ g/unit   L _____ g/unit   D_____ g/unit

6   To make insulin adjustments for consuming more or less carbohydrate, add the total carbohydrate and divide by the appropriate carbohydrate-to-insulin ratio.
    Total carbohydrate g _____ ÷ g/unit (ratio) _____ = _____units R

Practice

RO is going to eat a larger-than-usual dinner of a total of 90 grams of carbohydrate. Using step 6, calculate how much insulin will be needed for this meal.

Source: Adapted with permission from the American Dietetic Association. Carbohydrate counting: using carbohydrate/insulin ratios. Chicago: American Dietetic Association, 1995.

FIGURE 8.5. PROCEDURE FOR DETERMINING CARBOHYDRATE-TO-INSULIN RATIOS USING CARBOHYDRATE CHOICES (OR EXCHANGES)

Case Example

RO has kept food, activity, and blood glucose records for 2 weeks. Based on a consistent intake of carbohydrate (CHO) and appropriate insulin adjustments to meet target blood glucose levels, you observe the following:

> Breakfast: 8 units regular insulin for 4 CHO choices
> Lunch: 6 units regular insulin for 4 CHO choices (3 CHO choices for lunch, 1 CHO choice for midafternoon snack)
> Dinner: 7 units regular insulin for 5 CHO choices
> Use this information and follow the steps below to calculate RO's carbohydrate-to-insulin ratio.

1   Record the meal doses of regular (R) insulin that consistently meet target blood glucose levels based on blood glucose and food records.

Breakfast _____ units   Lunch _____ units   Dinner _____ units

2   Record the number of carbohydrate choices that are consistently eaten at each meal.

Breakfast_____   Lunch_____   Dinner_____
CHO choices   CHO choices   CHO choices

3   For each meal, determine the units of regular (R) insulin per carbohydrate choice by dividing the number of units by the number of carbohydrate choices.

units R insulin

CHO choices = _____ units/CHO choice

B_____units/CHO choice
L_____units/CHO choice
D_____units/CHO choice

4   If the answers to step 3 are different for one or more meals, use more than one ratio. The appropriate carbohydrate-to-insulin ratios are B _____ L _____ D _____units/CHO choice.

5   To make insulin adjustments for consuming more or less carbohydrate choices, add the total carbohydrate choices and multiply by the ratio units/CHO choice.

Total CHO choices _____ x _____ units/CHO choice = _____ units regular insulin

Practice

RO is going to eat a larger-than-usual dinner of a total of 6 carbohydrate choices. Using step 5, calculate how much insulin will be needed for this meal.

Source: Adapted with permission from the American Dietetic Association. Carbohydrate counting: using carbohydrate/insulin ratios. Chicago: American Dietetic Association, 1995.

5 Additional information that needs to be considered when using carbohy-drate-to-insulin ratios includes the following:

A Patients may have more than one carbohydrate-to-insulin ratio.[81] For example, a patient may have a ratio of 10 grams of carbohydrate to 1 unit of insulin at breakfast and a ratio of 15 grams to 1 unit at lunch and dinner.

B Carbohydrate-to-insulin ratios may change with changes in body weight or level of physical activity.

C Teach patients portion control to assure precise matching of insulin doses to anticipated carbohydrate intake.

D Teach patients that increased flexibility with carbohydrate amounts for meals and snacks and improving glycemic control places them at risk for weight gain. Reducing fat and total calorie intake can help main-tain desired weight.

E With the shorter duration of action of rapid-acting insulin (lispro), the dose taken with the preceding meal may not provide adequate cover-age of between-meal snacks. A lower carbohydrate snack may be needed or additional insulin at the time of a larger snack.

F The addition of large amounts of protein can produce an increase in blood glucose levels within 3.5 to 5 hours after the meal, requiring additional insulin prior to or following the meal.

G Because fat slows down gastric emptying time, delay in the timing of the premeal rapid- or short-acting insulin may be necessary to match the peak of the insulin with the peak postprandial blood glucose response.

H Dietary fiber, for the most part, is not digested and absorbed like other carbohydrates.[82] Therefore, paying close attention to the fiber content in foods will help the patient to more accurately match insulin to avail-able carbohydrate in high-fiber foods (those containing 5 grams or more dietary fiber). Total carbohydrate grams minus dietary fiber grams equals the available carbohydrate grams.

I Patients may identify specific carbohydrate foods or meals that pro-duce blood glucose responses greater or less than anticipated, which require changes in the carbohydrate-to-insulin ratios or timing of pre-meal insulin delivery.

- Pizza may require additional insulin.[83]
- Meals high in slowly absorbed carbohydrate (eg, cooked dried beans) may require delivery of premeal short-acting insulin closer to the consumption time or delivery of rapid-acting insulin after con-

sumption to match the peak insulin activity with the postprandial blood glucose peak.

KEY EDUCATIONAL CONSIDERATIONS

1   Emphasize the goals of meal planning for persons with either type 1 or type 2 diabetes. The goals are to prevent hyperglycemia and maintain euglycemia by balancing food intake with insulin taken by injection or insulin still being produced by the pancreas and with exercise. Strategies for improving blood glucose control for persons with type 2 diabetes that can be helpful include

   A   Moderate weight loss; the biggest improvement in blood glucose levels occurs with only a 10 to 20 lb (4.5 to 9.0 kg) weight loss

   B   Eating a hypocaloric diet through food selection (eg, decreasing fat intake) and eating smaller portion sizes

   C   Distributing carbohydrate and food intake throughout the day by eating smaller meals and snacks

   D   Increasing activity (exercise) level

   E   Improving eating behaviors (eg, eating breakfast and lunch instead of consuming all calories late in the day)

   F   Using blood glucose monitoring data to evaluate the effectiveness of food and meal and exercise changes

2   Emphasize to patients that they have not failed if meal planning strategies have not improved their blood glucose control. A change in therapy may be needed to meet blood glucose goals. Changing medications is a natural progression in the management of diabetes.

3   To encourage participation in nutrition education, show patients a list of the nutrition-related topics that are offered. Patients can check what they want to learn at the first session, second session, etc. This technique also removes the unrealistic burden from the educator of trying to teach everything in one visit.

4   Use blood glucose monitoring results to teach patients how to assess the relationships among food, exercise, medication, coping skills, etc.

5   Ask patients or use examples of former patients (without identifying information) to elicit a patient's past history with dietitians or with weight loss,

for example, "I worked with a woman who resisted making the initial appointment because her previous experience with dieting was in a program where she had to weigh in at every visit, measure her food at all times, and eat foods that she did not like. She was amazed that meal planning for blood glucose control could be so flexible. What's been your experience?"

6 Use the Nutrition Facts label on food packages to point out the grams of carbohydrate, protein, fat, and number of calories per serving. Help patients understand that carbohydrate servings are based on 15 g of carbohydrate and fat servings are based on 5 g of fat. Use an actual food label to illustrate that the serving size on the food label may differ from the exchange value. For example, a label for brown rice lists a serving size of 1 cup while the serving size from the starch list for brown rice is 1/3 cup.

7 Invite patients to teach the educator(s) about the ingredients in and preparation of cultural/ethnic foods. Combining the patient's cultural expertise with the diabetes and nutrition knowledge of the educator allows for a true exchange of information that will benefit the patient.

8 Use menus from local restaurants or fast-food chains to help patients plan a meal according to their meal plan. Using a menu allows for patient preferences and variety, and often brings some humor and realism to the teaching session. Through role playing, patients can also practice their assertiveness skills by asking their "waiter" partner questions about ingredients, preparation, and presentation of food.

9 Conduct a supermarket tour to teach flexibility and variety in meal planning. Participants can read the food labels, learn where to find the recommended foods in the supermarket, learn the aisles to avoid, and compare the nutritional content of different brands of foods.

10 Display a chart or test tubes showing the amounts of sucrose or fat in common foods.
  A Compare small portions of common foods such as a cookie, frozen yogurts, or ice milk, etc with the sucrose in a 12 ounce can of regular soft drink, Jello®, fruited yogurt, etc.
  B Point out that small portions of sucrose-containing foods can be used as a carbohydrate serving in the meal plan, but that the calorie and fat content of sucrose-containing foods also need to be considered.

11 Offer samples of products or coupons to encourage patients to try some new foods. Helping a patient change from the usual egg-and-bacon-on-a-roll breakfast may be more successful if the patient has tried and liked a new whole grain cereal.

12 The terms sugar-free, fat-free, lite, and dietetic on foods do not mean that these foods are "free." To teach this concept, use food labels to demonstrate the number of calories in and the fat and carbohydrate content of a common sugar-free or fat-free product, or use the American Diabetes Association's booklet, *A Guide to Fitting Foods with Sugar Substitutes and Fat Replacers into Your Meal Plan*. This booklet includes examples of food labels containing these products and is a guide to help individuals incorporate these foods into their meal plans.

13 To teach patients how to consider the total amount of carbohydrate when selecting a piece of cake, the educator can offer a rule of thumb that a 2-inch square contains ~30 g of carbohydrate and 5 g of fat (2 carbohydrate choices and 1 fat serving). One piece (1/6) of a frosted, two-layer cake, however, contains ~45 g of carbohydrate and 10 g fat (3 carbohydrate choices and 2 fat servings).

KEY EDUCATIONAL CONSIDERATIONS—LEVEL 1 CARBOHYDRATE COUNTING

1 Emphasize the importance of accurate portion skills. Encourage use of a food scale, measuring spoons, and measuring cups. Consider using food labs to improve your own skills as well as the patient's. Practice repeatedly. Teach patients that periodic measuring and weighing needs to be an ongoing activity for accurate carbohydrate counting.

2 Review measuring foods by weight (ounces) vs volume (cups) and the difference between a level and heaping measuring cup/tablespoon.

3 Clarify that the serving size listed by gram weight on a food label is not the same as the number of grams of total carbohydrate per serving.

4 Use the patient's records to demonstrate patterns in food, medication, activity, and blood glucose levels. Ask the patient what they think is happening. Initially, the educator can interpret the results. The patient can assume increasing responsibility for this over time.

Key Educational Considerations—Level 2 Carbohydrate Counting

1   Assess the patient's skills in using information from nutrition labels and reference books. Based on the assessment, review information if necessary.

2   Assess the patient's understanding of how to calculate the nutrient content of complex foods and restaurant meals, and the protein, fat, and fiber content in foods. Based on the assessment, review information if necessary.

3   Have the patient demonstrate an understanding of pattern management in a stepwise approach: step 1, study the records; step 2, find and interpret the records; and step 3, have the patient decide what to do on their pattern reading.

Key Educational Considerations—Level 3 Carbohydrate Counting

1   Make sure that the patient understands insulin adjustment and supplementation before introducing a new element that requires insulin dose adjustment such as carbohydrate-to-insulin ratios.

2   After determining individual carbohydrate-to-insulin ratios, provide ample opportunities for the patient to complete paper-and-pencil exercises that simulate situations in which insulin adjustments would be needed for larger- or smaller-than-usual meals or snacks. Examples include weekend brunch, pizza parties, or a light lunch.

3   Assess the patient's ongoing ability to accurately estimate carbohydrate amounts. If portion control or estimating skills are questionable, the patient may need to review Level 1 or Level 2 carbohydrate counting and continue practicing skills from those levels.

4   Periodically review the patient's food, blood glucose, and physical activity records to ascertain appropriate use of carbohydrate-to-insulin ratios.

5   Monitor the patient's weight. If weight gain is a problem, emphasize portion control, limiting protein and fat intake, and using weight-management behaviors.

SELF-REVIEW QUESTIONS

1   List four major goals of nutritional therapy for persons with diabetes.

2   How many calories per gram do carbohydrate, protein, fat, and alcohol contribute to the energy content of the diet?

3   State the approximate percentage of calories from protein in meal plans. The percentage of calories from carbohydrate and fat are dependent on what two factors?

4   Describe how foods containing sucrose are used in a meal plan.

5   Name three types of nonnutritive sweeteners currently available on the market and four nutritive sweeteners that are frequently substituted for sucrose in food products.

6   What are the two types of dietary fiber? List two examples of each type. What effects do each type of fiber have on metabolic parameters?

7   State the recommendation for the use of alcoholic beverages for persons with type 1 diabetes. How is this different for the person with type 2 diabetes?

8   List three types of fatty acids found in foods. List three examples of foods containing each type of fatty acid. What is the major effect of each type of fatty acid on blood lipid levels?

9   State two major factors in determining a meal plan.

10   List six considerations for an individualized meal plan.

11   List the exchange lists. Each list is based on how many calories and grams of carbohydrate, protein, and fat?

12   Distinguish between initial versus continuing nutrition education.

13   Determine the approximate range of caloric requirement per day for an inactive man weighing 195 lb (75 kg).

14   Determine the approximate range of caloric requirement per day for an inactive woman weighing 165 lb (75 kg).

15   List four meal planning tools that can be used to teach meal planning guidelines to persons with diabetes.

16   Define carbohydrate counting.

17   List three factors to consider in selecting patients for Level 1 carbohydrate counting.

18   List two primary principles of Level 1 carbohydrate counting.

19   Describe portion size tools that are recommended for Level 1 carbohydrate counting.

20   List at least three sources of carbohydrate information.

21   List at least four factors to consider when determining target carbohydrate range.

22 State the definition of a "free food" when using carbohydrate counting.

23 List at least three teaching strategies useful to assess a client's carbohydrate counting knowledge and skills.

24 List three factors to consider in assessing if a patient is ready for Level 2 carbohydrate counting.

25 List the complex areas of calculation a patient has to learn for Level 2 carbohydrate counting.

26 List the three steps that are useful to assess a patient's skill in pattern management.

27 List three prerequisites for determining carbohydrate-to-insulin ratios.

28 State two primary principles of carbohydrate-to-insulin ratios.

29 Explain how to figure carbohydrate-to-insulin ratios using the carbohydrate gram method.

30 Explain how to figure carbohydrate-to-insulin ratios using the carbohydrate choice method.

31 Calculate how much insulin would be needed to cover 90 grams of carbohydrate for someone using a carbohydrate-to-insulin ratio of 15 grams of carbohydrate per 1 unit of insulin.

32 Calculate how much insulin would be needed to cover 7 carbohydrate choices for a person using 1 unit of insulin per carbohydrate choice.

33 State why patients using carbohydrate-to-insulin ratios also need to be concerned about intake of dietary fat and protein.

CASE STUDY 1

AJ is a 45-year-old woman who was diagnosed with type 2 diabetes 5 years ago. She has not been in for a medical checkup for 3 years. She decided to return at this time because of chronic fatigue and blurry vision. Her glycosylated hemoglobin (HbA$_{1c}$) is 8.3% (normal = 4% to 6%), cholesterol 214 mg/dL (5.5 mmol/L), triglycerides are 275 mg/dL (3.1 mmol/L). Her current weight is 175 lb (79.5 kg) and height is 5'4" in. (160 cm). She states that she hasn't returned for any follow-up visits because the only advice she gets is to lose weight and not eat sugar, neither of which she is able to do.

QUESTIONS FOR DISCUSSION

1 How should you deal with AJ's negative feelings about diabetes meal planning?

2 What are possible initial educational topics for AJ?

3 What are short-term meal planning strategies for AJ?

4 What information and educational tools might be helpful for AJ at this time?

5 How can continued education and counseling be planned and provided for AJ?

DISCUSSION

1 Start the session by asking AJ about her concerns about diabetes and the symptoms she is experiencing. Ask how she believes you can be most helpful to her.

2 The initial educational approaches that can be discussed with AJ include reviewing strategies that can be implemented for glucose control as well as weight loss. Ask if she is willing to identify a strategy to implement, and then review blood glucose monitoring and blood glucose goals with her.

3 Short-term meal planning options for AJ include learning to count carbohydrate servings at meals and snacks, spreading her carbohydrate and food intake throughout the day, and beginning some type of regular exercise.

4 AJ was introduced to carbohydrate counting. A simplified educational tool was used to help her understand that foods are grouped into carbohydrate, meat, and fat choices. Average portion sizes for different types of food were discussed. She felt that three to four carbohydrate choices at meals (breakfast, lunch, dinner), one to two carbohydrate choices for snacks (morning, afternoon, evening), 1 to 2 oz of meat at lunch, 3 to 4 oz of meat at supper, and 1 to 2 fat servings per meal would be a reasonable food plan. She also stated she would like to begin a walking program.

    A AJ agreed to keep food and blood glucose records and return in 2 weeks for a follow-up visit. At that visit she will have the opportunity to identify problems she is having with the strategies she chose. The dietitian and AJ can also evaluate the effect of the food and exercise changes on her blood glucose levels. Changes will be made as needed.

    B At 3 months AJ is to return for a glycosylated hemoglobin and triglyceride laboratory test. At that time, the decision can be made as to whether medical nutrition therapy and exercise alone are adequate or if there is a need to add an oral agent or other medications.

C At each visit, the emphasis should be on reaching blood glucose goals and not on weight loss.

Case Study 2—for Level 2 Carbohydrate Counting

JD is a 52-year-old male diagnosed with type 2 diabetes 6 years ago. His glycosylated hemoglobin is 7.8% (normal = 4.4% to 6.1%). He has hypertension and is on antihypertensive medication, has elevated triglycerides, and has low HDL cholesterol. He is taking glipizide 2.5 mg, TID. JD has been asked to test his blood glucose before breakfast, dinner, and at bedtime. His blood glucose goals are 80 to 150 mg/dL (4.5 to 8.5 mmol/L). Results (Figure 8.3) show that he is meeting his goals during the day, but his glucose readings before dinner and at bedtime are above the target goals.

JD is 5'10" (178 cm) tall and weighs 200 lb (91 kg) (desirable body weight = 166 to 172 lb [75 to 78 kg]). His weight goal is 180 lb (82 kg). The nutrition assessment shows JD eats three meals daily, and a midafternoon and evening snack. His current estimated daily caloric intake is 2300 to 2500 calories, while his estimated daily calorie needs are 1800 calories for weight loss of 1 lb per week. He eats breakfast at home, eats a homemade lunch at work, and has his evening meal at home. He used to drink two to three beers per day but has been avoiding alcohol lately. His physical activity consists of his work as a school custodian and walks to and from work Monday through Friday, (2 miles round trip).

JD states that he has attended diabetes classes and has been introduced to Level 1 carbohydrate counting. He had tried to focus on carbohydrate consistency and has been keeping a record of food intake, blood glucose levels, and physical activity. He has difficulty at dinner and bedtime, when he often overeats. He states that his wife is a good cook.

FIGURE 8.3. EXAMPLE OF DIABETES DAILY RECORD

Name: JD
BG Goal: 80 to 150 mg/dL

Day/Date	Time	Med/Insulin Type/Dose	BG, mg/dL Premeal	BG, mg/dL Postmeal	Food Intake Amt.	Food Intake Type (food/drink)	Carbohydrate Info Choices	Carbohydrate Info Grams	Exercise Type/Amount
Tues. 4/15	5:30 PM	Glucotrol/2.5 mg	160		4 oz	Ground beef		0	Watch TV
					8 oz	Baked potato		43 g	
					1 c	Corn		30 g	
								73 g Total	
	9:00 PM			212					
Wed. 4/16	5:30 PM	Glucotrol/2.5 mg	141		2 c	Macaroni and cheese		60 g	Shop, walk in mall 1 hour
					1 c	Green peas		30 g	
					1 pc	Bread		12 g	
								102 g Total	
	9:00 PM			183					
Thurs. 4/17	5:45 PM	Glucotrol/2.5 mg	170		3 pc	Fried chicken		27 g	Walk 15 minutes
					1 c	Mashed potatoes		30 g	
					1/2 c	Gravy		6 g	
					3 oz	Biscuit		34 g	
								97 g Total	

QUESTIONS FOR DISCUSSION

1   What level of carbohydrate counting is appropriate for JD? What factors serve as predictors?

2   Which skills should you emphasize at the first nutrition visits?

3   What resources or tools should you recommend to JD to help him be successful with nutrition management?

4   How can you determine JD's interest in his wife's involvement and her willingness to alter her cooking habits?

5   What strategies might help JD deal with his evening bedtime overeating?

DISCUSSION

1   JD is ready for Level 2 carbohydrate counting because he appears to have mastered Level 1 (ie, he is able to determine carbohydrate values of food by reading food labels and carbohydrate reference books). He has demonstrated skills in portion control by correctly weighing and measuring foods in diabetes classes. He is willing to keep records of food intake, blood glucose levels, and activity necessary for using blood glucose pattern management with a focus on the influence of carbohydrate foods.

2   It will be beneficial if JD is willing and able to purchase a carbohydrate reference book, a food weighing scale, and measuring cups so he can better control portions by weighing and measuring foods at home. By carefully evaluating food content, he can adjust portions as needed to meet carbohydrate goals for meals and snacks. JD should also test and record blood glucose levels at least three times a day on weekdays: before breakfast and supper and at bedtime. On weekends he should also test before lunch. JD should walk 30 minutes each day, preferably at the time that he notes higher blood glucose levels. JD should modify his food plan if needed to improve blood glucose levels. JD should omit his bedtime snack if his blood glucose level is over 150.

3   JD indicates that his wife is willing to alter her cooking and that he needs her help and support. He decides to ask his wife to use lower fat cooking methods, cook at least one non-starchy vegetable for dinner or provide salad with a reduced calorie dressing, and cook smaller amounts of food at night so he will not be tempted to eat second helpings.

4 JD and his wife's ability to read food labels and to estimate carbohydrate amounts consumed should be reevaluated. Confirm his ability to control portions and use measuring tools by actually weighing and measuring items. Suggest that he review blood glucose levels, food intake, and activity records to identify patterns of blood glucose levels outside the target range; analyze probable causes; and identify possible solutions.

5 Work with JD and his wife to develop a list of dinner menus and bedtime snacks that are lower carbohydrate substitutes for current foods eaten. Arrange for a follow-up visit to again review records for one to two weeks; focus on the interval between afternoon snack and bedtime when blood glucose levels have previously been out of the target range.

CASE STUDY 3

RO is a 31-year-old female who has had type 1 diabetes for 5 years with no complications except for trace microalbuminuria. She and her husband are interested in starting a family within the next year. Her glycosylated hemoglobin was 8.6% to 9% on the last two tests (normal = 4.4% to 6.1%). Her preconception blood glucose goals are preprandial 70 to 100 mg/dL and postprandial at 1 h <140 mg/dL and at 2 h < 120 mg/dL. RO's blood glucose levels have ranged between 50 and 250 mg/dL for the past month. Her insulin regimen is 9 units regular at breakfast, 8 units regular at lunch, 10 units regular at dinner, and 9 units NPH (human insulin) at bedtime. She has been advised to test blood glucose >7x/day (before meals, after meals, at bedtime, plus before and after exercise and when hypoglycemic). She uses a meter with memory but does not keep blood glucose records.

RO is five feet four inches (163 cm) tall and weighs 140 lb (63 kg). She has a medium body frame with a desirable body weight of 120 to 130 lb (54 to 59 kg), she identifies her goal weight as 120 to 125 lb (54 to 57 kg). She eats three meals daily plus afternoon and bedtime snacks. Her lunches are fast food and her afternoon snacks are from a vending machine. The amount of food that she eats varies greatly depending on where she is eating. She uses candy bars to treat hypoglycemia, and she usually eats more healthful, low-fat foods when at home than when eating out.

RO's estimated daily calorie intake is 1500 to 2400 calories; estimated daily calorie need for gradual weight loss is 1500 calories. Based on your assessment, the following macronutrient distribution has been recommended: 60% carbohydrate, 14% protein, 26% fat. The recommended distribution of carbohydrate is as follows: breakfast, 60 to 65 gm; lunch, 50 to 55 gm; afternoon snack, 15 gm; dinner, 70 to 75 gm; and bedtime snack, 25 to 30 gm.

RO is a married college graduate and a sales representative for a large company. She travels frequently (about one out-of-town trip per week) to large metropolitan areas. Her finances are adequate.

RO has been experiencing problems with mid-morning and late-afternoon hypoglycemia. Safety factors are a concern since she spends 2 to 4 hours a day driving. She is also concerned about weight gain from treating insulin reactions. She recently switched from a split, mixed insulin regimen (NPH and regular twice a day) to the current MDI regimen. She is still not able to reach her blood glucose goals and continues to experience hypoglycemic reactions.

RO has been working on carbohydrate counting with her dietitian and has agreed to a plan for 1500 calories with specific carbohydrate goals for meals and snacks. RO has not kept 2 weeks of careful blood glucose levels, food intake, and activity records as requested. However, she states that she is interested in learning how to adjust insulin for varying amounts of food.

QUESTIONS FOR DISCUSSION

1   What level of carbohydrate counting is appropriate for RO's current skills?

2   What carbohydrate counting skills or activities should RO work on prior to carbohydrate-to-insulin ratios? Where should you start?

3   How could you determine that RO is ready to learn carbohydrate-to-insulin ratios?

DISCUSSION

1 RO needs flexibility with carbohydrate consumption at meals and snacks because her job involves frequent eating out and unpredictable meal times and locations. To achieve optimal glycemic control under these circumstances, she needs to learn how to adjust her premeal regular insulin for varying amounts of carbohydrate. But first RO must establish carbohydrate consistency in order for insulin doses to be adjusted around a constant intake. She must proceed from basic or Level 1 carbohydrate counting through intermediate or Level 2 before she can develop accurate carbohydrate-to-insulin ratios at Level 3.

2 Nutrition and behavior change options that can be presented to RO include recording blood glucose levels before each meal, 2 hours after meals whenever possible, and at bedtime. In addition, for the first few days, she should test blood glucose at 3 AM. She could test and record her blood glucose more frequently before driving and before and after exercise. Options can include:

    A Faxing her blood glucose records to her diabetes educator weekly so that they can discuss insulin adjustments and supplementation. She should use her individualized 1500 calorie meal plan consisting of three meals and a bedtime snack with an optional additional snack for exercise. She should focus on consistency of carbohydrate intake and include protein with meals to help prevent hypoglycemia between meals.

    B Practicing portion control by weighing and measuring food when at home for at least 2 weeks. She can buy a carbohydrate reference book that includes fast food and chain restaurant information to help with estimates when traveling.

    C Keeping a food intake, blood glucose, and physical activity record for 2 weeks prior to her visit to the dietitian to learn carbohydrate/insulin ratios.

    D Developing a carbohydrate-to-insulin ratio to use for adjusting insulin to anticipated food intake.

3 RO is very quick to grasp the principles of carbohydrate counting, and with adequate motivation and cooperation, she can probably follow a fast track through Levels 1 and 2 of carbohydrate counting.

4 At the initial visit and assessment (60 to 90 minutes), the dietitian and RO will develop a meal plan that includes food choices when eating away from home. The dietitian will explain the rationale for discipline with consistency in meal timing and carbohydrate portion sizes to facilitate insulin adjustments leading to greater freedom and flexibility later with carbohydrate-to-insulin ratios. The dietitian will also assess RO's skills in weighing, measuring, and estimating portion sizes, using measuring tools, food labels, and carbohydrate resources and references. The dietitian can emphasize that the possibility of developing carbohydrate-to-insulin ratios at the next visit depends on meeting carbohydrate goals and completeness of records. RO will also send food records to the dietitian for feedback between visits.

5 At a follow-up visit 2 to 3 weeks later, the dietitian and RO will review food intake, physical activity, insulin, and blood glucose records. If insulin doses have been adjusted around consistent and accurate carbohydrate intake and target blood glucose levels are met, then they are ready to figure carbohydrate-to-insulin ratios. RO can practice with sample meals and snacks using carbohydrate-to-insulin ratios to make insulin dosage adjustments. Areas to discuss can include glycemic effects of protein, fat, and fiber; any possible insulin adjustments needed for large amounts of these nutrients; and discuss continued need for portion control and control of fat intake to maintain weight control. The need for follow-up based on telephone contact to discuss records or additional visits for more practices needs to be determined based on the results of this visit.

REFERENCES

1 Delahanty LM, Halford BN. The role of diet behaviors in achieving improved glycemic control in intensively treated patients in the diabetes control and complications trial. Diabetes Care 1993;16:1453-58.

2 Franz MJ, Monk A, Barry B, et al. Effectiveness of medical nutrition therapy provided by dietitians in the management of non-insulin-dependent diabetes mellitus: a randomized, controlled clinical trial. J Am Diet Assoc 1995;95:1009-17.

3 American Diabetes Association. Standards of medical care for patients with diabetes mellitus. Diabetes Care 1998;21(suppl 1):S23-S31.

4 American Diabetes Association. Nutrition recommendations and principles for people with diabetes mellitus. Diabetes Care 1998;21(suppl 1):S32-S35.

5 Franz MJ, Horton ES Sr, Bantle JP, et al. Nutrition principles for the management of diabetes and related complications: a technical review. Diabetes Care 1994;17:490-518.

6 American Association of Diabetes Educators. Position statement. Medical nutrition therapy for people with diabetes mellitus. Diabetes Educ 1995;21:17-18.

7 Expert Panel on Detection, Evaluation, and Treatment of High Blood Cholesterol in Adults. Summary of the second report of the National Cholesterol Education Program (NCEP) Expert Panel on detection, evaluation, and treatment of high blood cholesterol in adults (Adult Treatment Panel II). JAMA 1993;269:3015-23.

8 Brownell KD, Wadden TA. Etiology and treatment of obesity: understanding a serious, prevalent, and refractory disorder. J Consult Clin Psychol 1992;60:505-17.

9 Foreyt JP. Issues in the assessment and treatment of obesity. J Consult Clin Psychol 1987;55:677-84.

10 Wing RR, Blair EH, Bononi P, et al. Caloric restriction per se is a significant factor in improvements in glycemic control and insulin sensitivity during weight loss in obese NIDDM patients. Diabetes Care 1994;17:30-36.

11 Kelley DE, Wing R, Buonocore C, Sturis J, Polonsky K, Fitzsimmons M. Relative effects of calorie restriction and weight loss in non insulin-dependent diabetes mellitus. J Clin Endocrinol Metab 1993;77:1287-93.

12 Watts NB, Spanheimer RG, DiGirolamo M, et al. Prediction of glucose response to weight loss in patients with non-insulin-dependent diabetes mellitus. Arch Intern Med 1990;150:803-6.

13 Wing RR, Koeske R, Epstein LH, et al. Long-term effects of modest weight loss in type II diabetic patients. Arch Intern Med 1987;147:1749-53.

14 Bjorntorp P. Metabolic implications of body fat distribution. Diabetes Care 1991;14:1132-43.

15 DeFronzo RA, Ferrannini E. Insulin resistance. A multifaceted syndrome responsible for NIDDM, obesity, hypertension, dyslipidemia, and atherosclerotic cardiovascular disease. Diabetes Care 1991;14:173-94.

16 Burton BT, Foster WR. Health implications of obesity: an NIH consensus development conference. J Am Diet Assoc 1985;85:1117-21.

17 Jenkins DJ, Ocana A, Jenkins AL, et al. Metabolic advantages of spreading the nutrient load: effects of increased meal frequency in non-insulin-dependent diabetes. Am J Clin Nutr 1992;55:461-67.

18 Bertelsen J, Christiansen C, Thomsen C, et al. Effect of meal frequency on blood glucose, insulin, and free fatty acids in NIDDM subjects. Diabetes Care 1993; 16:4-7.

19 Ruggiero L, Prochaska JO, eds. Readiness for change, application of the transtheoretical model to diabetes. Diabetes Spectrum 1993;6:21-60.

20 American Diabetes Association. Exercise and NIDDM: a technical review. Diabetes Care 1990;13:785-89.

21 American Diabetes Association. Position statement. Diabetes mellitus and exercise. Diabetes Care 1997;20(suppl 1):S51.

22 Monk A, Barry B, McClain K, et al. Practice guidelines for medical nutrition therapy provided by dietitians for persons with non-insulin-dependent diabetes mellitus. J Am Diet Assoc 1995;95:999-1006.

23 Henry RR. Protein content of the diabetic diet. Diabetes Care 1994;17:1502-13.

24 Joslin EP, Root HF, White P, Marble A. The treatment of diabetes mellitus. Philadelphia: Lea & Febiger, 1935.

25 The DCCT Research Group. Nutrition interventions for intensive therapy in the diabetes control and complications trial. J Am Diet Assoc 1993;93:768-72.

26 Peters AL, Davidson MB. Protein and fat effects on glucose responses and insulin requirements in subjects with insulin-dependent diabetes mellitus. Am J Clin Nutr 1993;58:555-60.

27 Nuttall FQ, Mooradian AD, Giannon MC, Billington C, Krezowski P. Effect of protein ingestion on the glucose and insulin response to a standardized oral glucose load. Diabetes Care 1984;7:465-70.

28 Gray RO, Butler PC, Beers TR, Kryshak EJ, Rizza RA. Comparison of the ability of bread versus bread plus meat to treat and prevent subsequent hypoglycemia in patients with insulin-dependent diabetes mellitus. J Clin Endocrinol Metab 1996;81:1508-11.

29 American Diabetes Association. Diabetic nephropathy: position statement. Diabetes Care 1998;21(suppl 1):S50-S53.

30 Brodsky IG, Robbins DC, Hiser E, et al. Effects of low-protein diets on protein metabolism in insulin-dependent diabetes mellitus patients with early nephropathy. J Clin Endocrinol Metab 1992;75:351-57.

31 Bantle JP, Swanson JE, Thomas W, Laine DC. Metabolic effects of dietary sucrose in type II diabetic subjects. Diabetes Care 1993;16:1301-5.

32 Peterson DB, Lambert J, Gerring S. et al. Sucrose in the diet of diabetic patients - just another carbohydrate? Diabetologia 1986;29:216-20.

33 Loghmani E, Rickard K, Washburne L, et al. Glycemic response to sucrose-containing mixed meals in diets of children with insulin-dependent diabetes mellitus. J Pediatrics 1991;119:531-37.

34 Franz MJ. Avoiding sugar: does research support traditional beliefs? Diabetes Educ 1993;19:144-46, 148, 150.

35 Nuttall FQ, Gannon MC, Burmeister LA, et al. The metabolic response to various doses of fructose in type II diabetic subjects. Metabolism 1992;41:510-17.

36 Butchko HH, Kotsonis FN. Acceptable daily intake vs actual intake: the aspartame example. J Am Coll Nutr 1991;10:258-66.

37 Hendra TJ, Britton ME, Roper DR, et al. Effects of fish oil supplements in NIDDM subjects: Controlled study. Diabetes Care 1990;13:821-29.

38 American Diabetes Association. Position statement. Role of fat replacers in diabetes medical nutrition therapy. Diabetes Care 1998;21:S64-S65.

39 Warshaw H, Franz M, Powers MA, Wheeler M. Fat replacers: their use in foods and role in diabetes medical nutrition therapy: a technical review. Diabetes Care 1996;19:1294-1301.

40 Tuck M, Corry D, Trujillo A. Salt-sensitive blood pressure and exaggerated vascular reactivity in the hypertension of diabetes mellitus. Am J Med 1990;88:210-16.

41 Mooradian AD, Failla M, Hoogwerf B, Maryniuk M, Wylie-Rosett J. Selected vitamins and minerals in diabetes mellitus: a technical review. Diabetes Care 1994; 17:464-79.

42 American Diabetes Association. Concensus statement. Magnesium supplementation in the treatment of diabetes. Diabetes Care 1996;19(suppl 1):S93-S95.

43 Franz MJ. Alcohol and diabetes: its metabolism and guidelines for occasional use, parts I and II. Diabetes Spectrum 1990;3:136-144, 210-16.

44 Koivisto VA, Tulokas S, Toivonen M, et al. Alcohol with the meal has no adverse effects on postprandial glucose homeostasis in diabetic patients. Diabetes Care 1993;16:1612-14.

45 Gin H, Morlat P, Ragnaud JM, Aubertin J. Short-term effect of red wine (consumed during meals) on insulin requirement and glucose tolerance in diabetic patients. Diabetes Care 1992;15:546-48.

46 Tinker LF, Heins JM, Holler HJ. Commentary and translation: 1994 nutrition recommendations for diabetes. J Am Diet Assoc 1994;94:507-11.

47 Diabetes Care and Education. Nutrition practice guidelines for type I diabetes mellitus. Chicago: American Dietetic Association, 1996.

48 Exchange lists for meal planning. Alexandria, Va and Chicago: American Diabetes Association and American Dietetic Association, 1995.

49 American Diabetes Association. Maximizing the role of nutrition in diabetes management. Alexandria, Va: American Diabetes Association, 1994.

50 Holler HJ, Pastors JG. Diabetes medical nutrition therapy: a professional guide to management and nutrition education resources. Chicago: American Dietetic Association, 1997.

51 Wheeler ML, Franz M, Barrier P, Holler H, Cronmiller N, Delahanty LM. Macronutrient and energy database for the 1995 exchange lists for meal planning: a rationale for clinical practice decisions. J Am Diet Assoc 1996; 96:1167-71.

52 US Department of Agriculture, US Department of Health and Human Services. Nutrition and your health: dietary guidelines for Americans. 4th ed. Hyattsville, MD: USDA Human Nutrition Information Service, 1995.

53 National Dairy Council. Guide to good eating. Rosemont, Il: National Dairy Council, 1992.

54 US Department of Agriculture. The food guide pyramid. Hyattsville, Md: USDA Human Nutrition Information Service, 1992.

55 The first step in diabetes meal planning. Alexandria, Va and Chicago: American Diabetes Association and American Dietetic Association, 1995.

56 Healthy food choices. Alexandria, Va and Chicago: American Diabetes Association and American Dietetic Association, 1986.

57 Healthy eating for people with diabetes. Minneapolis: International Diabetes Center, 1997.

58 Single-topic diabetes resources. Alexandria, Va and Chicago: American Diabetes Association and American Dietetic Association, 1996.

59 Month of meals 1, 2, 3, 4, 5: menu planner. Alexandria, Va: American Diabetes Association, 1989, 1990, 1992, 1993, 1994.

60 Carbohydrate counting: adding flexibility to your food choices. Minneapolis: International Diabetes Center, 1994.

61 Carbohydrate counting: getting started (level 1). Alexandria, Va and Chicago: American Diabetes Association and American Dietetic Association, 1996.

62 Carbohydrate counting: moving on (level 2). Alexandria, Va and Chicago: American Diabetes Association and American Dietetic Association, 1996.

63 Carbohydrate counting: using carbohydrate/insulin ratios (level 3). Alexandria, Va and Chicago: American Diabetes Association and American Dietetic Association, 1996.

64 My food plan. Mi plan de comidas. Minneapolis: International Diabetes Center, 1996.

65 Facilitating lifestyle change: a resource manual. Alexandria, Va and Chicago: American Diabetes Association and American Dietetic Association, 1996.

66 Schafer RG, Bohannon B, Franz M, et al. Translation of the diabetes nutrition recommendations for health care institutions: a technical review. Diabetes Care 1997;20:96-105.

67 American Diabetes Association. Translation of the diabetes nutrition recommendations for health care institutions. Diabetes Care 1998;21(suppl 1): S66-S68.

68 Coulston AM, Mandelbaum D, Reaven GM, Dietary management of nursing home residents with non-insulin-dependent diabetes mellitus. Am J Clin Nutr 1990;51:67-71.

69 American Diabetes Association. Food labeling. Diabetes Care 1998;21(suppl 1):S64-S65.

70 Wheeler ML, Franz MJ, Heins J, et al. Food labeling: a technical review. Diabetes Care 1994;17:480-87.

71 Kittler PG, Sucher KP. Diet counseling in multicultural society. Diabetes Educ 1990;16:127-34.

72 Joslin EP. The diabetic diet. J Am Diet Assoc 1927;(3):89-92.

73 Nuttall FQ. Carbohydrate and dietary management of individuals with insulin-requiring diabetes. Diabetes Care 1993;16:1039-42.

74 Nuttall FQ, Gannon MC. Plasma glucose and insulin response to macronutrients in nondiabetic and NIDDM subjects. Diabetes Care 1991;14:824-38.

75 Dinneen S, Gerich J, Rizza R. Carbohydrate metabolism in non-insulin-dependent diabetes mellitus. N Engl J Med 1992;327:707-13.

76 West JB, ed. Regulation of carbohydrate metabolism. In: Best and Taylor's physiological basis of medical practice. Baltimore, Md: Williams & Wilkins, 1991:729-40.

77 American Diabetes Association. Position statement. Nutrition recommendations and principles for people with diabetes mellitus. J Am Diet Assoc 1994;94:504-6.

78 Daly A, Barry B, Gillespie S, Kulkarni K, Richardson M. Carbohydrate counting: getting started. Alexandria, Va and Chicago: American Diabetes Association and American Dietetic Association, 1995.

79 Daly A, Barry B, Gillespie S, Kulkarni K, Richardson, M. Carbohydrate counting: moving on. Alexandria, Va and Chicago: American Diabetes Association and American Dietetic Association, 1995.

80 Daly A, Barry B, Gillespie S, Kulkarni K, Richardson, M. Carbohydrate counting: using carbohydrate/insulin ratios. Alexandria, Va and Chicago: American Diabetes Association and American Dietetic Association, 1995.

81 Geil PB. Complex and simple carbohydrates in diabetes therapy. In: Powers MA, ed. Handbook of diabetes medical nutrition therapy. Gaithersburg, Md: Aspen Publishers Inc, 1996:303-19.

82 Wursch P. Dietary fiber and unabsorbed carbohydrates. In: Gracey M, Kretchmer N, Rossi E, eds. Sugars in nutrition. Vol. 25. New York: Raven, 1991:153-68.

83 Ahern JA, Gatcomb PM, Held NA, Petit WA Jr, WA, Tamborlane WV. Exaggerated hyperglycemia after a pizza meal in well-controlled diabetes. Diabetes Care 1993;16:578-80.

SUGGESTED READINGS

American Diabetes Association. Maximizing the role of nutrition in diabetes management. Alexandria, VA: American Diabetes Association, 1994.

Babione L. SMBG: the underused nutrition counseling tool in diabetes management. Diabetes Spectrum 1994;7:196-97.

Beebe CA, Pastors JG, Powers MA, Wylie-Rosett J. Nutrition management for individuals with non insulin-dependent diabetes mellitus in the 1990s: a review by the Diabetes Care and Education Dietetic Practice Group. J Am Diet Assoc 1991;91:196-207.

Brackenridge B. Carbohydrate counting for diabetes nutrition therapy. In: Powers MA, ed. Handbook of diabetes medical nutrition therapy. Gaithersburg, Md: Aspen Publishers Inc, 1996:255-67.

Brackenridge B. Carbohydrate counting: managing your nutrition. In: Walsh J, Roberts R. Pumping insulin: everything in a book for successful use of an insulin pump. San Diego, Calif: Torrey Pines Press 1994:35-45.

Connell JE, Thomas-Dobersen D. Nutritional management of children and adolescents with insulin-dependent diabetes mellitus: a review by the Diabetes Care and Education Dietetic Practice Group. J Am Diet Assoc 1991;91:1556-64.

Daly A. A graduated approach to carbohydrate counting. Practical Diabetol 1996;15(1):19-23.

Daly A, Gillespie S, Kulkarni K. Carbohydrate counting: vignettes from the trenches. Diabetes Spectrum 1996;9:114-17.

Diabetes Care and Education Practice Group. Nutrition practice guidelines for type 1 and type 2 diabetes mellitus. Chicago: American Dietetic Association, 1996.

Fagen C, King JD, Erick M. Nutrition management in women with gestational diabetes mellitus: a review by ADA Diabetes Care and Education Dietetic Practice Group. J Am Diet Assoc 1995; 95:460-67.

Foster-Powell K, Miller JB. International tables of glycemic index. Am J Clin Nutr 1995;62:871S-893S.

Franz MJ. Exchanges for all occasions. Minneapolis, Minn: International Diabetes Center, 1997.

Franz MJ, Etzwiler DD, Joynes JO, Hollander P. Learning to live well with diabetes. Minneapolis: Chronimed Inc, 1991.

Fredrickson L, ed. The insulin pump therapy book. Insights from the experts. Los Angeles: MiniMed Technologies, 1995.

Gillespie S, Kulkarni K, Daly A. Using carbohydrate counting in diabetes clinical practice. Submitted for publication J Am Diet Assoc.

Gregory RP, Davis DL. Use of carbohydrate counting for meal planning in type I diabetes. Diabetes Educ 1994;20:406-9.

Lyon RB, Vinci SM. Nutritional management of insulin-dependent diabetes mellitus in adulthood: a review by the Diabetes Care and Education Dietetic Practice Group. J Am Diet Assoc 1993;93:309-314, 317.

Maryniuk M. Nutrition education: taking it one step at a time. Diabetes Educ 1990;16:26-28.

Pastors JG. Alternatives to the exchange system for teaching meal planning to persons with diabetes. Diabetes Educ 1992;18:57-64.

Powers MA, ed. Handbook of diabetes nutritional management. Rockville, Md: Aspen Publishers Inc, 1996.

Tinker LF, Heins JM, Holler HJ. Commentary and translation: 1994 nutrition recommendations for diabetes. J Am Diet Assoc 1994;94:507-11.

Wasserman DH, Zinman B. Exercise in individuals with IDDM: a technical review. Diabetes Care 1994;17:924-37.

Woodyatt RT. Objects and method of diet adjustment in diabetes. Arch Intern Med 1921;28:125-42.

Carbohydrate Counting Resource Books

Exchange lists for meal planning. Alexandria, Va and Chicago: American Diabetes Association and American Dietetic Association, 1995.

Franz M. Exchanges for all occasions. 4th ed. Minneapolis: Chronimed Publishing, 1997.

Holzmeister LA. The diabetes carbohydrate and fat gram guide. Alexandria, Va and Chicago: American Diabetes Association and American Dietetic Association, 1997.

Kraus B. Calories and carbohydrates. 11th ed. New York: Plume, 1996.

Netzer C. The complete book of food counts. New York: Dell Publishing Co, 1997.

Netzer C. The Corinne T. Netzer carbohydrate gram counter. New York: Dell Publishing, 1994.

Pennington J. Food values of portions commonly used. New York: JB Lippincott Company, 1994.

Eating Out, Convenience, and Fast Food Guides

Franz M. Fast food facts. 5th ed. Minneapolis: Chronimed Publishing, 1998.

Monk A. Convenience food facts. Minneapolis: Chronimed Publishing, 1996.

Month of meals, 1, 2, 3, 4, 5: menu planner. Alexandria, Va: American Diabetes Association, 1989, 1990, 1992, 1993, 1994.

Nutrition in the fast lane. Indianapolis: Franklin Publishing Inc, 1996.

Warshaw H, Ob A. American Diabetes Association's guide to healthy eating in family and chain restaurants. Alexandria, Va: Am Diabetes Association, 1997.

THERAPIES

Exercise

Joy A. Kistler, MS, CDE
Joslin Diabetes Center
Boston, Massachusetts

INTRODUCTION

1 The beneficial effects of exercise in treating diabetes were recognized as early as the ancient times.[1] Centuries later in the 1920s, exercise was first recommended as a therapeutic tool for lowering blood glucose levels.[2,3]

2 Today, exercise is regarded as a primary component of diabetes management.

3 Much of the morbidity and mortality among persons with diabetes is attributed to cardiovascular disease. Epidemiological evidence[4] suggests that regular exercise and physical fitness are associated with decreased cardiovascular disease in the general population, as well as a decreased occurrence of type 2 diabetes.

4 Because individuals with diabetes are living longer, the prevalence of diabetes in the elderly and the number of people with diabetic complications are increasing. Consequently, the role of exercise becomes even more significant.

5 This chapter focuses on the benefits, effects, risks, and precautions of exercise for persons with diabetes. Also discussed are exercise options for special populations, strategies for enhancing exercise, and guidelines for developing exercise prescriptions and strategies for self-directed exercise programs.

OBJECTIVES

Upon completion of this chapter, the learner will be able to

1 State the benefits of exercise.
2 Describe the physiologic response to exercise in individuals with and without diabetes.
3 Identify the risks associated with exercise and ways to minimize them.
4 Explain the principles of an exercise program for people with diabetes.
5 Identify appropriate exercise therapies for special populations.
6 Describe strategies for self-directed exercise programs.

BENEFITS OF EXERCISE

1   Exercise generally is regarded as having a salutary effect for everyone. The benefits are many and may be even more favorable for the person with diabetes.

2   Most of the benefits result from chronic (regular, long-term), aerobic (cardiovascular) exercise.

3   Resistance exercise to increase muscle strength is an important means of preserving and increasing muscular strength and endurance, and of preventing falls and increasing mobility among the elderly.[5]

4   Because persons with diabetes have an increased risk of cardiovascular disease, the role of exercise in reducing modifiable risks has primary importance. The potential benefits of exercise for persons with diabetes include[6,7]

   A   Improved functioning of the cardiovascular system

   B   Improved strength and physical work capacity

   C   Decreased risk factors for coronary artery disease (CAD)
- Reduction in plasma cholesterol, triglycerides, and low-density lipoproteins (LDL)
- Increase in high-density lipoproteins (HDL), particularly in the presence of weight loss

   D   Increased insulin sensitivity[7,8]

   E   Reduced hyperinsulinemia, a proposed risk factor for atherosclerosis[9-11]

   F   Enhanced fibrinolysis
- Hypercoagulability frequently is present in persons with diabetes
- Chronic exercise can enhance fibrinolysis and affect other mechanisms responsible for this hypothesized risk factor for atherosclerosis[12,13]

   G   Favorable changes in body composition (reduction of body fat and weight, and increase in muscle mass)

   H   Adjunct therapy for controlling hypertension

   I   Improved quality of life and self-esteem, and reduced psychological stress[14]

5   The chronic effects of exercise appear to benefit the person with type 2 diabetes by reducing HbA$_{1c}$, improving insulin sensitivity, assisting in attainment and maintenance of desirable body weight, and decreasing CAD risk factors.[15]

A Several long-term studies[16-19] demonstrate a sustained improvement in glucose control while a regular exercise program is maintained.

B Thus, exercise is an essential component of diabetes self-management education for all individuals with type 2 diabetes.

6 Exercise is also a critical part of the overall diabetes self-management education of type 1 diabetes, especially in light of the increased risk for macrovascular disease in this patient population.

A Regular exercise in type 1 has not been shown consistently to result in improved diabetes control as evidenced by HbA$_{1c}$.[20-22] This finding may be due to the difficulty of balancing insulin adjustments with food in concordance with physical activity.

B It may be possible, however, for select patients to obtain a sustained decrease in HbA$_{1c}$.[23-26]

C Recommendations for the prevention of exercise-induced hypoglycemia must be included in the exercise plan and educational program.

7 Because of its effects on self-esteem and stress reduction, the addition of a regular exercise program can serve as the first step in self-directed behavior change for many patients.

PHYSIOLOGY OF EXERCISE IN INDIVIDUALS WITHOUT DIABETES

1 Plasma glucose levels in individuals without diabetes who exercise remain relatively stable due to an intricate regulation between the increase in glucose uptake by exercising muscles and increased hepatic glucose production.[27]

2 The contribution of carbohydrate (stored as glycogen in the liver and muscles) and fat (stored as triglyceride in adipose tissue) depends on exercise intensity, duration, fitness level, and time and content of the last meal.[6,28] This regulation involves a hormonal balance between decreased insulin secretion and increased action of catecholamines, glucagon, growth hormone, and cortisol (counterregulatory hormones).

A At the onset of exercise, fuel utilization by muscles progresses from fat (extracted from the bloodstream as free fatty acids [FFA] at rest) to high energy phosphate compounds, such as adenosine triphosphate (ATP) and phosphocreatine (CP), to glucose utilization from intramuscular stores of glucose and triglycerides.

- The immediate fuel sources available for muscle contraction are ATP and CP. The breakdown of these high-energy phosphate compounds contributes to the immediate resynthesis of ATP (the primary fuel source for muscle contraction).
- ATP and CP stores are limited and can only supply the energy needs of quick, powerful movements, such as sprinting for time periods of 8 to 12 seconds.
- As exercise moves from the quick, initial muscle action to an extended exercise session, the fuel supply for the contracting muscles shifts from the immediate high energy phosphate groups to the second system from which ATP is produced (glycolysis).[29]

B During the first few minutes of exercise, intramuscular glucose is broken down anaerobically (without oxygen present). Although this pathway does not provide an abundant quantity of ATP, this pathway is important at the onset of exercise when oxygen availability is limited. As exercise continues, an adequate supply of oxygen becomes available for the breakdown of carbohydrates, fats, and proteins, if necessary, for the resynthesis of ATP.

- During sustained exercise, carbohydrate, protein, and fat continually recharge the phosphate pool.
- After the first 5 to 10 minutes, glycogen breakdown decreases, as circulating glucose from the liver becomes a major fuel source (hepatic glycogenolysis).[30]

C As exercise continues beyond 20 to 30 minutes, the muscle glycogen stores are depleted. Plasma glucose is maintained as glucose is broken down from the liver (hepatic glycogenolysis) and free fatty acids (FFA) (triglycerides mobilized from adipose tissue) are utilized.

- At the beginning of exercise, hepatic glucose production is mainly derived from glycogenolysis.
- As exercise continues, gluconeogenesis becomes increasingly important in providing glucose. The main substrates for hepatic gluconeogenesis during exercise are lactate, amino acids, and glycerol.

D As exercise duration increases, the contribution of FFA as a fuel increases relative to glucose, from about 35% at 40 minutes of exercise to nearly 70% at 4 hours of exercise.[6,30]

- Exercise of low-to-moderate intensity relies primarily on FFA as the oxidative fuel for muscle.[6]

- The oxidation of fat-derived fuels cannot replace the utilization of glucose. When carbohydrate is limited, fat is not completely oxidized and ketone bodies are formed.

E Hormonal response to exercise determines substrate utilization during exercise (Table 9.1).

- Secretion of counterregulatory hormones increases and helps maintain glucose homeostasis.[26,31]
- Insulin secretion is decreased during exercise as a result of increased activity of the sympathetic nervous system.[31,32]
- The suppression of insulin secretion facilitates hepatic glucose production and lipolysis, which allows blood glucose to be maintained.[28,30,34]

F An ongoing increased uptake of glucose by muscle occurs during the postexercise period as one means of replenishing glycogen stores.

- Replenishment of glycogen stores may take 24 to 48 hours.[6,35]
- The postexercise recovery, particularly after exhaustive work, is characterized by enhanced insulin sensitivity.[36,37]

TABLE 9.1. HORMONAL RESPONSE AND METABOLIC EFFECTS DURING EXERCISE IN INDIVIDUALS WITHOUT DIABETES

Hormone	Response During Exercise	Metabolic Effect
Insulin	⬇	• Facilitates hepatic glucose and FFA production
Glucagon	⬆	• Increases hepatic glucose production, increases blood glucose
Epinephrine	⬆	• Stimulates FFA production which provides glycerol as a substrate for glucogenesis
Norepinephrine	⬆	• Stimulates hepatic and muscle glycolysis, stimulates lipolysis
Growth hormone/cortisol	⬆	• Increases lipolysis, decreases insulin-stimulated glucose uptake, increases gluconeogenic substrates

G Trained athletes demonstrate the following responses:
  • A reduction in fasting insulin secretion in response to a glucose load
  • An increase in muscle sensitivity to insulin despite reduced insulin secretion[28,38]
  • Less of a generalized secretion of counterregulatory hormones than sedentary individuals[32]
  • Less glucose utilization than sedentary individuals during exercise that is of similar intensity and duration and, as a result, a slower rate of duration and, as glycogen usage as well as a greater reliance on fats for fuel, which are associated with greater endurance[31,32]

PHYSIOLOGY OF EXERCISE IN INDIVIDUALS WITH DIABETES

1 A person with diabetes who exercises may have a decreased need for, or better utilization of, insulin; the result may be a decrease in diabetes medications needed to reach glucose goals.

  A Acute effects of exercise generally cause a reduction in plasma glucose.

  B Chronic exercise results in improved insulin sensitivity and glucose tolerance, because of changes in body composition and the additive effects of daily exercise.

  C The hormonal response to exercise depends on the degree of diabetes control, medication, time and content of the last meal, fitness level, and type of exercise.
  • Because the person with type 1 diabetes does not have a normal compensatory decrease in insulin secretion with exercise, metabolic abnormalities may occur.[9,27,32,34,39]

2 Hypoglycemia is the most commonly encountered problem in individuals with diabetes who exercise and are treated with insulin or sulfonylureas.

  A Normally, plasma insulin decreases with exercise in individuals without diabetes. This decrease, along with increases in plasma counterregulatory hormones, allows hepatic glucose production and lipolysis to match glucose utilization.

  B In persons with diabetes taking insulin, the plasma insulin concentration does not decrease. Because the insulin is exogenous in origin, the plasma insulin concentration actually may increase due to increased sensitivity or mobilization from subcutaneous depots (Table 9.2).

Table 9.2. Factors That Contribute to Hypoglycemia in Type 1 Diabetes

- Accelerated absorption of insulin
- Nonsuppressible plasma insulin levels
- Increased insulin sensitivity
- Possible impaired counterregulatory hormonal response

- A high plasma insulin level during exercise may enhance glucose uptake and further stimulate glucose oxidation in the exercising muscle.[7]
- A high plasma insulin level inhibits hepatic glucose production and FFA mobilization.[34] As a result, hepatic glucose production does not keep pace with peripheral glucose utilization and the blood glucose concentration falls.
- Hypoglycemia also can result from exercise in patients with type 2 diabetes treated with sulfonylureas.[40] These individuals are less prone to exercise-induced hypoglycemia, although it still can occur, and very rarely develop hyperglycemia with ketosis. Improvements in insulin sensitivity, insulin secretion, and glucose disposal rates have been well documented in type 2 diabetes as a result of regular exercise, although the mechanisms underlying these improvements have not been clearly explained.[7,41] Changes in body composition (decrease in fat weight and increase in muscle mass) contribute to increasing sensitivity to endogenous and exogenous insulin. The potential result is a reduction in exogenous insulin and/or oral hypoglycemic agents.

3 Another major concern for persons with diabetes who are taking insulin or sulfonylureas, particularly those with type 1 diabetes, is *post-exercise, late-onset hypoglycemia* (PEL), hypoglycemia occurring 4 or more hours following exercise.

   A PEL generally occurs following exercise of moderate to high intensity with a duration greater than 30 minutes.

   B PEL results from increased insulin sensitivity, ongoing glucose utilization, and repletion of glycogen stores.[42]

4   In type 1 individuals with hyperglycemia and/or ketosis, acute exercise may result in a worsening of metabolic control.[7,33]   A certain amount of insulin is required for glucose uptake.   In the absence of adequate insulin, exercise raises plasma glucose, FFA, and ketones (Table 9.3).

5   Exercise of a high intensity can also cause blood glucose levels to be higher after exercise than before, even though blood glucose levels are in the normal range before beginning exercise. This hyperglycemia can also extend into the postexercise state and is mediated by the counterregulatory hormones. Hepatic glucose production no longer matches, but in fact, exceeds the rise in glucose use.[43-45]

TABLE 9.3. CONSEQUENCES OF INSUFFICIENT INSULIN

- Impaired peripheral glucose utilization
- Excessive counterregulatory hormones
- Enhanced hepatic glucose production, lipolysis, and ketogenesis
- Rapid rise in already elevated blood glucose level and increased ketosis

---

SPECIAL CONSIDERATIONS AND PRECAUTIONS OF EXERCISE

1   The primary side effect of acute exercise is hypoglycemia. Occasionally, hyperglycemia and ketosis also occur in individuals with type 1 diabetes (Table 9.4).

    A   Blood glucose response to exercise is affected by the type, amount, and intensity of exercise; the timing and type of previous meal and medication; the preexercise blood glucose level; and the fitness level.[8,29,30]

    B   Hypoglycemia is a significant threat to persons who exercise while taking insulin or sulfonylureas; persons who use meal planning and exercise alone to control type 2 diabetes are not at risk of hypoglycemia when exercising.

    C   General guidelines to either increase carbohydrate consumption or decrease medication(s) are based on planned vs unplanned exercise. Provide initial guidelines, then adjust them based on the individual's response to the exercise program.

TABLE 9.4. RISKS OF EXERCISE IN PERSONS WITH DIABETES

Hypoglycemia (if diabetes is treated with insulin or sulfonylureas)
- Exercise-induced hypoglycemia
- Postexercise, late-onset hypoglycemia (PEL)

Hyperglycemia after very strenuous exercise

Hyperglycemia and ketosis in insulin-deficient patients

Precipitation or exacerbation of cardiovascular disease
- Presence of silent heart disease: arrhythmia, cardiac dysfunction
- Excessive increases in blood pressure with exercise
- Angina pectoris
- Myocardial infarction
- Sudden death

Worsening of long-term complications
- Proliferative retinopathy: vitreous hemorrhage, retinal detachment
- Nephropathy: increased proteinuria
- Peripheral neuropathy: soft tissue and joint injury, foot ulcers, orthopedic injury
- Autonomic neuropathy: decreased cardiovascular response to exercise, decreased maximum aerobic capacity, impaired response to dehydration, orthostatic hypotension, impaired counterregulatory response

Source: Adapted from Horton ES. *Prescription for exercise.* Diabetes Spectrum 1991;4:250-57.

2   Exercise-induced hypoglycemia can be largely prevented by implementing certain guidelines.

   A   During planned exercise/activity, the following self-management tasks can reduce the risk of hypoglycemia.

- Adjustments are needed to prevent hypoglycemia in the insulin-treated individual because hepatic glucose production is blocked or partially inhibited by exogenous insulin.[29,34] The physiological decrease in circulating insulin levels that occurs with exercise cannot take place in patients treated with insulin.
- A reduction of the short-acting insulin of 30% to 50% has been demonstrated to decrease the risk of hypoglycemia.[46]
- Also effective would be to decrease the insulin acting during the time of exercise by 10% of the total daily insulin.
- When using rapid-acting insulin, such as lispro insulin, exercising 2 to 3 hours after a meal will prevent hypoglycemia.[47]
- The insulin dose may need to be reduced substantially, by as much as 50%, for vigorous or prolonged exercise.[3]

- The recommendation to change the injection site to a part of the body not involved in the activity to prevent hypoglycemia was based on published reports in the 1970s.[48] These studies demonstrated an increase in serum insulin levels in patients who exercised shortly after an insulin injection. The recommendation to inject in the arm or abdomen instead of the leg if the activity was jogging or cycling emerged from these studies. Despite the increased absorption rate, subsequent research[49] demonstrated that simply changing the insulin injection site was not effective for preventing hypoglycemia. If the level of circulating insulin is elevated for any reason, hypoglycemia is likely to occur. Dose reductions should accompany any exercise that is performed during the peak action of the insulin.[50]
- Teach patients to avoid intramuscular injection of insulin because muscle contractions accelerate the absorption of insulin into the circulation.[50]
- Blood glucose monitoring before and after exercise provides needed feedback for the patient who is learning to adjust insulin and/or carbohydrate (CHO) with exercise.
- Tailor any adjustments to the specific exercise response of each individual (Table 9.5). The choice between decreasing medication or increasing carbohydrate will depend on the patient's goals.

TABLE 9.5. EXERCISE ADJUSTMENTS

	Patient Goals
Insulin Adjustment	• Weight loss • Improved control • Planned, regularly scheduled exercise
CHO Replacement	• Long duration of exercise • Unplanned exercise

B During unplanned exercise/activity, carbohydrate replacement may be necessary to prevent hypoglycemia when insulin adjustments are not made or when exercise occurs several hours after a meal.

- The amount of additional carbohydrate needed depends on the time of exercise in relation to medication and previous meal; the type, intensity, and duration of exercise (Table 9.6); and the preexercise blood glucose level.
- Exercise performed 1 to 3 hours after a meal may not require any additional carbohydrate supplement.
- Moderate intensity exercise (<50% maximum oxygen uptake) increases glucose uptake by the muscle 2 to 3 mg/kg/body weight/min above resting levels. For example, a 154 lb (70 kg) individual would require an additional 140 to 210 mg of glucose for every minute of moderate exercise. This would mean an additional 8.4 to 12.6 g of glucose is required for every hour of exercise.
- For high intensity exercise, the rate of glucose utilization by the muscle may increase to as much as 5 to 6 ml/kg/body weight/min or an additional 350 to 420 mg of glucose for every minute of exercise. Even though the rate of glucose utilization increases, the demand on glucose stores and risk of hypoglycemia is less, because exercise of this intensity cannot be sustained for long periods of time.[39]
- A preexercise snack is needed when the blood glucose level is less than approximately 100 to 120 mg/dL (5.6 to 6.7 mmol/L).
- If blood glucose is 100 to 150 mg/dL (5.6 to 8.3 mmol/L), exercise can be initiated and, if needed, a carbohydrate supplement can be taken following a session.
- Preexercise snacks have been demonstrated to prevent post-exercise hypoglycemia when taken 15 to 30 minutes before exercise of short duration (less than 45 minutes).[51]

TABLE 9.6. CARBOHYDRATE REPLACEMENT DURING EXERCISE[52]

Intensity	Duration	CHO Replacement	Frequency of Snack
Mild-to-moderate	<30	May not be needed	—
Moderate	30 to 60	15 g	Each hour
High	60+	30 to 50 g	Each hour

C   For individuals participating in extended periods of exercise (longer than 2 hours), reducing insulin may be easier than continually supplementing with carbohydrate. It may be necessary to reduce the dose of both regular and intermediate- or long-acting insulin depending on the time and type of exercise.

D   Hypoglycemia remains a risk with exercise, for persons using continuous subcutaneous insulin infusion (CSII).
   • The chances of developing hypoglycemia may be less for insulin pump users due to the steady infusion of insulin.
   • The amount of insulin decrease or the amount of carbohydrate supplement depends on a person's fitness level and the duration and intensity of the exercise.[46,53]
   • Options for insulin pump users to maintain euglycemia with exercise include reducing the basal infusion rate, consuming additional carbohydrates, or temporarily suspending pump use.[46,51,53,54]

E   A link between the time of day when exercise is performed and the risk of exercise-induced hypoglycemia has not been confirmed with research.
   • The risk for hypoglycemia with exercise is low when the level of circulating insulin is low. For example, exercise performed prior to the morning insulin injection presents a low risk of hypoglycemia.
   • The risk for nocturnal hypoglycemia is increased when exercise is performed during the evening hours. However, decreasing the evening insulin dose can reduce this risk.

F   The likelihood of exercise-induced hypoglycemia can be decreased by avoiding exercise when the injected insulin is reaching the peak level. An insulin adjustment usually is required because it is difficult to avoid exercise when medication is peaking.

3   Postexercise, late-onset hypoglycemia (PEL) occurs several hours following an exercise session and is a significant concern to persons treated with insulin; it also can occur in persons treated with oral hypoglycemic agents.

A   PEL can be the result of acutely increased insulin mobilization and sensitivity, increased glucose utilization, replenishment of glycogen stores, and defective counterregulatory mechanisms.[27,42]

B   Options to minimize the occurrence of PEL include
   • Providing patient education to increase awareness
   • Reducing the insulin that peaks during the postexercise period
   • Supplementing carbohydrate during the postexercise phase

- Avoiding exercise prior to bedtime
- Monitoring blood glucose frequently during the postexercise period[42]

4 Exercise-induced hyperglycemia can occur in individuals with type 1 diabetes.

   A Hyperglycemia and worsening of ketosis can result if exercise is initiated when the blood glucose level is greater than 240 to 300 mg/dL (13.3 to 16.7 mmol/L).[33]

- Teach patients to avoid exercise until ketones are negative.
- If a type 1 patient has a blood glucose level greater than 240 to 300 mg/dL (13.3 to 16.7 mmol/L) due to a dietary indiscretion, an insulin deficiency may not be indicated. Exercise under this condition generally will cause a drop in blood glucose levels.
- Negative urine ketones confirm the absence of insulin deficiency.

   B Occasionally, high-intensity, short-term, exhaustive exercise causes an acute rise in blood glucose levels in persons with well-controlled diabetes.[43-45]

- Participation in highly competitive sports frequently results in postexercise hyperglycemia. This phenomenon may be due to excess sympathetic stimulation as a result of high-intensity exercise; catecholamines are released that act on the liver to produce glucose. This has been observed to cause initial increases, followed by declines, in blood glucose levels.
- An extra injection of insulin should not be administered in response to the hyperglycemia. The insulin action will coincide with the postexercise increase in insulin sensitivity and potentially result in severe hypoglycemia.

OTHER SAFETY PRECAUTIONS

1 Teach all persons with diabetes who are treated with insulin or sulfonylureas to carry some type of carbohydrate with them while exercising.

2 Blood glucose monitoring, both pre- and postexercise, is the key to safety and understanding of how exercise affects blood glucose.

3 Advise persons with diabetes to wear some form of diabetes and personal identification.

4 Avoid vigorous exercise if the environment is extremely hot, humid, smoggy, or cold.

5 Proper equipment and exercise shoes appropriate for the activity will reduce the likelihood of injury.

6 Include a warm-up and cool-down sessions with each workout. Stretching exercises performed following the cool-down enhance flexibility and prevent injury.

7 Certain medications can impair exercise tolerance. β-blockers alter the heart-rate response to exercise as well as mask hypoglycemia and the body's counterregulatory response.

8 Maintain adequate hydration should be maintained while exercising.

9 Stop exercise if pain, light-headedness, or shortness of breath occurs.

10 The American Diabetes Association recommends an exercise stress electrocardiogram in all people over age 35 years who want to begin exercising.[41] Direct special attention during assessments toward identifying a history of cardiac disease (including silent heart disease), the presence of complications, medications, medical and family history, and degree of diabetes control. Physical activity assessments are useful for patients and educators when planning exercise.

EXERCISE PROGRAMS

1 There are two types of exercise, aerobic and anaerobic.

    A *Aerobic exercise*, is defined as exercise that involves repetitive, submaximal contraction of major muscle groups (eg, swimming, cycling, jogging) and requires oxygen to sustain muscular effort.[41,55] Aerobic exercise provides the greatest benefits for people with diabetes in terms of blood glucose control and cardiovascular status. The health-related benefits of exercise do not appear to be dependent on the type of aerobic exercise.

    B *Anaerobic exercise* is defined as exercise that does not require sustained oxygen to meet the energy demands and generally does not induce the same health benefits as an aerobic program.

- Anaerobic exercise may cause excessive rises in blood pressure, cardiac workload, and intraocular pressure. These reactions could be potential problems in persons with diabetes and vascular disease or complications.
- Studies[56,57] suggest that properly designed resistance programs may improve indices of cardiovascular function, glucose tolerance, strength, and body composition provided the person with diabetes does not have contraindications to weight training.

2 The duration of exercise is inversely related to the intensity of the exercise: lower-intensity exercise needs to be conducted over a longer period of time than higher intensity exercise for maximum benefit. The duration of exercise to meet the required weekly energy expenditure is 20 to 60 minutes per session.[15]

A All workouts should include a 5- to 10-minute warm-up and cooldown.
- The warm-up increases core body temperature and prevents muscle injury; the cool-down prevents blood pooling in the extremities and facilitates removal of metabolic by-products.
- Initiate exercise to be performed in the training phase in the warm-up and conclude in the cool-down phase.[58]

B New studies have shown similar cardiorespiratory gains to occur when physical activity is done in shorter bouts (~10 minutes) accumulated throughout the day, as when activity of similar duration and intensity occurs for one prolonged session (~30 minutes).[5,58]
- These findings, although beneficial in terms of cardiorespiratory gains, have not been studied in the diabetes population.
- It may be necessary for severely deconditioned individuals to exercise in multiple sessions of short duration (~10 minutes).[58]

3 To achieve the desired fitness level, exercise needs to be done five times per week or three to four times per week for maintenance.[41]

A The duration of glycemic improvement after the last exercise session usually is greater than 12 hours but less than 72 hours.[18]

B To improve glycemic control, exercise needs to be done at least every other day, on at least 3 nonconsecutive days, and ideally 5 days per week.

C Obese individuals may need to exercise more frequently (5 to 7 days per week) to optimize weight loss.

D Exercise that is limited to 2 days per week generally does not produce a meaningful change in maximal uptake.

E The minimum physical conditioning for health benefits requires expending at least 700 calories per week.

F For maximum health benefits, 2000 calories per week are required; there is limited substantial health benefit to expending greater than 2000 calories per week.[58]

4 The intensity of exercise should be 60% to 85% of the maximal age-adjusted heart rate (comparable to 50% to 70% of maximal oxygen uptake or VO_2 max).

A Training intensity can be calculated accurately using the results of an exercise stress test.

B When stress testing is not possible, the following heart-rate (HR) reserve formula is commonly used to calculate target heart-rate zone: target heart-rate range = $[(HR_{MAX} - HR_{REST}) \times 0.50$ and $0.85] + HR_{REST}$.

- Select a range between 50% to 85% based on the individual's fitness level, duration of diabetes, degree of complications, and patient's goals.

C The following equation can be used to estimate the true maximal heart rate when the actual rate is unknown: $HR_{MAX} = 220 -$ patient's age.

- This procedure may overestimate the maximal heart rate of some type 2 patients, particularly those with autonomic neuropathy.[41,58]
- Due to the high prevalence of occult cardiovascular disease, caution is required when applying standard heart-rate formulas to the diabetes population.

D Exercise performed at low levels (<50% HR_{MAX}) has less effect on glucose disposal than exercise performed at higher intensities. The effect on glucose disposal during high-intensity exercise is roughly proportional to the total work performed (time x intensity). However, high-intensity exercise may result in transient hyperglycemia and cause an excessive rise in blood pressure.

E When initiating an exercise program, it may be necessary to begin at low levels (50%) with brief rest intervals and progress weekly to higher-intensity, continual exercise.[58]

5 Exercise components of duration, frequency, and intensity will help achieve aerobic training effects.

A Individual factors such as fitness level, age, and health status can affect the attainment of these goals.

B Medications (eg, β-blockers) and the presence of secondary complications may affect the exercise plan and individual tolerance (Table 9.7).

TABLE 9.7. SUMMARY OF EXERCISE RECOMMENDATIONS

Screening	• Presence of vascular and neurological complications, silent heart disease, stress ECG (GXT*) in patients >35 y
Exercise Prescription	*Type* • Aerobic preferred; anaerobic allowed if no secondary limitations *Intensity* • 60% to 85% of maximal heart rate (50% to 70% of maximum aerobic capacity) *Duration* • 20 to 60 min *Frequency* • 3 to 5 times per week; schedule every other day
Safety Precautions	• Warm-up/cooldown • Careful selection and progression of exercise program • Patient education • Monitor blood glucose pre-/postexercise • Adjust guidelines to prevent hypoglycemia • Management by healthcare personnel

*GXT = graded exercise test.
Source: Adapted from the American Diabetes Association. *Exercise and NIDDM: a technical review.*[41]

---

6 It has been recommended that strength-developing exercises be included with cardiorespiratory endurance activities in order to improve musculoskeletal health, maintain independence in performing daily activities, and reduce the possibility of injury.[5,59] The acute components of a resistance-training program include the following:

A The choice of which exercises to perform is based upon what the individual wants to achieve with the strengthening program.

- If an individual wants to achieve specific strength gains, then the resistance program is planned to target the particular action and muscular components that are essential in the desired activity.

- Individuals who are interested in basic fitness, can select exercises that use each of the major muscle groups of the body (shoulders, back, chest, abdomen, and legs).[60]

B Advise patients to exercise in a specific order to use the larger muscle groups first and then move to the smaller muscle groups.
  - By working the larger muscle groups and then proceeding to the smaller groups, the demanding exercises are performed early in the workout while the energy supply is the greatest and the individual has an abundance of energy.
  - If one chooses to perform the exercises in an alternative manner, the exercises which have a small energy demand will start to deplete energy stores, leaving the individual with a reduced energy supply to complete more debilitative exercises (exercises including the larger muscle groups).[61]

C For individuals with diabetes and no known cardiac disease, it is important to find out what physical attributes are necessary to attain their goal before determining the appropriate resistance. Once these parameters have been identified, the resistance and repetition load can be determined.
  - The resistance used is determined though the individual's *repetition maximum* (RM), which is defined as the amount of weight that allows for successful completion of a specified number of repetitions (no more, no less).[61]
  - Studies have shown repetitions of eight RM or less to produce the greatest strength gains, and muscular endurance is maximized through the use of resistance that allows for the performance of more than 12 repetitions.
  - For an individual who wants to achieve both muscular strength and endurance, 8 to 12 repetitions would be the most appropriate range.
  - When working with individuals with cardiac disease, particular attention must be focused on blood pressure and heart-rate response to the resistance training. It is recommended that these individuals start at lighter resistance loads and perform exercises that utilize a smaller amount of muscle mass, which in turn will decrease the myocardial oxygen demand on the heart.[61] The heart rate and blood pressure need to remain within the limits established by the exercise tolerance test, and therefore should be monitored throughout the training session.

D Performing one to two sets of each exercise has been proven to be beneficial to increase general muscle strength and endurance.

- Instruct individuals with a low fitness level or little training experience to complete just one set of each exercise for the first 4 to 6 weeks. Once they are comfortable with the exercise and have demonstrated good technique, the number of sets can be increased.

E Rest for an adequate amount of time between sets to allow for successful completion of the next set.

- For individuals training at lower intensities, rest periods are short (15 seconds to 1 minute).
- Individuals training at higher intensities will take longer to recover and may take up 2 minutes to regain enough energy to successfully complete the next set.[60]

7 Special precautions need to be taken by patients with diabetes prior to starting a resistance-training program.

A Before starting the exercise sessions teach the individual proper weight lifting technique:

- Keep the body properly aligned.
- Breathe properly, exhaling during the phase in which the muscle is exerting its force against the apparatus and inhaling while lowering the weight.
- Control the lifting movement.
- Obtain the adequate range of motion.
- Make sure the equipment is adjusted to fit the body frame.

B Individuals with long-term microvascular or macrovascular complications will require program modifications to decrease the strain on their cardiovascular systems due to the resistive exercises.

- Teach patients with proliferative retinopathy or nephropathy to avoid resistive training. Resistive exercises may be harmful due to the excessive systolic pressure responses experienced.[61]
- Individuals with diabetes who also have cardiovascular disease should possess an ejection fraction of $\geq 45\%$ and a cardiorespiratory fitness level of ≥ 7 metabolic equivalents (METs), without ischemic ST segment depression on their electrocardiogram, hypo- or hypertensive responses, serious ventricular arrhythmias, or symptoms of cardiovascular disease, prior to beginning a resistance training program.[62]

- Patients with any complications that may be exacerbated by resistance training should always receive approval from their physician before starting a program.

EXERCISE CONSIDERATIONS FOR THE ELDERLY

1 Age-associated changes in body composition in the elderly account for decreases in basal metabolic rate, muscle strength, activity levels, and a decreased energy expenditure.

   A Reductions in lean body mass occur primarily as a result of loss of skeletal muscle mass and increase in body fat. This decrease in muscle mass is a direct cause of the decrease in muscle strength seen in older adults.

   B Research[63] has provided evidence that muscle mass, not muscular function, is the major determinate of age- and gender-related differences in strength. As physical activity levels decline with advancing age, muscle power and strength become critical elements in walking ability.

   C The capacity of the elderly to respond to an exercise program is often underrated. Individuals over the age of 60 years have demonstrated greater benefits from aerobic and strength training in fitness capacity, strength, functional capacity, and glucose tolerance than comparable younger groups.

   D Special attention needs to be directed toward potential hazards for the elderly population.[64,65]

   - A thorough physical exam is required prior to initiation of an exercise program. Emphasis is placed on detecting occult heart disease, cardiovascular and/or peripheral vascular disease, joint/bone disease, and secondary complications.

   - Strength training improves performance activities of daily living and counteracts muscle weakness. Teach patients to train each major muscle group two to three times per week. Muscular toning can be accomplished via free weights, strap-on ankle/wrist weights, and traditional strengthening machines (eg, Nautilus®). The appropriate intensity is in the range of one set of 8 to 12 repetitions "somewhat hard" on the perceived exertion rating (12 to 13).[58]

   - Aerobic fitness is beneficial for older persons (Table 9.8). Because of the progressive decline in oxygen transport and functional capacity, an effective training stimulus for this age group may be much less than is needed in a younger person.[64]

E Teach individuals with degenerative joint disease or osteoarthritis to avoid orthopedic or musculoskeletal stress. Vary exercise so that it is primarily weight-bearing one day and nonweight-bearing on alternate days.[58]

F Sedentary individuals have an increased risk for cardiac arrest and cerebral vascular accidents if exercise is too vigorous. Teach these patients to initiate exercise at lower levels, progress slower, and gradually increase in duration and frequency to reach their desired fitness level.

TABLE 9.8. GUIDELINES FOR AEROBIC EXERCISE IN THE ELDERLY

Beneficial aerobic activities include cycling, brisk walking, swimming, dancing, rowing.

Intersperse initial exercise with brief rest periods; continuous exercise is achieved over time.

Adding 2 to 5 minutes per week to the workout usually is appropriate for achieving the following desired goals[64]:
- Duration of 30 to 40 minutes
- Frequency of five to six times per week
- Intensity based on graded exercise test (GXT), risk factors, medical history (typical training heart rate in the elderly is 60% to 75% of maximal heart rate)

Assess progress and reevaluate the exercise plan in about 4 to 6 weeks.

EXERCISE CONSIDERATIONS FOR OBESE PERSONS

1 Combined programs of exercise, meal planning, and behavior change are effective for obese persons.

A The therapeutic approach that emphasizes increased levels of physical activity offers the advantage of enhancing caloric expenditure and providing the benefits of exercise in terms of influencing blood lipids, blood glucose control, blood pressure, mood, and attitude.[55]

B Often, the initial fitness goal of the obese person is to simply increase the amount of physical activity from an inactive state.

C A combination of meal planning plus exercise has been shown to be more effective at long-term weight control than either meal planning or exercise alone. The addition of exercise to a weight-control program may facilitate more permanent weight loss than total reliance on caloric restriction.[8]

D Regular exercise during a weight-control program helps to maintain muscle mass while promoting fat loss. Weight loss achieved by caloric restriction alone may lead to loss of lean muscle mass and less loss of fat.

E Continuous aerobic exercise has the greatest impact on weight loss because of enhanced caloric expenditure.

- Walking is an effective choice for continuous aerobic exercise. Alternative types of exercise include cycling and water exercise.
- Less effective options are swimming (less likely to induce weight loss or provide aerobic effects) and running (too much knee stress for obese individuals).

F As the duration of exercise increases, so does the utilization of fat as a fuel. A longer duration (eg, greater than 45 minutes) has been shown to have a greater calorie-burning and fat-mobilization effect than shorter exercise periods.[6,58]

G Intensity should be at the low end of the target heart-rate range.

- The duration of exercise should be sufficient to expend 200 to 300 kcal per session.
- This calorie expenditure may be accomplished with low-intensity exercise of long duration (40 to 60 minutes) such as walking.[58]

H Frequency of exercise should be a minimum of three times per week. An exercise frequency of five times per week is recommended for increased weight loss and facilitation of blood glucose goal attainment.

EXERCISE CONSIDERATIONS FOR PERSONS WITH DIABETES COMPLICATIONS

1 Persons with chronic complications of diabetes often do not take part in activity programs. Yet, it is useful for this group to undertake an exercise program to improve or maintain their functional capacity, strength, and flexibility.[66] Since persons with diabetes have an increased risk of cardiovascular disease, comprehensive assessments may be necessary to determine the most appropriate exercises.

2 Patients with established cardiovascular disease usually require supervision in a cardiac rehabilitation program.

A Hypertension and a hypertensive response to exercise (SBP >260 mmHG, DBP > 25 mgHG) frequently are seen in persons with diabetes.[58]

- Exercise should be performed at an intensity that avoids a hypertensive response.

- If the patient is hypertensive, advise them to avoid exercises that involve heavy lifting, straining, and Valsalva-like maneuvers.
- Exercise that involves the upper body and arms generally induces larger increases in systolic blood pressure than similar workloads performed by the legs alone.

B Rhythmic exercises using the lower extremities are recommended, such as walking, light jogging, and cycling. Weight training should involve low resistance with high repetitions.[58]

3 Patients with peripheral vascular disease will experience ischemic pain during physical activity as a result of insufficient oxygen supply and demand for the active muscles.

A A walking program for intermittent claudication may improve collateral circulation and muscle metabolism and, in turn, decrease pain.[67]

B An interval training program of walk/rest periods results in greater exercise tolerance of pain-limited work capacity.
- The distance and duration of the walk is determined by a pain-limited threshold.
- Advise patients to keep the intensity low because higher intensity demands a greater blood supply and induces claudication pain.[65]
- Teach patients that conversation, music, etc. can divert attention from the discomfort and pain.
- Discontinue exercise when the discomfort or pain accelerates from moderate to intense discomfort, and the individual's attention cannot be diverted.[58]

C Weight-bearing activities are preferred, although nonweight-bearing activities may allow for longer duration and higher intensity exercise.

D Pain at rest and during the night are indications of severe peripheral vascular disease, which is an absolute contraindication for a walking exercise program.[68]

E Daily exercise will maximize tolerable pain.[58]

4 Patients with retinopathy have significant restrictions on exercise participation.

A Provide exercise recommendations based on the severity and stage of diabetic retinopathy. In general, exercise has not been shown to accelerate retinopathy.

B In the early stages of retinopathy, there are limited restrictions on exercise.
  • Exercise may actually reduce the risk of developing proliferative diabetic retinopathy (PDR) and diabetic macular edema by its effect on blood pressure and HDL, which are associated with retinopathy.
  • For patients with active PDR, strenuous activity may precipitate vitreous hemorrhage or traction retinal detachment; clearance for exercise must be provided by the patient's ophthalmologist.
C The level of retinopathy determines which activities are appropriate and which activities are to be avoided (Table 9.9).[69]

TABLE 9.9. EXERCISE GUIDELINES FOR PERSONS WITH DIABETIC RETINOPATHY

Level of Retinopathy	Exercise Recommendation(s)
No diabetic retinopathy	• No exercise limitations.
Mild nonproliferative	• No exercise limitations.
Moderate nonproliferative	• Avoid activities that dramatically elevate blood pressure (eg, power lifting).
Severe to very severe nonproliferative	• Limit increase in systolic blood pressure (eg, Valsalva maneuvers), and avoid activities that jar the head. Heart rate should not exceed that which elicits a systolic blood pressure response greater than 180 mmHg (eg, boxing and intense competitive sports).[66]
Proliferative	• Avoid strenuous activity, high-impact activities, Valsalva maneuvers, and activities that jar the head (eg, weight lifting, jogging, high-impact aerobic dance, racquet sports, strenuous trumpet playing, and competitive sports). • Encourage activities that are low-impact, aerobic, and stress cardiovascular conditioning (eg, swimming without diving, walking, low-impact aerobic dance, stationary cycling, and endurance exercising).[69]

5 For persons with recent visual impairment, and for some with long-standing visual loss, aerobic capacity may be reduced due to loss of independent mobility.

   A Suitable options for exercise include swimming (using lane guides), stationary cycling, treadmill walking, tandem cycling, and folk dancing (using the sighted person as an anchor).

   B Various teaching adaptations and organizations have broadened sports participation (snow skiing, track-and-field competition) for visually impaired individuals.[66]

6 Nearly all known risk factors for coronary artery disease are found in persons with end-stage renal disease, thus underscoring the need for a properly planned exercise program.

   A Although aerobic activities are preferred, the ability to perform this type of exercise depends on the degree of kidney impairment. These individuals usually have low functional and aerobic capacity.

   B Recommend beginning any aerobic activity at a low level, perhaps using interval work, followed by a gradual, progressive exercise plan.[70] Brisk walking, swimming, and cycling are beneficial choices.

7 Peripheral neuropathy can result in sensory losses of pain, touch, and balance. For example, neuroarthropathy (Charcot's foot) can lead to disarticulations and injury in sensory-impaired individuals.

   A Exercise cannot reverse the symptoms of neuropathy, but it can prevent further loss of muscle strength and flexibility that commonly is seen in patients with sensory polyneuropathy. Adaptive shortening of connective tissue can occur due to immobilization or limited proprioception. Thus, daily range-of-motion exercises are recommended.

   B Extra care is needed to avoid injury and overstretching by sensory-impaired individuals.[66]

- Weight-bearing activities usually are not recommended because of the increased likelihood of soft tissue and joint injury.
- Because avoiding orthopedic stress is important, exercises such as cycling and swimming are beneficial choices.
- If balance is not impaired, brisk walking may be another alternative.[55]
- Jogging is contraindicated because it places a threefold increase on the foot compared with walking.

C Proper footwear and inspection of the feet after exercise are strategies to prevent blisters and detect injuries. For persons with limited mobility, chair exercises may improve flexibility and strength.

8 Exercise in people with autonomic neuropathy should be approached with caution because of the role of the autonomic nervous system in hormonal and cardiovascular regulation during exercise.

A Symptoms of angina are not reliable indicators of coronary artery disease due to the higher frequency of silent ischemia and myocardial infarction among people with diabetes.[27]

B Physical working capacity is reduced.

C High-intensity exercise should be avoided.

D Because dehydration may be a risk in individuals who have difficulty with thermoregulation, exercise in hot or cold environments should be avoided. Hypotension and hypertension following vigorous exercise are possibilities.

E Recumbent cycling and water aerobics are options for persons with orthostatic hypotension.

F Frequent blood glucose monitoring also is recommended during exercise for people with defective counterregulatory mechanisms.[66]

EXERCISE PARTICIPATION

1 Little is known about how to increase and maintain participation in exercise programs.

A Only 22% of American adults participate in an exercise program that has been recommended for health benefits (light-to-moderate physical activity sustained for at least 30 minutes). About 54% are somewhat active but do not meet this objective, and 24% or more are completely sedentary.[71-73]

B More is known about exercise relapse than effective interventions. Approximately 50% of people who join an exercise program drop out during the first 3 to 6 months.

2 The transtheoretical model for change has been applied to exercise participation, weight loss, smoking cessation, and mammography screening.[74,75]

A A perception of the pros (benefits) versus the cons (demands) of exercising determine the transition from consideration to participation to maintenance of an exercise program .

B The stages of change can be used to tailor intervention strategies and exercise outcomes to include both readiness and behavioral changes (see Chapter 5, Behavior Change, for more information).

3 Stage-matched interventions are the most effective. These interventions provide strategies for overcoming barriers to participation at each stage.

A In the precontemplation stage, exercise is not even a consideration. People in this stage lack confidence in their ability to begin or continue an exercise program and avoid reading, talking and thinking about it.
- Asking that they begin to exercise will have a negative effect.
- Building a trusting relationship and providing information are needed at this stage.

B Individuals in the contemplation stage think about exercise and perceive the advantages and disadvantages to be equal, but they do not exercise.
- Be supportive of these patients; they are looking for assistance and validation.
- It is important not to criticize any ambivalence about exercise but rather to encourage discussion of concerns, questions, and personal reasons to exercise.

C In the preparation stage, the individuals have thought about exercise and are ready to begin.
- The patient is ready to set goals and develops a self-exercise plan.
- This stage is probably the most rewarding time for patients.

D In the action stage, the individuals are exercising. They have achieved a regular level of exercise at least 20 minutes three times per week. There is a high risk of relapse because the behavior is new.

E In the maintenance stage, the rewards of exercise are more subtle after 6 months more. However, as the potential for relapse still exists, the educator's role is to keep activities interesting and assist the individuals in progressing with their program.

F Most people are not successful with their first try; they may need three or four attempts before exercise becomes a long-term habit. When relapse does occur, feelings of failure, embarrassment, guilt, or shame may surface. Fifteen percent of people become demoralized and resist trying again, so support is important in all stages.
- Eighty-five percent will try again.
- Sixty percent of all New Year's resolutions are repledged the following year.

- People progress through the stages as they learn from their mistakes and try something different the next time.
- The more action taken, the better chance of progressing forward.

SELF-DIRECTED EXERCISE PROGRAMS

1 Anecdotal reports suggest that personally designed programs enhance enjoyment and are more likely to be sustained. Patients who choose an activity that they enjoy are more likely to participate in it on a regular basis. Exercise is more likely to occur when it is convenient (eg, close to home or work).

2 The transtheoretical model for change has been applied to exercise participation, weight loss, smoking cessation, and mammography screening.[74,75]

   A The patient's perception of the pros (benefits) versus the cons (demands) of exercising determine the transition from consideration to participation to maintenance of an exercise program.

   B The stages of change can include both readiness and behavioral changes (see Chapter 5, Behavior Change, for more information).

3 Asking patients if they are thinking about exercising and their feelings about it provide cues for how to provide information.

4 It is important for patients to establish realistic and practical goals at the beginning of an exercise program. Goals that are too vague, too ambitious, or too distant do not provide enough self-motivation to maintain long-term interest.

   A This is probably the most rewarding time for patients.

   B Ask patients to identify barriers and develop strategies to overcome possible interruptions in their regular exercise schedule (eg, inclement weather, seasonal change, vacations, and holidays).

   C Teach patients strategies to optimize social support from the family, exercise class members, or a buddy system.

   D Suggest to patients that they develop stimulus control strategies to initiate and continue exercise participation (eg, write exercise in appointment books, set watch alarms for exercise time).

    E Suggest patients compare the time it takes to walk 2 miles at the beginning of their exercise program with the time required to walk this distance after they have been exercising for a period of time.

    F One method of feedback for people with diabetes is to keep a log of pre- and postexercise blood glucose levels or to chart HbA$_{1c}$ for the duration of the training program.

5 Most people need three or four attempts before exercise becomes a long-term habit. when relapse does occur, feelings of failure, embarrassment, guilt, or shame may surface. Fifteen percent of people become demoralized and resist trying again.

    A Asking patients what they learned from their experiences with exercise can provide patients with information to use for future planning and goal-setting.

    B Eighty-five percent will try again. Sixty percent of all New Year's resolutions are repledged the following year.

    C The more action taken, the better chance of progressing forward.

Key Educational Considerations

1 Assist patients in designing an exercise plan that will help them to safely achieve their goals. Reevaluate the exercise goals and plan between 5 and 7 weeks to establish new goals, as necessary, that reinforce the effects, benefits, and principles of the exercise program.

2 Assist patients to identify barriers to the exercise program and determine options for overcoming the barriers. For example, to overcome fear of hypoglycemia, discuss ways to make adjustments to prevent hypoglycemia.

3 Ask the patient to check blood glucose levels pre- and postexercise and record the results along with information about medication, nutritional intake, and the type and time of any symptoms that develop during or after exercise. By reviewing these records with the patient, the educator can discuss the effects of exercise and offer ideas about needed adjustments in management. Furthermore, record keeping may provide reinforcement for the exercise program.

4 Ask patients to perform self-assessments to evaluate exercise results. Compare current level of physical activity to the amount of exercise performed at the beginning of the exercise program. Other parameters that can be monitored that reflect progress with the exercise program include weight, blood glucose, and lipid levels.

5 Assist patients who may be self-conscious because of their weight or fitness level to find a group or class of similar status and with comparable goals. A significant deterrent for many overweight people is joining an exercise class that consists of people who are lean and relatively fit.

Self-Review Questions

1 List the benefits of regular exercise for individuals with diabetes.

2 Discuss the mechanisms for exercise-induced hypoglycemia.

3 Describe precautions that can be taken to help prevent exercise-induced hypoglycemia, including postexercise, late-onset hypoglycemia.

4 For persons with type 1 diabetes, describe when and why can exercise result in a worsening of hyperglycemia and ketosis.

5 Describe components and give examples of aerobic exercise.

6 Discuss strategies to improve adherence to an exercise program.

7 State the potential risks of exercise for persons with type 1 and type 2 diabetes.

8 Briefly discuss and identify exercise that would be appropriate or contraindicated for persons with retinopathy and neuropathy.

9 Describe the importance of self-directed goals for exercise.

Case Study

AB is a 41-year-old female with a 26-year history of type 1 diabetes. She has come to the diabetes center because she wants to start an exercise program. She is very enthusiastic about using some new exercise equipment, but she wants to know where to begin. During the assessment she tells you, "I have nonproliferative retinopathy and my feet are a little numb, but otherwise my diabetes is well controlled." AB is 5 feet 4 inches tall, weighs 170 lb (76.5 kg), and her HbA_{1c} is >11% (normal = < 6.2%). She is on a split dose of regular and NPH insulins at breakfast and dinner. She checks her blood glucose levels in the morning, and her results are around 180 mg/dL (10.8 mmol/L). She states that she hasn't seen her doctor in awhile.

QUESTIONS FOR DISCUSSION

1 What questions would you ask AB about her diabetes management?

2 What does AB need to know before beginning her exercise program?

3 What kind of program is safe for AB (eg, exercise type, intensity, duration, restrictions)?

DISCUSSION

1 Although AB states that her diabetes is fine, she has an elevated glycosylated hemoglobin level. This finding, together with her comments about her eyes and feet, indicate to the diabetes educator certain key facts about AB's diabetes.

A Her diabetes probably is not adequately controlled.

B Complications could be well established.

C AB may not be adequately informed regarding diabetes and its management.

2 Since AB has not seen her physician for some time, she is encouraged to do so prior to initiating an exercise program.

3 Based on the American College of Sports Medicine guidelines for her age and duration of diabetes, a graded exercise stress electrocardiogram test (GXT) is warranted prior to initiating an exercise program. The results of the GXT allow accurate and safe determinations of exercise tolerances and limitations.

4 A medical exam also is necessary and should include a plasma lipid profile and blood chemistries, kidney function tests, and a comprehensive eye exam. These assessments are important in view of AB's history and are necessary before she can safely exercise.

5 Results of the GXT show no cardiac dysfunction during exercise but reveal a poor tolerance for exercise, indicating a deconditioned state. When AB walked on the treadmill, her exercise systolic blood pressure was >200 mmHg when her heart rate was 145 beats per minute. Maximal exercise heart rate was 165 beats per minute.

6 Further assessments showed elevated lipids and a low HDL:LDL ratio (risk factors for CAD), slight proteinuria, and stable nonproliferative retinopathy.

7 AB and her doctor decide that she will continue with the same insulin regimen, perform more frequent blood glucose monitoring, reevaluate her meal plan with the assistance of a dietitian, and begin an exercise program. AB is referred to an exercise specialist.

8 The goals of an exercise program AB identifies are a weight loss of about 10 to 15 lb (4.5 to 6.8 kg) (combined with a meal plan), improved lipid profile, improved aerobic capacity, improved overall diabetes control (combined with an education program), and increased feelings of control and self-worth.

9 An aerobic exercise program is established with AB.

   A Because treadmill walking at a heart rate of 145 beats per minute resulted in an elevated systolic blood pressure, AB's recommended intensity will be based on blood pressure response to exercise.

   B Due to the correlation of elevated blood pressure to increased proteinuria and retinopathy, the exercise will be performed at an intensity that does not induce large systolic changes.

   - AB's training intensity is 165 (HR_{MAX}) x 0.60 to 0.85 = 99 to 140 beats per minute.

   - At 132 beats per minute, her systolic blood pressure was 160 mmHg, which is an appropriate training intensity.

   - Because AB has been inactive and is obese, she will need to initiate her exercise program at a lower training intensity (eg, 110 beats per minute).

   - Initially, she may need some brief rest periods during the workout, performing only 15 minutes of exercise at a time.

   - Alternating weekly additions of time and intensity to the workout will help accomplish the ultimate goal (within 6 to 8 weeks) of continual exercise for 45 to 60 minutes at a heart rate of 130 beats per minute.

   C AB decides to exercise five times per week. Focusing on increasing duration instead of only intensity will aid in fat mobilization and favorably alter the lipid profile.

D Prior to initiating the exercise prescription, her blood glucose profile showed late-afternoon hyperglycemia.

- Consequently, the best time for AB to exercise is between 2 PM and 4 PM, when her blood glucose levels are high. This is also AB's preferred time because her work is finished and her children are not yet home from school.
- Exercising at this time will control her late-afternoon hyperglycemia.
- Her NPH insulin may be peaking at this point or even waning if she takes human insulin. Therefore, AB will monitor pre- and post-exercise blood glucose levels at this time of day to determine her blood glucose response to exercise. Her late afternoon blood glucose level may improve, in which case she can adjust her insulin to prevent hypoglycemia. If her blood glucose levels do not improve and remain elevated, this may be suggestive of underinsulinization and an increase in insulin may be needed.

10 AB's feet are a little numb, therefore jogging, stair climbing, or heavy weight-bearing exercises are not appropriate exercise choices.

A Cycling, walking, or water walking could be suggested as alternatives.

REFERENCES

1 Sushruta SCS. Vaidya jadavaji trikamji acharia. Bombay, India: Sagar, 1938.

2 Allen FM, Stillman E, Fitz R. Total dietary regulation in the treatment of diabetes. Exercise 1919; Monograph 11.

3 Lawrence RH. The effects of exercise on insulin action in diabetes. Br Med J 1926;1:648-52.

4 Helmrich SP, Ragland DR, Leung RW, Paffenbarger RS Jr. Physical activity and reduced occurrence of non-insulin-dependent diabetes mellitus. N Engl J Med 1991;325:147-52.

5 U.S. Department of Health and Human Services. Physical activity and health: a report of the surgeon general. Atlanta: US Department of Health and Human Services, Centers for Disease Control and Prevention, National Center for Chronic Disease Prevention and Health Promotion.

6 Astrand P, Rodahl K. Textbook of work physiology. St Louis: Macmillan, 1977.

7 Horton ES. Role and management of exercise in diabetes mellitus. Diabetes Care 1988;11:201-11.

8 Bogardus C, Ravussin E, Robbins DC, Wolfe RR, Horton ES, Sims EAH. Effects of physical training with diet therapy on carbohydrate metabolism in patients with glucose intolerance and non-insulin-dependent diabetes mellitus. Diabetes 1984;33:311-18.

9 Stout RW. Insulin and atheroma: 20 year perspective. Diabetes Care 1990;13:631-54.

10 Fontbonne AM, Eschwege EM. Insulin and cardiovascular disease: Paris prospective study. Diabetes Care 1991; 14:461-69.

11 Schneider SH, Ruderman NB. Exercise and physical training in the treatment of diabetes mellitus. Compr Ther 1986; 12:49-56.

12 Colwell JA. Effects of exercise on platelet function, coagulation and fibrinolysis. Diabetes Metab Rev 1986;1:501-12.

13 Hornsby WG, Boggess KA, Lyons TJ, Barnwell WH, Lazarchick J, Colwell JA. Hemostatic alterations with exercise conditioning in NIDDM. Diabetes Care 1990;13:87-92.

14 Rodin J. Physiological effects of exercise. In: William RS, Wallace AG, eds. Biological effects of physical activity. Champaign, Ill: Human Kinetics, 1990.

15 Schneider SH, Amorosa LF, Khachadurian AK, Ruderman NB. Studies on the mechanism of improved glycemic control during regular exercise in type II diabetes. Diabetologia 1984;26:355-60.

16 Eriksson KF, Lindgarde F. Prevention of type II diabetes mellitus by diet and physical exercise. The 6-year Malmo Feasibility Study. Diabetologia 1991; 34:891-98.

17 Heath GW, Wilson RH, Smith J, Leonard BE. Community-based exercise and weight control: diabetes risk reduction and glycemic control in Zuni Indians. Am J Clin Nutr 1991;53:S1642-46.

18 Schneider SH, Khachadurian AK, Amorosa LF, Clemow L, Ruderman NB. Ten-year experience with an exercise-based outpatient lifestyle modification program in the treatment of diabetes mellitus. Diabetes Care 1992; 15(suppl 4):1800-10.

19 Vanninen E, Uusitupa M, Siitonen O, Laitinen J, Lansimies E. Habitual physical activity, aerobic capacity, and metabolic control in patients with newly diagnosed type II diabetes mellitus: effect of a 1-year diet and exercise intervention. Diabetologia 1992;35:340-46.

20 Stratton R, Wilson DP, Endres RK, Goldstein DE. Improved glycemic control after supervised 8-wk exercise program in insulin-dependent diabetic adolescents. Diabetes Care 1987;10:589-93.

21 Landt KW, Campaigne BN, James FW, Sperling MA. Effects of exercise training on insulin sensitivity in adolescents with type 1 diabetes. Diabetes Care 1985;8: 461-65.

22 Wallberg-Henrikssonn H, Gunnarsson R, Henriksson J, et al. Increased peripheral insulin sensitivity and muscle mitochondrial enzymes but unchanged blood glucose control in type 2 diabetics after physical training. Diabetes 1982;31:1044-50.

23 Peterson CM, Jones RL, Dupuis A, Levine BS, Bernstein R, O'Shea M. Feasibility of improved blood glucose control in patients with insulin-dependent diabetes mellitus. Diabetes Care 1979;2:329-35.

24 Wallberg-Henriksson H, Gunnarsson R, Henriksson J, Ostman J, Wahren J. Influence of training on formation of muscle capillaries in type 1 diabetes. Diabetes 1984;33:851-57.

25 Zinman B, Zuniga-Guajardo S, Kelly D. Comparison of the acute and long-term effects of exercise on glucose control in type 1 diabetics. Diabetes Care 1984;7: 515-19.

26 Stratton R, Wilson DP, Endres RK. Acute glycemic effects of exercise in adolescents with insulin-dependent diabetes mellitus. Physician Sports Med 1988;16:150-57.

27 Vitug A, Schneider SH, Ruderman NB. Exercise in type 1 diabetes. In: Terjung RI, ed. Exercise and sport sciences reviews. New York: Macmillan, 1988: 285-304.

28 Vranic M, Berger M. Exercise and diabetes. Diabetes 1979;28:147-63.

29 Tzankoff SP, Norris AH. Longitudinal changes in basal metabolism in man. J Appl Physiol 1978;45:536-93.

30 Franz MJ. Exercise and diabetes: fuel metabolism, benefits, risks and guidelines. Clin Diabetes 1988;6:58-60.

31 Winder WW. Regulation of hepatic glucose regulation during exercise. In: Terjung RL, ed. Exercise and sport sciences reviews. New York: Macmillan, 1985:1-32.

32 Hartley LH, Mason JW, Hogan RP, et al. Multiple hormonal responses to graded exercise in relation to physical training. J Appl Physiol 1972;33:602-6.

33 Berger M, Berchtold P, Cuppers HJ, et al. Metabolic and hormonal effects of muscular exercise in juvenile type diabetics. Diabetologia 1977;13:355-65.

34 Zinman B, Vranic M, Albisser AM, Leibel BS, Marliss ED. The role of insulin in the metabolic response to exercise in the diabetic man. Diabetes 1979;28(suppl 1):76-81.

35 Wahren J. Glucose turnover during exercise in healthy men and in patients with diabetes mellitus. Diabetes 1979;29(suppl 1):82-88.

36 Ahlborg G, Felig P. Lactate and glucose exchange across the forearm, legs and splanchnic bed during and after prolonged leg exercise. J Clin Invest 1982;69:45.

37 Richter EA, Garetto LP, Goodman M, Ruderman N. Muscle glucose metabolism following exercise in the rat: increased sensitivity to insulin. J Clin Invest 1982;69:785-93.

38 Mondon CE, Dolkas CB, Reaven GM. Site of enhanced insulin sensitivity in exercise-trained rats at rest. Am J Physiol 1980;239(Endocrinol Metab 2):E169-177.

39 Wasserman DH, Zinman B. Exercise in individuals with IDDM. Diabetes Care 1994;17:924-37.

40 Kemmer FW, Tacken M, Berger M. Mechanism of exercise-induced hypoglycemia during sulfonylurea treatment. Diabetes 1987;36:1178-82.

41 American Diabetes Association. Exercise and NIDDM: a technical review. Diabetes Care 1990;13:785-89.

42 MacDonald MJ. Postexercise late-onset hypoglycemia in insulin dependent diabetic patients. Diabetes Care 1987; 10:584-88.

43 Mitchell TH, Abraham G, Schiffrin A, Leiter A, Marliss EB. Hyperglycemia after intense exercise in IDDM subjects during continuous subcutaneous insulin infusion. Diabetes Care 1988;11:311-17.

44 Calles J, Cunningham JJ, Nelson L, et al. Glucose turnover during recovery from intensive exercise. Diabetes 1983;32: 734-38.

45 Purdon C, Brousson M, Nyveen SL, et al. The roles of insulin and catecholamines in the glucoregulatory response during intense exercise and early recovery in insulin-dependent diabetic and control subjects. J Clin Endocrinol Metab 1993; 76:566-73.

46 Schiffrin A, Parikh S. Accommodating planned exercise in type I diabetic patients on intensive treatment. Diabetes Care 1985;8:337-42.

47 Tuominen JA, Karonen SL, Melamies L, Bolli G, Koivisto VA. Exercise-induced hypoglycaemia in IDDM patients treated with a short-acting insulin analogue. Diabetologia 1995;38:106-11.

48 Koivisto VA, Felig P. Effects of leg exercise on insulin absorption in diabetic patients. N Engl J Med 1978;298:79-83.

49 Kemmer FW, Berchtold P, Berger M, et al. Exercise-induced fall of blood glucose in insulin-treated diabetics unrelated to alteration in insulin mobilization. Diabetes 1979;28:1131-37.

50 Frid A, Ostman J, Linde B. Hypoglycemia risk during exercise after intramuscular injection of insulin in thigh in IDDM. Diabetes Care 1990;13:473-77.

51 Nathan D, Madnek SF, Delahanty L. Programming preexercise snacks to prevent postexercise hypoglycemia in intensively treated insulin dependent diabetics. Ann Intern Med 1985; 102:483-86.

52 Franz MJ. Nutrition: can it give athletes with diabetes a boost? Diabetes Educ 1991;17(3):163-72.

53 Sonnenberg GE, Kemmer FW, Berger M. Exercise in type I diabetic patients treated with continuous subcutaneous insulin infusion. Diabetologia 1990;33:696-703.

54 Beaser RS. Outsmarting diabetes. Minneapolis, Minn: Chronimed, 1994.

55 Durstine JL, King AC, Painter PL, Roitman JL, Zwiren LD, Kenney WL, eds. American College of Sports Medicine. Resource manual for guidelines for exercise testing and prescription. 2nd ed. Philadelphia: Lea & Febiger, 1993.

56 Durak EP, Jovanovic-Peterson L, Peterson CM. Randomized crossover study of effect of resistance training on glycemic control, muscular strength and cholesterol in type I diabetic men. Diabetes Care 1990;13:1039-43.

57 Goldberg AP. Aerobic and resistive exercise modify risk factors for coronary heart disease. Med Sci Sports Exer 1989;21:669-74.

58 Kenney WL, Humphrey RH, Bryant CX, et al, eds. American College of Sports Medicine. Guidelines for exercise testing and prescription. 5th ed. Baltimore: Williams & Wilkins, 1995.

59 National Institutes of Health. NIH consensus statement: physical activity and cardiovascular health. Bethesda, Md: Department of Health and Human Services, Public Health Service, 1995:13(3).

60 Kraemer WJ, Fleck SJ. Resistance training: exercise prescription. Physician Sportsmedicine 1988;16(6):69-81.

61 Soukup JT, Maynard TS, Kovaleski JE. Resistance training guidelines for individuals with diabetes mellitus. Diabetes Educ 1994;20:129-37.

62 Franklin B, Bonzheim K, Gordon S, Timmis G. Resistance training in cardiac rehabilitation. J Cardiopulmonary Rehabil 1991;11:99-107.

63 Frontera WR, Hughes VA, Lutz KJ, Evans WJ. A cross-sectional study of upper and lower extremity muscle strength in 45- to 78- year-old men and women. J Appl Physiol 1991;71:644-50.

64 Graham C. Exercise and aging: implications for persons with diabetes. Diabetes Educ 1991;17:189-95.

65 Schwartz RS. Exercise training in treatment of diabetes mellitus in elderly patients. Diabetes Care 1990;13(suppl 2):77-85.

66 Graham C, Lasko-McCarthey P. Exercise options for persons with diabetic complications. Diabetes Educ 1990;16:212-20.

67 Hiatt WR, Regensteiner JG, Hargarten ME, Wolfel EE, Brass EP. Benefit of exercise conditioning for patients with peripheral arterial disease. Circulation 1990;81:602-9.

68 Levin, ME. The diabetic foot. In: Ruderman NB, Devlin JT, eds. The health professional's guide to diabetes and exercise. Alexandria, Va: American Diabetes Association, 1995.

69 Aiello LM, Cavallerano J, Aiello LP, Bursell SE. Retinopathy. In: Ruderman NB, Devlin JT, eds. The health professional's guide to diabetes and exercise. Alexandria, Va: American Diabetes Association, 1995.

70 Painter P. Exercise in end-stage renal disease. In: Terjung RL, ed. Exercise and sport sciences reviews. New York: Macmillan, 1988:305-40.

71 Pate RR, Pratt M, Blair SN, et al. Physical activity and public health: a recommendation from the Centers for Disease Control and Prevention and the American College of Sports Medicine. JAMA 1995;273:402-7.

72 Marcus BH, Rakowski W, Rossi JS. Assessing motivational readiness and decision making for exercise. Health Psychol 1992;11:257-61.

73 Dishman RK, Sallis JF, Orenstein DR. The determinants of physical activity and exercise. Public Health Rep 1985; 100:158-71.

74 Marcus BH, Simkin LR. The transtheoretical model: applications to exercise behavior. Med Sci Sports Exerc 1994;26: 1400-4.

75 Marcus BH, Selby VC, Niaura RS, Rossi JS. Self-efficacy and the stages of exercise behavior change. Res Q Exerc Sport 1992;63:60-66.

SUGGESTED READINGS

General Exercise Physiology
Albright, AL. American College of Sports Medicine. Exercise management for persons with chronic diseases and disabilities: Diabetes. Champaign, Ill: Human Kinetics, 1997:94-100.

McArdle, WD, Katch F, Katch V. Exercise physiology. 4th ed. Philadelphia: Lea & Febiger, 1996.

Exercise and Diabetes
Fleck, SJ, Kraemer, WJ. Designing resistance training programs. Champaign, Ill. Human Kinetics, 1987.

Franz M. Exercise and diabetes. In: Haire-Joshu D, ed. Management of diabetes mellitus: perspectives of care across the life span. 2nd ed. St. Louis: Mosby Year Book, 1996:162-201.

Horton ES. NIDDM-the devastating disease. Diabetes Res Clin Pract 1995;28:S3-S11.

Maynard T. Exercise: part I. Physiological response to exercise in diabetes mellitus. Diabetes Educ 1991;17:196-206.

Maynard T. Exercise: part II. Translating the exercise prescription. Diabetes Educ 1991;17:384-95.

Ruderman NB, Devlin JT, eds. The health professional's guide to diabetes and exercise. Alexandria, Va: American Diabetes Association, 1995.

Wallberg-Henriksson H. Exercise and diabetes mellitus. In: Holloszy JO, ed. Exercise and sport sciences reviews. Baltimore: Williams & Wilkins, 1992:339-68.

THERAPIES

Pharmacologic Therapies   **10**

John R. White, Jr., RPh, PharmD
Washington State University
Spokane, Washington

R. Keith Campbell, RPh, MBA, CDE
Washington State University
Spokane, Washington

Peggy C. Yarborough, RPh, MS, CDE
Campbell University and
Wilson Community Health Center
Wilson, North Carolina

INTRODUCTION

1 For some people with diabetes, nonpharmacologic interventions will suffice to attain an optimal level of blood glucose control:

A Regular physical activity

B Medical nutrition therapy

C Blood glucose monitoring

D Attention to relevant clinical educational and psychosocial needs

2 For the majority of people with diabetes, however, treatment will also require pharmacologic intervention. Approximately 90% of patients with type 1 or type 2 diabetes require oral antidiabetes medications, insulin injections, or both, to reach glucose goals.[1]

3 In addition to antidiabetes drugs, the pharmacologic therapies for a person with diabetes often include other agents to treat the myriad of associated comorbid conditions or complications of diabetes. These pharmacologic therapies are considered part of standard diabetes care even though they are not used for the purpose of altering blood glucose levels.

4 Diabetes educators must be cognizant of the total range of therapies that are available for comprehensive diabetes care, not just the therapies that are used for glycemic control. They also need to be able to advise patients about the effects of other drugs on blood glucose levels, diabetes complications, and other aspects of self-management.

5 This chapter will provide an update of the pharmacologic therapies for glycemic control and an overview of the impact of other drugs on diabetes management. The goal is for the educator to understand and be able to teach patients some of the intricacies of the pharmacologic interventions that are necessary for comprehensive diabetes self-management.

OBJECTIVES

Upon completion of this chapter, the learner will be able to

1 Explain the physiologic effects of insulin.

2 Differentiate insulin preparations based upon species/source, type, purity, and concentration.

3 Describe proper administration and storage guidelines for insulin.

4 Explain the limitations for insulin mixing.

5 Explain the similarities and differences of potential insulin therapy regimens, including the use of subcutaneous infusion pumps, and indications for specific insulin products.

6 Explain the mechanism(s) of action of sulfonylureas, meglitinides, biguanides, alpha-glucosidase inhibitors, and thiazolidinediones.

7 Describe the clinical use of acarbose, metformin, sulfonylureas, repaglinide, and troglitazone.

8 Explain the use of combination therapy in patients with type 2 diabetes.

9 Explain the clinical use of glucagon.

10 Identify three categories of drug-related effects on diabetes.

11 List two or more classes of medications that commonly are prescribed for patients with diabetes, and describe potential drug-disease, drug-drug or drug-food interactions.

12 List suggestions the diabetes educator may offer to help patients prevent, minimize, or be prepared for a drug-related problem.

PHYSIOLOGIC EFFECTS OF INSULIN AND INDICATIONS FOR ITS USE

1 The following describes the physiologic actions and release of endogenous insulin:

   A Insulin is a hormone produced in the β-cells of the Islets of Langerhans in the pancreas; it is formed from a substance called proinsulin (Figure 10.1).

   • When the pancreas is stimulated, primarily by an elevated blood glucose level, the proinsulin is cleaved at two sections of the molecule - at the glycine position identified as the #1 amino acid of the "A" chain and at the alanine position identified as the #30 amino acid of the "B" chain (see Figure 10.1). When the proinsulin molecule is thus broken apart, insulin and the connecting peptide (C-peptide) are both secreted and enter the bloodstream in equimolar amounts. Some uncleaved proinsulin also enters the blood.

   • Once in the blood stream, the half-life of free insulin has been reported to be in the order of 5.2 +/-0.7 minutes and may be increased in persons with diabetes who have high insulin antibody titers.

   • Normal daily insulin secretion in a healthy, nonpregnant, nonobese adult is approximately 0.5 to 0.7 unit insulin per kg per day.

FIGURE 10.1. BIOCHEMICAL FORMATION OF HUMAN INSULIN FROM PROINSULIN

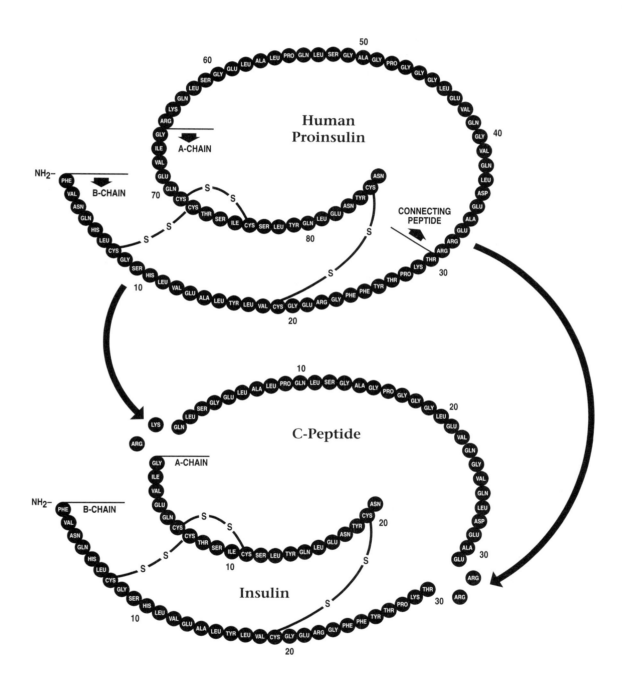

- Since insulin and C-peptide are jointly secreted, a measurement of C-peptide level can be used as a clinical monitor of endogenous insulin production and to determine type of diabetes. Direct measurement of insulin secretion is difficult, except under controlled or research conditions, because insulin is rapidly removed from the blood as it exerts its pharmacologic action.
- Demonstration of measurable levels of C-peptide may also be used to rule out factitious insulin administration as a cause of unexplained hypoglycemia in a person without insulin-requiring diabetes.
- Because insulin and C-peptide have different biologic durations, a measurement of C-peptide level may not accurately reflect the endogenous insulin level at that period of time.

B Insulin exerts varied effects on body tissues.
- Stimulates entry of amino acids into cells, enhancing protein synthesis.
- Enhances fat storage (lipogenesis) and prevents the mobilization of fat for energy (lipolysis and ketogenesis).
- Stimulates the entry of glucose into cells for utilization as an energy source and promotes the resultant storage of glucose as glycogen (glycogenesis) in muscle and liver cells.
- Inhibits production of glucose from liver or muscle glycogen (glycogenolysis).
- Inhibits formation of glucose from noncarbohydrates, such as amino acids (gluconeogenesis).

C The major untoward effect of insulin therapy is hypoglycemia. Virtually all persons who inject insulin will experience hypoglycemia at some time.
- Frequent causes of hypoglycemia include too much (excessive dosage of) insulin; delayed, missed, or insufficient caloric intake; or too much (unplanned) exercise.
- Strategies to reduce the risk of hypoglycemia include routine self-monitoring of blood glucose levels; observing for, and responding quickly to early symptoms of hypoglycemia; ingesting appropriate quantities and choices of a pre-exercise carbohydrate supplement; and using a consistent meal plan and pattern.
- Instruct all insulin-using patients concerning the symptoms, prevention, and treatment of hypoglycemia. In addition, teaching patients to routinely carry a source of carbohydrate can help to prevent mild reactions from becoming severe.

D *Endogenous insulin* is defined as insulin that is supplied from the pancreas, while *exogenous insulin* is defined as injected pharmaceutical insulin.

2   There are several hormones in the body which exert antagonistic effects to the hypoglycemic actions of insulin. These hormones are collectively referred to as *counterregulatory hormones*. Blood glucose management in diabetes needs to take into account, and make compensation for, the release of one or more of these hormones throughout the day in response to a variety of stimuli. The primary counterregulatory hormones include

   A Glucagon: produced in the alpha cells of the pancreas

   B Epinephrine

   C Norepinephrine

   D Growth hormone

   E Cortisol

3   Insulin is indicated for specific patients with diabetes or in certain medical conditions.

   A All individuals with type 1 diabetes require exogenous insulin to sustain life. In type 1 diabetes, production of insulin by beta cells is completely or largely lost.

   B Individuals with type 2 diabetes may need insulin if other forms of therapy do not adequately control blood glucose levels or during periods of physiological stress such as surgery or infection.

   C Women with gestational diabetes may need insulin if medical nutrition therapy alone does not adequately control blood glucose levels.

   D Diabetic or non-diabetic patients receiving parenteral nutrition or high-caloric supplements to meet an increased energy need may require exogenous insulin to maintain normal glucose levels during periods of insulin resistance or increased insulin demand.

   E Insulin is necessary in the treatment of diabetic ketoacidosis (DKA).

   F Insulin is often needed in the treatment of hyperosmolar hyperglycemic nonketotic syndrome (HHNS).

   G Individuals with secondary diabetes may require insulin, such as diabetes secondary to pancreatitis or other disease that severely diminishes β-cell production of insulin.

Insulin Species/Source, Type, Purity, and Concentration

1 Insulin preparations are differentiated by specific product characteristics (Table 10.1).

2 The species/sources for insulin are beef, pork, and human. The six product types include pork and beef-pork combinations, which are isolated from animal pancreas glands; biosynthetic human insulin derived from bacteria, (*E coli*) or fungal cells (*Saccharomyces cerevisiae*); semisynthetic human insulin; and biosynthetic human insulin analog.

   A Beef insulin differs from human insulin at three amino acid sites, while pork insulin differs at only one amino acid site (Table 10.2). Because of this difference, beef insulin induces more antigenic reactions than pork insulin. Beef-pork combination products are generally thought to induce the most antigenic reactions. Beef insulin alone is not available in the US.

   B Human insulin and the human insulin analog lispro are manufactured by using recombinant-DNA technology (biosynthetic). Human insulin is also manufactured by chemical conversion of pork insulin to human insulin (semisynthetic). Human insulin and lispro insulin are less antigenic than beef insulin and slightly less antigenic than pork insulin.

   C Human biosynthetic NPH, Lente and Ultralente insulins appear to be absorbed faster and therefore act more quickly than animal-derived insulins, even though they have similar pharmacologic effects. Commercially prepared human insulins are effective and chemically identical to endogenous human insulin.

   D Patients who change from animal insulin to human insulin may require dosage adjustment because of the shorter duration of action and lower antigenicity (eg, less potential for antibody production) of human insulin.

   E Human insulin provides an option for vegetarians, Moslems, Orthodox Jews, or Hindus who prefer not to use pork or beef insulins. There are virtually no contraindications to human insulin, although there are rare instances of hypersensitivity.

   F Animal-derived insulins may induce insulin antibody formation to a greater degree than human insulins or lispro. When insulin is bound to insulin-antibodies the predictability of the insulin's peak effect and duration of action will be altered.

TABLE 10.1. INSULINS AVAILABLE IN THE UNITED STATES

	Product	Manufacturer	Strength
Short-Acting	**Pork**		
	Iletin® II regular	Lilly	U-100, U-500
	Purified Pork regular	Novo Nordisk	U-100
	Beef/Pork		
	Iletin® I regular	Lilly	U-100
	Human		
	Humulin® R (regular)	Lilly	U-100
	Novolin® R (regular)	Novo Nordisk	U-100
	Velosulin® BR (regular)	Novo Nordisk	U-100
Rapid-Acting	**Human Insulin Analog**		
	Humalog® lispro	Lilly	U-100
Intermediate-Acting	**Pork**		
	Iletin® II Lente	Lilly	U-100
	Iletin® II NPH	Lilly	U-100
	Purified Pork Lente	Novo Nordisk	U-100
	Purified Pork NPH	Novo Nordisk	U-100
	Beef/Pork		
	Iletin® I NPH	Lilly	U-100
	Iletin® I Lente	Lilly	U-100
	Human		
	Humulin® L (Lente)	Lilly	U-100
	Humulin® N (NPH)	Lilly	U-100
	Novolin® L (Lente)	Novo Nordisk	U-100
	Novolin® N (NPH)	Novo Nordisk	U-100
Long-Acting	**Human Insulin Analog**		
	Humulin® U (Ultralente)	Lilly	U-100
Fixed Combination (all are U-100 insulins)			**NPH/reg Ratio**
	Human		
	Humulin® 70/30	Lilly	70/30
	Novolin® 70/30	Novo Nordisk	70/30
	Humulin® 50/50	Lilly	50/50

3 Insulin is generally classified according to peak effect and duration of action (Table 10.3). The currently available *rapid-acting insulin* is lispro, the *short-acting insulin* is regular, the *intermediate-acting insulins* are NPH and Lente, and the *long-acting insulin* is Ultralente.

TABLE 10.2. AMINO ACID SEQUENCE DIFFERENCES BETWEEN VARIOUS INSULIN SPECIES

Species	A Chain		B Chain		
	A-8	A-10	B-30	B-29	B-28
Bovine	Alanine	Valine	Alanine	Lysine	Proline
Porcine	Threonine	Isoleucine	Alanine	Lysine	Proline
Human	Threonine	Isoleucine	Threonine	Lysine	Proline
Analog	Threonine	Isoleucine	Threonine	Proline	Lysine

Source: Adapted from Insulin. In: Waife SO, ed. Diabetes mellitus. Indianapolis: Lilly Research Laboratories, 1980:37.

A Regular insulin and lispro are the only clear insulins or solution of insulin; all of the others are suspensions. Regular insulin is the only insulin product routinely used for intravenous administration, although lispro may be given intravenously.

- Lispro is an insulin analog identical to human insulin in its structure, with the exception of the juxtaposition of lysine and proline in positions 28 and 29 on the B chain (see Figure 10.1). This molecular alteration yields an insulin with a faster rate of absorption than regular human insulin.[2]
- A dose of lispro insulin peaks in half the time and in double the concentration of a comparable subcutaneous injection of regular insulin.[3]
- Lispro insulin can generally be used in place of regular insulin to provide better coverage of postprandial glycemic excursions.
- Lispro insulin can be injected immediately prior to eating (generally less than 15 minutes preprandially); injecting lispro insulin 30 to 60 minutes prior to meals may result in profound hypoglycemia.
- Lispro insulin is available in the US only by prescription.

B NPH contains protamine and some zinc to prolong the duration of action.

C Lente and Ultralente insulins have high zinc levels to prolong the duration of action.

D Both protamine and zinc have occasionally been implicated as the causative agents of immunologic reactions such as urticaria at the injection site.

TABLE 10.3. ONSET, PEAK, AND DURATION OF DIFFERENT INSULINS

Insulin	Onset, h	Peak, h	Duration Therapeutic*	Pharmaceutic†
Rapid-acting (lispro insulin)	15 to 30 min	1 to 2	3 to 4	
Short-acting (regular)	1/2 to 1	2 to 4	6 to 8	5 to 12
Intermediate-acting (NPH, Lente)	1 to 4	8 ± 2	10 to 16	16 to 24
Long-acting (Ultralente)	4 to 6	18	24 to 36	36+

* Therapeutic or effective duration of action = the amount of active insulin needed to keep blood glucose levels in normal limits.
† Pharmaceutic or pharmacokinetic duration of action = the action of insulin on "entrance" into and "exit" from the body.

Source: Adapted from Campbell RK. Diabetic management: insulin, oral agents and intensified insulin therapy (module 9). Chicago: American Association of Diabetes Educators Continuing Education Self-Study Program, 1985: table 3; and Care and control of your diabetes. Wichita, Kan: St Joseph Medical Center, Diabetes Treatment Center, 1988:59.

4   Purity of animal-source insulin is expressed as parts per million (ppm) of proinsulin, the primary contaminant after extraction from the pancreas. Concern about purity is a less significant issue in insulin therapy today than previously, as all insulins are now highly purified.

5   The concentrations of insulin currently available in the US are U-100 and U-500, indicating 100 units per cubic centimeter (cc) or 500 units per cubic centimeter (cc), respectively. U-100 insulin is the insulin of choice for nearly all patients. U-100 insulin is not available worldwide; instruct patients to take extra supplies when traveling to foreign countries.

   A   Patients requiring large doses of insulin may benefit by using U-500 regular insulin. The onset and duration of action of U-500 is not the same as U-100 regular.

   B   U-500 regular insulin is available in the US only by prescription.

6   Velosulin® Human BR insulin is usually recommended for insulin pump use because it contains phosphate buffers that may minimize crystallization or aggregation of insulin in the infusion tubing. The chemical and

gest that it would be an efficacious choice for insulin pump use; however, results from clinical trials are needed before the product labeling can reflect this indication.

ADMINISTRATION AND STORAGE GUIDELINES

1   Effective use of insulin requires the correct equipment, insulin preparation, and consistent use of proper technique.

2   Teach patients to store insulin according to the manufacturer's recommendations.

  A   Generally, insulin should be refrigerated at 36° to 46° F (2° to 8° C).
    • Unopened insulin products may be stored under refrigeration until the expiration date noted on the product label.

  B   To reduce local irritation at the injection site that may occur when injecting cold insulin, advise patients to roll the prepared syringe between the palms, bring the bottle of insulin to room temperature before withdrawing the dose, or store the insulin at room temperature. Opened or unopened vials of insulin may be stored at a controlled room temperature of 59° to 86° F (15° to 30° C) for a period of one month; unused insulin should be discarded after that time.[4-6]

  C   Storage guidelines differ for use and storage of used (punctured) or unused cartridge insulin (Penfill®) and disposable prefilled insulin pens.[5]
    • Lispro or regular insulin cartridges or regular prefilled insulin pens may be kept unrefrigerated for 28 days (1.5 or 3.0 ml cartridges)
    • 70/30 insulin cartridges or prefilled insulin pens may be kept unrefrigerated for 10 days.
    • NPH insulin cartridges or prefilled insulin pens may be kept unrefrigerated for 14 days.

  D   Keep extemporaneously prepared, prefilled syringes of either single formulations or mixtures of insulins refrigerated and use within 21 to 30 days.[7,8]

  E   Availability of insulin and supplies may vary; teach patients to carry insulin and supplies when traveling. Due to variance of temperature, insulin should not be left in a car or checked through in airline baggage.

  F   Instruct patients to examine vials of insulin for sediment or other visible changes before withdrawing the insulin into the syringe. Cloudiness or discoloration of clear insulin, clumping of insulin suspensions, or flocculation (frosting) of insulin suspensions indicates that the insulin has lost potency and should not be used but returned to the pharmacy for exchange. The incidence of frosting may be minimized if temperature is stabilized through refrigeration and if agitation or shaking of the vial is minimized.

3 Insulin administration equipment

    A Disposable insulin syringes with attached needles for U-100 insulin are available in different syringe sizes, chosen according to the dose of insulin to be injected: 0.25 cc (for doses <25 units), 0.3 cc (for doses <30 units), 0.5 cc (for doses <50 units) or 1 cc (for doses 50-100 units). Needle length may be 5/16-inch or ½-inch. The "short needle" (5/16-inch length) is appropriate only for individuals with normal or near-normal body mass index (BMI <27 kg/m²).

    B In most circumstances, and with proper training, syringes and needles may be safely reused,[8] however reuse may carry an increased risk of infection for some individuals. Advise patients who choose to reuse syringes that the markings on the syringe may rub off and that the needle becomes dull with repeated use. Instruct patients to safely recap the needle and store at room temperature.

    C Alternative equipment to the traditional syringe-needle unit is available. The variety of injection devices includes automatic needle injectors, automatic needle and insulin injectors, pen injectors, and needle-free jet injectors. The needle-free jet injectors propel insulin through the skin by air pressure.

    D Insulin pumps, also known as continuous subcutaneous insulin infusion (CSII) devices, are programmed to deliver a continuous infusion of insulin subcutaneously; before each ingestion of food, the patient programs the device to administer a bolus (rapid release) of insulin. This method provides a more physiologic pattern of insulin delivery than attained by multiple injections of insulin.

        • Frequent blood glucose monitoring provides patients and professionals with the data needed for decision-making and flexibility.

        • Because of the expense of pumps, patients need to consider pump therapy carefully in collaboration with their healthcare team.

        • Insulin pumps currently available for daily use utilize an open-loop system. A continuous basal dose is programmed, and the patient then adjusts bolus doses of insulin based on blood glucose levels, food intake and activity levels.

4 Teach patients to follow a specific routine for insulin injections, including consistent technique, accurate dosage, and site rotation.

  A Injections are given into the subcutaneous tissue. Most individuals are able to lightly grasp a fold of skin and inject at a 90° angle. Thin individuals or children may need to pinch the skin and inject at a 45° angle to avoid intramuscular injection.[8]

  B Commonly used injection sites are shown in Figure 10.2. These sites are chosen because of the low potential for adverse reactions as well as general patient acceptability and accessibility.

  • Areas for injection must be determined individually, allowing for scar tissue, areas with less subcutaneous fat, and patient preference.

  • Both the patient and the health professional need to examine injection areas at regular intervals to detect bruising, redness, infection, lipoatrophy, or lipohypertrophy.

  • Teach patients to rotate injection sites to prevent local irritation. Some advocate rotating injections within one anatomical area, then moving to another area, to provide each area several weeks of "rest" between uses.

  C Insulin absorption may vary depending upon several parameters.

  • Abdominal injection provides the most rapid absorption followed by the arm, leg, and hip sites.[9,10] Deeper intramuscular (IM) injections induce faster absorption and shorter duration of action. High levels of insulin antibodies can also inhibit insulin action following injection.

  • Massage of the injection site may induce more rapid absorption and action from a dose of insulin by increasing the rate of blood flow through the tissue around the site, so it is seldom recommended.[11]

5 Various problems or complications may arise from insulin impurity, species source, and improper injection technique.

  A Insulin impurity can cause lipodystrophies (atrophy and hypertrophy).

  • *Atrophy,* which is a concavity or pitting of the fatty tissue, is an immune phenomenon that occurs in a small number of patients and is related to species source or purity. Use of highly purified insulins such as human insulin or purified pork reduces the occurrence of atrophy. Patients who develop this problem may benefit from injecting human or highly purified insulin around the periphery of the atrophied areas.[12]

FIGURE 10.2. INJECTION SITES

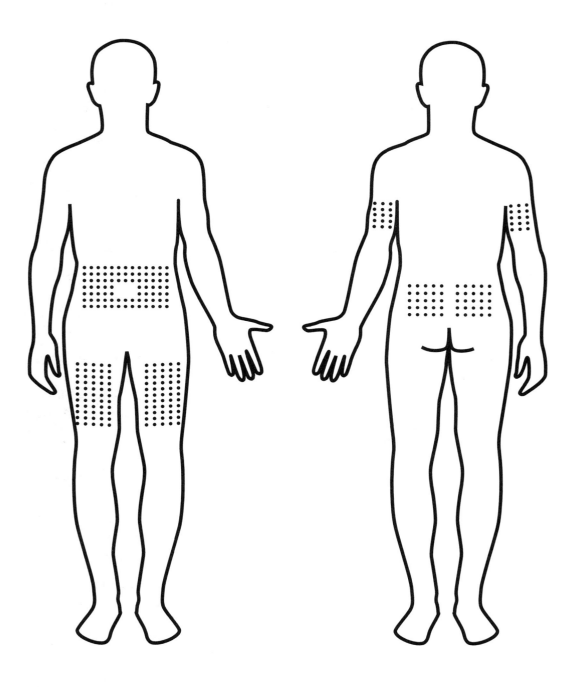

Adapted from: Michigan Diabetes Research and Training Center, University of Michigan, 1988.

- *Hypertrophy*, which is a fatty thickening of the lipid tissue, is best prevented by rotation of injection sites.

B Allergies to insulin are rare. Insulin allergy may occur as local reactions (rash, urticarial cutaneous reaction) or systemic reactions (serum sickness, anaphylaxis).

- Prior to insulin purification, local cutaneous reactions were more common.
- Zinc or protamine in the insulin, preservatives, and rubber or latex stoppers have all been implicated in inducing allergic reactions.
- Both local and systemic reactions appear to be immunologically mediated through induction of high titers of IgG and IgE antibodies.
- When allergic reactions occur, a change from animal insulin to a purified or human insulin may resolve the problem. If systemic reaction occurs, desensitization to the insulin will also be necessary.

MIXING INSULINS

1 Organizing the necessary materials prior to insulin injection will limit errors.

2 Guidelines for extemporaneous insulin mixtures are listed in Table 10.4. These standards are based on published data.[13]

A Varying the time delay for injecting after mixing may result in a different insulin action.

B As a general rule, the two insulins being mixed should be of the same brand.

C Regular or lispro insulin is usually drawn up first, followed by the intermediate-acting insulin. This practice limits the potential for contamination which may result in dose variance.

3 Commercially-available premixed insulins (70/30 and 50/50) are manufactured and stabilized by altered buffering. These products may be advantageous for individuals unable to mix insulins accurately or reliably.

INSULIN THERAPY PROGRAMS

1 Insulin dosing schedules vary among individuals (see Chapter 12, Pattern Management).

A Physiologically, insulin is released throughout the day in frequent bursts in response to a variety of stimuli such as the glycemic rise from ingestion of food or the release of counterregulatory hormones. Insulin release in response to food intake is referred to as a "bolus" secretion; insulin release to counteract ongoing hormonal or other glycemic influences is referred to as "basal" secretion. Thus, the physiologic insulin profile is one of peaks (boluses) and valleys (basal) of insulin release throughout the day (Figure 10.3).

B A goal of insulin therapy is to mimic, as nearly as possible, the physiologic profile of insulin secretion (eg, the peaks and valleys). Such a pattern is difficult to achieve with infrequent injections of insulin.

C To optimize glycemic control, the pharmacology and pharmacokinetics of insulin require that a person receive small amounts of insulin continuously (basal), with boluses of insulin before meals and snacks.

D The evolution of insulin management in the US is clearly moving from single injection therapy with intermediate-acting insulin to multiple injection therapy with human insulin.[14]

E The kinetics of various insulin products are shown in Table 10.3.

2 The starting dose and schedule of insulin administration is based on the clinical assessment of insulin deficiency and suspected insulin resistance, and the person's preferences for eating times, exercise, and waking/sleep patterns.[15]

A Type 1 diabetes or individuals within 20% of ideal body weight: usually 0.5-1.0 Unit/kg body weight/day.
- Insulin requirements will be higher (even double) in the presence of intercurrent illness or other metabolic instability.
- Insulin requirements will be less (0.2-0.6 Unit/kg body weight/day) during the "honeymoon phase," the period of relative remission early in the course of the disease.

B Type 2 diabetes: varies considerably, and may range from as little as 5 to 10 U/day to as much as several hundred units per day.[16] This variability may be attributed to interpatient variability of insulin deficiency and insulin resistance.

C Gestational diabetes: 0.3-0.7 Units/kg body weight/day, with increasing doses as the pregnancy progresses (may even triple).

Table 10.4. Guidelines for Mixing Insulin and/or Prefilling Syringes

Regular and NPH	• Mixture stable in any ratio • Mixture of choice, if regular and intermediate combination is needed • Extemporaneously prepared syringes that are refrigerated are stable for at least one month • Prefilling is acceptable
Regular and Lente	• Binding of regular begins immediately • Binding continues for 24 hours • Activity of regular is blunted • Velosulin should not be mixed with Lente insulins • If mixed or prefilled, the interval between mixing the insulins and administering the insulin should be standardized
Commercially Prepared Premixed Insulins	• Prefilling is acceptable
Lente and Ultralente	• Mixture stable in any ratio • Mixture stable for 18 months • Prefilling is acceptable
Lispro Insulin with NPH or Ultralente	• Mixture stable in any ratio • Administer immediately after mixing

Source: Adapted from White J, Campbell RK. Guide to mixing insulins. Hosp Pharm, 1991;26:1046-48.

Figure 10.3. Time Action of Physiologic (Endogenous) Insulin*

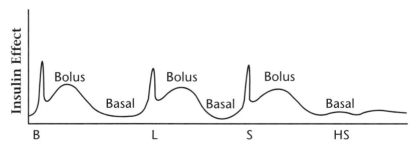

B = breakfast, L = lunch, S = supper, HS = bedtime.

"Bolus" secretion: The biphasic release of insulin in response to food intake.
"Basal" secretion: The release of insulin to counteract ongoing hormonal or other glycemic influences.

*Schematic representation only

D Establish target blood glucose levels for test times before meals, after meals, and during sleep. Setting targets *with* the patient (rather than *for* the patient) enhances patient understanding and decision making as the person observes changes in blood glucose levels in relation to changes in diet, exercise, stress, or illness.

E Subsequent adjustments in dose or timing of the insulin are based on self-monitoring of blood glucose (SMBG) and clinical signs and symptoms of hypoglycemia or hyperglycemia.

F Other parameters used to refine the insulin dose and schedule include glycosylated hemoglobin levels, achievement of weight or lipid goals, and variability of lifestyle or activities from day to day.

3 Regimens for insulin monotherapy vary as needed, to meet the needs of the individual's daily habits with regard to meals, exercise, medications, work or activity schedule, and emotional factors. *Note:* The following regimens assume that the patient's lifestyle includes a waking time in the morning, meals spaced consistently during the day and waking hours, with a late evening bedtime. Appropriate alterations can be made in the insulin program to accommodate a midnight or rotating work schedule or other lifestyle preferences. Combination therapy using insulin with antidiabetes oral agents is discussed later.

A Single Daily Injection Regimen: usually administered in the morning or sometimes at bedtime (Figure 10.4).
   * Not indicated for type 1 diabetes.
   * Usually utilizes an intermediate-acting insulin, but could include a combined dose of a rapid- or short- and intermediate-acting product.
   * Bedtime administration may offer the advantage of improved fasting blood glucose control by suppressing nocturnal hepatic glucose production or increasing the basal-metabolic clearance of glucose.[17]
   * Single daily doses of intermediate-acting insulin may be used when doses are < 30 U/day; for larger daily doses, two or more doses will likely be needed.

B Two Injection Regimens: administered in the morning and before the evening meal (Figure 10.5).
   * Could include only intermediate-acting insulin, or may be mixed doses of regular or lispro insulin with intermediate-acting insulin at one or both injection times. Mixed doses in the morning and before the evening meal is often called a "split-mixed regimen" and is considered conventional insulin therapy.

Figure 10.4. Time Action of Insulin*; One Daily Injection

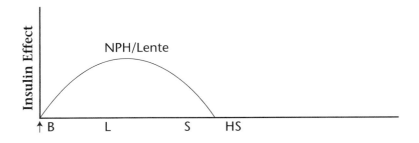

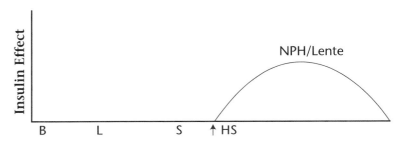

B = breakfast, L = lunch, S = supper, HS = bedtime.

*Schematic representation only

Adapted with permission: University of Kansas School of Medicine at Wichita.

- Usually two thirds of the total daily dose of insulin is given before breakfast (using a ratio of 1 part rapid- or short-acting insulin to 2 parts intermediate-acting insulin) and one third is given before the evening meal (using a ratio of 1:1 or 1:2, rapid- or short-acting to intermediate insulin).

C Three Injection Regimens: administered in the morning, before the evening meal, and at bedtime, or before each meal. Multiple injections of insulin (three or more) are one component of the system called intensive insulin therapy (Figure 10.6).

- Combination of rapid- or short- and intermediate-acting insulin before breakfast, short-acting insulin alone before the evening meal, and intermediate-acting insulin at 10 PM (Figure 10.6-A) The intermediate-acting insulin at 10 PM.

FIGURE 10.5. TIME ACTION OF INSULIN*, TWO DAILY INJECTIONS

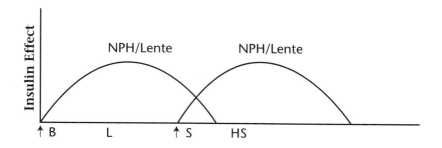

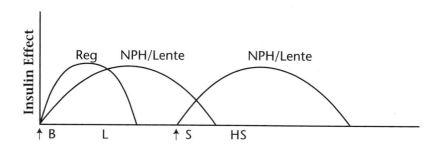

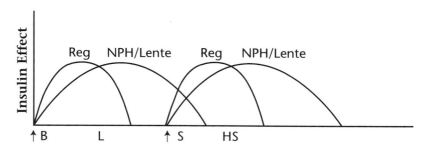

B = breakfast, L = lunch, S = supper, HS = bedtime, Reg = regular insulin.

*Schematic representation only

Adapted with permission: University of Kansas School of Medicine at Wichita.

— reduces the risk of nocturnal (2-4 AM) hypoglycemia,

— allows better insulin coverage for early morning (5-10 AM) hyperglycemia from the release of growth hormone (the dawn phenomenon), and

— may accommodate "sleeping in" in some cases

• Ultralente insulin combined with regular insulin or lispro insulin before breakfast and before the evening meal, and regular or lispro

Figure 10.6. Time Action of Insulin*, Three Daily Injections

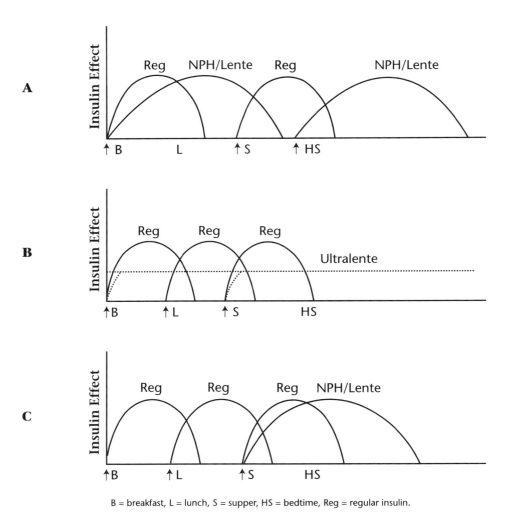

B = breakfast, L = lunch, S = supper, HS = bedtime, Reg = regular insulin.

*Schematic representation only

Adapted with permission: University of Kansas School of Medicine at Wichita.

insulin alone before lunch (Figure 10.6-B). This protocol is particularly useful for individuals with unusual schedules.

• Regular or lispro insulin alone before breakfast and lunch, and regular or lispro insulin with intermediate-acting insulin before the evening meal (Figure 10.6-C).

FIGURE 10.7. TIME ACTION OF INSULIN*, FOUR DAILY INJECTIONS

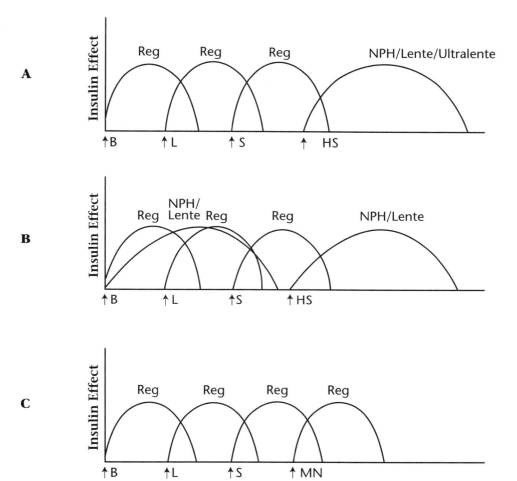

B = breakfast, L = lunch, S = supper, HS = bedtime, MN = midnight, Reg = regular insulin.

*Schematic representation only

Adapted with permission: University of Kansas School of Medicine at Wichita.

D Four Injection Regimens: administered in the morning, before lunch, before the evening meal, and at 10 PM (Figure 10.7).
  • Regular or lispro insulin alone before breakfast, lunch, and dinner, and an intermediate- or long-acting insulin (NPH, Lente, or Ultralente) at 10 PM (Figure 10.7-A).

- Regular or lispro insulin with an intermediate-acting insulin in the morning, regular or lispro insulin alone before lunch and before the evening meal, and an intermediate-acting insulin at 10 PM (Figure 10.7-B).
- The rapid- or short-acting insulin provides postmeal glycemic control, while the intermediate- or long-acting dose ensures a low, steady rate of insulin throughout the day.
- Four injections of regular insulin given about 6 hours apart may be indicated for some patients. This program may be effective during an illness or if ketoacidosis is imminent. Formulas for calculating dosages vary, but about one third of the total daily dose is given before breakfast, a slightly smaller amount at lunchtime, about 30% preceding the evening meal, and about 15% at midnight (Figure 10.7-C).

E Continuous Subcutaneous Insulin Infusion: a continuous basal amount of insulin (0.5 to 1.0 u/h) is usually administered in addition to bolus doses given prior to meals (Figure 10.8).

ORAL ANTIDIABETES AGENTS IN THE MANAGEMENT OF DIABETES

1 Currently, there are five chemical classes of oral agents available in the US for the management of diabetes.

A Sulfonylureas (oral hypoglycemic agents)

B Meglitinides: repaglinide (oral hypoglycemic agent)

C Biguanides: metformin ("insulin sensitizer")

D Thiazolidinediones: troglitazone ("insulin sensitizer")

E Alpha-glucosidase inhibitors: acarbose

2 These agents may be used as monotherapy for the treatment of type 2 diabetes or secondary diabetes with substantial capacity for insulin production, or may be used in combination with each other or with insulin.[18]

3 Oral antidiabetes agents may be used in type 1 diabetes only as an adjunct to insulin therapy.

4 These agents are not routinely advised for use during preconception care, pregnancy (pregestational diabetes or gestational diabetes) nor for children.

FIGURE 10.8. TIME ACTION OF INSULIN*; CONTINUOUS SUBCUTANEOUS INSULIN INFUSION (INFUSION PUMP THERAPY)

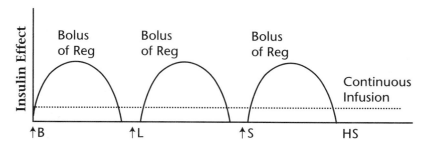

B = breakfast, L = lunch, S = supper, HS = bedtime.

The insulin pump is programmed to deliver a determined rate of insulin throughout the day; prior to each meal, the patient activates the pump to deliver a bolus of insulin to control the glycemic response to food intake.

*Schematic representation only

5 Generally, monotherapy with any of these agents is associated with a reduction in HbA$_{1c}$ of approximately 0.5 to 1.5%. This does not mean, however, that any agent will be equally efficacious for all patients; matching the pharmacologic action of a given agent with the patient's pathophysiologic basis(es) of hyperglycemia is a major determinant in therapeutic efficacy.

6 When combination therapy is utilized (two or more oral antidiabetes agents or an oral agent combined with insulin) an additive effect is observed, as demonstrated by a further decrease in HbA$_{1c}$.

7 Combination therapies:
  A Frequently used and/or well-studied
  - Sulfonylurea with metformin
  - Sulfonylurea with insulin
  - Sulfonylurea with alpha-glucosidase inhibitor
  - Troglitazone with insulin
  - Troglitazone with sulfonylurea

B Less frequently used and/or less well-studied, or not studied
- Sulfonylurea with metformin with insulin
- Metformin with alpha-glucosidase inhibitor
- Metformin with insulin
- Alpha-glucosidase inhibitor with insulin
- Repaglinide with metformin

SULFONYLUREAS

1 Available agents: Sulfonylureas can be classified as first- and second-generation oral hypoglycemic agents as shown in Table 10.5. The first-generation agents are further divided into rapid-, intermediate-, and long-acting products.

2 Pharmacologic actions:
  A Hypoglycemic agent: the major pharmacologic action has the potential to reduce blood glucose level below normal (ie, cause hypoglycemia).
  B Primary effect: Increases release of insulin from the pancreas, especially at the onset of therapy.
  C Secondary effects:
    - Enhances performance and increased numbers of insulin receptors on muscle and fat cells
    - Accelerates glucose transport into cells at the postinsulin receptor site
    - Reduces hepatic glucose production

3 Pharmacokinetics:
  A Absorption is generally rapid, fairly complete, and unaffected by food except for short-acting glipizide, which is most effective when taken on an empty stomach.
  B Metabolism and excretion of these agents varies greatly. Most sulfonylureas are metabolized in the liver to active or inactive metabolites except for chlorpropamide, which is partially excreted unchanged in the urine. Biliary excretion is significant with glyburide and to a lesser extent with glipizide.[19]

C   Increases release of insulin from the pancreas; the effect is glucose-dependent and diminishes at low blood glucose concentrations

3   Pharmacokinetics[24]:
A   Absorption from the GI tract is rapid and complete; food slightly decreases absorption
B   Protein binding and binding to serum albumin: >95%
C   Rapid hepatic metabolism to inactive metabolites; half-life of the drug is ~1 hour. Less than 1% of the parent drug is excreted by the kidneys. Because of the short half-life, the potential for accumulation is minimal with normal dosing regimens.

4   Significant contraindications or precautions to repaglinide therapy:
A   Not recommended for use during pregnancy, for breast-feeding women, or children
B   Diabetic ketoacidosis
C   Severe infection
D   Surgery, trauma, or other severe metabolic stressor
E   Impaired hepatic function: use cautiously. Titrate doses upward very gradually, with careful monitoring, to detect accumulation of parent drug and/or metabolites.
F   Elderly, debilitated or malnourished patients, and those with adrenal, pituitary or hepatic insufficiency are particularly susceptible to the hypoglycemic effects of glucose-lowering agents.
G   Refer to package labeling for additional contraindications and precautions.

5   Adverse effects associated with repaglinide therapy:
A   Gastrointestinal disturbances (~4%)
B   Upper respiratory infection or problems
C   Arthralgia or back pain
D   Headache

6   Treatment failure occurs when an individual is insensitive to the effects of repaglinide.
A   Primary failure: no response to the initial repaglinide therapy
B   Secondary failure: no or diminished response to the repaglinide, after an initial therapeutic response

7 Clinically important drug interactions with repaglinide are listed in Table 10.6.

8 Role of repaglinide in the treatment of diabetes mellitus:

    A Use as monotherapy only in type 2 diabetes or secondary diabetes with substantial capacity for insulin production.

- Typical candidate for initial repaglinide monotherapy: type 2 diabetes, without dyslipidemia, with or without renal failure, not overweight, and fasting plasma glucose level >20 mg/dL above the target concentration.

    B Therapy initiated at a low, single daily dose, with gradual increases to reach glucose goals.

- Instruct patients to take 15 minutes (0-30 minutes) before each meal. The number of daily doses taken is determined by the number of meals eaten. The "meal-based" dosing frequency may offer advantages for patients who vary frequency of daily meals, or for those who choose to eat only two meals a day and need to avoid persisting hypoglycemic activity between the meals.
- Initial dose for patients not treated previously with glucose-lowering drugs or with HbA_{1c} <8%: 0.5 mg with each meal.
- Initial dosage does not need to be adjusted for patients with renal dysfunction; however, upward titration should proceed cautiously.
- Initial dose for patients previously treated with glucose-lowering drugs and with HbA_{1c} >8%: 1 or 2 mg with each meal
- At one week intervals, each preprandial dose may be doubled, up to 4 mg, until desired effect is attained.
- Maximum dose: 16 mg daily

    C Combination therapy, or transition to insulin monotherapy, is considered when repaglinide therapy approaches the maximum dose.

BIGUANIDES

1 Available agent: Metformin (Glucophage®): 500 mg, 850 mg dosage units

2 Pharmacologic actions:

    A Not a hypoglycemic agent: the major pharmacologic action does not increase insulin secretion and thus does not increase the risk of hypoglycemia. This agent may best be described as an anti-hyperglycemic agent or an insulin sensitizer.

- The slight (2 to 5 kg) weight loss seen with metformin therapy is likely due to its insulin-sparing property.

B Primary effects:

- Reduces hepatic glucose production primarily by reduction in glycogenolysis.[25]
- Enhances insulin-stimulated glucose transport in adipose tissue and skeletal muscle, thus reversing or partially reversing insulin resistance.[26]

C Decreases intestinal absorption of glucose (minor effect)

D Causes a reduction in triglyceride concentrations (16%), LDL cholesterol (8%), and total cholesterol (5%), and is associated with an increase in HDL cholesterol (2%).[27]

3 Pharmacokinetics:

A Oral bioavailability: 50% to 60%. Food decreases the extent and slightly delays the absorption of metformin.

B Does not bind to liver or plasma proteins

C Major excretion is by the kidneys, largely unchanged, through an active tubular process.

4 Significant contraindications or precautions to metformin therapy:

A Generally not indicated during pregnancy, for breast-feeding women, or children.

B Renal dysfunction with serum creatinine levels >1.5 mg/dL in males or > 1.4 mg/dL in females. Metformin is excreted renally and can accumulate in patients with renal dysfunction.

C Hepatic dysfunction (lactate metabolism is carried out in the liver)

D Acute or chronic lactic acidosis

E History of alcoholism or binge ingestion of alcohol

F Metformin should be temporarily withheld in any situation which would predispose the individual to acute renal dysfunction or tissue hypoperfusion, including

- Cardiovascular collapse
- Acute myocardial infarction
- Acute exacerbation of congestive heart failure
- Use of iodinated contrast media
- Major surgical procedure

G Refer to package labeling for additional contraindications and precautions.

5 Adverse effects associated with metformin therapy:

    A Metformin monotherapy is not associated with hypoglycemia.

- Patients using combination therapy (metformin with insulin or metformin with sulfonylureas) may experience hypoglycemia secondary to the hypoglycemic agent.

    B Gastrointestinal effects (up to 30%): abdominal bloating, nausea, cramping, feeling of fullness, diarrhea

- Usually self-limiting, transient (7 to 14 days), and can be minimized by taking the medication with food, starting with a low dose, and slow upward titration of dosage.

    C Miscellaneous: agitation, sweating, headache, and metallic taste.

    D Associated with a reduction in vitamin B-12 levels, although no cases of anemia have been reported in the US.

    E Lactic acidosis can occur with the administration of metformin but is rare (0.03 cases per 1000 patient years). Lactic acidosis is primarily associated with its use in patients who have contraindications to the drug or in cases of overdose.

6 Clinically important drug interactions with metformin are listed in Table 10.6.

7 Role of metformin in the treatment of diabetes mellitus:

    A Use as monotherapy only in type 2 diabetes or secondary diabetes with substantial capacity for insulin production.

- Typical candidate for initial metformin monotherapy: type 2 diabetes, with dyslipidemia, with obesity or genetic factors favoring insulin resistance, and fasting plasma glucose level >20 mg/dL above the target concentration.[21]

    B Therapy initiated at a low dose, with gradual increases to obtain desired control.

- Usual initial dose: 500 mg or 850 mg qd or 500 mg bid, with doses taken prior to a meal.
- Titrate dose upward as tolerated (to GI effects) to reach glucose goals. Increases usually occur at 7-14 day intervals.
- Maximum daily dose: 2550 mg (850 mg tid). Note, however, that the greatest reduction in fasting plasma glucose is seen at 2000 mg/day (1000 mg bid).

    C Combination therapy, or transition to insulin monotherapy, is considered when metformin therapy approaches the maximum dose.

THIAZOLIDINEDIONES

1   Available agent: Troglitazone (Rezulin®): 200 mg, 300 mg, 400 mg dosage units

2   Pharmacologic actions:

   A   Not a hypoglycemic agent: the major pharmacologic action does not increase insulin secretion and thus does not increase the risk of hypoglycemia. This agent may best be described as an anti-hyperglycemic agent or insulin sensitizer.[28]

   B   Enhances insulin action at the receptor and postreceptor level in hepatic and peripheral tissues, thus reversing or partially reversing insulin resistance.

3   Pharmacokinetics:

   A   Oral bioavailability is increased by 30% to 85% when administered with food.

   B   Extensively bound (>99%) to serum albumin.

   C   Extensively metabolized in the liver to inactive metabolites.

   D   Metabolites eliminated primarily in the feces, and minor amounts in the urine.

4   Significant contraindications or precautions to troglitazone therapy:

   A   Generally not indicated during pregnancy, for breast-feeding women, or children.

   B   Troglitazone should be used with caution in patients with hepatic dysfunction. Rare cases of severe idiosyncratic hepatocellular injury have occurred. Serum transaminase levels should be monitored routinely during the first year of therapy.

   C   In premenopausal anovulatory women with insulin resistance, troglitazone therapy may result in resumption of ovulation, with a subsequent risk of pregnancy.

   D   Refer to package labeling for additional contraindications and precautions.[29]

5   Adverse effects associated with troglitazone therapy:

   A   Elevated hepatic enzymes. Rare cases of severe idiosyncratic hepatocellular injury have occurred. Hepatic injury is generally reversible, but rare cases of hepatic failure, including death, have been reported.[29]

   B   Plasma volume expansion, resulting in small reductions in hemoglobin, hematocrit, and neutrophil counts.

C Other considerations include incidences similar to that of placebo: GI discomfort, headache, peripheral edema, pharyngitis.

D Small increases in HDL and LDL may occur; this alteration in lipid concentration is thought to be clinically insignificant. The HDL/LDL ratio remains unchanged.

6 Clinically important drug interactions with troglitazone are listed in Table 10.6

  A Troglitazone inhibits several of the major hepatic P450 isozymes. Exhaustive studies have not been performed to assess the interactions of troglitazone with all drugs metabolized by these enzymes. Only those combinations which have been noted thus far are included in Table 10.6. Caution should be exercised whenever troglitazone is used with a drug known to be metabolized by one of the P450 isozymes.

7 Role of troglitazone in the treatment of diabetes mellitus:

  A Use as monotherapy only in type 2 diabetes or secondary diabetes with substantial capacity for insulin production.
  - Typical candidate for initial troglitazone monotherapy: type 2 diabetes, with obesity or genetic factors favoring insulin resistance, and fasting plasma glucose level >20 mg/dL above the target concentration.

  B Therapy initiated at a low dose, with gradual increases to reach glucose goals. Instruct patients to take with main meal of day for maximum absorption.
  - Usual initial dose: 200 mg qd, doses given with a meal.
  - Titrate dose upward until desired therapeutic effect is reached. Dose increases should not occur less often than 2 to 4 weeks.
  - Maximum recommended daily dose: 600 mg qd (usually divided into 300 mg bid)

  C Combination therapy, or transition to insulin monotherapy, is considered when troglitazone therapy approaches the maximum dose.

  D When troglitazone is added as an adjunct to insulin therapy, the insulin dose is decreased by 10% to 25% when the fasting plasma glucose drops below 120 mg/dL.

ALPHA-GLUCOSIDASE INHIBITORS

1   Available agent: Acarbose (Precose®): 25 mg, 50 mg, 100 mg dosage units

2   Pharmacologic actions:

    A   Not a hypoglycemic agent—the major pharmacologic action does not increase insulin secretion and thus does not increase the risk of hypoglycemia. This agent may best be described as an anti-hyperglycemic agent.

    B   Inhibits alpha-glucosidase enzymes in the brush border of the small intestine[30] and pancreatic alpha-amylase,[31] leading to a reduction in carbohydrate-mediated postprandial blood glucose elevation.

       • Alpha-glucosidase enzymes (maltase, isomaltase, glucoamylase, and sucrase) hydrolyze oligosaccharides, trisaccharides, and disaccharides to glucose and other monosaccharides in the brush border of the small intestine.

       • Alpha-amylase hydrolyzes complex starches to oligosaccharides in the lumen of the small intestine.

       • Inhibition of these enzyme systems reduces the rate of digestion of complex carbohydrate and the subsequent absorption of glucose.

3   Pharmacokinetics:

    A   Oral bioavailability: Negligible absorption of unchanged drug; about 35% of the intestinal metabolites of acarbose are absorbed.

    B   Acarbose is metabolized within the GI tract by intestinal bacteria and by digestive enzymes.

    C   Excretion of absorbed parent drug and metabolites is by the kidneys.

    D   Acarbose plasma levels are elevated in patients with creatinine clearance (ClCr) <25 mL/min, suggesting accumulation of acarbose. However, dosage adjustment in this setting is not feasible because acarbose acts locally.

4   Significant contraindications or precautions to alpha-glucosidase inhibitor therapy:

    A   Generally not indicated during pregnancy, for breast-feeding women, or children.

    B   Inflammatory bowel disease, colonic ulceration, or obstructive bowel disorders; chronic intestinal disorders of digestion or absorption; or any medical condition that might deteriorate with increased intestinal gas formation.[31]

C Cirrhosis of the liver.

D Not recommended in patients with serum creatinine levels >2.0 mg/dL since studies have suggested increases in drug or metabolite plasma concentrations with renal dysfunction, and long term studies have not been carried out in this population.[31]

E Refer to package labeling for additional contraindications and precautions.

5 Adverse effects associated with alpha-glucosidase inhibitor therapy:

A Alpha-glucosidase inhibitor monotherapy is not associated with hypoglycemia.[31,33]

- Patients using combination therapy (alpha-glucosidase inhibitor with insulin or alpha-glucosidase inhibitor with sulfonylureas) may experience hypoglycemia secondary to the insulin or sulfonylurea.

- Hypoglycemia in this situation can be managed with oral glucose (if the patient is conscious) or intravenous glucose or glucagon (if the patient is unconscious). Because these drugs blunt the digestion of complex sugars to glucose, oral sugar sources other than glucose or lactose (eg, glucose tablets, milk) are unsuitable for rapid correction of hypoglycemia.

B Gastrointestinal effects, occurring primarily at initiation of therapy or when dosage is increased: diarrhea, abdominal pain, and flatulence (about 30%, 10 to 20%, and 42 to 77%, respectively).

- Usually self-limiting, transient, and can be minimized by starting with a low dose, and slow upward titration of dosage.

C Elevation of serum transaminases (AST or ALT) may occur, but is generally dose-related and/or related to low body weight (<60 kg). At doses greater than 100 mg tid, elevations (three times the upper limit of normal) in serum transaminase levels were two to three times more frequent than observed with placebo. For this reason, the maximum recommended dose for patients >60 kg is 100 mg tid. For patients <60 kg, the maximum recommended dose is 50 mg tid.[29]

D Other considerations include small reductions in hematocrit with no accompanying change in hemoglobin have been observed; reductions in serum calcium and vitamin B-12 have been observed in patients treated with acarbose but were considered either spurious or not clinically significant.[29]

6 Clinically important drug interactions with alpha-glucosidase inhibitors are listed in Table 10.6.

7 Role of alpha-glucosidase inhibitors in the treatment of diabetes mellitus

    A Use as monotherapy only in type 2 diabetes or secondary diabetes with substantial capacity for insulin production.

- Typical candidate for initial alpha-glucosidase inhibitor monotherapy: type 2 diabetes, with dyslipidemia or obesity, and symptoms suggesting, or blood glucose profile demonstrating, significant postprandial hyperglycemia.
- Individuals demonstrating significant premeal hyperglycemia without a significant premeal-to-postmeal glucose rise would not be expected to respond optimally to alpha-glucosidase inhibitor monotherapy.

    B Therapy initiated at a low dose to minimize GI side effects, with gradual increases to reach glucose goals.

- Usual initial dose: 25 mg qd. Instruct patients to take with the first bite of the meal for the drug to be effective.
- Titrate dose upward as patient tolerance (to GI effects) allows, until desired therapeutic effect is reached.
  - 25 mg qd for 1-2 weeks
  - 25 mg bid for 1-2 weeks
  - 25 mg tid for 1-8 weeks
  - Maintenance dose: 50 or 100 mg tid (50 mg tid if patient <60 kg)
- Maximum daily dose: 50 mg tid if patient <60 kg; 100 mg tid if patient >60 kg.

    C Combination therapy, or transition to insulin monotherapy, is considered when the maximum dose is reached.

USE OF GLUCAGON INJECTION FOR SEVERE HYPOGLYCEMIA

1 Available agent: Glucagon injection: 1 mg lyophilized powder in a single dose vial, with 1 ml diluent contained in a disposable syringe/needle to allow rapid reconstitution of the powder and administration of the dissolved drug. (Glucagon Emergency Kit)

    A The dose is mixed by adding the diluent from the prefilled syringe in the emergency kit to the contents of the vial.

B A 10 mg Glucagon injection is commercially available, but is not intended for use as a glucose elevating agent; this product is used as a diagnostic aid in gastrointestinal examinations.

2 Pharmacologic actions:
  A Primary effects: Raises blood glucose level by accelerating hepatic glycogenolysis and stimulating hepatic gluconeogenesis.
  B Other effects: stimulates catecholamine and insulin release
  C Glucagon is effective if adequate hepatic glycogen (stored glucose) is available, but may not be beneficial in patients with inadequate glycogen stores (eg, patients with alcoholic hepatic disease, starvation, adrenal insufficiency or chronic hypoglycemia).

3 Pharmacokinetics:
  A Bioavailability: 100%; may be injected intramuscularly, intravenously, or subcutaneously.
  B Degraded in the liver, kidney, and plasma. Plasma half-life is 3 to 6 minutes.

4 Significant contraindications or precautions for glucagon:
  A Insulinoma: marked hypoglycemia may occur following the initial increase in blood glucose
  B Pheochromocytoma: marked hypertension may occur
  C Safety during pregnancy or for breast-feeding women is not known
  D Refer to package labeling for additional contraindications and precautions

5 Adverse effects associated with glucagon use:
  A Nausea, vomiting (most common side effect)
  B Generalized allergic reactions including urticaria, respiratory distress, and hypotension

6 Clinically important drug interactions with glucagon:
  A Oral anticoagulants: hypoprothrombinemic effects may be increased, possibly with bleeding, which may occur after several days. Appears to be dose-related, and occurs minimally with a single 1 mg dose for hypoglycemia.

7 Role of glucagon injection in diabetes mellitus:

A Indicated for the treatment of severe hypoglycemia, in situations when the individual requires assistance from another person (see Chapter 14, Hypoglycemia for more information). For example,

- Patient is unconscious or uncooperative
- Patient cannot take oral fluids
- Emergency staff are not available to treat the hypoglycemia with an injection of 50% dextrose.
- If a hospitalized patient develops severe hypoglycemia, is unconscious, and an intravenous line is not running, glucagon may be administered until intravenous access can be obtained.

B Dosage: based upon patient's age and clinical condition

- Adults and children over 5 or 6 years of age (>20 kg): 1.0 mg SC or IM
- Children under 5 years of age (<20 kg): 0.5 mg SC or IM
- Infants: should probably be given 0.25 mg SC or IM

C Blood glucose response usually occurs in 5 to 20 minutes. If response is insufficient, an additional dose may be needed.

- Liquids containing glucose are needed when the patient becomes conscious to restore hepatic glycogen stores and to prevent secondary hypoglycemia.
- Instruct patients to eat a snack containing carbohydrate and protein when nausea subsides. The snack may need to be repeated because glycogen reserves can take 8 to 12 hours to be replenished.

D Protect patients from injury or aspiration if convulsions occur. A common side effect of glucagon is nausea and possibly vomiting as the patient returns to consciousness.

USE OF OTHER DRUGS IN DIABETES CARE

1 A variety of drugs other than hypoglycemic or antihyperglycemic agents are commonly used in the care of people with diabetes.

A Medications are used for the treatment or prevention of the following complications of diabetes:

- Autonomic neuropathy
- Cardiovascular disease
- Problems of peripheral circulation
- Distal symmetric polyneuropathy
- Hyperlipidemia

- Nephropathy
- Periodontal disease
- Circulation abnormalities

B Medications are used for the treatment of the following conditions or diseases that occur frequently in people with diabetes:
- Hypertension
- Glaucoma
- Cataracts
- Hypothyroidism
- Infections (eg, vaginitis)
- Certain forms of joint disease

C Medications are used for the treatment of the following conditions of diseases that are unrelated to the diabetes:
- Colds
- Coughs
- Birth control/hormone replacement therapy
- Smoking cessation
- Arthritis
- Depression/anxiety
- Sunburn
- Acid indigestion
- Allergies
- Contact dermatitis
- Others

2 Because of the number of drugs that may be used for various concurrent problems, it is important to examine the overall potential consequences when one or more drugs are added to or removed from the drug regimen for a person with diabetes (for more information, see chapters on Complications).

POTENTIAL EFFECTS OF OTHER DRUGS

1 Certain drugs have an effect on blood glucose levels. The following types of interactions can occur:

A A *drug-disease* or pharmacodynamic interaction is defined as a desirable or undesirable alteration of blood glucose level by a drug prescribed for a purpose other than its glycemic effect (Table 10.6). This interaction has an intrinsic physiologic effect.

B A *drug-drug interaction* is defined as a desirable or undesirable effect of a drug on the efficacy or toxicity on the hypoglycemic or antidiabetes drug(s) (Table 10.6).

C A *drug-food interaction* is defined as a desirable or undesirable effect of food on the efficacy or toxicity of the hypoglycemic or antidiabetes drugs(s) (Table 10.7).

2 Certain drugs have an effect on the complications of diabetes (Table 10.9).

A A complication or comorbid condition may be worsened when certain drugs are added to or removed from the overall diabetes treatment program.

B Potential effects can be best anticipated by carefully examining the pharmacologic action or side effects of a drug that are described in the package labeling (insert) or other therapeutic reference.

C The following are examples of drugs that have an effect on the complications of diabetes.

- An antacid with a side effect of constipation may aggravate constipation associated with diabetic autonomic neuropathy.
- An oral decongestant with vasoconstriction side effects may aggravate peripheral vascular problems such as intermittent claudication.
- An antihypertension medication with a side effect of impotence may worsen diabetes-related sexual dysfunction.

3 Certain drug side effects have an impact on diabetes self-management (Table 10.8).

A Patients are taught to be attentive to particular signs and symptoms that may indicate impending hypoglycemia or hyperglycemia. In addition, certain procedures and aspects of diabetes care require the patient to be alert, coordinated, and capable of making self-management decisions. A drug that mimics a patient's usual warning signs of hypoglycemia or hyperglycemia, or one that impairs a patient's ability to perform necessary self-care tasks, may adversely affect glycemic control.

- Frequent urination or nocturia from initiation of diuretic therapy may be mistakenly interpreted as a symptom of hyperglycemia.
- Central nervous system side effects such as dizziness, headache, fatigue, weakness, loss of energy, or tingling of extremities may be mistaken for symptoms of hypoglycemia.

TABLE 10.6. DRUG-DISEASE AND DRUG-DRUG INTERACTIONS

Interacting Drug	Type of Interaction							Net Effect on Blood Glucose		Notes
	Drug-disease (Intrinsic-Effect)	Drug-drug interaction						↑BG	↓BG	
		SU	Repag	Met	Trog	a-G Inh	Ins			
Allopurinol		X							X	Decreased renal tubular secretion of chlorpropamide
Androgens/anabolic steroids	X								X	Mechanism unknown
Anticoagulants, oral (Dicumarol)		X							X	Interfere with metabolism of tolbutamide, chlorpropamide
Asparaginase I	X	X**						X*	X**	* Hyperglycemia associated with inhibition of insulin synthesis. ** Hypoglycemia reported occasionally.
Aspirin	X*	X**							X	* Large daily doses (approx 4 gm/d): Increased basal and stimulated release of insulin ** Displace sulfonylurea from protein binding. Decrease urinary excretion of sulfonylurea.
β-adrenergic antagonists	X							X	X	Both hypo- and hyperglycemic response has been reported. May alter physiologic response to, and subjective symptoms of, hypoglycemia. May reduce hyperglycemia-induced insulin release or decrease tissue sensitivity to insulin
Calcium channel blockers	X							X	X	Hypoglycemia reported with verapamil Hyperglycemia reported with diltiazem, nifedipine
Cholestyramine					X*	X**		X*	X**	* Cholestyramine reduces absorption of coadministered drugs. ** Cholestyramine may enhance effects of acarbose. Interactions may be avoided by administering cholestyramine 2 hr apart from other medications
Chloramphenicol			X						X	Decreased hepatic metabolism and/or protein-binding displacement of tolbutamide, chlorpropamide
Chloroquine	X								X	Mechanism unknown

TABLE 10.6. DRUG-DISEASE AND DRUG-DRUG INTERACTIONS

Interacting Drug	Drug-disease (Intrinsic-Effect)	SU	Repag	Met	Trog	a-G Inh	Ins	↑ BG	↓ BG	Notes
Cimetidine/possible other H₂ antagonists		X*		X**					X	* Increased absorption and/or decreased clearance of glipizide, glyburide, tolbutamide. ** Decreased renal tubular secretion of metformin. Other drugs excreted via renal tubular transport may similarly interfere with metformin clearance.
Clofibrate	X*	X**							X	* Intrinsic hypoglycemic effect: mechanism unknown ** Displace certain sulfonylureas from protein binding
Corticosteriods	X							X		Increased gluconeogenesis; transient insulin resistance
Cyclosporine	X							X		
Diazoxide	X							X		Inhibition of insulin secretion
Dicumarol		X							X	Inhibits hepatic metabolism of tolbutamide, chlorpropamide
Disopyramide	X								X	Most susceptible: Elderly or patients with renal or liver impairment
Diuretics	X							X		Mechanism not known
Estrogen products	X							X		
Ethanol	X	X***						X**	X*	* Intrinsic hypoglycemic effect; imparis gluconeogenesis and increases insulin secretion. Effect is potentiated if alcohol consumed without food or in fasting state. ** Chronic alcohol ingestion may increase metabolism of sulfonylurea. ** Alcohol ingestion, especially with carbohydrate-based drink (beer, mixed drink) has caloric effect. *** Disulfiram-like reaction may also occur, especially with chlorpropamide. Not noted with second-generation sulfonylureas

TABLE 10.6. DRUG-DISEASE AND DRUG-DRUG INTERACTIONS

Interacting Drug	Type of Interaction							Net Effect on Blood Glucose		Notes
	Drug-disease (Intrinsic-Effect)	SU	Repag	Met	Trog	a-G Inh	Ins	↑BG	↓BG	
Fluoxetine	X								X	Hypoglycemia and hyperglycemia have been reported
Fluconazole		X							X	Reported with glipizide
Gemfibrozil	X							X		
Guanethidine	X*	X**							X	* Intrinsic glycemic effect ** Protein-binding displacement of certain sulfonylureas
NSAIDS (non-steroidal anti-inflammatory drugs)	X*	X**							X	* Possible intrinsic hypoglycemic effect ** Protein-binding displacement (tolbutamide, tolazamide)
Isoniazid	X							X		Increases glycogenolysis
Metformin						X		X		Acarbose reduces metformin bioavailability by ~35% when coadministered. Separate doses to avoid
Monoamine Oxidase Inhibitors	X*	X**							X	* May stimulate insulin secretion (beta-adrenergic stimulation) or may be secondary to hepatotoxicity ** May interfere with metabolism of sulfonylurea
Nicotinic Acid (Niacin)	X							X		Dose dependent, when lipid-lowering doses are used. Insignificant effect at vitamin supplement dose
Octreotide	X							X		Hypoglycemia and hyperglycemia have been reported
Oral contraceptives	X**				X*			X**		* Troglitazone reduces plasma concentratins of oral contraceptive by ~30%. A higher dose of oral contraceptive or altenative method of contraception may be needed ** Mechanism not known for hyperglycemic effect
Pancrelipase/pancreatic enzymes						X		X		Do not administer these agents concurrently with acarbose
Pentamidine	X								X	Initially, hypoglycemia; hyperglycemia may occur days or even months after initiation of therapy

TABLE 10.6. DRUG-DISEASE AND DRUG-DRUG INTERACTIONS

Interacting Drug	Drug-disease (Intrinsic-Effect)	SU Repag	Met	Trog	a-G Inh	Ins	↑ BG	↓ BG	Notes
Phenothiazines	X						X	X	Hypoglycemia observed with some phenothiazines, hyperglycemia with others.
Phenytoin	X						X		Decreased insulin secretion
Probenecid	X*	X**						X	* Intrinsic glycemic effect ** Decrease urinary excretion of chlorpropamide
Protease inhibitors	X						X		
Rifampin	X*	X**					X**	X*	* Possible intrinsic hypoglycemic effect ** Increased metabolism of chlorpropamide, glyburide, tolbutamide
Salicylates	X*	X**						X	* Large daily doses (apprx 4 gm/d): Increase basal and stimulated release of insulin ** Displace sulfonylurea from protein binding. Decrease urinary excretion of sulfonylurea.
Sulfonamides, highly protein-bound		X						X	Various effects upon chlorpropamide, tolbutamide kinetics: displacement from protein binding, decreased urinary excretion, and/or altered metabolism.
Sympathomimetics	X						X		Increases glycogenolysis and gluconeogenesis
Tacrolimus	X						X		
Thyroid products	X						X		Once euthyroid status is achieved, diabetes medications may need to be adjusted to compensate for glycemic effect of thyroid product.
Urinary Acidifiers		X						X	Interfere with chlorpropamide excretion

This listing is not intended to be inclusive. Before any new medication is initiated, consult the package labeling (insert) or other reference. In general, these interactions are based on moderate to severe clinical significance and/or possible or established documentation.

Table 10.7. Drug-Food Interactions of Diabetes Medications

Sulfonylurea Agents	• Administration of most sulfonylurea agents with food only slightly alters absorption characteristics. • Patients are often advised to take these agents 1/2 to 1 hour prior to eating to allow the onset of action to occur more closely with the postprandial glucose rise. • When sulfonylurea-induced gastric distress occurs, patients may be advised to take these agents with food to minimize stomach upset. • Glipizide (short-acting) is the only sulfonylurea specifically recommended to be taken on an empty stomach.
Repaglinide	• Food only slightly affects absorption; however, patients are advised to take repaglinide 15 minutes before eating so that the rapid action of the drug matches the timing of glucose rise following the meal.
Metformin	• Food decreases the extent of, and slightly delays, the absorption of metformin. • Taking metformin with or after food is usually advised to reduce stomach upset.
Troglitazone	• Food increases extent of absorption by 30% to 85%. • Taking troglitazone with food ("main meal of the day") is advised to maximize absorption of drug.
Acarbose	• No reported food interactions. • Acarbose must be taken with the meal ("first bite of the meal") to attain optimal therapeutic effect.
Insulin	• Not applicable because insulin must be taken by injection. • Timing of injection prior to eating may be an important factor in postprandial glycemic control. • Lispro insulin is injected no more than 5 to 15 minutes prior to eating to avoid preprandial hypoglycemia.

• Side effects of drowsiness, tiredness, lethargy, or depression could be mistaken for symptoms of hyperglycemia or may affect diabetes control by interfering with the patient's ability or desire to exercise or carry out other self-management activities.

• Blurred vision as a side effect of another agent may lead to a dosing error in insulin administration.

- Drug-induced night blindness may aggravate night blindness from previous retinal photocoagulation or autonomic neuropathy.

TABLE 10.8. ADVERSE DRUG EFFECTS RELATED TO DIABETES

Specific Drugs or Drug Classes *(see Table 10.6 for blood glucose effects)*
Drugs within a drug class often share adverse effects, although to varying degrees. Certain drug classes warrant particular attention to effects that may have an impact upon complications or comorbidity conditions for specific patients.

Alpha-1 antagonists (prazosin, terazosin, doxazosin)	Impotence; constipation (aggravates chronic constipation from autonomic neuropathy); diarrhea (aggravates diarrhea from autonomic neuropathy); dizziness, headache, weakness (may be confused for signs of hypoglycemia); blurred vision, drowsiness, xerostomia (may be confused for signs of hyperglycemia)
Antihistamines, anticholinergic	Contraindicated in neurogenic bladder (may occur in diabetic autonomic neuropathy); blurred vision; constipation, abdominal pain
Anti-hypertensives in general	Impaired sexual function; constipation (selected agents)
Anti-inflammatory agents	Nonsteroidal: renal effects; hypertensive effects Steroidal: osteoporosis; hypertension; weight gain/increase in appetite may worsen diabetes control; diminished wound healing; thin fragile skin; glaucoma
β-blockers	Mask signs/symptoms of hypoglycemia; impaired sexual function; reduced peripheral circulation and cold extremities
Calcium channel blockers	Constipation (selected agents aggravate chronic constipation from autonomic neuropathy); orthostatic hypotension (aggravate diabetes-related orthostatic hypotension); glycemic effects (selected agents)
Chemotherapeutic agents	Nausea, vomiting, stomatitis, anorexia, alterations in taste (makes diabetes nutrition therapy difficult or inconsistent); diarrhea
Clonidine	Urinary retention; constipation; diminished sexual function; orthostatic hypotension; nocturia, lethargy, xerostomia, drowsiness (may be confused for signs of hyperglycemia)
Codeine (as cough suppressant) or opiate analgesics	Constipation (aggravate chronic constipation from autonomic neuropathy)

Diuretics	Changes in lipid profile; total body potassium loss; (unless potassium-sparing diuretic or formulation); diuresis mimics polyuria/nocturia which may interfere with use of these signs as a warning sign of hyperglycemia; diminished effectiveness in decreasing renal function; aggravate diabetes-related orthostatic hypotension
Sorbitol, as compounding ingredient and/or sweetening agent	Loose stools, diarrhea, flatulence (aggravate diarrhea from autonomic neuropathy)
Sympathomimetics	Hypertension; peripheral vasoconstriction

Specific Side Effects/Adverse Reactions

The package labeling (insert) or product information usually provides a list of side effects by body system affected and in the order of frequency of occurrence. Certain adverse effects should arouse suspicions or raise questions about the potential for drug-related problems in patients with diabetes.

Gastrointestinal (GI)	• Nausea, vomiting, constipation, diarrhea, bloating, gas: additive problem with various forms of autonomic neuropathy • Dry mouth: could be mistakenly interpreted as a symptom of hyperglycemia
Genitourinary (GU)	• Impotence, failure to ejaculate, reduced libido: additive problem with diabetes-related impotence
Renal	• Glycosuria listed as a side effect: carefully read the package insert to ascertain if this side effect refers to a lowered threshold for glucose or an indication of hyperglycemia • Frequent urination, nocturia, polyuria: could be mistakenly interpreted as a symptom of hyperglycemia; could lead to hypovolemia and problems with orthostatic hypotension • Elevations of creatinine or BUN: may pose problems in patient predisposed to renal dysfunction
Central nervous system (CNS)	• Dizziness: additive problem with orthostatic hypotension, hypoglycemia • Headache, fatigue, weakness, loss of energy, blurred vision, tingling of extremities: could be mistakenly interpreted as symptom of hypoglycemia • Drowsiness, tiredness, lethargy, depression: could be mistaken for symptom of hyperglycemia; could affect diabetes control by interfering with ability and desire to exercise

	• Numbness/tingling of extremities, paresthesias, neuropathy: additive problem with diabetes-related neuropathy
Dermatologic	• Pruritus, rash, dry skin: aggravate the dry skin and itching associated with peripheral neuropathy and venostasis
Ophthalmic	• Night blindness: may aggravate night blindness resulting from retinal photocoagulation
General	• Elevated cholesterol or triglyceride levels: may pose problems in patient predisposed to lipid disorders • Hypoglycemia, hyperglycemia: may require adjustment of diabetes treatment plan • Peripheral edema: aggravate problems in patient with impaired peripheral circulation and venous return

SIGNIFICANCE OF DRUG-RELATED EFFECTS

1 Some problems have *major clinical significance*, which means an event is relatively well-documented (established documentation) and has the potential of being harmful to the patient.

2 Some problems have *moderate clinical significance*, which means more documentation is needed (possible documentation) and/or the potential harm to the patient is less.

3 Some problems have *minor clinical significance*, which means an event may occur but may be less significant because of poor documentation, minimal potential harm to the patient, or low incidence of the interaction.

4 It is important to note that the classification of "major" versus "minor" significance is not solely a matter of the degree of documentation. *The individual patient characteristics must be considered in making this determination.* For example, in the following situations the first would represent a problem of minor significance whereas the second could be major:

A A 37-year-old man with type 2 diabetes, who is relatively healthy otherwise, has been taking an oral hypoglycemic agent for the past 2 years. Today his provider has added a diuretic. If this individual experiences hypoglycemia during the first few days of diuretic therapy, it is unlikely that the potential diuresis, hypovolemia, or dizziness from the diuretic would exaggerate the dizziness/weakness of hypoglycemia to a dangerous state.

B   An 87-year-old widow with type 2 diabetes, osteoporosis, sporadic nutrition and fluid ingestion, and occasional disequilibrium, has been taking an oral hypoglycemic agent for the past 2 years. She lives alone. Today her provider has added a diuretic. If this patient experiences hypoglycemia *at the same time she experiences* dizziness from the diuretic, the drug-related problem may have major significance: a fall, broken hip, and no one in the house to render assistance.

CAVEATS TO DRUG INTERACTIONS AND DRUG-RELATED PROBLEMS

1   Drug interactions may be beneficial or detrimental.

A   Administering troglitazone with the largest meal of the day is advantageous because the absorption of the drug is enhanced by food (drug-food interaction).

B   Using a drug with intrinsic hypoglycemic activity may be detrimental for a patient with hypoglycemia unawareness (drug-disease interaction, and an effect on a diabetes complication).

2   Drug interactions are not necessarily predictable because they do not always happen to all people.

3   Drug interactions are usually dose dependent.

4   A specific combination of interacting drugs can have a different interaction profile depending on the order in which the drugs are initiated.

A   Adding a diuretic to an established dose of sulfonylurea can reasonably be expected to raise the blood glucose level, thus lessening the apparent effectiveness of the sulfonylurea.

B   When a sulfonylurea is added to an established dose of a diuretic, the blood glucose would not be expected to rise further.

5   The severity of an interaction is different for different people (variable responses) depending on the following individual variables:

A   Current metabolic control

B   Self-monitoring practices

C   Lability/stability of complications and concurrent conditions

D   Duration/dosage of proposed therapy

E   Potential for administration error

Ways to Help Prevent, Minimize or Prepare for Potential Drug-Related Problems

1   Inform the patient if a drug-related problem is likely to occur, and the usual signs and symptoms to watch for.

2   If possible, inform the patient as to when the interaction/drug problem would be expected to occur. Some interactions may occur after the first dose while others may not occur until the problem drug has reached steady state or has accumulated in the body.

3   Devise a strategy by which the patient can determine if the anticipated problem has occurred.

   A   Recommend blood glucose monitoring at specific times of day or at more frequent intervals until the patient's response to the drug is established.

   B   Stress the importance of additional monitoring or observation.

4   Provide an action plan for the patient to use if the suspected drug-related problem has occurred. This action plan is based on the drug and the severity of the interaction/problem.

   A   For problems of major clinical significance, instruct the patient to notify the provider as soon as possible. Specify whether the drug should be stopped or continued while attempting to reach the health professional.

   B   For problems of moderate clinical significance, the problem may be resolved by making appropriate compensations. A member of the healthcare team may need to be contacted for assistance.

   C   For problems of minor clinical significance, the problem is primarily an inconvenience or is self-limiting and does not generally require any specific action.

5   Prepare a backup plan should problems arise. Determine alternatives the patient might use if the drug problem occurs.

SELF-REVIEW QUESTIONS

1 Describe the effects of insulin on fat, protein, and glucose utilization.

2 List four categories of patients who are candidates for insulin therapy.

3 What concentrations of insulin are available and which concentration is most commonly used in the United States?

4 Describe the guidelines for insulin storage.

5 Compare and contrast the sulfonylureas, meglitinides, biguanides, thiazolidinediones, and acarbose as to side effects and contraindications.

6 How should metformin therapy be initiated and titrated?

7 How should acarbose therapy be initiated and titrated?

8 Which antidiabetes oral medication which must be taken with a meal ("first bite of the meal") to attain its therapeutic effect?

9 Which antidiabetes oral medication should be taken with food ("main meal of the day") to maximize absorption of the drug?

10 Which antidiabetes oral medication is specifically recommended to be taken on an empty stomach?

11 List the indications for use of glucagon.

12 List three chronic complications of diabetes for which some type of pharmacologic therapy will be needed to prevent or treat that complication.

13 Name the two complications or conditions associated with diabetes which may be aggravated by administration of certain oral decongestants (sympathomimetics).

14 List three drugs with intrinsic hyperglycemic activity.

15 List three drugs with intrinsic hypoglycemic activity.

16 List three side effects of various drugs which may mimic symptoms of hypoglycemia and cause confusion in the perception of hypoglycemia.

17 List two side effects of various drugs which may mimic symptoms of hyperglycemia and cause confusion in the perception of hyperglycemia.

18 Define the following terms (a) Major clinically significant problem, (b) Moderate clinically significance problem, (c) Minor problem.

Key Educational Considerations

1 Oral agents are not a substitute for meal planning and exercise, but will work best when all aspects of therapy are combined.

2 Many patients assume that sulfonylureas are "oral insulin" and become confused by what they hear about insulin.

3 It is common for patients who take oral agents to believe that they have a "touch of sugar" or "mild diabetes." If this information is obtained as part of the educational assessment, it can prompt the educator to ask additional questions about the patient's perceptions and beliefs about diabetes and then to provide relevant content.

4 The recognition and treatment of hypoglycemia is essential information for all patients taking insulin, sulfonylureas or repaglinide.

5 Teach patients to inform all healthcare providers about their diabetes and their medications so that the potential for drug interactions will be recognized.

6 Address the potential problems of using alcohol with certain sulfonylureas with those patients for whom it is appropriate.

7 The dosage of metformin or acarbose may be titrated over weeks in order to minimize side effects. Written dosage instruction handouts may help patients minimize side effects.

8 Type 2 diabetes patients taking oral agents often assume that when they must start insulin, it is a signal that they are "getting worse" or that it is because they have not "followed the diet right." Explain that over time, the oral agents do not lower the blood glucose as well as they did originally.

9 Type 2 diabetes patients who change from oral agents to insulin sometimes assume that they no longer have to be concerned about the amounts of food eaten because the insulin will regulate the blood glucose. It should be explained that the insulin is being started to meet the patient's physiologic insulin requirement, not to replace meal planning related to amounts, timing, and consistency of eating.

10 Inform patients and families that with weight loss, nutrition changes, and/or increased physical activity some individuals may no longer require therapeutic agents (including insulin). However, that applies *only* to people with type 2 diabetes. The current treatment for type 1 diabetes requires lifelong insulin therapy.

11 Most insulin-requiring individuals will need two or more daily insulin injections, often using two types of insulin in each injection to provide insulin in a more physiologic manner.

Case Study 1

LR is a 22-year-old woman with type 1 diabetes that was diagnosed 5 years ago. She has cared for her diabetes with two insulin injections daily for the past 15 months as follows:

AM: 20 units NPH insulin and 8 units Regular insulin
PM: 10 units NPH insulin and 4 units Regular insulin

She has hypertension, for which she is taking 50 mg hydrochlorothiazide daily. She has also been taking an oral contraceptive for 3 months. Today she comes to the clinic expressing concern about her glucose levels. Her SMBG record averages for the past 3 weeks are as follows:

SMBG Levels

	7 AM mg/dL (mmol/L)	11 AM mg/dL (mmol/L)	4 PM mg/dL (mmol/L)	9 PM mg/dL (mmol/L)
Previous month	107(6.0)	112(6.2)	129(7.1)	120(6.6)
Week 1	151(8.3)	168(9.2)	112(6.3)	176(9.7)
Week 2	158(8.7)	167(9.2)	142(7.9)	168(9.2)
Week 3	167(9.2)	172(9.5)	141(7.8)	171(9.4)

She reports that her activity, weight and dietary intake are unchanged.

Questions for Discussion

1 What other information do you need?

2 What possible explanations could be given for her blood glucose levels?

3 What therapeutic options are available for LR?

DISCUSSION

1   An initial review of these data suggests that further information is needed.

   A   Your assessment reveals that LR's insulin administration routine is accurate, including storage of insulin, injection sites, timing, and technique.

   B   She reports no significant change in her caloric intake or the introduction of new food products.

   C   There has been no change in her activity level, daily habits, level of stress or coping methods.

2   Potential explanations are either the hydrochlorothiazide or the estrogen-containing contraceptive is causing a drug interaction that is inducing an increase in blood glucose level. LR has been taking hydrochlorothiazide for 3 years with no previous problem. The contraceptive has produced no problem thus far.

3   A trial period of other medications for hypertension and/or contraception might be indicated.

   A   Unless the HCTZ was specifically chosen for diuresis as well as antihypertensive effects (ie, the patient has problems with peripheral edema or other fluid accumulation) an angiotensin-converting-enzyme inhibitor (ACE-inhibitor) is the drug of choice for hypertension in diabetes. Unlike HCTZ, an ACE-inhibitor does not have a potential for causing hyperglycemia or lipid abnormalities.

   B   A "low dose" contraceptive agent may be considered.

4   Adjustments in insulin are also an option, such as

   A   The evening dose of intermediate-acting insulin could be increased by 1 to 2 units, or LR could eat less carbohydrates or calories for supper or exercise in the evening to reduce her 7 AM glucose concentration.

   B   The AM regular insulin could be increased by 1 or 2 units, or LR could eat less carbohydrates or calories for breakfast to reduce her 11 AM glucose concentration.

   C   Evaluate the 9 PM level based on when LR eats her evening meal.

   D   Her 4 PM level may be improved by reducing the morning glucose levels.

   E   If LR is open to the idea of three daily injections, the evening dose could be changed to regular insulin at the evening meal and NPH at bedtime. Administering her NPH at bedtime would help to lower her fasting glucose.

5 Any changes in insulin doses needs to be made slowly, and by altering one dose at a time.

Case Study 2

AH is a 57-year-old male referred to the diabetes clinic for evaluation of his glycemic control. He was diagnosed with type 2 diabetes about 15 months ago. He remains overweight in spite of numerous attempts to lose weight. His fasting blood glucose concentrations have risen lately and range from 170 to 185 mg/dL (9.4 to 10.3 mmol/L) over the last few weeks. He complains of weakness, fatigue, increased urination, and increased thirst.

Past Medical History
Hypertension x 10 y
Type 2 diabetes mellitus

Family History
(+) Diabetes
(+) Hypertension

Social History
Smokes, 1/2-1 packs per day
Alcohol, none

Current Medications
Hydrochlorothiazide (HCTZ) 50 mg qd
KCL 40 mEq q AM
propranolol 40 mg qid

Physical Examination
Weight 198 lb (90 kg), up 3 kg
Height 5'8"
BP 154/94 (previous BP ranged from 150/92 to 160/96)
Pulse 88 regular
RR 14

QUESTIONS FOR DISCUSSION

1 How do the antihypertensive agents affect AH's blood glucose level?

2 Which class of oral agent might be appropriate for AH?

DISCUSSION

1 It would be appropriate to begin by substituting different drugs for those that worsen glucose tolerance (HCTZ and propranolol).

   A This patient's hypertension might be better treated with an ACE-inhibitor or a calcium channel blocker.

   B If the HCTZ is discontinued or an ACE-inhibitor is initiated the potassium supplement should probably be discontinued as well.

2 The effects of HCTZ and propranolol on glucose tolerance may take a number of weeks to resolve. In the interim, his hyperglycemia should be treated with oral agents or low dose insulin in order to relieve his symptoms. Metformin may be a good choice for AH because he is overweight and probably insulin resistant. Metformin could lower his blood glucose levels, weight, and lipid levels (if elevated).

3 Prior to initiation of any new therapy, evaluation for potential contraindications (particularly hepatic or renal dysfunction) or drug allergies is needed.

4 Other considerations include cost, patient convenience, patient preference and lifestyle concerns.

   A Many of the sulfonylurea agents are available generically, which are generally less expensive than the brand or newer products.

   B A once-a-day agent such as glyburide, glipizide long-acting, glimepiride, or troglitazone may offer the advantage of being easier to take correctly and consistently.

   C If hypoglycemia poses a particular risk for AH (eg, due to work or living situation), a non-hypoglycemic agent such as acarbose, metformin, or troglitazone may offer an advantage.

   D The patient's willingness or ability to self-monitor blood glucose levels may influence the type of agent chosen or blood glucose goals.

5   As the effects of the propranolol and HCTZ wane following their discontinuance, AH may no longer need an antidiabetes agent.

6   Assess the patient's level of interest in meal planning for glucose control and referral to a dietitian.

Case Study 3

MC is a 79-year-old female with type 2 diabetes who resides in a nursing home. You are the nursing home consultant. You notice that 10 days ago MC developed a urinary tract infection (UTI), which was initially treated with co-trimoxazole (Septra DS®). After the second dose of Septra DS, intense pruritus and a rash appeared on her arms and upper chest. The Septra was discontinued and ampicillin was prescribed. Diphenhydramine (Benadryl®) and a methylprednisolone dose pack (Medrol®) were given for the sulfonamide reaction.

Over the next several days, you notice that symptoms of increased urination, incontinence, and mental confusion are documented in the nursing notes. After reading the notes and talking with the staff, you learn that these observations were attributed to her advancing age and deteriorating mental status, so no action was taken.

You suspect that the changes observed are related to drug problems rather than changes in patient's mental status.

Questions for Discussion

1   What information would you need to help determine if this reaction is a drug-related problem?

2   What possible explanations could be given for what has happened to MC?

3   Assuming your suspicions are correct and MC has experienced a drug-related reaction, what recommendations could you make to resolve MC's problem?

4   What could be done to prevent this from occurring in the future?

DISCUSSION

1 The following information is needed to help determine the causes of MC's problem:

   A Current drug profile (Is she taking oral agents? Insulin? Have other drugs been recently initiated that would cause symptoms of polyuria or mental confusion?)

   B Recent blood glucose results (Have her blood glucose levels been increasing recently, and did the increase coincide with the onset of UTI symptoms? Did the blood glucose levels increase further when the steroid was initiated?)

   C Ongoing blood glucose patterns and HbA$_{1c}$ (Has chronic hyperglycemia predisposed this patient to infection?)

   D Description of MC's mental status during the period of the UTI and treatment

   E Lab results and vital signs to assess if the UTI is responding to therapy

   F Blood chemistries to assess for possible hyperglycemic hyperosmolar nonketotic syndrome (HHNS)

2 A urinary tract infection is an example of physical stress that can raise blood glucose concentrations (release of counterregulatory hormones). If MC's diabetes was previously poorly controlled or "brittle" (blood glucose fluctuating dramatically with changes in her meal plan, exercise, illness, stress) the hyperglycemic effect of illness would be more exaggerated.

3 Subsequent hyperglycemic factors include the allergic reaction (causing endogenous release of corticosteroid) and the initiation of methylprednisolone (intrinsic hyperglycemic activity).

4 The increased urination, incontinence, and mental confusion may be symptoms of the resulting hyperglycemia; depending upon severity of neurologic symptoms and blood chemistries, HHNS may be developing.

5 Diphenhydramine in an elderly person may substantially alter mental alertness or cause urinary retention resulting in overflow incontinence.

6 The following measures can be taken to resolve MC's symptoms:

   A Assure adequate hydration

   B Insulin may be needed temporarily in place of oral antidiabetes agents; if MC is already on insulin, doses need to be increased temporarily

   C Monitor blood glucose more frequently until control is re-established

   D Continue to follow signs and symptoms of UTI to assure resolution of infection

   E Discontinue diphenhydramine. Institute shorter-acting or non-sedating antihistamine if antipruritic agent still needed. Topical steroid creams may provide relief.

   F Discontinue methylprednisolone as soon as feasible. A slow taper is not necessary.

7 The following preventive recommendations could be instituted:

   A The nursing home could establish standard policies regarding detection and management of acute loss of glycemic control in residents with diabetes.

     • Blood glucose testing is essential even for residents with well-controlled diabetes. An increase in blood glucose levels often precedes the clinical manifestations of infection and may thus serve as a warning that illness may be developing.

   B Blood glucose testing (at least qd or bid) is performed under the following conditions:

     • When infection is suspected or confirmed, more frequent testing is needed until blood glucose results return to preinfection levels.

     • Upon initiation of drugs with intrinsic hyperglycemic or hypoglycemic activity, more frequent testing is needed until the drug interaction is resolved.

     • Upon initiation of drugs with potential side effects that mimic hyperglycemia or hypoglycemia, more frequent testing is needed until the patient's response to the drug is determined.

REFERENCES

1   Fertig BJ, Simmons DA, Martin DB. Diabetes in America. 2nd edition. National Diabetes Data Group eds. Bethesda, Md: National Institute of Diabetes and Digestive and Kidney Diseases, NIH publication no. 95-1468; 1995:519-40.

2   Betz JL. Fast-acting human insulin analogs: a promising innovation in diabetes care. Diabetes Educ 1995;21: 195-200.

3   Howey DC, Bowsher RR, Brunelle RL, Woodworth JR. [Lys(B28), Pro(B29)]-human insulin, a rapidly absorbed analogue of human insulin. Diabetes 1994;43:396-402.

4   Product information and recommendations. Indianapolis: Eli Lilly and Company, 1987.

5   Product information and recommendations. Princeton, NJ: Novo Nordisk Pharmaceuticals, 1993.

6   Anderson JH, Campbell RK. Mixing insulins in 1990. Diabetes Educ 1990;16:380-87.

7   White JR, Campbell RK. Guide to mixing insulins. Hosp Pharm. 1991;26:1046-48

8   American Diabetes Association. Position statement. Insulin Administration. Diabetes Care 1998;21 (suppl 1): S72-S75.

9   Kovisto VA, Felig P. Alterations in insulin absorption and in blood glucose control associated with varying insulin injection sites in diabetic patients. Ann Intern Med 1980;92:59-61.

10 White JR Jr, Campbell RK. Pharmacologic therapies in the management of diabetes mellitus. In: Haire-Joshu D, ed. Management of diabetes mellitus. 2nd ed. St. Louis: Mosby Year Book,1996:202-33.

11 Linde B. Dissociation of insulin absorption and blood flow during massage of a subcutaneous injection site. Diabetes Care 1986;9:570-74.

12 Bolognia JL, Braverman IM. Skin and subcutaneous tissues. In: Lebovitz HE. ed. Therapy for diabetes mellitus and related disorders. 2nd ed. Alexandria, Va: American Diabetes Association, 1994:213.

13 White JR Jr, Hartman J, Campbell RK. Drug interactions in diabetic patients. Postgrad Med 1993;93:131-39.

14 Hirsch I B, Farkas-Hirsch R, Skyler JS. Intensive insulin therapy for treatment of type I diabetes. Diabetes Care 1990;13:1265-83.

15 Insulin treatment. In: Santiago JV, ed. Medical management of insulin-dependent (type I) diabetes. 2nd ed. Alexandria, Va: American Diabetes Association, 1994:35.

16 Pharmacologic intervention. In: Raskin P, ed. Medical management of non-insulin-dependent (type II) diabetes. 3rd ed. Alexandria, Va: American Diabetes Association, 1994;35.

17 Seigler DE, Olsson GM, Skyler JS. Morning versus bedtime isophane insulin in type 2 (non-insulin dependent) diabetes mellitus. Diabetic Med 1992;9:826-33.

18 White JR Jr. Combination oral agent/insulin therapy in patients with type II diabetes mellitus. Clinical Diabetes 1997; 15:102-12.

19 Lebovitz H. Sulfonylureas. In: Lebovitz HE, ed. Therapy for diabetes mellitus and related disorders. 2nd ed. Alexandria, Va: American Diabetes Association, 1994;116.

20 Halter JB. Geriatric patients. In: Lebovitz HE, ed. Therapy for diabetes mellitus and related disorders. 2nd ed. Alexandria, Va: American Diabetes Association, 1994:164

21 White JR Jr. The pharmacologic management of patients with type II diabetes mellitus in the era of new oral agents and insulin analogs. Diabetes Spectrum 1996;9:227-34.

22 Gerich JE. Oral hypoglycemic agents. N Engl J Med 1989; 321:1231-45.

23 Stenman S, Melander A, Groop P, Groop LC. What is the benefit of increasing the sulfonylurea dose? Ann of Intern Med 1993;118:169-172

24 Prandin® package insert. Princeton, NJ: Novo Nordisk, 1997.

25 DeFronzo RA, Barzilai N, Simonson DC. Mechanism of metformin action in obese and lean non-insulin dependent diabetic subjects. J Clin Endocrinol Metab 1991;73:1294-1301.

26 Bailey CJ. Metformin, an update. Gen Pharmaco 1993;24:1299-1309.

27 DeFronzo RA, Goodman AM, and the Multicenter Metformin Study Group. Efficacy of metformin in patients with NIDDM. N Engl J Med 1995;333:541-49.

28 Suter S, Nolan JJ, Wallace P, Gumbiner B, Olefsky JM. Metabolic effects of new oral hypoglycemic agent CS-045 in NIDDM subjects. Diabetes Care 1992;15: 193-203.

29 Rezulin® package insert. Morris Plains, NJ: Parke Davis, 1997.

30 Santeusanio F, Compagnucci P. A risk-benefit appraisal of acarbose in the management of non-insulin-dependent diabetes mellitus. Drug Safety 1994; 11:432-444.

31 Precose® package insert. West Haven, CT: Bayer Pharmaceuticals, 1996.

32 Lebovitz H. alpha-glucosidase inhibitors in treatment of hyperglycemia. In: Therapy for diabetes mellitus and related disorders. 2nd ed. 1994. Lebovitz H. ed. Alexandria, Va: American Diabetes Association, 1994.

33 Coniff RF, Shapiro JA, Seaton TB, Bray GA. Multicenter, placebo-controlled trial comparing acarbose (BAY g 5421) with placebo, tolbutamide, and tolbutamide-plus-acarbose in non-insulin-dependent diabetes mellitus. Am J Med 1995; 98:443-51.

SUGGESTED READINGS

ADA Vital Statistics. American Diabetes Association. Alexandria, Va. 1996.

American Diabetes Association. Consensus statement. The pharmacologic treatment of hyperglycemia in NIDDM. Diabetes Care 1996: 19(supp 1):S54-S61.

Ahrens ER, Gossain VV, Rovner DR. Human insulin: its development and clinical use. Postgrad Med 1986;80:181-187.

Bailey TS, Mezitis NHE. Combination therapy with insulin and sulfonylureas for type II diabetes. Diabetes Care 1990;13:687-95.

Bell DH, Mayo MS. Outcome of metformin-facilitated reinitiation of oral diabetic therapy in insulin-treated patients with non-insulin-dependent diabetes mellitus. Endocr Pract 1997;3:73-6.

Belgrade MJ, Lev BI. Diabetic neuropathy. Helping patients cope with their pain. Postgrad Med 1991;90:263-70.

Bohannon NJ. Benefits of lispro insulin. Postgrad Med 1997;101:73-80. Fleming DR, Jacober SJ, Vandenberg MA, Fitzgerald JT, Grunberger G. The safety of injecting insulin through clothing. Diabetes Care 1997;20:245-48.

Bressler P, DeFronzo RA. Drugs and diabetes. Diabetes Reviews 1994; 2:53-84.

Garber AJ, Duncan TG, Goodman AM et al. Efficacy of metformin in type II diabetes: results of a double-blind, placebo-controlled, dose-response trial. Am J Med, 1997. 103:491-497.

Genuth S. Insulin use in NIDDM. Diabetes Care 1990;13:1240-64.

Hollander P. Pre-mixed insulins. Postgrad Med 1991;89:52-61.

Kasiske BL, Kalil RS, Ma JZ, Liao M, Keane WF. Effect of antihypertensive therapy on the kidney in patients with diabetes: a meta-regression analysis. Ann Int Med 1993;118:129-38.

Krosnick A. Newer insulin, insulin allergies, and the clinical use of insulins. In: Bergman M, ed. Principles of diabetes management. New Hyde Park, NY: Medical Examination Publishing Co, 1987;123-35.

Lewis EJ, Hunsicker LG, Bain RP, Rohde RD. The effect of angiotensin-converting enzyme inhibition on diabetic nephropathy. N Engl J Med 1993;329:1456-62.

O'Byrne S, Feely S. Effects of drugs on glucose tolerance in non-insulin-dependent diabetics, Part I and II Drugs 1990;40:6-18, 203-19.

Peragallo-Dittko, V. Buyer's guide to injection devices. Diabetes Self-Manage 1990;7(1):6-12

Peragallo-Dittko, V. Straight shooting: a critical look at injection technique. Diabetes Self-Manage 1992;9(3):8-10

Skyler JS. Algorithms for adjustment of insulin dosage by patients who monitor blood glucose. Diabetes Care 1981;4:311-18.

Skyler JS. Insulin therapy in type II diabetes. Postgrad Med 1997;101: 85-96.

Yarborough PC. Recommending cold and cough products for people with diabetes. Diabetes Spectrum 1988;1:6.

Young DS. Effects of drugs on clinical laboratory tests. 4the ed. Washington, DC: American Association of Clinical Chemistry Press, 1995:274-281.

White JR Jr, Campbell RK, Hirsch I. Insulin analogues. Postgrad Med 1997;101:58-70.

THERAPIES

Monitoring   **11**

Virginia Peragallo-Dittko, RN, MA, CDE
Diabetes Education Center
Winthrop-University Hospital
Mineola, New York

INTRODUCTION

1   Regular monitoring is an essential component of any diabetes management program.

2   Monitoring by the patient includes self-monitoring of blood glucose (SMBG), urine ketones, and urine glucose, if recommended.

3   Monitoring of metabolic control by the healthcare team involves assessing glycosylated hemoglobin and fructosamine, reviewing blood glucose patterns, assessing growth and patterns of weight change, and monitoring the development and progression of long-term complications, including urinary protein measurements. This area of diabetes care clearly combines the diabetes educator's skills of management and education.

OBJECTIVES

Upon completion of this chapter, the learner will be able to

1   List factors that affect the accuracy of self-monitoring of blood glucose (SMBG) results.

2   Describe the most common user error related to SMBG.

3   Identify three critical uses of SMBG data by patients.

4   Describe two ways that educators use SMBG results to teach an abstract principle of diabetes management.

5   Identify two psychosocial adaptations related to SMBG.

6   Identify the SMBG needs of special populations.

7   Explain the measurement methods and target ranges for glycosylated hemoglobin, fructosamine, and urinary protein.

8   List the indications for urine tests of ketones and glucose.

9   Identify how to use documentation of weight patterns as a monitoring tool.

SELF-MONITORING OF BLOOD GLUCOSE

1   Self-monitoring of blood glucose (SMBG) is an important component of the treatment plan for patients with diabetes mellitus because it provides immediate feedback and data for:

   A   Achieving and maintaining a specific glycemic goals.

   B   Preventing and detecting hypoglycemia and avoiding severe hypoglycemia.

C Adjusting care in response to changes in lifestyle of individuals who require pharmacologic therapy.

D Determining the need for insulin therapy in gestational diabetes mellitus.[1]

2 Two types of blood glucose meters are used for SMBG: color reflectance meters and those that use sensor technology.

A With reflectance meters, the glucose in a drop of blood reacts with an enzyme on the test strip and changes the color of the strip. The meter accurately measures the color of the strip and gives a numeric readout. In general, the darker the test area, the higher the glucose content.

B Sensor-type meters measure the electronic charge generated by the reaction of the glucose and the enzyme.

3 It is essential to ensure the accuracy of the blood glucose monitoring values because these values are used to make treatment decisions concerning medication dosage adjustment, food-intake or timing and exercise timing.

A The reagents (strips or sensors) are one source of potential error.

- The reagents must be stored according to the manufacturer's guidelines to yield accurate results. These guidelines also refer to avoiding exposure to heat, cold, and humidity during shipping.

- Teach patients to check the expiration date of the reagents, especially when a mail-order shipment could include reagents that expire within a few months and need to be used immediately. Because reagents are costly, patients are commonly tempted to use expired reagents. This may lead to inaccurate readings.

- Control solution is a product that is provided by manufacturers to verify that the meter and reagent are working together properly. This underused method of verifying accuracy operates the same way that the patient monitors a drop of blood. Every manufacturer provides at least one control solution and some have low-, normal- and high-level control solutions to test the meter at extremes.

- Other factors that may influence the results of SMBG systems include variations in the hematocrit (newer systems are accurate with hematocrit ranges of 20% to 60%), altitude, environmental temperature and humidity, hypotension, hypoxia, and triglyceride concentrations.[1]

B Calibrating the meter is another way to ensure the most accurate results. Newer meter technology automatically calibrates the reagent with the meter, whereas older meter technology requires setting a code or inserting a chip or strip to calibrate the meter.

C With some reflectance meters, the blood sample intended for the strip may come in contact with the meter and soil the optic window. This will yield inaccurate results. The manufacturers provide instructions for cleaning the meter.

D User error is the most common reason for inaccurate results. Despite improvements in technology such as the inclusion of error codes, not putting enough blood on the reagent is frequently the cause of inaccurate results and errors in subsequent treatment decisions. Patients should be asked at every opportunity to demonstrate their technique for using their meters. This demonstration gives the educator an opportunity to verify technique, provide advice, or clean a soiled unit.

- Some patients have difficulty securing a drop of blood and may require guidance in choosing a lancing device or meter. Providing individualized guidance for each patient's needs minimizes waste of reagents and eases patient frustration with blood glucose monitoring.

E Patients should be taught specific directions for securing an adequate blood sample.[2] For example:

- Vigorously wash hands with warm water to increase circulation to fingertips.
- Try hanging the hand at your side for 30 seconds so the blood can pool in your hand.
- Shake the hand to be pricked as though you were shaking down a thermometer.
- Use a lancing device endcap that will allow a deeper puncture.
- After your finger is punctured, gently milk the blood from the bottom to the tip of your finger until the blood drop is the correct size. Milking the finger works better than just squeezing the fingertips.

4 Many patients are trained in the mechanics of using a meter but not how to use the data. This inadequacy may be related to patient education. Harris and associates[3] found that the frequency of monitoring was related to having attended a diabetes patient education class. Diabetes patient education was associated with an almost threefold greater probability that subjects monitored their blood glucose at least once per day.

TABLE 11.1. PATIENT USES OF SMBG DATA

- Identifying and treating hypoglycemia
- Making decisions concerning food intake or medication adjustment when exercising
- Determining the effect of food choices or portions on blood glucose levels
- Pattern management
- Managing intercurrent illness
- Managing hypoglycemia unawareness

A The critical uses of SMBG data by patients are shown in Table 11.1.

B Self-monitoring of blood glucose provides reliable data for problem-solving and decision-making.

- While some decisions (eg, treating hypoglycemia or determining the need for a snack), require instantaneous feedback for decision making, most decisions require reviewing numerous readings to identify a pattern (eg, adjusting medication dosages, changing the meal plan or recognizing the impact of exercise).
- The memory feature of many meters is not intended to replace the logbook, but rather provide the option of recording readings at a later date.
- Although a written record and graph of blood glucose readings yields important information, jotting down comments or explanations can be more helpful for teaching the impact of certain decisions related to medication, exercise, or food.

C Educators and clinicians rely on SMBG to teach problem-solving skills, which are the essence of diabetes self-management, and complex management skills such as blood glucose pattern awareness and insulin dose adjustment (see Chapter 12, Pattern Management, for examples).

D Diabetes educators use SMBG as the tool that links abstract principles of management with daily decision making.

- Educators can use blood glucose results to teach the concept of postexercise, late-onset hypoglycemia, and the behaviors necessary to prevent this condition.
- Behavior change concerning food choices or portions is facilitated by relating the food or portion to the postprandial blood glucose result.[4,5]

- For patients with type 2 diabetes who are asymptomatic for hyperglycemia, the need for behavior change becomes personally relevant when they monitor and record blood glucose levels.

E Self-monitoring of blood glucose is used by educators to identify and influence psychosocial adaptations.

- Self-monitoring of blood glucose can influence self-efficacy.[6] For example, patients report increased confidence in their problem solving abilities as a result of using SMBG.

- The act of monitoring can also hold emotional consequences when patients are confronted with an unacceptable number. This phenomenon, called *monitor talk*[7] can help identify psychosocial needs and direct future learning. Educators can discourage value judgment and replace the notion of good and bad readings with the terms *in range* or *out of range*. Reference to blood glucose tests can be replaced with the terms *checks* or *measurements*.

- Identified barriers to monitoring include the discomfort of fingersticks, elevated or labile readings, reminder of the diagnosis of diabetes, cost of reagents, and the inconvenience of record keeping. By identifying barriers, the educator can provide direction and support the patient's choice in using this valuable tool.

- Self-monitoring of blood glucose can be used to allay anxiety about hypoglycemia, especially parental anxiety and is a critical tool for treating fear of hypoglycemia.[8]

- Although the influence of stress and stress management techniques on glycemic control is controversial, individuals may benefit from identifying a physical marker for their psychological distress.

F The frequency of SMBG is determined by how the data will be used.

- More frequent monitoring is beneficial during insulin dose adjustment, whereas periodic postprandial checks may benefit someone with type 2 diabetes who is learning about the glycemic effect of food portions.

- Monitoring schedules are based on the patient's needs, desires, and use of the data. Although some insurers and clinicians have not yet been convinced of the merit of SMBG for patients with non-insulin treated diabetes, the value of SMBG cannot be overemphasized as a teaching tool, a motivator, a reinforcer and as an aid in prescribing appropriate dosages of the various combinations of blood glucose lowering agents.

G Guidelines for teaching patients how to use a blood glucose meter are listed in Table 11.2.

TABLE 11.2. GUIDELINES FOR TEACHING PATIENTS HOW TO USE A BLOOD GLUCOSE METER

- Use universal precautions: change lancets, endcaps, and gloves for each patient.[9]
- Demonstrate how to check blood glucose using control solution first and then using the patient's blood.
- After demonstrating this technique, ask the patient to provide a return demonstration before teaching about control solution, calibration, cleaning, and using the logbook.
- Explain how to dispose of lancets in an appropriate sharps container.
- Evaluate the patient's technique at every opportunity.

---

5 Educators are frequently asked to provide consultation regarding the choice of a meter for a hospital or other facility. Although the scientific literature contains numerous reports of the statistical accuracy of systems for SMBG, most determine accuracy in ways that may not be clinically useful for these settings. The Error Grid Analysis[10] provides a useful methodological contribution for evaluating accuracy of glucose meters and clinical relevancy of statistical data related to SMBG.

6 Methods for noninvasive blood glucose monitoring are being developed. Noninvasive monitoring involves measuring the concentration of glucose in the blood without puncturing the finger to obtain a drop of blood.[11]

7 Data management systems allow for downloading the memory stored in the meter to a remote computer (either directly or by modem) for plotting the results on a graph. Data summarization alone, however, does not identify the relationship that leads to the observed outcomes (eg, the four bread servings at breakfast that led to postprandial hyperglycemia).

8 The Joint Commission for the Accreditation of Health Care Organizations (JCAHO) and the Health Care Financing Administration (HCFA) require hospitals and other facilities to have quality assurance programs for bedside blood glucose monitoring.[12] Proficiency testing, use of control solutions, staff training, and correlational studies comparing bedside results with hospital laboratory values are essential elements of the quality assurance process.

A The Clinical Laboratory Improvement Act of 1988 (CLIA '88)[13] placed additional restrictions on blood glucose monitoring performed outside the hospital setting. Blood glucose meters must have verified accuracy, and the provider's office must complete additional paperwork and submit fees for a waivered test that provides exemption from the requirements.

9 Certain populations of people with diabetes have unique needs relating to SMBG.

A Elderly people with diabetes remain an underserved population despite the prevalence of diabetes in the elderly and the validity of SMBG as a management tool.

- Age should not be the sole criterion for decisions concerning SMBG. The elderly are a heterogeneous population requiring personalized therapy and monitoring schedules.

- Educators need to consider the unique needs of some elderly patients that may influence the choice of products, such as potential limitations in manual dexterity, slowed reaction time, or fluctuating vision[14] (for more information, see Chapter 19, Diabetes in the Elderly).

B Children also have unique needs that influence product choice.

- Children especially benefit from reagents that require a small sample size of blood, and lancing devices that hide the lancet and minimize discomfort.

- Parents benefit from meters that quickly yield results and store at least the last reading in the memory. This latter feature is particularly important because after a fingerstick, parents are focused on comforting their child and the meter may turn off before the parent can write down the result (for more information see Chapter 17, Childhood and Adolescence).

C Visually impaired persons with diabetes, including those with fluctuating vision to nonfunctional vision, need products that are fully accessible to the visually impaired person; current products fall short of this need. Equipment features that would be of benefit include tactile markings on the reagent, durable reagents not damaged by touching, clear speech output on a small, portable meter, and a method of consistent placement of the blood sample[15] (for more information, see Chapter 21, Eye Disease and Adaptive Education for Visually Impaired Persons).

Long-Term Monitoring of Metabolic Control

1 Glycosylated hemoglobin (HbA₁c), the most abundant minor hemoglobin component in the red blood cell, increases in proportion to the blood glucose level over the preceding 3 to 4 months in persons with diabetes. It is an accurate, objective measure of chronic glycemia in diabetes.

   A *Glycosylation* occurs as glucose in the plasma attaches itself to the hemoglobin component of the red blood cell; this process is irreversible.

- The more glycosylation, the higher the values.

- Because the red blood cell has a life span of 120 days, this test reflects the blood glucose concentration over that period of time.

- The glycosylated hemoglobin does not reflect the simple mean but reflects the weighted mean over a long period of time.[16] The traditional idea that glycosylated hemoglobin reflects the simple mean and is referred to as the average of the blood glucose is inaccurate. For example, in a HbA₁c measured on May 1, 50% of the HbA₁c level is determined by the plasma glucose level during the preceding one-month period (April), 25% of its level is determined by the plasma glucose level during the one-month period before that (March) and the remaining 25% is determined by the plasma glucose level during the two-month period before the past two months (February and January).

   B Glycosylated hemoglobin can be measured by many different methods. Accurate interpretation requires knowledge of the method used to determine the glycosylated hemoglobin level, the component measured, and the normal range for the particular assay.[17]

- Affinity chromatography and colorimetric assay methods measure total glycated hemoglobin (GHb), including all fractions of the hemoglobin molecule: HbA₁a, HbA₁b, and HbA₁c.[17] Upper normal values of GHb may be in the range of 8% to 9%.

- Ion-exchange chromatography, high-performance liquid chromatography (HPLC), and immunoassay methods are used to measure HbA₁c.[17] The normal value is usually in the range of 4% to 6%.

- It has been suggested that all glycosylated hemoglobin assays be standardized and reported in values equivalent to the HbA[1c] as measured in the Diabetes Control and Complications Trial (DCCT).[18]
- Interfering factors (sickle-cell hemoglobin and other hemoglobinopathies) may affect measurement of HbA[1c] depending upon the method.[19]

B Regular measurements of HbA[1c] permit timely detection of departures from the target range. In the absence of well-controlled studies that suggest a definite testing protocol, the Standards of Medical Care for Patients with Diabetes Mellitus[20] suggest glycosylated hemoglobin testing at least one or two times a year in patients with a history of stable glycemic control, and at least quarterly assessments in patients whose therapy has changed or who are in poor control.

C Glycemic targets should be individualized for each patient.

- The DCCT[18] conclusively demonstrated, however, that the risk of retinopathy, nephropathy, and neuropathy in patients with type 1 diabetes is reduced by intensive treatment regimens compared with conventional treatment regimens. These benefits were observed with an average HbA[1c] of 7.2% (normal range = 4.0% to 6.0%) in the intensively treated group of patients. The reduction in risk of these complications correlated continuously with the reduction in HbA[1c] produced by intensive therapy.[20]
- A glycosylated hemoglobin result within the nondiabetic reference range (Table 11.3) may reflect frequent hypoglycemia. The glycosylated hemoglobin is a strong indicator of blood glucose control when compared with SMBG results.

TABLE 11.3. GLYCEMIC TARGETS FOR NONPREGNANT INDIVIDUALS WITH DIABETES[20]

Biochemical Index	Nondiabetic Reference Range	Goal	Suggested Action Range
HbA[1c], %	4.0 to 6.0	7.0	>8.0

Action suggested depends on individual patient circumstances. Such actions may include enhancement of diabetes self-management education, co-management with a diabetes team, referral to an endocrinologist, change in pharmacological therapy, initiation of increased SMBG, or more frequent contact with the patient.

D Glycosylated hemoglobin is a teaching tool as well as a marker of metabolic control. If a patient monitors only fasting blood glucose levels and finds values in the normal range with a HbA1c result of 9.8% (normal range = 4.0% to 6.0%), the educator can encourage the patient to monitor at other times of the day (especially postprandial readings) to uncover periods of elevated blood glucose and identify the factors that may be associated with the elevations.

2 Glycosylated albumin (fructosamine), a glycated serum protein test, measures glycemic control over 2 to 3 weeks.[21] Normal ranges vary among the different methods of measurements. Fructosamine values are used in short-term follow-up of interventions that have been recently implemented to lower blood glucose.[17]

Urine Tests

1 Monitoring for the presence of urinary ketones remains an essential component of diabetes care. Patients with type 1 diabetes are ketosis-prone whereas patients with type 2 diabetes are generally ketosis-resistant.

A Urinary ketones measured with dipsticks or tablets should be tested routinely during illness by all patients with diabetes. Patients with type 2 diabetes can become ketotic during severe stress precipitated by infections or trauma.[22]

- Patients with type 1 diabetes should test urinary ketones when their blood glucose is consistently elevated (>240 mg/dL [>13.3 mmol/L]). For patients using an insulin pump, ketonuria in the presence of hyperglycemia may indicate failure of the insulin delivery system.

- Pregnant women with diabetes (including gestational diabetes) are advised to monitor urinary ketones every morning. These measurements are useful for detecting inadequate dietary intake (starvation ketosis) and providing warning of impending metabolic decompensation (for more information see Chapter 18, Pregnancy).[23]

- Urinary ketones also should be measured on a regular schedule in patients actively trying to lose weight by calorie restriction. Because ketones are a waste product of fat metabolism, ketonuria in the presence of euglycemia can indicate weight loss, not metabolic decompensation.

- Patents with type 1 diabetes who are restricting calories to lose weight require decreased dosages of insulin to prevent hypoglycemia. Too much of a reduction of insulin will result in hypglycemia, ketonuria and, if not corrected, metabolic decompensation to ketoacidosis.

B Three ketone bodies are formed from the conversion of free fatty acids in the liver: acetone, acetoacetate, and beta-hydroxybutyrate.

- Urinary ketones are detected by the nitroprusside reaction in the treatment of acute diabetic ketoacidosis. The nitroprusside reagent predominantly reacts with acetoacetate and does not react with beta-hydroxybutyrate.

- Following the institution of insulin therapy, the concentration of acetoacetate increases and beta-hydroxybutyrate decreases. This shift accounts for the clinical observation that urine ketone test results may become more positive during the early phase of therapy and indicate clinical improvement rather than deterioration.

2 The ability to detect low levels of albumin in the urine (microalbuminuria) represented an important advance in the diagnosis and treatment of diabetic nephropathy. The presence of microalbuminuria represents an early phase of nephropathy and is important for prompt diagnosis and intervention.

A Annual urine protein screening in individuals with type 1 diabetes should begin at puberty and after 5 years duration of diabetes. Because of the difficulty in precise dating of type 2 diabetes, urinary protein screening should begin at the time of diagnosis.[20]

B The albustix reagent does not screen for microalbuminuria because it does not become positive until the albumin excretion rate (AER) exceeds 300 mg/dL (200 (g/min).

C In healthy individuals, small amounts of albumin can be found in the urine with a mean albumin excretion rate of 10 ± 3 mg/day (7 ± 2 (g/min).[25]

D Screening for microalbuminuria should be avoided if the patient has a urinary tract infection or hematuria, has recently performed strenuous exercise, is experiencing acute illness or fever, and during menstruation.[23]

TABLE 11.4. DEFINITION OF MICROALBUMINURIA[25]

	Urinary AER mg/24hr	Urinary AER mg/min
Normoalbuminuria	<30	<20
Microalbuminuria	30 to 300	0 to 200
Macroalbuminuria	>300	>200

AER = Albumin Excretion Rate.
Source: Adapted with permission. DeFronzo. In: Ellenberg and Rifkin's diabetes mellitus: theory and practice. 5th ed. Appleton and Lange, 1997.

3 Urine glucose testing was the original method of monitoring glycemic control, but blood glucose monitoring is the preferred method. Urine glucose testing provides retrospective information and does not reflect current blood glucose. Urine glucose testing is used only if the patient is unable or unwilling to perform blood glucose monitoring or if the only goal is avoiding symptomatic hyperglycemia.[20]

A The results of urine glucose testing should be reported in percent values not plus (+) values for continuity of results from one method to another.

B The advantages of urine testing for glucose are that it is less expensive than blood glucose monitoring and is noninvasive.

C Urine testing for glucose offers several distinct disadvantages.

- Elevated renal thresholds (blood glucose >180 mg/dL [>10 mmol/L]) that occur with age and during pregnancy will give false negative results.
- Since urine testing gives a delayed picture of what is happening in the blood, it is not indicated in intensive diabetes management.[17]
- False results (negative or positive) may occur with ingestion of certain medications (cephalosporins, large amounts of ascorbic acid).
- Urine testing can be awkward to do especially when away from home.

ASSESSMENT OF GROWTH AND WEIGHT

1 Monitoring also involves assessing of growth in children and weight in all patients with diabetes.

2 Documentation of weight is considered another indicator for diabetes management.

    A Weight gain may reflect improvement in glycemic control, increased caloric consumption, frequent episodes of hypoglycemia, fluid retention and eating disorders, among other conditions.

    B Similarly, weight loss may reflect elevated blood glucose levels, decreased caloric consumption or eating disorders.

    C Fluctuations in weight can occur depending upon the scale used and time of day.

SUMMARY

1 Since self-monitoring of blood glucose is one of the essential tools of self-management, diabetes educators have the unique opportunity and responsibility to provide instruction concerning not only monitoring techniques but use of the data.

2 Diabetes educators can also teach patients to approach monitoring as feedback (ie, helpful information) rather than evaluation (ie, punishment).

3 Teach patients that the meaning of the results from the methods used to monitor metabolic control provides more than feedback; it reinforces their active role in self-management and their position as the center of the healthcare team.

KEY EDUCATIONAL CONSIDERATIONS

1 A variety of meters are available for monitoring blood glucose, and each one is unique.

    A It is important to carefully assess the patients visual acuity and dexterity skills before recommending a specific meter. Let the patient practice using the meter. Demonstration meters and supplies are available from the manufacturer's representative.

    B Diabetes educators, are pivotal in guiding patient's to select the meter that is most appropriate for them and one for which they easily can obtain supplies. Some insurers only reimburse for certain meters and reagents.

2 Ask patients to bring their meters and all supplies to each visit.

    A The meter can be cleaned, the reagents and control solution can be tested, codes can be verified, and an actual blood glucose measurement can be performed.

    B Comparing the meter results to a lab test can be additional verification of accuracy. Expect the results from venous serum blood glucose to be 10% to 15% higher than the results from capillary whole blood glucose samples[26] except for meters that are plasma/serum referenced.

3 Provide patients with the toll-free customer service number for the manufacturer of their meter. Experts are available at this number 24-hours per day to answer questions and provide assistance.

4 Careful and safe disposal of used lancets is critical. Teach patients to dispose of used lancets in an appropriate sharps container (regulations vary from state to state). When monitoring blood glucose away from home, patients can place their used lancets in an empty pill container or 35 mm film canister.

5 Consider the cost of supplies when considering with patients the frequency of monitoring. Be familiar with local suppliers who charge reasonable prices. Refer patients to a social worker or community agency when appropriate.

6 Some patients benefit from having a second meter that is compact, quick, and simple to use for easily checking their blood glucose level away from home or before driving.

7 Postprandial monitoring is effective for teaching the impact of food portions on blood glucose levels. For example, a patient may choose a large portion of frozen yogurt and have an elevated blood glucose reading 2 hours later, whereas after a medium portion of frozen yogurt the postprandial reading may be in the goal range.

8 Use patient records or logbooks that list glucose levels for a certain time of day in a linear and vertical fashion. This format allows simple visual interpretation of the results.

9 Recording blood glucose levels on a graph, as well as having a numerical listing, provides a useful visual aid for teaching the concept of blood glucose patterns. Computer software marketed by meter manufacturers can be very helpful in providing graphs and other visual representations of the data.

10 Actual blood glucose records of common patterns should be used when teaching self-management.

11 Provide patients with the opportunity to practice urine testing for ketones during their teaching appointment.

12 A supply sheet, signed by the healthcare provider, can be an effective organizational aid for the patient and the pharmacist and may serve as a prescription.

13 Teaching the concept of glycosylated hemoglobin can be challenging. This test can be referred to as a "smart" blood test that represents blood glucose levels over the last 3 months. HbA_{1c} can be thought of as a long-term monitoring method as opposed to the day-to-day self-monitoring measurements that are performed with a home meter.

14 Avoid referring to HbA_{1c} as an average of blood glucose levels. Besides being technically inaccurate, patients often confuse HbA_{1c} with the average in their meter memory.

15 The educator can use a picture of a pyramid or a thermometer to outline the various HbA_{1c} levels, then demonstrate the goal range and the patient's most recent result. Ask patients what they think about the results and what they'd like to do about it rather than offering judgments.

Self-Review Questions

1 List the factors that affect the accuracy of SMBG results.

2 Describe the most common user error related to SMBG.

3 List tips that can be followed to secure an adequate blood sample.

4 Define the critical uses of SMBG data by patients.

5 Describe ways educators can use SMBG to link the principles of diabetes management with daily decision making.

6 Describe common psychosocial adaptations related to SMBG.

7 Describe how monitoring schedules are determined.

8 Define a reliable method for evaluating the accuracy of blood glucose meters.

9 List the elements of quality assurance regarding blood glucose meters.

10 Describe the unique SMBG needs of the elderly, children, and visually impaired persons with diabetes.

11 Define glycosylated hemoglobin and the target ranges.

12 Define fructosamine and when this assessment is used.

13 List the advantages and disadvantages of urine glucose testing.

14 Describe what groups of patients should monitor urine for ketones.

15 List two methods of screening for microalbuminuria and the target ranges.

16 List when time testing for microalbuminuria should be avoided.

17 Describe the role of documenting weight changes in the management of diabetes.

Case Study 1

AD sees the diabetes educator regularly following a visit with his physician. At each visit with the educator, he brings both of his meters (from two different manufacturers) and presents different scenarios concerning the discrepancies between the two meters or between the lab and each meter. He keeps no records and barely checks his blood glucose because "he is not confident of the results." The diabetes educator dutifully verifies the accuracy of the meters and spends the entire visit defending the meters. When reviewing the documentation of these visits, the diabetes educator realizes that there has been no diabetes education and looks to colleagues for advice.

QUESTIONS FOR DISCUSSION

1   What are the dynamics of these visits?
2   What are possible explanations for the patient's behavior?
3   How can the educator alter the pattern of the visits?
4   What content is generally included when teaching about blood glucose monitoring?

DISCUSSION

1   AD may be using the meters as an effective smoke screen.

   A   If AD organizes the visits around the meters then nothing else is discussed. He may have lost confidence in the meters, but verifying accuracy and defending the meters is not helping him regain his confidence.

   B   When interactions with patients become frustrating, reflecting on the experience and seeking the advise of colleagues often helps to bring a different perspective to the situation. As a result of her thoughts and discussions, the educator recognizes her role in perpetuating this pattern. While she knows she cannot change AD's behavior, she can change her own.

2   To alter the pattern of visits, the educator decides to develop a specific plan of action. When making the plan, she realizes that she needs to be sure that it is designed to meet AD's needs and includes strategies that keep him in control of the visit, such as asking questions and seeking his options rather than just offering advice. The important thing is to create a different, more functional partnership with him.

   A   Because this might represent avoidance behavior, the educator needs to assess what AD is trying to avoid in order to more effectively meet his needs. This task will no doubt be challenging, but one technique for inviting discussion is to say, "It seems like we spend all of our time on this topic and I am concerned that you are not getting what you need from me. Could we start with your other concerns?"

   B   If he is unable to identify concerns, you could share the barriers to self-care that others have identified and ask if he has had similar experiences or if there are other things about his diabetes care that are hard for him.

C   Another option would be to ask AD if the physician made any treatment changes during the last visit, offer to review these changes with AD and use them as a springboard for teaching new content. The issues surrounding monitoring still need to be discussed, but focusing on another area of AD's concerns may decrease frustration for him and the educator.

3   Generally, once the patient's technique in using the meter has been assessed (including reagent storage, expiration date, etc.), teach how to record blood glucose readings, target ranges, and, most importantly, how to use the data.

Case Study 2

MN has quarterly visits with a diabetes educator whose job includes providing diabetes education and management. At this visit, MN presents with a 7 pound (3.2 kg) weight gain and her BaNc is 9.6% (reference range = 4.0% to 6.0%). Her HbA_{1c} was 7.2% three months ago. MN brought her meter and used the memory feature to review the readings. "The numbers are up and down. I know I've been eating more but I'm disgusted." The educator recognizes that the dosage of the oral agent is too low and changes the dose and type of medication. After MN is given information about the new prescription, she begins to leave but the educator is not finished.

Questions For Discussion

1   What does the educator still need to assess?
2   What clues are provided by the elevated BaNc and weight gain?

Discussion

1   It would be helpful to either download the meter memory using computer software (if possible) or use the memory feature to create a written log. Organizing the readings according to the time of day may help the patient recognize patterns, for example that the blood glucose readings are high in the morning and lower at night.

2 The educator can use the logbook to ask MN what she thinks is happening. When MN describes her evening snacking behaviors, the educator and MN discover that MN is eating all evening because of her fear of a low blood glucose at night.

3 Further questioning may reveal that MN has had frequent episodes of symptomatic hypoglycemia in the late afternoon and that she frequently skips lunch to save calories because she eats all evening.

4 Based on this assessment, the educator may decide to delay changing the medication and work with the patient on the following issues:
   A Avoiding the nocturnal hypoglycemia that she fears
   B Reinforcing the benefits of eating lunch
   C Teaching the benefit of recording blood glucose readings in a logbook

5 Beginning with future visits a discussion of the monitoring records and what the patient believes is affecting her levels may help increase the educator's efficiency and effectiveness.

REFERENCES

1 American Diabetes Association. Consensus statement. Self-monitoring of blood glucose. Diabetes Care 1996;19(suppl 1):S62-66.

2 Peragallo-Dittko V. Buyer's guide to blood glucose meters. Diabetes Self-Manage 1994;11(3): 6-14.

3 Harris MI, Crowe CC, Howie LJ. Self-monitoring of blood glucose by adults with diabetes in the United States population. Diabetes Care 1993; 16:1116-23.

4 Babione L. SMBG: the underused nutrition counseling tool in diabetes management. Diabetes Spectrum 1994;7: 196-97.

5 Ahern JA, Gatcomb PM, Held NA, Petit WA, Jr, Tamborlane WV. Exaggerated hyperglycemia after a pizza meal in well-controlled diabetes. Diabetes Care 1993;16:578-80.

6 Rubin RR, Peyrot M, Saudek CD. The effect of a diabetes education program incorporating coping skills training on emotional well-being and diabetes self-efficacy. Diabetes Educ 1993;19:210-14.

7 Price MJ. Qualitative analysis of the patient-provider interactions: the patient's perspective. Diabetes Educ 1989;15:144-48.

8 Cox DJ, Irvine A, Gonder-Frederick L, Nowacek G, Butterfield J. Fear of hypoglycemia: quantification, validation and utilization. Diabetes Care 1987; 10:617-21.

9 American Association of Diabetes Educators. Position statement. Prevention of transmission of blood-borne infectious agents during blood glucose monitoring. Diabetes Educ 1988; 14:425-26.

10 Clarke WL, Cox D, Gonder-Frederick LA, Carter W, Pohl SL. Evaluating clinical accuracy of systems for self-monitoring of blood glucose. Diabetes Care 1987; 10:622-28.

11 Klonoff DC. Noninvasive blood glucose monitoring. Diabetes Care 1997;20:433-37.

12 Walker EA. Quality assurance for blood glucose monitoring. Nurs Clin North Am 1993;28:61-70.

13 American Diabetes Association. CLIA guidelines implemented. Diabetes Rev 1993;1:130.

14 Peragallo-Dittko V. Clinical and educational usefulness of SMBG with the elderly. Diabetes Spectrum 1995;8:17-19.

15 Bernbaum M, Albert SG, Brusca S, et al. Effectiveness of glucose monitoring systems modified for the visually impaired. Diabetes Care 1993;16:1363-66.

16 Tahara Y, Shima K. Kinetics of BaNc, glycated albumin, and fructosamine and analysis of their weight functions against preceding plasma glucose level. Diabetes Care 1995;18;440-47.

17 Farkas-Hirsch R, ed. Intensive diabetes management. Alexandria, Va: American Diabetes Association, 1995:80-87.

18 The Diabetes Control and Complications Trial Research Group. The effect of intensive treatment of diabetes on the development and progression of long-term complications of insulin-dependent diabetes. N Engl J Med 1993;329:77-86.

19 Goldstein DE, Little RR. More than you ever wanted to know (but need to know) about glycohemoglobin testing. Diabetes Care 1994;17:938-39.

20 American Diabetes Association. Position statement. Standards of medical care for patients with diabetes mellitus. Diabetes Care 1998;21 (suppl 1): S23-S3.1

21 Negoro H, Morley JE, Rosenthal MJ. Utility of serum fructosamine as a measure of glycemia in young and old diabetic and non-diabetic subjects. Am J Med 1988;85:360-64.

22 Fajans SS. Classification and diagnosis of diabetes. In: Porte D, Jr, Sherwin RS, eds. Ellenberg and Rifkin's diabetes mellitus: theory and practice. 5th ed. Stamford, Conn: Appleton and Lange, 1997: 357-72.

23 Metzger BE, Phelps RL, Dooley SL. The mother in pregnancies complicated by diabetes mellitus. In: Porte D, Jr, Sherwin RS, eds. Ellenberg and Rifkin's diabetes mellitus: theory and practice. 5th ed. Stamford, Conn: Appleton and Lange, 1997: 887-915.

24 Morgensen CE, Vestbo E, Poulsen PL, et al. Microalbuminuria and potential confounders. Diabetes Care 1995;18: 572-81.

25 DeFronzo RA. Diabetic nephropathy. In: Porte D, Jr, Sherwin RS, eds. Ellenberg and Rifkin's diabetes mellitus: theory and practice. 5th ed. Stamford, Conn: Appleton and Lange,1997:971-1008.

26 Tietz N. Fundamentals of clinical chemistry. Philadelphia: WB Saunders, 1976: 242-44.

Suggested Readings

1 Atkin SH, Dasmahapatra A, Jaker MA, Chorost MI, Reddy S. Fingerstick glucose determination in shock. Ann Intern Med 1991;114:1020-24.

2 Nettles A. User error in blood glucose monitoring: The National Steering Committee for Quality Assurance Report. Diabetes Care 1993;16:946-48.

3 Wedman B, Michael SR. Tool chest: glycosylated hemoglobin models. Diabetes Educ 1988;14:280-82.

For a listing of currently available meters, refer to Diabetes Forecast: Buyers Guide (Annual Issue) and Diabetes Self-Management.

MANAGEMENT

MANAGEMENT

Pattern Management of Blood Glucose 　　　　　**12**

Deborah A. Hinnen RN, MN, ARNP, CDE
Via Christi Regional Medical Center
Wichita, Kansas

Diana W. Guthrie RN, ARNP, FAAN, CDE
University of Kansas School of Medicine
Wichita, Kansas

Belinda P. Childs RN, MN, ARNP, CDE
Mid-America Diabetes Associates
Wichita, Kansas

Richard A. Guthrie MD, CDE
Mid-America Diabetes Associates
Via Christi Regional Medical Center
University of Kansas School of Medicine
Wichita, Kansas

INTRODUCTION

1   Pattern management is the application of a systematic analysis of data by both patients and health professionals in the daily and long-term management of blood glucose levels.

2   It is often used with intensive management programs to achieve euglycemia with the ultimate goal of preventing the chronic complications of diabetes.[1-3]

3   This chapter addresses pattern management as a way to analyze the data collected through self-monitoring of blood glucose (SMBG) in a logical and methodical way, thus allowing carefully planned changes to the treatment program.

OBJECTIVES

Upon completion of this chapter, the learner will be able to

1   List concepts of pattern management.

2   Identify strategies utilized in pattern management.

3   Describe algorithms for making insulin adjustments.

4   Describe changes in the timing of injections to accommodate specific situations (eg travel, shift work).

5   Identify that combination therapy may result from pattern management and contribute to intensive diabetes management for patients with type 2 diabetes.

CONCEPTS OF PATTERN MANAGEMENT

1   Pattern management is a comprehensive approach to blood glucose management that includes all aspects of current diabetes therapy.[4] While this approach is typically identified with intensive insulin therapy, pattern management can actually include utilization of many pharmacological combinations for blood glucose control.

2   Combinations of multiple oral agents can be used to address the specific pathophysiologic problems of insulin resistance in hyperinsulinemia which further enhances the opportunity to personalize and intensify diabetes management for type 2 patients.

3 Improvements in monitoring tools increase the potential for gathering the information necessary to appropriately apply medical nutritional therapy, exercise, and medications to attain blood glucose goals established by the patient and the diabetes care team (see Chapter 11, Monitoring, for standard blood glucose goals for adults and Chapter 17, Childhood and Adolescence, for target ranges for children).

4 Elements of pattern management include:

A Self-identified desire to be an active participant in care.

B Identification of personal blood glucose goals by the patient and diabetes care team.

C Self-adjustment of food intake, exercise, and medication to achieve goals.

D Frequent SMBG to provide data for making adjustments.

E Multiple injections of insulin, combinations of oral medications or oral medications and insulin, or continuous subcutaneous insulin infusion (CSII) therapy.

F Frequent interaction between patients and the diabetes care team.
- Telephone, fax, and e-mail can be used to discuss glucose values between visits.

G Self-management education
- Comprehensive and interactive coverage of the 15 content areas identified by the National Standards for Diabetes Self-Management Education.[5,6]
- Relationship of glucose levels, food, activity, and medications.
- Impact of elements of control on personal glucose levels.
- Purpose, strategies, and value of pattern management for intensive therapy to achieve blood glucose goals.
- Decision making and problem solving.
- Personal diabetes and health-related goods.
- Understanding of personal belief system related to the value of health and intensive diabetes management.

H Support systems to provide emotional and management support
- Diabetes care team with on-call nursing support
- Family or care partners
- Support groups
- Other community diabetes educational activities and offerings

STRATEGIES FOR PATTERN MANAGEMENT

1   Pattern management involves reviewing several days of glucose records and making adjustments in diabetes management based on trends, rather than reacting to a single, high or low blood glucose reading. Adding supplemental or sliding scale insulin at the time of the elevated glucose level solves the problem only for that particular point in time but does not prevent the problem from occurring again.

2   If blood glucose readings are high for several days at a specific time, potential causes for the elevated levels are examined so the problem can be corrected. This method of managing diabetes has been used since the 1930s, originally with children and later among adults with type 1 and type 2 diabetes.[7-9] Options for pattern management have included sliding scale approaches or long-term algorithms.

3   Pattern management includes a review of all parameters of intensive management (nutrition, exercise, stress, and illness) not just insulin adjustment.[10] (See Table 12.1)

TABLE 12.1. QUESTIONS TO ASK WHEN EVALUATING BLOOD GLUCOSE READINGS

1   Is there a pattern appearing upon examination of 3-5 days of blood glucose readings?

2   Is there something happening at the same time every day, like an insulin reaction, high glucose after breakfast, etc.?

3   Are there blood glucose readings representing all "times" of the day?

4   Are there blood glucose readings representing the "peak" times of each medication (insulins and oral agents)?

5   Are there readings to represent peak glucose readings from all meals?

6   Are there "other notes" or "changes" such as mealtimes, calorie or carbohydrate variances, exercise changes, unusual hours of work or school, etc.?

7   Is prevention of weight gain important for the patient? If so, consideration must be given to trying to reduce the use of hypoglycemic medications (ie, insulin or sulfonylureas), especially if low blood glucose levels are occurring routinely.

4 Timing of glucose monitoring is variable depending on the pharmacological therapy and glucose goals.

    A SMBG is done at the peak effect of the medication so that the appropriate insulin or medication can be adjusted (see the Problem-Solving Practice section of this chapter for examples).

        • Premeal glucose measurements are needed to monitor basal insulin dose (eg, NPH or Ultralente) and to determine the dose/timing of the bolus insulin. (Tables 12.2, 12.3)

        • Two-hour postprandial glucose readings are needed to titrate regular insulin for multiple injections. (Tables 12.4, 12.5, 12.6)

        • Two-hour post injection SMBG readings are needed to titrate lispro insulin.

        • The effectiveness of metformin, troglitazone, acarbose, glipizide, glucotrol, repaglinide, and others is tested using 2-hour postprandial readings.

    B CSII therapy requires SMBG levels 4 to 6 times per day to determine the effectiveness of the basal dose and the amount of the bolus dose.

    C Pregnancy requires frequent SMBG (eg, 5 to 6 times per day) in order to make the adjustments needed for tight blood glucose control (see Chapter 18, Pregnancy).

    D During acute illness, premeal testing is needed to determine the need for and dose of any supplemental insulin.

    E Elevated fasting glucose levels require 3 AM testing at least once a week to rule out the Somogyi (rebound) syndrome or the dawn phenomenon.

    F Asymptomatic hypoglycemia requires regular testing on a daily basis, particularly at peak insulin times and before driving as a method for recognizing low blood glucose levels.

    G Unusual schedules present special challenges where use of pattern management can help to maintain blood glucose levels.

        • Travel across time zones, working night shifts or swing shifts, farming, business schedules, and college student schedules all can make blood glucose levels difficult to control. Food intake varies and may not be able to be scheduled. Eating out makes it difficult to estimate calories or carbohydrate content. Exercise opportunities are also variable.

- Each situation requires flexibility and individual planning. Understanding medications and their actions is critical, especially insulin action. Start with the patient's plan and factor in the special situation as it relates to food intake, meal patterns, medication, and activity. SMBG is critical and may be required 6 to 8 times per day until insulin doses are adequately titrated and glucose goals are attained.

5 Objective summary assessment of glycemia is needed in addition to SMBG data.

  A Glycosylated hemoglobin is measured quarterly until goals are reached, then at least two times per year.[11]

  B Glycosylated albumin (fructosamine) can be used for biweekly testing during in pregnancy[12] and for others needing a more rapid assessment of overall glycemic control.

6 Insulin therapy options for pattern management can include sliding scale or long term algorithm approaches.

  A The sliding scale approach tries to solve the problem only for a particular point in time but does not prevent the problem from occurring again.

    - Sliding scale doses are given in addition to the usual insulin dose.

    - A typical program suggests a preset amount of insulin based on glucose readings, regardless of age or weight. The result is often a roller coaster-like shift between hypoglycemia and hyperglycemia, a situation that does nothing to contribute to overall health or feelings of well-being for the patient.

    - If a sliding scale is used, it is based on past patterns of the individual patient.

  B The algorithm approach to insulin therapy is used to provide variation in the usual insulin dose; supplemental insulins are often utilized. Algorithm approaches may be compensatory or anticipatory.

    - Compensatory—This supplement is additional insulin used to correct unusual hyperglycemia in response to an unanticipated event (eg, acute illness). One example of formulas used to compensate for a high blood sugar is the 1500 rule for regular insulin and the 1800 rule for lispro insulin. Use of this formula provides a starting point for bringing down glucose elevations.

- 1500 rule: 1500 ÷ current total daily insulin dose = sensitivity factor (sensitivity factor defines how much a unit of insulin will lower blood glucose); supplemental dose = actual blood glucose minus goal blood glucose ÷ sensitivity factor. The 1800 rule is calculated in the same manner, substituting 1800 for 1500.
- Anticipatory—This supplement is additional insulin administered before expected increases in carbohydrate or calorie intake. Various formulas are available for calculating carbohydrate/insulin ratios (see Chapter 8, Nutrition, for more information on carbohydrate counting). One unit of lispro or regular insulin per 10 to 15 grams of carbohydrate is a common starting point.
- Also, if the pre-meal glucose is low, the appropriate insulin dose may be decreased.

COMBINATION THERAPIES

1 In the 1980s, combination therapy was limited to insulin and sulfonylurea combinations. The recent availability of multiple oral agents for the treatment of type 2 diabetes has created many new therapeutic options.

2 A common combination is initiating monotherapy with either a sulfonylurea or metformin and adding the other agent when the doses approach maximum therapeutic limits. This combination requires specific clinical considerations.

A Careful patient selection regarding liver and renal function (metformin)

B Possible hypoglycemia (with sulfonylureas and rapaglinide)

C Need for postprandial SMBG for dose titration

D Differences in when to take agents in relation to meals (eg, sulfonylureas taken 30 minutes prior to the meal, metformin taken with the meal to reduce gastrointestinal disturbances and enhance medication action).[13]

3 Acarbose may be added as a third agent or used as monotherapy; taking with meals enhances medication action and reduces gastrointestinal side effects.

4 Troglitazone was initially approved for use in combination with insulin. Recent studies[14-17] have demonstrated its effectiveness for other indications.

A Because the time to therapeutic response can be 6 to 8 weeks, other agents must be available to control hyperglycemia.

B After the glycemic benefit occurs, doses of insulin or the other oral agent may be titrated downward.

- The Diabetes Prevention Program (DPP) sponsored by the National Institutes of Health (NIH) is evaluating the effectiveness of troglitazone for patients with impaired glucose tolerance.

- Troglitazone appears to be more effective when it is used in combination with other agents (see Chapter 10, Pharmacologic Therapies, for additional information).

5 Repaglinide provides an additional option for combination therapies.

Table 12.2. Pattern Management—Pre-meal Monitoring

Insulin (3 injections per day)

Regular or lispro/NPH insulin, (or 70/30) AM dose
Regular or lispro insulin, PM dose
NPH insulin, bedtime dose

Evaluate Blood Glucose (BG) Patterns

1 Adjust insulin based on 2- to 3-day BG patterns.
2 Determine which insulin is responsible for the pattern.
3 Adjust insulin 10% to 20%.
4 2 hr pp blood glucose tests needed for lispro titration.
5 If using lispro, 1 injection of NPH may not provide 24 hr basal coverage in insulinopenic patients.

AM	Below Target Blood Glucose	Above Target Blood Glucose
Dose affecting	*hs NPH insulin*	*hs NPH insulin*
	1 Consider increasing total calories or carbohydrate content of the evening snack.	1 Consider decreasing total calories or carbohydrate content of the evening snack.
	2 Determine if low blood glucose is occurring during or after exercise.	2 Evaluate nocturnal hypoglycemia or hyperglycemia (check 3 AM BG).
	3 Evaluate nocturnal hypoglycemia (check 3 AM BG).	3 Evaluate nocturnal hypoglycemia (check 3 AM BG).
	4 Consider decreasing hs NPH.	4 Consider increasing hs NPH.

Midday Lunch	Below Target Blood Glucose	Above Target Blood Glucose
Dose affecting	AM *regular or lispro insulin*	AM *regular or lispro insulin*
	1 Consider increasing total calories or carbohydrate content of midmorning snack.	1 Consider decreasing total calories or carbohydrate content of the midmorning snack.
	2 Determine if low blood glucose is occurring during or after exercise.	2 Consider adjusting exercise times or adding exercise.
	3 Consider decreasing AM regular or lispro insulin.	3 Consider increasing AM regular or lispro insulin.

PM Supper	Below Target Blood Glucose	Above Target Blood Glucose
Dose affecting	AM *NPH insulin*	AM *NPH insulin*
	1 Consider increasing total calories or carbohydrate content of afternoon snack.	1 Consider decreasing total calories or carbohydrate content of the afternoon snack.
	2 Determine if low blood glucose is occurring during or after exercise.	2 Consider adjusting exercise times or adding exercise.
	3 Consider decreasing AM NPH insulin.	3 Consider increasing AM NPH.

hs Bedtime	Below Target Blood Glucose	Above Target Blood Glucose
Dose affecting	PM *regular or lispro insulin*	PM *regular or lispro insulin*
	1 Consider increasing total calories or carbohydrate content of supper.	1 Consider decreasing total calories or carbohydrate content of supper.
	2 Determine if low blood glucose is occurring during or after exercise.	2 Consider adjusting exercise times or adding exercise.
	3 Consider decreasing PM regular or lispro insulin.	3 Consider increasing PM regular or lispro insulin.

Table 12.3. Pattern Management—Premeal Monitoring

Insulin (4 injections per day)

Regular or lispro insulin, AM dose
Regular or lispro insulin, midday dose
Regular or lispro insulin, PM dose
NPH insulin, bedtime dose or ultralente, supper dose

Evaluate Blood Glucose (BG) Patterns

1. Adjust insulin based on 2- to 3-day BG patterns.
2. Determine which insulin is responsible for the pattern.
3. Adjust insulin 10% to 20%.
4. 2 hr pp blood glucose testing needed for lispro titration.
5. If using lispro, 1 injection of NPH may not provide 24 hr basal coverage in insulinopenic patients.

AM	Below Target Blood Glucose	Above Target Blood Glucose
Dose affecting	*hs NPH insulin or supper ultralente*	*hs NPH insulin or supper ultralente*
	1. Consider increasing evening snack. 2. Evaluate nocturnal hypoglycemia (check 3 AM BG). 3. Consider decreasing hs NPH or ultralente insulin.	1. Consider decreasing evening snack. 2. Evaluate nocturnal hypoglycemia or hyperglycemia (check 3 AM BG). 3. Consider increasing hs NPH or ultralente insulin.

Midday Lunch	Below Target Blood Glucose	Above Target Blood Glucose
Dose affecting	*AM regular or lispro insulin*	*AM regular or lispro insulin*
	1. Consider increasing total calories or carbohydrate content of midmorning snack. 2. Determine if low blood glucose is occurring during or after exercise 3. Consider decreasing AM regular or lispro insulin.	1. Consider decreasing total calories or carbohydrate content of the midmorning snack. 2. Consider adjusting exercise times or adding exercise. 3. Consider increasing AM regular or lispro insulin.

PM Supper	Below Target Blood Glucose	Above Target Blood Glucose
Dose affecting	*Midday regular or lispro insulin*	*Midday regular or lispro insulin*
	1. Consider increasing total calories or carbohydrate content of the afternoon snack. 2. Determine if low blood glucose is occurring during or after exercise. 3. Consider decreasing insulin.	1. Consider decreasing total calories or carbohydrate content of the afternoon snack. 2. Consider adjusting exercise times or adding exercise. 3. Consider increasing insulin.

hs Bedtime	Below Target Blood Glucose	Above Target Blood Glucose
Dose affecting	*PM regular or lispro insulin*	*PM regular or lispro insulin*
	1. Consider increasing total calories or carbohydrate content of supper. 2. Determine if low blood glucose is occurring during or after exercise. 3. Consider decreasing PM regular or lispro insulin.	1. Consider decreasing total calories or carbohydrate content of supper. 2. Consider adjusting exercise times or adding exercise. 3. Consider increasing PM regular or lispro insulin.

TABLE 12.4. PATTERN MANAGEMENT—2 HOURS POSTMEAL MONITORING

Insulin (2 injections per day)

Regular or lispro insulin/NPH AM dose
Regular or lispro insulin/NPH PM dose

Evaluate Blood Glucose (BG) Patterns

1 Adjust insulin based on 2- to 3-day BG patterns.
2 Determine which insulin is responsible for the pattern.
3 Adjust insulin 10% to 20%.
4 2 hr pp blood glucose testing needed for lispro titration.
5 If using lispro, 1 injection of NPH may not provide 24 hr basal coverage for insulinopenic patients.

2 hr pp Breakfast	Below Target Blood Glucose	Above Target Blood Glucose
Dose affecting	AM *regular or lispro insulin* 1 Consider increasing total calories or carbohydrate content of breakfast. 2 Determine if low blood glucose is occurring during or after exercise. 3 Consider decreasing AM regular or lispro insulin.	AM *regular or lispro insulin* 1 Consider decreasing carbohydrate content at breakfast or adding solid protein. 2 Consider adjusting exercise times or adding exercise. 3 Consider giving regular injection 45 minutes before meal. 4 Consider increasing AM regular or lispro insulin.

2 hr pp Lunch	Below Target Blood Glucose	Above Target Blood Glucose
Dose affecting	AM *NPH insulin* 1 Consider increasing total calories or carbohydrate content of lunch. 2 Determine if low blood glucose is occurring during or after exercise. 3 Consider decreasing AM NPH insulin.	AM *NPH insulin* 1 Consider decreasing total calories, or carbohydrate content of lunch. 2 Consider adjusting exercise times or adding exercise. 3 Consider increasing AM NPH insulin.

2 hr pp Supper	Below Target Blood Glucose	Above Target Blood Glucose
Dose affecting	PM *regular or lispro insulin* 1 Consider increasing total calories or carbohydrate content of supper. 2 Determine if low blood glucose is occurring during or after exercise. 3 Consider decreasing PM regular or lispro insulin.	PM *regular or lispro insulin* 1 Consider decreasing total calories or carbohydrate content of supper. 2 Consider adjusting exercise times or adding exercise. 3 Consider giving regular injection 45 minutes before meal. 4 Consider increasing PM regular or lispro insulin.

TABLE 12.5. PATTERN MANAGEMENT—2 HOURS POSTMEAL MONITORING

Insulin (3 injections per day)

Regular or lispro/NPH insulin, AM dose
Regular or lispro insulin, PM dose
NPH insulin, bedtime dose

Evaluate Blood Glucose (BG) Patterns

1 Adjust insulin based on 2- to 3-day BG patterns.
2 Determine which insulin is responsible for the pattern.
3 Adjust insulin 10% to 20%.
4 2 hr pp blood glucose testing needed for lispro titration.
5 If using lispro, 1 injection of NPH may not provide 24 hr basal coverage for insulinopenic patients.

2 hr pp Breakfast	Below Target Blood Glucose	Above Target Blood Glucose
Dose affecting	AM *regular or lispro insulin*	AM *regular or lispro insulin*
	1 Consider increasing total calories or carbohydrate content of breakfast.	1 Consider decreasing carbohydrate content at breakfast or adding solid protein.
	2 Determine if low blood glucose is occurring during or after exercise.	2 Consider adjusting exercise times or adding exercise.
	3 Consider decreasing AM regular or lispro insulin.	3 Consider giving regular injection 45 minutes before meal.
		4 Consider increasing AM regular or lispro insulin.

2 hr pp Lunch	Below Target Blood Glucose	Above Target Blood Glucose
Dose affecting	AM *NPH insulin*	AM *NPH insulin*
	1 Consider increasing total calories or carbohydrate content of lunch.	1 Consider decreasing total calories, or carbohydrate content of lunch.
	2 Determine if low blood glucose is occurring during or after exercise.	2 Consider adjusting exercise times or adding exercise.
	3 Consider decreasing insulin.	3 Consider increasing insulin.

2 hr pp Supper	Below Target Blood Glucose	Above Target Blood Glucose
Dose affecting	PM *regular or lispro insulin*	PM *regular or lispro insulin*
	1 Consider increasing total calories or carbohydrate content of supper.	1 Consider decreasing total calories or carbohydrate content of supper.
	2 Determine if low blood glucose is occurring during or after exercise.	2 Consider adjusting exercise times or adding exercise.
	3 Consider decreasing regular or lispro insulin.	3 Consider giving regular injection 45 minutes before meal.
		4 Consider increasing PM regular or lispro insulin.

TABLE 12.6. PATTERN MANAGEMENT—2 HOURS POSTMEAL MONITORING

Insulin (4 injections per day)

Regular or lispro insulin, AM dose
Regular or lispro insulin, midday dose
Regular or lispro insulin, PM dose
NPH insulin, bedtime dose or ultralente, supper dose

Evaluate Blood Glucose (BG) Patterns

1 Adjust insulin based on 2- to 3-day BG patterns.
2 Determine which insulin is responsible for the pattern.
3 Adjust insulin 10% to 20%.
4 2 hr pp blood glucose testing needed for lispro titration.
5 If using lispro, 1 injection of NPH may not provide 24 hr basal coverage for insulinopenic patients.

2 hr pp Breakfast	Below Target Blood Glucose	Above Target Blood Glucose
Dose affecting	AM *regular or lispro insulin*	AM *regular or lispro insulin*
	1 Consider increasing total calories or carbohydrate content of breakfast.	1 Consider decreasing carbohydrate content at breakfast or adding solid protein.
	2 Determine if low blood glucose is occurring during or after exercise.	2 Consider adjusting exercise times or adding exercise.
	3 Consider decreasing AM regular or lispro insulin.	3 Consider giving regular injection 45 minutes before meal.
		4 Consider increasing AM regular or lispro insulin.

2 hr pp Lunch	Below Target Blood Glucose	Above Target Blood Glucose
Dose affecting	Midday *regular or lispro insulin*	Midday *regular or lispro insulin*
	1 Consider increasing total calories or carbohydrate content of lunch.	1 Consider decreasing total calories, or carbohydrate content of lunch.
	2 Determine if low blood glucose is occurring during or after exercise.	2 Consider adjusting exercise times or adding exercise.
	3 Consider decreasing midday regular or lispro insulin	3 Consider giving regular injection 45 minutes before meal.
		4 Consider increasing midday regular or lispro insulin.

2 hr pp Supper	Below Target Blood Glucose	Above Target Blood Glucose
Dose affecting	PM *regular or lispro insulin*	PM *regular or lispro insulin*
	1 Consider increasing total calories or carbohydrate content of supper.	1 Consider decreasing total calories or carbohydrate content of supper.
	2 Determine if low blood glucose is occurring during or after exercise.	2 Consider adjusting exercise times or adding exercise.
	3 Consider decreasing PM regular or lispro insulin.	3 Consider giving regular injection 45 minutes before meal.
		4 Consider increasing PM regular or lispro insulin.

PROBLEM-SOLVING PRACTICE

This section is designed to provide practice in pattern management through the evaluation of blood glucose logs and determination of problems, possible causes, and options for adjustments. Use the following as a guide for all of these situations.

Goals when well: Blood sugars in target range without insulin reactions; no ketones

1   Monitor fasting and 2-hour post prandial blood glucose levels

2   Analyze records once or twice per week.

3   For type 1 diabetes, aim for 75% to 85% in the target range; for type 2 diabetes, aim for 95% to 100% in the target range.

4   Increase or decrease food as the first change.

5   Evaluate exercise amount and timing.

6   Change insulin dose in amounts of one step or 10%.

7   Evaluate sites and timing of injections.

8   Evaluate the need for stress management.

9   If blood glucose levels are erratic due to Somogyi (rebound) syndrome, do not change dose.

Sean:

Type 1 patient taking:

- AM—12 units lispro/8 units NPH
- Lunch—3 units lispro
- Supper—14 units lispro
- HS—11 units NPH
- 2600 calories—3 meals, 1 snack

Time	Mon	Thurs	Sun
Fasting	100 mg/dL	110 mg/dL	103 mg/dL
After breakfast	322	284	250
Before lunch			
After lunch	280	246	150
Before supper			
After supper	148	131	133
Changes			
Diet	+2 milk	pancakes, OJ	+1 toast
Insulin/Pills			
Reactions			
Activity	⬆		
Remarks	7pm football		

Key: Diet changes/time   Activity   Reaction/Illness
       +1 = 1 point food extra   ⬆ increased activity   M = mild   S = severe
       −1 = 1 point food less   ⬇ decreased activity   Mo = moderate

PROBLEM

- Patterned high blood glucose

POSSIBLE CAUSES

- Too much carbohydrate or too many calories at breakfast/lunch
- Not enough insulin at breakfast/lunch

OPTIONS

- Change something in routine before the high tests:
  - —Decrease total calories or carbohydrate at breakfast/lunch
  - —Include exercise
  - —Increase breakfast/lunch insulin

Ethel:

Type 2 patient taking:
- Glipizide 10 mg bid
- Metformin 1000 mg bid
- 1400 calories

Time	Mon	Wed	Sat
Fasting	72 mg/dL	60 mg/dL	71 mg/dL
After breakfast	100	53	67
Before lunch			
After lunch	64	55	90
Before supper			
After supper	80	66	91
Changes			
Diet	+1/2 OJ	+1/2 milk	+1/2 honey
Insulin/Pills			
Reactions	2:30 PM **M**	9:15 AM **M**	11:30 AM **M**
Activity		Usual	Usual
Remarks	Yardwork	Picking beans	

Key: Diet changes/time   Activity   Reaction/Illness
         +1 = 1 point food extra   ↑ increased activity   M = mild   S = severe
         –1 = 1 point food less   ↓ decreased activity   Mo = moderate

PROBLEM
- Reactions too often throughout the day

POSSIBLE CAUSES
- Too much medication
- Inadequate carbohydrate or total food intake

OPTIONS
- Decrease sulfonylurea until blood glucose is >100 mg/dL for adults or those who don't want to gain weight, or
- Increase food 100 to 200 calories (growing children or adults who want to gain weight). *Example:* 100 calories = 1½ bread or 1½ meat. Distribute throughout the day.

Mark (college student):

Type 1 patient taking:

- AM—34 units 70/30
- Supper—6 units R
- HS—11 units NPH
- 1900 calories—3 meals, 3 snacks

Schedule	Tues	Thurs	Sat
Fasting	106 mg/dL	110 mg/dL	117 mg/dL
After breakfast	175	341	148
Before lunch			
After lunch	151	150	229
Before supper			
After supper	135	153	210
Changes			
Diet	No change	No change	No change
Insulin/Pills			
Reactions			
Activity	Usual	Usual	Usual
Remarks			

Key: Diet changes/time   Activity   Reaction/Illness
       +1 = 1 point food extra   ▲ increased activity   M = mild   S = severe
       −1 = 1 point food less   ▼ decreased activity   Mo = moderate

PROBLEM

- Erratic blood glucose levels

POSSIBLE CAUSES

- Injection sites
- Stress
- Somogyi, (rebound, over insulinization)

OPTIONS

- No change in dose, as 75% are in normal range

Melissa:

Type 1 patient taking:

- AM—3 units lispro/2 units Ultralente
- Lunch—2 units lispro
- Supper—4 units lispro/2 units Ultralente
- 1600 calories

Schedule	Thurs	Sat	Sun
Fasting	110 mg/dL	150 mg/dL	163 mg/dL
After breakfast	132	191	198
Before lunch			
After lunch	163	161	185
Before supper			
After supper	128	230	236
Changes			
Diet			
Insulin/Pills			
Reactions			
Activity	Usual	Usual	Usual
Remarks			

Key: Diet changes/time   Activity   Reaction/Illness
+1 = 1 point food extra   ⬆ increased activity   M = mild   S = severe
−1 = 1 point food less   ⬇ decreased activity   Mo = moderate

PROBLEM

- Gradual increase in overall blood glucose levels

POSSIBLE CAUSES

- Out of "honeymoon"
- Pregnancy
- Insulin losing potency
- Illness
- Puberty

OPTIONS

- For adults: Decrease food intake 100 to 200 calories and/or increase exercise.
- For growing children: Increase insulin 1 to 2 steps. Take this dose for 2 to 3 days. Increase again if blood glucose is still high. An increase in food intake may also be needed. If 3 dose changes do not decrease levels, instruct patient to call the diabetes care team.

Mary:

Type 2 patient taking:

- 300 mg Rezulin (for 1 week)
- 1400 calories

Schedule	Tues	Thurs	Sat
Fasting	314 mg/dL	288 mg/dL	301 mg/dL
After breakfast	282	214	285
Before lunch			
After lunch	296	322	274
Before supper			
After supper	252	297	244
Changes			
Diet	Birthday party 8 pm	Church lunch	Very careful
Insulin/Pills	X	X	After breakfast
Reactions			
Activity	Shopping		
Remarks		Tired	

Key: **Diet changes/time** **Activity** **Reaction/Illness**
+1 = 1 point food extra ↑ increased activity M = mild   S = severe
−1 = 1 point food less ↓ decreased activity Mo = moderate

PROBLEM

- Blood glucose too high

POSSIBLE CAUSE

- Rezulin not taken long enough

OPTIONS

- Add another antidiabetes agent
- Add sulfonylurea or insulin for 4 to 6 weeks, then reevaluate

John:

Type 2 patient taking:

- AM—20 mg Glucotrol, 1000 mg Metformin
- PM—20 mg Glucotrol, 1000 mg Metformin
- 1600 calories

Schedule	Mon	Wed	Sat
Fasting	180 mg/dL	192 mg/dL	219 mg/dL
After breakfast	145	154	138
Before lunch			
After lunch	162	143	121
Before supper			
After supper	129	116	95
Changes			
Diet	1800		
Insulin/Pills	X	X	X
Reactions			
Activity	Work at airplane factory	Work	"honey do" list and football
Remarks			

Key: Diet changes/time   Activity   Reaction/Illness
    +1 = 1 point food extra   ↑ increased activity   M = mild   S = severe
    −1 = 1 point food less   ↓ decreased activity   Mo = moderate

PROBLEM

- High fasting blood glucose levels

POSSIBLE CAUSES

- Too much carbohydrate or total calories at dinner or bedtime snack
- Inadequate medication in evening or at bedtime

OPTIONS

- Evaluate meal plan (dinner and hs snack)
- Add hs NPH dose

Summary

1 Diabetes therapy in the next century will become more specific to the physiologic problems causing hyperglycemia.

2 New agents are emerging that allow treatment of the specific cause of the hyperglycemia, insulin resistance, and insulinemia.
   A Insulin analogs allow very precise treatment based on lifestyles and variables in eating and exercise routines.
   B CSII therapy is changing due to use of these insulin analogs.

3 The success of this complex therapy depends on the skill and expertise of the educator in presenting and verifying understanding of self-management skills for the patient with diabetes.

4 Practitioners will require continuing education, protocols, and support from diabetes experts if these new therapies are to be effective for improving patient outcomes and quality of life.

Key Educational Considerations

1 Pattern management can be used by both type 1 and type 2 patients. Careful assessment of the patient's readiness to participate actively in such a program is critical to the success of pattern management.

2 Comprehensive self-management education is essential to achieve success in pattern management techniques. Particular emphasis for education includes
   A Monitoring and recording blood glucose results
   B Medications and appropriate blood glucose testing times to validate efficacy
   C Medical nutrition therapy
   D Exercise
   E Hypoglycemia
   F Sick-day care
   G Team care
   H Psychosocial implications
   I Role of patient in self-management

3 Engage patients in problem-solving situations during instruction to teach pattern recognition and application of appropriate options.

4 Assure patients that they will be able to access their healthcare team when necessary to establish confidence that self-initiated changes can be made safely.

Self-Review Questions

1 If a patient's fasting blood glucose level is elevated, what would you do to determine the cause?

2 If you determined that a patient's elevated fasting glucose level is due to low blood glucose levels during the night, what therapy changes could be made?

3 If a patient is taking the maximum dose of an oral sulfonylurea and insulin therapy is recommended, what other options might you suggest?

4 If a patient has persistently elevated glucose readings at midmorning or prelunch, what adjustment could be made?

5 If a patient's presupper glucose level is elevated, what options are available to normalize that blood glucose?

Case Study 1

KS, a 14-year-old adolescent with type 1 diabetes, is going to try out for volleyball. Her games are at 5:30 PM. KS takes her insulin (70/30) at 4:30 PM, eats dinner, and then plays volleyball. However, KS is having low blood sugars during every game. Her fasting glucose levels (at 7 AM) are always above 170 mg/dL. She usually takes her morning injection of 70/30 insulin at 7:30 AM.

Questions for Discussion

1 What are reasons for KS's fasting glucose levels to be elevated?

2 What could you suggest that would provide increased flexibility and help KS meet her glycemic goals?

DISCUSSION

1 KS has a hectic schedule and would likely benefit from splitting the evening 70/30 injection into regular or lispro at suppertime and NPH at 10 PM. Her suppertime insulin could be given after the volleyball game.

2 Giving the NPH at 10 PM would shift its peak to early AM. That single change may correct her elevated fasting level. If not, the bedtime NPH dose could be increased by 1 to 2 units every 2 to 3 days until the fasting blood glucose level is within range.

3 The rationale behind KS's current use of 70/30 insulin must be explored as there may be personal, emotional, or developmental issues in conflict with KS's pursuit of other options that are available for improved glycemic control.

CASE STUDY 2

SA is taking 40 mg of glipizide. Her doctor tells her she could stop taking this medication if she could lose 75 pounds. At her annual physical last week, the doctor said her laboratory values were good, except for her fasting blood glucose of 248 mg/dL and her HbA$_{1c}$ of 11.3. He recommends insulin injections, but SA does not want to give herself injections.

QUESTIONS FOR DISCUSSION

1 Are there other oral agents that might be effective?
2 What lab work is needed prior to initiating troglitazone or metformin?

DISCUSSION

1 SA might be a candidate for metformin. If her creatinine is <1.4 she might start with 500 mg at breakfast, with weekly increases of 500 mg at supper, then breakfast and so on until she reaches her blood glucose goals.

2 SA may also be a candidate for adding troglitazone if her transaminase levels are within normal limits. However, it may take 6 to 8 weeks starting at 300 to 400 mg/day to demonstrate a glycemic response.

3 Repaglinide before meals may also be a consideration in lieu of glyburide. While not a sulfonylurea, it increases first phase insulin release for patients who still have endogenous insulin producing ability.

References

1 The Diabetes Control and Complications Trial Research Group. The effect of intensive treatment of diabetes on the development and progression of long-term complications in insulin-dependent diabetes mellitus. N Engl J Med 1993;329: 977-86.

2 Turner R, Cull C, Holman R. United Kingdom Prospective Diabetes Study 17: a 9-year update of a randomized, controlled trial on the effect of improved metabolic control on complications in non-insulin-dependent diabetes mellitus. Ann Intern Med 1996;124:136-45.

3 Ohkubo Y, Kishikawa H, Araki E et al. Intensive insulin therapy prevents the progression of diabetic microvascular complications in Japanese patients with non-insulin-dependent diabetes mellitus: a randomized prospective 6-year study. Diabetes Res Clin Pract 1995;28:103-17.

4 Hirsch I. Implementation of intensive diabetes therapy for IDDM. Diabetes Rev 1995;3:288-307.

5 American Diabetes Association. National standards for diabetes self-management education programs and American Diabetes Association review criteria. Diabetes Care 1998;21(suppl1):595-98.

6 Guthrie DW, Guthrie RA, eds. Nursing management of diabetes mellitus. 4th ed. New York: Springer, 1997.

7 Jackson RL, Kelly HG. Growth of children with diabetes mellitus in relationship to level of control of the disease. J Pediatr 1946; 29:316.

8 Jackson RL, Guthrie RA. Physiologic management of diabetes in children. New York: Medical Examination Publishers, 1986:80-157.

9 Shagan BP. Does anyone here know how to make insulin work backwards? Why sliding-scale insulin coverage doesn't work. Practical Diabetol 1990; 9(3):1-4.

10 Guthrie DW, Guthrie RA. Approach to management. Diabetes Educ 1990;16: 401-6.

11 American Diabetes Association. Standards of medical care for patients with diabetes mellitus. Diabetes Care 1998; 21(suppl 1):S23-31.

12 American Diabetes Association. Tests of glycemia in diabetes. Diabetes Care 1998; 20(suppl 1):S69-71.

13 Childs BP, Guthrie RA, Carr M, McDaniel J, Rhiley D. Incorporating new diabetes oral agents into clinical practice. Diabetes Spectrum 1996;9:266-68.

14 Troglitazone Study Group. The metabolic effects of troglitazone in non-insulin-dependent diabetes (NIDDM). Diabetes 1997; 46(suppl 1): 149A.

15 Valiquett T, Haung S, Whitcomb R. Effects of troglitazone monotherapy in patients with NIDDM: a 6-month multicenter study. Diabetes 1997; 46(suppl 1):43A.

16 Ghazzi M, Radke-Mitchell L, Venable T, Whitcomb R, The Troglitazone Study Group. Troglitazone improves glycemic control in patients with type 2 diabetes who are not optimally controlled on sulfonylurea. Diabetes 1997; 46(suppl 1):44A.

17 Inzucchi SE, Maggs DG, Spollett GR, Page SL, Rife FS, Shulman GI. Efficacy and metabolic effects of troglitazone and metformin in NIDDM. Diabetes 1997; 46(suppl 1):34A.

Suggested Readings:

Brackenridge BP. Carbohydrate gram counting: a key to accurate meal time boluses in intensive diabetes therapy. Practical Diabetology 1992;11(2):22-28.

Hirsch IB. Technological advances in diabetes care. Where are we going? Diabetes Spectrum 1996;9:225-250.

Intensive diabetes management. Alexandria, Va: American Diabetes Association, 1996.

Pampanelli S, Torlone E, Talli C, Del Sindaco P, et al. Improved postprandial metabolic control after subcutaneous injection of a short-acting insulin analog in IDDM of short duration with residual pancreatic β-cell function. Diabetes Care 1995;18:1452-59.

Peragallo-Dittko V. Tight control: a guide to getting started. Diabetes Self-Manage 1996;13(5):20-24.

Pieber TR, Brunner GA, Schnedl WJ, Schattenbert S, et al. Evaluation of a structured outpatient group education program for intensive insulin therapy. Diabetes Care 1995;18:625-30.

Skyler JS, Skyler DL, Seigler DE, O'Sullivan MJ. Algorithms for adjustment of insulin dosage by patients who monitor blood glucose. Diabetes Care 1981;4:311-18.

Tuttleman M, Lipsett L, Harris MI. Attitudes and behaviours of primary care physicians regarding tight control of blood glucose in IDDM patients. Diabetes Care 1993;16:765-72.

Ziegher O, Kolopp M, Louis J, et al. Self-monitoring of blood glucose and insulin dose alteration in type I diabetes mellitus. Diabetes Res Clin Pract 1993; 21:51-59.

MANAGEMENT

Hyperglycemia 13

Mayer B. Davidson, MD
Cedars-Sinai Medical Center
Los Angeles, California

Stephanie Schwartz, MPH, RN, CDE
Children's Mercy Hospital
Kansas City, Missouri

INTRODUCTION

1 Prolonged hyperglycemia can lead to two types of metabolic crises, *diabetic ketoacidosis* (DKA) and *hyperglycemic hyperosmolar nonketotic syndrome* (HHNS). Either of these life-threatening conditions may result in an altered mental state, loss of consciousness, or possibly death. Prompt medical attention is necessary to avoid adverse outcomes.

2 DKA is a complication that results from an absolute or relative deficiency in insulin. Occurring most frequently in type 1 diabetes, DKA can occur in type 2 patients as well.[1] DKA is characterized by hyperglycemia, ketosis, acidosis, and dehydration.

3 HHNS is a life-threatening emergency with a high mortality rate.[2] This metabolic crisis is usually seen in the elderly or undiagnosed person with type 2 diabetes and is characterized by four main clinical features:
  A Severe hyperglycemia (blood glucose >800 mg/dL [44.4 mmol/L])
  B Absence of ketoacidosis
  C Profound dehydration
  D Neurologic signs ranging from depressed sensorium to frank coma

4 Despite improved monitoring and treatments, DKA and HHNS still remain significant problems. Prevention through patient education, early recognition of symptoms, and prompt efficacious treatment must be emphasized.

OBJECTIVES

Upon completion of this chapter, the learner will be able to
1 Identify the precipitating factors in DKA.
2 Describe the pathophysiology of DKA.
3 State presenting signs and symptoms of DKA.
4 Describe possible variations in initial laboratory values.
5 State three goals in the treatment of DKA.
6 Identify precipitating factors in HHNS.
7 Describe the pathophysiology of HHNS.
8 State presenting signs and symptoms of HHNS.
9 State the major or primary component of treatment for HHNS.
10 Explain the major differences between laboratory values found in DKA and HHNS.

Diabetic Ketoacidosis

1   The characteristics of diabetic ketoacidosis (DKA) are hyperglycemia, ketosis, dehydration, and electrolyte imbalance.

2   Precipitating factors of DKA vary from individual to individual.

A   Illness and infection are the precipitating factors in approximately 25% to 30% of cases. Illness and infection increase production of glucocorticoids by the adrenal gland, promoting gluconeogenesis (production of new glucose by the liver). Epinephrine and norepinephrine levels are also increased, which in turn cause an increase in glycogenolysis (breakdown of glycogen into glucose).

B   Inadequate insulin dosage (either provider- or patient-directed) may lead to DKA and is the major factor in approximately one half of the cases.

• Patients with gastrointestinal (GI) symptoms often decrease or omit their insulin doses in the mistaken belief that less insulin is needed when food intake is decreased.

• Because GI signs and symptoms are prominent features of DKA, decreasing insulin dosages can be dangerous.

C   The initial manifestation of type 1 diabetes may be DKA.

D   Emotional stress may be a precipitating factor, particularly among adolescents. Neglect or mismanagement may be a deliberate call for help. Insulin doses may be omitted in attempts to lose weight.

Pathophysiology of DKA

1   DKA is caused by profound insulin deficiency. Although small amounts of insulin may be circulating, the presence of large amounts of stress hormones (glucagon, catecholamines [eg, epinephrine and norepinephrine], cortisol, and growth hormone) render the insulin less effective. Carbohydrate, protein, and fat metabolism are all markedly affected (Figure 13.1).

A   After eating, insulin deficiency impairs glucose uptake in the peripheral tissues (mainly muscle) and liver, leading to hyperglycemia. During fasting, insulin deficiency results in excess hepatic glucose production that can also lead to hyperglycemia.

B   Insulin deficiency causes impaired protein synthesis and excessive protein degradation.

FIGURE 13.1. DKA—HHNS PATHWAYS

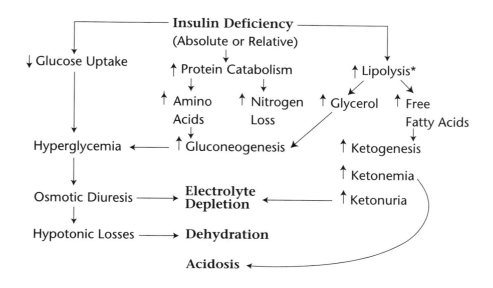

*not increased in HHNS

Source: Adapted with permission from Davidson.[3]

- The resulting increase in the gluconeogenic amino acids leads to increased hepatic glucose production (by means of gluconeogenesis) and finally hyperglycemia.
- The failure to build new protein and the increased breakdown of already formed protein are the reasons for the loss of lean body mass in uncontrolled diabetes.

C Severe insulin deficiency causes excessive hydrolysis of triglycerides, the stored form of fat, yielding increased amounts of glycerol and free fatty acids (FFA). This metabolic pathway is called *lipolysis.*

- Glycerol is an important gluconeogenic precursor that leads to increasing hepatic glucose production and further hyperglycemia.
- Excessive amounts of ketone bodies (acetoacetic acid and beta-hydroxybutyric acid) are formed in the liver from the FFA.
- Low levels of insulin permit ketogenesis, not only by providing more FFA but also by enhancing certain critical hepatic enzymes that change FFA into ketone bodies.

2 Hyperglycemia leads to an osmotic diuresis, which causes hypotonic fluid losses and dehydration as well as electrolyte depletion.

    A Ketone bodies are weak acids that can be used by most tissues only to a limited extent. When this capacity is exceeded, the ketone bodies must be neutralized (buffered). As ketones continue to accumulate, the buffering capacity of the body is exhausted and acidosis supervenes.

    B The excretion of ketone bodies in the urine, a process called *ketonuria*, leads to more electrolyte depletion because cations must be eliminated along with the anionic ketone bodies to maintain electrical neutrality.

    C Twelve to 24 hours of insulin deficiency in patients with type 1 diabetes (depending on the hyperglycemic state) causes profound fluid and electrolyte losses.

       • Fluids, sodium, potassium, and chloride must be vigorously replaced in the initial hours of treatment.

       • There is controversy concerning the need for magnesium and phosphate replacement.[3]

Signs and Symptoms of Hyperglycemia

1 The symptoms of hyperglycemia may mimic other diseases or conditions.

    A Manifestations of hyperglycemia are polyuria, polydipsia, blurred vision, polyphagia, if insulin deficiency is present long enough (days to weeks), and weight loss.

    B Nonspecific symptoms include weakness, lethargy, malaise, and headache.

    C Gastrointestinal symptoms are nausea, vomiting, and abdominal pain. The cause of these symptoms is unclear, but they are probably related to the ketosis and/or acidotic state.

    D Respiratory symptoms may include an inability to "catch one's breath," and a very deep, sometimes rapid, breathing unrelated to exertion termed *Kussmaul's respiration*. This hyperventilation produces a respiratory alkalosis in a partial, but not completely successful, attempt to correct the metabolic acidosis.

2 There are no specific signs of DKA; rather, a constellation of evidence should suggest the possibility of DKA.

    A Hypothermia is often found; therefore, the presence of fever suggests associated infection.

B Hyperpnea (deep respirations) is always present in DKA and reflects a pulmonary response to acidosis.

C Acetone breath may be present. Acetoacetate, one of the ketone bodies, is converted to *acetone*, which is excreted by the lungs. It has a fruity odor that can sometimes be detected on the breath of the patient.

D Dehydration (intravascular volume depletion) is a common sign.

- Dehydration can be assessed by observing for decreased neck vein filling from below when the patient is lying absolutely flat.

- *Orthostatic hypotension* (a fall of systolic blood pressure of 20 mm Hg after 1 minute of standing) may occur as a result of decreased intravascular volume from dehydration.

- Poor skin turgor and "soft eyeballs" are late signs of profound dehydration in adults. Poor skin turgor is seen earlier in children.

E *Acute abdomen* is a common condition marked by tenderness to palpation, diminished bowel sounds, and some muscle guarding, especially in children. A few patients may have more severe signs (absent bowel sounds, rebound tenderness, boardlike abdomen) that suggest a surgical emergency. However, in virtually every case, these signs are due to profound DKA and disappear after treatment.

F *Mentation changes* may be present. Patients may be alert, obtunded, stuporous, or in frank coma. Mentation seems to correlate best with serum osmolality, less well with glucose concentrations, and least with pH changes.

G *Hyporeflexia*, or decreased reflexes, if not present initially may occur during treatment as the potassium level falls.

H *Hypotonia*, uncoordinated ocular movements, and fixed, dilated pupils are all late signs that suggest a poor prognosis.

INITIAL LABORATORY VALUES OF DKA

1 After the diagnosis of DKA is made by clinical impression and bedside testing (a fingerstick blood glucose and blood/urine test for ketone bodies), initial laboratory tests should be obtained before therapy is begun (Table 13.1).

2 Normal values may vary in relation to the methodology of the test procedure used in an institution.

TABLE 13.1. INITIAL LABORATORY VALUES FOR PATIENTS EXPERIENCING DKA

Test	Result	Remarks
Glucose level	Usually >250 mg/dL (>13.9 mmol/L)	Concentration not related to severity of DKA
Ketone bodies	Strong at least in undiluted plasma	Measures only acetoacetate, not beta-hydroxybutyrate
Bicarbonate concentration	0-15 mEq/L (0-15 mmol/L)	
pH	<7.2	
Sodium concentration	Low, normal, or high	Total body depletion
Potassium concentration	Low, normal, or high	Total body depletion; heart responsive to extracellular concentration
Phosphate level	Usually normal or slightly elevated, occasionally slightly low	Associated with phosphaturia; marked decrease in levels of both serum and urine phosphates following treatment
Creatinine, BUN* concentrations	Usually mildly increased	May be prerenal; spurious increases in creatinine level by acetoacetate in some automated methods
White blood cell count	Usually increased	Possibility of leukemoid reaction (even in absence of infection); >10% band forms usually signify severe infection
Amylase value	Often increased	Predominant form is of salivary gland origin
Hemoglobin, hematocrit, total protein values	Often increased	Secondary to contracted plasma volume
AST (SGOT),† ALT (SGPT),‡ alkaline phosphatase values	Can be elevated	Nonspecific and reversible

*BUN = blood urea nitrogen.
†AST = aspartate aminotransferase (previously SGOT, serum glutamic oxaloacetic transaminase).
‡ALT = alanine aminotransferase (previously SGPT, serum glutamic pyruvic transaminase).

Source: Adapted with permission from Davidson.[3]

A Glucose concentrations are usually >250 mg/dL (>13.9 mmol/L). This value is not a good index of the severity of DKA. Lower glucose levels are not uncommon, especially in children, pregnant women, and patients who have been vomiting frequently.

B The test for ketone bodies is semiquantitative and involves the development of a purple color when serum or plasma is added to the reagent nitroprusside.

- Typically, the serum is serially diluted until a dilution is found in which no purple color is seen. The result is usually expressed as the last dilution that produces a 1+ reaction (eg, 1:8).

- Nitroprusside reacts only with acetoacetate, not with beta-hydroxybutyrate. These two ketones exist in equilibrium, with the latter in excess by three- to fivefold in DKA.

- This test for ketones can only be used to diagnose DKA; it is not useful in monitoring response to therapy because the excess beta-hydroxybutyrate is converted back to acetoacetate as the patient improves biochemically.

C The serum bicarbonate (HCO_3) concentration will be low, usually less than 15 mEq/L, reflecting acidosis.

D The pH is obtained on an arterial blood gas determination and will be low (less than 7.20), reflecting acidosis.

E The carbon dioxide pressure (PCO_2) is obtained by an arterial gas determination and will be low (less than 35 mm Hg), reflecting the hyperventilatory response to the metabolic acidosis.

F Even though loss of total body sodium (Na^+) is profound, the serum sodium level can be low, normal, or high because the sodium level depends on the amount of total body water (H_2O).

- The sodium concentration at a particular time will reflect the relative amounts of water and sodium lost and replaced up to that point.

- If the deficit of water is greater than that of sodium, the sodium level will be high; if the deficit of sodium is greater than that of water, the sodium level will be low; if the deficits are approximately equal, the sodium level will be normal.

G The serum potassium (K^+) level can also be low, normal, or high despite a profound loss of potassium.

- The potassium level does not reflect the relative amounts of water lost but depends on the balance between the amount of potassium lost in the urine and other factors that raise the potassium level, such as the lack of insulin, which allows potassium to remain in the circulation rather than enter cells.

- If potassium entrance from the cells into the circulation exceeds excretion, serum potassium level may be high.
- Total body depletion of potassium always occurs regardless of the initial serum level.

H Phosphate concentrations are usually high or high-normal initially, and decrease, sometimes markedly, to very low levels over the next day or two.

I Creatinine and blood urea nitrogen (BUN) concentrations are usually mildly increased because of the dehydration and prerenal azotemia. After rehydration, elevated creatinine and BUN levels indicate the presence of renal insufficiency prior to DKA.

J Hemoglobin, hematocrit, and total protein values are often mildly elevated, reflecting the decreased plasma volume (dehydration).

K White blood cell (WBC) counts are usually increased, occasionally to very high levels. This increase does not necessarily reflect an ongoing infection, since DKA itself often causes a rise in white count. However, if a differential count is performed, >10% band forms (immature WBC) almost always denote a severe infection, whereas <10% band forms usually do not.

L Amylase values are usually increased. This increase does not reflect pancreatitis because in DKA, salivary glands, not the pancreas, release most of the amylase.

M Liver function tests often produce mildly elevated values. This elevation does not necessarily reflect acute or chronic liver damage because the values usually return to normal in several weeks (see Table 13.1).

TREATMENT OF DKA

1 The goals of treatment of DKA are to (1) correct fluid and electrolyte disturbances, (2) provide adequate insulin to restore and maintain normal glucose metabolism and correct acidosis, (3) prevent complications resulting from the treatment of DKA, and (4) provide patient and family education and follow-up.

2 The treatment of mild DKA (ie, patients who can ingest and retain oral fluids without difficulty) should focus on rehydration, euglycemia, and education. If the patient or family can provide accurate blood glucose values and results of urine ketone tests, therapy provided by a knowledgeable healthcare professional over the phone may prevent a hospitalization or emergency room visit.

A Oral hydration, 3 to 5 oz per hour, is recommended if the patient is not vomiting.

- Fluids may be given in small quantities every 20 to 30 minutes.

- Although sugar-free fluids may be offered if the blood glucose levels are above 250 to 300 mg/dL (13.9 to 16.7 mmol/L), some programs advocate the use of sugar-containing liquids regardless of the blood glucose level. It is more important to prevent or treat the dehydration than the hyperglycemia (although the latter will maintain an osmotic diuresis that leads to continued loss of fluid if not eventually controlled).

B Patients with mild DKA require supplemental insulin. If the hyperglycemia is unaccompanied by ketosis, a proportionately smaller amount of insulin is required.

- Insulin doses for children should be supplemented with 0.25 to 0.5 units/kg of regular insulin every 4 to 6 hours or rapid-acting (lispro) insulin every 3 to 4 hours as needed.

- The supplemental dose of insulin for adults will vary between 4 to 10 units or 10% to 20% of the usual total daily dose. The actual dose will depend on the patient's known sensitivity to insulin.

C Education regarding self-management during illness and stress management is essential to prevent DKA (see Chapter 15, Illness and Surgery).

3 Moderate DKA (ie, patients who cannot retain oral fluids) and severe DKA (ie, patients with altered mentation) require immediate emergency treatment.

A In the rare situation in which a cardiac or respiratory arrest has occurred, the first step is to ensure an adequate airway and to assess and maintain respiratory function (and oxygen delivery). In all cases, circulation should be maintained by ensuring appropriate fluid volume replacement.[3,4]

B Diagnosis is established by testing for one or a combination of the following: the presence of urine ketones, serum ketones, lowered serum bicarbonate level, and/or a lowered arterial pH. The presence of hyperglycemia can be established by bedside measurement of the capillary blood glucose level.

C A preliminary history and rapid physical examination (eg, vital signs, weight, blood pressure in the supine and upright positions, and pulse rate) may be obtained to confirm clinical findings and to identify other emergency measures that may be needed.

D Baseline laboratory data should be obtained without delay, including measurements of serum electrolyte values; BUN and creatinine levels; calcium, phosphorus, and serum ketone body concentrations; arterial blood gas determination; and a complete blood cell (CBC) count.

E After the preliminary evaluation has been made and therapy initiated, a more thorough examination needs to be performed. Precipitating causes may be identified.

4 General principles of treatment apply to almost all patients in a compromised hyperglycemic state.

A Bladder catheterization is generally not desirable. A patient who is alert will usually cooperate with voiding as required.
- If patients cannot produce urine initially, they are often successful after several hours of rehydration.
- If there is no urine flow after 4 hours of appropriate rehydration, bladder catheterization is usually warranted.
- In small infants and children, urine may be obtained through the use of urine-collection bags.

B In most patients, hypovolemia is the most acute and critical problem. The largest practical intravenous line for the rapid administration of saline must be started and its potency maintained.

C An electrocardiogram (ECG) is important, especially with leads II, V_1, or V_2. The T-wave configuration aids in determining serum potassium status on admission and usually allows for earlier decisions regarding potassium therapy (Figure 13.2).
- Hypokalemia causes low or flattened T- or U-waves.
- Hyperkalemia causes peaked T-waves and, if markedly elevated, a widened QRS interval.
- Serial ECG tracings will reflect changes in potassium levels as therapy proceeds. This information is available immediately before values are returned from the laboratory.

D Placement of a nasogastric tube should be considered in a patient who is stuporous or comatose, or who has signs of gastric dilatation, to prevent aspiration should the patient vomit.

FIGURE 13.2. T-WAVE CONFIGURATION

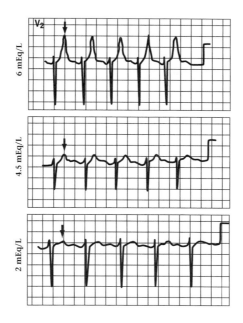

Relationship between serum concentration of potassium (K) and T-wave configurations.

Source: Reproduced with permission from Davidson.[3]

E A flowsheet of pertinent lab values and actions taken is an absolute necessity to provide parameters that can be followed sequentially and in an organized fashion by different observers.

5 Fluid and electrolyte replacement is based on specific needs.

  A Adequate fluid replacement is critical for lowering glucose concentrations. Hyperglycemia will persist (even with appropriate insulin therapy) if fluid replacement is inadequate.

  B Considerations should include maintenance needs, replacement requirements, and ongoing losses.

  C Initial fluid replacement should be made with one-half normal (0.45%) or normal (0.9%) saline.

    • For adults, the initial fluid replacement level depends on the degree of dehydration and cardiovascular status. In general, 1 to 2 liters should be delivered in the first 1 to 2 hours, then the patient's status should be reassessed.[3-5]

- The quantities for adults are not appropriate for children. Many specialists prefer to state all values for children on the basis of kilograms of body weight. The usual calculation for fluid replacement in children is 20 mL/kg of body weight in the first hour. If no urination occurs, 20 mL/kg of body weight of fluid is given during the second and third hours as well, followed by routine fluid replacement calculated on maintenance plus deficit.

D As soon as the serum glucose level is decreased to approximately 300 mg/dL (16.7 mmol/L), intravenous fluids should be changed to contain glucose (usually D5/.45NS). *Acidosis almost always persists longer than marked hyperglycemia during treatment.* Therefore, adequate amounts of insulin must continue to be given (and glucose concentrations supported) until the acidosis is treated appropriately.

E Hypokalemia, if not treated properly, can lead to death.

- Potassium (K^+) should be given immediately if hypokalemia is present as determined by ECG changes or initial laboratory findings. Because of the total body potassium depletion associated with DKA, all patients with urine flow eventually need potassium repletion.

- Potassium may be added in the second to fourth hour of treatment or sooner, depending on T-wave changes confirmed by laboratory values.

- Potassium replacement is based on serum potassium levels. Potassium is administered at concentrations of 20 to 40 mEq/L depending on the serum potassium level. One half is sometimes given as potassium chloride and the other half as potassium phosphate. Some treatment regimens use only potassium chloride for potassium replacement, especially if the initial phosphate (PO_4) level is high or high-normal on admission, as is most often the case.

- As therapy is begun, potassium concentrations can decline rapidly from those initially obtained because of the expansion of the intravascular volume and increased renal excretion due to improved perfusion of the kidneys, both secondary to rehydration. Increased potassium entry into cells also occurs secondary to insulin administration. When the serum potassium level is <3.0 mEq/L (<3.0 mmol/L), potassium replacement using a solution of potassium >40 mEq/L (>40 mmol/L) may be used, but the patient must be placed on a cardiac monitor.

- Patients should be carefully observed for clinically significant signs of hypokalemia including skeletal weakness progressing to paralysis, rapid diminution or absence of deep tendon reflexes, arrhythmias, and shallow, gasping respirations (in contrast to Kussmaul's deep ventilation).

- Continuous, frequent monitoring of ECG status and serum potassium concentration is essential to guide therapy.

F Phosphate (PO_4) levels should be measured. Some experts recommend replacing phosphate when PO_4 is low or low-normal by using potassium phosphate. Doses exceeding 1.5 mEq/L (1.5 mmol/L)/kg of body weight per 24 hours may cause hypocalcemia.

G Treatment with sodium bicarbonate ($NaHCO_3$) is controversial and is not recommended by most diabetologists.

- Some experts recommend sodium bicarbonate in severe metabolic acidosis, as indicated by an arterial pH of 7.0 or less or a serum bicarbonate level of less than 5 mEq/L (5 mml/L). Even in this situation, a clinical benefit has not been shown with sodium bicarbonate therapy,[5] and potassium levels will drop faster and must be monitored closely.

- Rapid infusions, or large amounts of sodium bicarbonate over a short time span, should never be routinely ordered (even if potassium levels are elevated) and are used only in acute cardiorespiratory arrest situations or to treat hyperkalemia-induced cardiac arrhythmias. Potassium values may drop quickly and to low levels, resulting in dangerous hypokalemic-induced arrhythmias.

- If sodium bicarbonate is used, it should be given by slow intravenous infusion over several hours. It should never be given as a bolus injection except in a cardiac arrest.

6 All patients with diabetic ketoacidosis need insulin.

A It takes longer to reverse the acidosis than to treat the hyperglycemia with insulin. Short-acting or rapid-acting insulin should always be used, producing relatively fast results in reducing glucose levels.

B Insulin treatment protocols may be varied based on provider preference. However, a popular method to use is intravenous, low-dose, continuous infusion of insulin.

- The benefits of low-dose infusions include a reduced risk of hypoglycemia and hypokalemia because decreases in glucose and potassium levels are predictable. Additionally, the theoretical risk of cerebral edema is decreased, and the need to estimate doses and administer repeated intramuscular injections is eliminated.

C An example of a protocol for giving a low-dose insulin infusion is shown in Figure 13.3.

7 Response to therapy can be predicted in most instances. Glucose levels should fall at the rate of approximately 75 to 100 mg/dL/h. Ketosis should be reversed in 12 to 24 hours, although occasionally urinary ketone bodies may be present for several days.

A The time-course for the reversal of acidosis has not been well studied because serial pH measurements are not carried out. However, as most patients recover from DKA, they experience a transient state of hyperchloremic acidosis.[3]

- Hyperchloremic acidosis is manifested by bicarbonate levels plateauing at approximately 15 to 20 mEq/L (15 to 20 mmol/L), usually between 12 to 24 hours after treatment is started.
- Chloride levels are elevated, pH has returned to normal, and serum ketone bodies are low or absent.
- The transient state does not require the administration of additional insulin, and recovery to a normal acid-base status occurs naturally.

B Mortality is less than 10%, with most deaths occurring in older patients primarily because of medical complications other than DKA.[4] Older age and depth of coma are the most accurate prognostic indicators. Death is usually due to infection, arterial thrombosis, or unrelenting shock.

- Even in the most controlled environment, complications in the treatment of DKA can occur. These complications can include aspiration, unrecognized renal tubular necrosis, pulmonary edema, and unsuccessfully treated precipitating causes.
- Cerebral edema occurs rarely, but is the primary cause of death in children who succumb to DKA. When the patient's mental function begins to improve and then deteriorates while the metabolic condition continues to return to normal, cerebral edema should be suspected. One factor contributing to the development of cerebral edema may be that the rate of falling blood glucose levels is too rapid.
- The addition of intravenous glucose to the regimen is important once the serum glucose level reaches about 300 mg/dL.
- Treatment of cerebral edema, if it occurs, should include IV osmotic diuretics (mannitol) and possibly high-dose glucocorticoids (dexamethasone). The earlier the treatment, the better the prognosis.

FIGURE 13.3. SAMPLE APPROACH FOR LOW-DOSE INSULIN INFUSION FOR DKA

1 Administer the insulin through a piggyback system into the existing intravenous (IV) line. It is preferable to use an infusion pump to assure accurate delivery of dosages.

2 Attach IV tubing and preflush with at least 50 mL of infusion to allow insulin to bind to the plastic tubing if larger volume containers are used. This procedure ensures that the infusion entering the circulation contains the correct amount of insulin. It is not necessary to use albumin.

3 Some providers give 0.1 to 0.2 units/kg of body weight of regular insulin intravenously as a bolus. However, no benefit of this method has been documented.[6]

4 In children, give 0.1 to 0.2 units/kg of body weight of regular insulin per hour as a continuous infusion. In adults, the rate should be 5 to 10 units per hour as a continuous infusion.

5 The glucose level should drop approximately 75 to 100 mg/dL/hr with proper rehydration and insulin therapy. Administering insulin alone without appropriate fluid replacement will not be very effective in lowering glucose concentrations.

6 Monitor blood glucose levels after 1 hour and then every 1 to 2 hours. Double the insulin infusion rate if the glucose level has not dropped by 10% over 2 hours and the patient is being adequately hydrated. Check electrolyte values every 2 to 4 hours as needed. Because urinary ketone bodies may take several days to clear, their presence is not useful for management decisions.

7 Subcutaneous insulin may be started when the patient is able to eat. Administer four to 10 cc short-acting insulin before stopping the insulin infusion to maintain blood glucose in a safe range.

8 Frequent errors made in the management of DKA include delay in diagnosis or misdiagnosis, delay in instituting therapy, and inadequate fluid replacement. Patients may be misdiagnosed as having gastroenteritis or appendicitis.

  A Hypokalemia and cerebral edema may also go unrecognized, causing critical delays in beginning appropriate therapy for these conditions.

B It is essential to assess mental status frequently (every 1 to 2 hours), especially in children, who are more susceptible to cerebral edema than adults. Treatment of cerebral edema at early stages may be beneficial but is usually ineffective at later stages.

9 DKA can be prevented by thorough patient education, strategic planning, and rapid action (see Chapter 15, Illness and Surgery, for more information on self-management guidelines for patients).

A Evaluate the patient's knowledge and sick-day management skills following an episode of DKA. Omitting insulin when unable to eat, not monitoring glucose levels frequently enough, and failing to test urine for ketones are common misjudgments. Ask the patient and family what they might specifically do differently next time. Review potential positive and negative consequences of actions they choose.

B A multidisciplinary team approach, including psychosocial intervention, is critical when caring for patients with recurrent episodes of DKA.

HYPERGLYCEMIC HYPEROSMOLAR NONKETOTIC SYNDROME

1 Hyperglycemic hyperosmolar nonketotic syndrome (HHNS) is sometimes overlooked and often confused with other illnesses or conditions.

A HHNS occurs in elderly patients with type 1 or type 2 diabetes.

B HHNS occurs in elderly patients who are being treated with medical nutrition therapy with or without oral antidiabetic agents and who may be inadequately monitored (eg, nursing home residents, those who live alone, elderly hospitalized patients who are not receiving adequate fluid intake or adequate monitoring of blood glucose and are often unable to communicate their needs). HHNS is often precipitated by illness or other stresses.

C The symptoms that normally signal the onset of HHNS may go unrecognized for several weeks in the elderly. The absence of significant ketosis (<2+ in a nitroprusside test in a 1:1 dilution of plasma) differentiates HHNS from DKA.

D The mortality rate in HHNS is greater than in DKA because of severe metabolic changes, delay in diagnosis, or other medical complications in elderly patients.

2 Some precipitating factors for HHNS are massive fluid loss from prolonged osmotic diuresis secondary to hyperglycemia, severe burns, severe diarrhea, hemodialysis, peritoneal dialysis, and the use of thiazide or other diuretics.

   A Other causes are infections, myocardial infarction, gastrointestinal hemorrhage, uremia, and arterial thrombosis.

   B Hypertonic feeding (prolonged parenteral nutrition via IV infusion, high-protein or gastric tube feeding) and pharmacologic agents (eg, thiazides, propranolol, phenytoin, steroids, furosemide, chlorthalidone) may precipitate the onset of HHNS.

Pathophysiology of HHNS

1 HHNS is considered to be a syndrome with four primary features: severe hyperglycemia, absence of ketosis, profound dehydration, and neurologic manifestations.

   A HHNS is similar to DKA except that insulin deficiency is probably less profound so increased lipolysis does not occur (Figure 13.1).

   B Absence of ketosis and acidosis decreases gastrointestinal symptoms so that patients do not seek medical care as quickly. Consequently, the prolonged osmotic diuresis and dehydration secondary to hyperglycemia lead to decreased renal blood flow and allow glucose concentrations to reach a very high level.

   C Impaired thirst mechanism or impaired ability to replace fluids, especially in the elderly, exacerbate the tendency toward HHNS. Patients lose fluids over a longer time, so they may be more dehydrated than with DKA. Thus, BUN and creatinine levels may be higher.

   D Because HHNS patients are more dehydrated, mentation changes are more commonly seen than in DKA.

Signs and Symptoms of HHNS

1 The signs and symptoms of HHNS are similar to DKA, with several important exceptions. The gastrointestinal symptoms are usually milder than those found in DKA.

2 Kussmaul's respiration is seldom observed because of a lack of severe acidosis.

3 Decreased mentation (eg, lethargy and mild confusion) is common in HHNS. Frank coma is unusual. As in DKA, mentation correlates best with serum osmolality.

4 Patients with HHNS may also have focal neurological signs (hemisensory deficits, hemiparesis, aphasia, and seizures) that mimic a cerebrovascular accident. These signs will abate as biochemical status is restored to normal. A comparison of DKA and HHNS is shown in Table 13.2.

TABLE 13.2. DIABETIC KETOACIDOSIS (DKA) AND HYPERGLYCEMIC HYPEROSMOLAR NONKETOTIC SYNDROME (HHNS): COMPARISON OF SOME SALIENT FEATURES

Feature	Conditions	
	DKA	HHNS
Age of patients	Usually <40 y	Usually >60 y
Duration of symptoms	Usually <2 d	Usually >5 d
Glucose level	Usually <600 mg/dL (<33.3 mmol/L)	Usually >800 mg/dL (>44.4 mmol/L)
Sodium concentration	More likely to be normal or low	More likely to be normal or high
Potassium concentration	High, normal, or low	High, normal, or low
Bicarbonate concentration	Low	Normal
Ketone bodies	At least 4+ in 1:1 dilution	<2+ in 1:1 dilution
pH	Low	Normal
Serum osmolality	Usually <350 mOsm/kg (<350 mmol/kg)	Usually >350 mOsm/kg (>350 mmol/kg)
Cerebral edema	Often subclinical; occasionally clinical	Subclinical has not been evaluated; rarely clinical
Prognosis	3% to 10% mortality	10% to 20% mortality
Subsequent course	Insulin therapy required in virtually all cases	Insulin therapy not required in many cases

Source: Adapted with permission from Davidson.[3]

Initial Laboratory Values of HHNS

1 Appropriate laboratory tests such as a complete blood cell count (CBC), roentgenogram, and cultures (blood, urine, and sputum) may help identify the precipitating cause of HHNS.

2 The glucose level is usually >800 mg/dL (>44.4 mmol/L).

3 Ketone bodies are not present in the blood or urine except in small amounts.

4 Osmolality is markedly elevated.

Treatment of HHNS

1 The primary treatment goal is rehydration to restore circulating plasma volume and correct electrolyte deficits. Additional treatment goals are similar to those for DKA:

   A Provide adequate insulin to restore and maintain normal glucose metabolism.

   B Prevent complications due to treatment of HHNS.

   C Treat any underlying medical condition.

   D Provide patient/family education and follow-up.

2 Treatment is based on fluid and electrolyte replacement and administration of insulin.[1,7]

3 As in DKA, fluid replacement depends on the patient's state of hydration and cardiovascular status. Use caution when hydrating elderly patients to avoid fluid overload.

   A Because older patients are more likely to have a compromised cardiovascular status, fluid replacement with saline needs to be done cautiously.

   B Observe patients frequently to ensure that they are not developing congestive heart failure.

   C Patients with a previous history of cardiovascular disease should be monitored by central venous pressure (CVP) or Swan-Ganz catheter.

4 Although glucose levels will not decrease appreciably without adequate rehydration, insulin administration is also an important treatment of HHNS.

    A In general, the same guidelines for DKA apply.

    B Glucose and electrolyte levels need to be evaluated every 2 to 4 hours until they are stable.

    C Because treatment of acidosis is not part of HHNS, insulin can be decreased when glucose values reach acceptable levels.

5 To prevent HHNS from occurring, identify high-risk patients, encourage adequate hydration, and educate patients and family about warning signs and symptoms.

    A Older adults need information about sick-day care.

    B Keep fluids within reach or offer fluids every 2 hours to hospital/nursing home residents.

KEY EDUCATIONAL CONSIDERATIONS

1 The importance of recognizing the signs and symptoms of hyperglycemia, not omitting insulin, and maintaining adequate fluid intake need to be emphasized at diagnosis and reinforced regularly. Teach patients and their significant others when, whom, and how to call for help; reinforce this information frequently.

2 Effective teaching methods can include the use of analogies (particularly for explaining the physiology of the signs and symptoms) and the use of practice through simulation and situational problem solving.

3 Review the proper use of fluids (sugared and sugar-free), supplemental insulin when experiencing hyperglycemia and/or ketonemia, and blood glucose levels to serve as guidelines for "take-action" times.

4 After an acute episode of DKA or HHNS, assess the patient and family's use of sick-day guidelines. Review specific precipitating factors and use the information to develop a plan with the patient to prevent reoccurrence. Children and adolescents who experience repeated episodes of DKA, may need supervision of insulin injections.

5   Elderly patients (especially those living alone) may need to have a family member or friend check frequently for signs of hyperglycemia or a change in mentation to ensure prompt medical care if symptoms develop. Provide education to the patient and/or care provider about the risk, possible symptoms, and actions to take if the blood glucose rises to dangerous levels whenever patients are started on new medications that may exacerbate hyperglycemia.

Self-Review Questions

1   List the precipitating factors in the development of DKA.
2   Describe the pathophysiology of DKA.
3   List three presenting signs and symptoms of DKA.
4   What laboratory values indicate DKA?
5   List the three major treatment goals for DKA.
6   List the two precipitating factors of HHNS.
7   Describe the pathophysiology of HHNS.
8   List the presenting signs and symptoms of HHNS.
9   What is the primary treatment for HHNS.
10 What are two differences in laboratory values between DKA and HHNS?

Case Study

CR is an 8-year-old female with known type 1 diabetes since the age of 6 years. She presents for her third admission to the ICU with a pH of 7.11, HCO_3 of 7, and a blood glucose of 310 mg/dL. Over the past month, her total daily insulin dose has increased 2.6 U/kg/day, yet her blood glucose levels have remained in the 300 to 400 mg/dL range. She has continually had small to moderate ketones in her urine.

For the past week, CR has supplemented her usual insulin dose with an extra 3 to 4 units of lispro insulin every 4 to 6 hours. Despite this additional insulin, her urine showed large ketones at the time of admission. Her oral intake of food and fluids has been increasingly poor over the 3 days prior to arrival. Insulin was omitted on the day of admission because she had no oral intake that day. Her parents report no emesis at home, but she did have one episode of large emesis on arrival to the emergency room. Her only physical complaint was abdominal pain. Her parents report there has been no change in her usual meal-planning patterns. She has been administering her own insulin injections, despite a request by the diabetes educator for the parents to do so. The physical exam reveals a temperature of 36.3° C, pulse 140, respirations 25 and slightly labored, BP 137/69, and a weight of 59 lb (26.8 kg) (down from 27.9 kg 14 days prior). Her lips and mucosa are dry, and the rest of the exam is unremarkable.

QUESTIONS FOR DISCUSSION

1   How should treatment proceed?

2   What interventions could the diabetes care team initiate?

3   What are possible reasons for CR's DKA?

DISCUSSION

1   History and symptoms are classic for DKA.

2   An IV was started and CR was given an infusion of D5/.45 normal saline solution with 20 mEq/L potassium chloride and 20 mEq/L potassium phosphate at a rate of 67 cc/hour. An additional infusion of one half normal saline was run at 33 cc/hour.

3   An insulin infusion was begun at a rate of 3 units/hour.

4   Blood glucose levels and electrolyte levels were checked hourly, and the insulin drip and IVs were adjusted accordingly. On the day following admission, CR's blood glucose level normalized. The insulin drip was continued until adequate hydration and oral intake were established.

5   CR then started to eat her usual meal plan. Subcutaneous insulin administration was initiated 30 minutes prior to discontinuing the insulin drip and the dose was adjusted over the next several days.

6   During her hospital stay, CR and her parents met with the diabetes nurse educator and the dietitian. Since both of CR's parents expressed frustration about CR's insulin routine and the many hospitalizations, along with the concern that CR was not receiving all of her prescribed insulin, the opportunity to consult with a psychologist was offered.

7 The following suggestions were offered to help prevent future hospitalizations: continue to monitor blood glucose closely, explore reasons for parental reluctance to give insulin injections, and call daily for further insulin dose adjustment and problem solving. Further discussions with CR and her parents are also needed. Ask CR's parents what they believe to be the cause of her DKA and what they are willing to do to prevent future occurrences. Asking CR what it's like for her at home and school might provide insights about possible precipitating factors.

8 Outpatient follow-up was scheduled with the diabetes team 2 weeks following hospital discharge.

9 CR's saga is a typical one. Recurrent episodes of DKA are not the norm in children with diabetes. Most often, when there are repeated episodes, the diabetes educator needs to assess for a psychosocial etiology. Children often "like" being in the hospital; when they are "ill," their parents give them undivided attention and concern. However, repeated DKA episodes can have disastrous outcomes. CR will need the support of her diabetes care team, including her parents, on an ongoing basis if further episodes of DKA are to be prevented.

References

1   The Expert Committee on the Diagnosis and Classification of Diabetes Mellitus. Report of the expert committee on the diagnosis and classification of diabetes mellitus. Diabetes Care 1998;21(suppl 1):S5-22.

2   Marshall SM, George K, Alberti MM. Hyperosmolar hyperglycemic nonketotic coma. In: DeFronzo RA, ed. Current therapy of diabetes mellitus.   St. Louis: Mosby, 1998:27.

3   Davidson MB. Diabetic ketoacidosis and hyperosmolar non-ketotic coma. In: Davidson MB, ed. Diabetes mellitus: diagnosis and treatment. 3rd ed. New York: Churchill Livingstone, 1991:175-212.

4   Siperstein MD. Diabetic ketoacidosis and hyperosmolar coma. Endocrinol Metab Clin North Am 1992;21:415-32.

5   Lebovitz HE. Diabetic ketoacidosis. Lancet 1995;345:767-72.

6   Krane EJ. Diabetic ketoacidosis and cerebral edema (http://pedsccm.wusl. edu/FILE-CABINET/Metab/DKA-Cedema.html)

7   Howton JC. Management of hyperosmolar coma: a review. (http://gema.library. uscfedu:8081/originals/howton.html)

Suggested Readings

DeFronzo RA, Matsuda M. Diabetic ketoacidosis: a combined metabolic nephrologic approach to therapy. Diabetes Rev 1994;2:204-38.

Ennis ED, Stahl EJ vonB, Kreisberg RA. The hyperosmolar hyperglycemic nonketotic syndrome. Diabetes Rev 1994;1:115-26.

Fosler DW, McGarry JD. The metabolic derangement and treatment of diabetic ketoacidosis. N Engl J Med 1983;309:159-69.

MANAGEMENT

Hypoglycemia 14

Linda A. Gonder-Frederick, PhD
University of Virginia
Behavioral Medicine Center
Charlottesville, Virginia

INTRODUCTION

1   It is extremely difficult to duplicate normal blood glucose metabolism with insulin therapies. Therefore, blood glucose levels in patients taking insulin tend to fluctuate between abnormally high (hyperglycemia) and abnormally low (hypoglycemia) levels due to under- and over-insulinization relative to food intake and metabolic needs.

2   Almost every patient using insulin therapy, especially those with type 1 diabetes, eventually experiences hypoglycemic episodes. Patients with type 2 diabetes using insulin, a sulfonylurea or meglitinide alone or in combinations are at risk for hypoglycemia.

3   Hypoglycemia tends to occur suddenly and almost always requires immediate treatment to prevent blood glucose levels from continuing to fall to a dangerously low range.

4   Hypoglycemia is associated with a number of negative consequences for the patient:
   A   Unpleasant physical symptoms
   B   Impaired cognitive function
   C   Embarrassment
   D   Emotional trauma
   E   Accidents
   F   Bodily injury, including death

5   The problem of hypoglycemia has become even more significant as patients strive to maintain their blood glucose levels in a near-normal range by using more intensive insulin therapies as recommended by the Diabetes Control and Complications Trial.[1] As blood glucose levels are normalized, the frequency of hypoglycemic episodes greatly increases. For this reason, hypoglycemia has been called the major barrier to optimal control of type 1 diabetes.[2]

Objectives

Upon completion of this chapter, the learner will be able to

1   Define and describe mild and severe hypoglycemic episodes, including the symptoms associated with varying levels of severity.

2   Explain the physiological changes that occur with hypoglycemia.

3   Describe hypoglycemic symptomatology, the effects of hypoglycemia on emotions and behavior, and factors underlying symptom idiosyncrasy.

4   Identify causes of hypoglycemia and possible risk factors for individual patients.

5   Explain the treatment for different levels of hypoglycemia, including guidelines for when the patient is unable to self-treat due to a severe hypoglycemic episode.

6   Identify psychosocial sequelae of hypoglycemia.

7   Develop general education plans for teaching patients about hypoglycemia, as well as more specific assessment and intervention plans for patients experiencing frequent or severe hypoglycemic episodes.

Definition of Hypoglycemia

1   *Hypoglycemia* can be defined as any blood glucose (BG) level of 70 mg/dL (3.9 mmol/L) or lower. However, hypoglycemic episodes vary greatly in their severity. Currently, severity of hypoglycemia is not defined by any particular blood glucose level per se, but rather is defined symptomatically.

   A   Mild hypoglycemia is characterized by symptoms such as sweating, trembling, difficulty concentrating, and lightheadedness. These symptoms are usually alleviated quickly by drinking or eating carbohydrates.

   B   Severe hypoglycemia is characterized by an inability to self-treat due to mental confusion, lethargy, or unconsciousness. Because the patient is unable to self-treat, others must provide treatment to raise the blood glucose level out of a dangerously low range.

2   Absolute blood glucose levels cannot be used to describe the severity of hypoglycemic episodes because glycemic thresholds for the onset of symptoms, as well as symptom magnitude, differ greatly across individual patients and from episode to episode, depending on various mediating variables.

A Some patients remain alert with only a few symptoms at a blood glucose level of 40 mg/dL (2.2 mmol/L), while others become stuporous at the same glucose concentration.

B An individual patient may tolerate a blood glucose level of 40 mg/dL (2.2 mmol/L) with few symptoms on one occasion, but become completely incapacitated at the same glucose concentration on another occasion.

3 The classification of hypoglycemic episodes as previously stated is based exclusively on whether patients can treat themselves. Thus, the term *mild* does not necessarily mean that the symptoms experienced by the patient are mild or easily tolerated. In fact, a patient can be quite symptomatic (eg, sweating profusely, nauseous, disoriented, and uncoordinated) and still manage to self-treat. Therefore, even mild hypoglycemic episodes can be aversive and distressing from the patient's perspective.

4 Hypoglycemic episodes caused by oral antidiabetes medications are just as potentially dangerous as episodes caused by insulin.

A Although the frequency of severe hypoglycemia from the use of oral medications is lower than that from insulin, the mortality rate is significant (10%). In survivors of these episodes, there is a 5% rate of permanent brain damage.

B Different rates of hypoglycemia appear to be associated with different oral medications.

- The risk is highest with sulfonylureas
- Of the sulfonylureas, the highest rates are found with glyburide and chlorpropamide.
- The half-life of sulfonylureas is quite long and, when hypoglycemia occurs, it can be quite significant and prolonged.
- Monotherapy with metformin, troglitizone or acarbose is not associated with hypoglycemia.
- Meglitinides may cause hypoglycemia.

C Factors that increase the risk for hypoglycemia in patients with type 2 diabetes include

- Advanced age
- Poor nutrition
- Hepatic or renal disease

HYPOGLYCEMIC SYMPTOMS

1 Two biological mechanisms are responsible for most hypoglycemic symptoms.

   A Hormonal counterregulation involves autonomic symptoms caused by hormonal reactions that increase the glucose level to counteract hypoglycemia.

   B Neuroglycopenia involves disruptions in mental and motor function secondary to depletion of glucose that is available to the central nervous system.

2 The symptoms that result from these biological mechanisms are typically the first warning signs that blood glucose levels are too low, and thus play a critical role in the treatment of hypoglycemia and the prevention of severe episodes.[3]

3 Some of the most common hypoglycemic symptoms are shown in Table 14.1.

   A The autonomic symptoms are generally adrenergically-based, although sweating appears to be cholinergic.

   B Because hypoglycemia causes such widespread physiological changes in hormonal and central nervous system (CNS) function, many different symptoms can occur; the list presented in Table 14.1 is not intended to be exhaustive.

   C Hypoglycemic symptoms appear to be similar for type 1 and type 2 diabetes patients.

   D There do not appear to be differences in symptomatic or hormonal response to hypoglycemia induced by human and porcine insulin.

4 Autonomic symptoms provide early warning signs of hypoglycemia.

   A In the nondiabetic person, the primary counterregulatory hormones are glucagon, which enhances the release of glucose that is stored in the liver, and epinephrine, which increases the liver's production of glucose and inhibits glucose utilization.[4]

   B After only a few years of diabetes duration (2 to 5 years), glucagon secretion is impaired in most type 1 patients and epinephrine secretion becomes the primary mechanism for raising low blood glucose levels.

TABLE 14.1. HYPOGLYCEMIC SYMPTOMS

Type of Symptom	Symptom
Autonomic	• Trembling/shaking • Sweating • Pounding heart • Fast pulse • Changes in body temperature • Tingling in extremities • Heavy breathing
Neuroglycopenic	• Slow thinking • Blurred vision • Slurred speech • Uncoordination • Numbness • Trouble concentrating • Dizziness • Fatigue/sleepiness
Unknown Etiology	• Hunger • Nausea • Weakness • Headache • General feeling of something not right

C If the epinephrine response to hypoglycemia is adequate, blood glucose levels will either stop falling or increase slightly before they become dangerously low. With prolonged hypoglycemia, growth hormone and cortisol may also play a role in recovery, although these hormones do not appear to contribute to early warning symptoms.

D Over the course of type 1 diabetes, defective hormonal counterregulation can cause the epinephrine response to hypoglycemia to be diminished or delayed.[5] The result is that epinephrine secretion may not occur until blood glucose levels are quite low or the amount of epinephrine released is inadequate to stop blood glucose levels from falling further.

E Defects in hormonal counterregulation also delay or diminish the onset of autonomic symptoms, resulting in reduced hypoglycemic symptom awareness. Because the blood glucose level drops further before the patient recognizes that treatment is needed, the risk of becoming severely hypoglycemic increases greatly.

F Hormonal counterregulation and autonomic symptoms can disappear almost completely, resulting in what is called *hypoglycemia unawareness.* This term is somewhat misleading because even patients with significantly reduced hypoglycemia awareness typically still have some symptoms such as those associated with neuroglycopenia.[6]

G Patients with reduced hypoglycemia awareness are at increased risk of severe hypoglycemia and should be encouraged to test their blood glucose more frequently, especially at times when blood glucose levels are likely to be low.

H Several clinical risk factors associated with defective hormonal counterregulation and reduced hypoglycemia awareness[7,8] are shown in Table 14.2; all appear to increase the frequency of hypoglycemia.

TABLE 14.2. CLINICAL RISK FACTORS THAT INCREASE THE FREQUENCY OF HYPOGLYCEMIA

1 Use of intensive insulin therapies
2 Near normal glycosylated hemoglobin level
3 Autonomic neuropathy
4 History of frequent/recurrent episodes of severe hypoglycemia

---

I The clinical risk factors listed in Table 14.2 result in what has been called hypoglycemia-associated autonomic failure.[9] Research suggests that this autonomic failure may be reversible. For example, when patients with defective counterregulation meticulously avoid low blood glucose fluctuations over a period of several weeks, epinephrine response improves and autonomic symptoms increase in magnitude.[10,11]

J Research has shown that the occurrence of only one mildly low blood glucose episode can cause temporary deficits in epinephrine response and a reduction in autonomic symptoms for the next 24 hours.[12]

- If another low blood glucose episode occurs during the subsequent 24 hours, glucose levels will drop much lower before hormonal counterregulation and autonomic symptoms occur.
- Consequently, patients need to be taught the importance of testing their blood glucose levels more frequently and monitoring themselves for symptoms more carefully for the next day or so after a hypoglycemic episode.

5 Neuroglycopenic symptoms provide early warning signs of hypoglycemia.

   A Traditionally, autonomic symptoms were considered to be the most reliable early warning signs of hypoglycemia. Neuroglycopenic symptoms, in contrast, were believed to have little utility as early warning signs. These symptoms were assumed to not appear until blood glucose levels were quite low and the patient was too mentally compromised to recognize the low blood glucose level.

   B More recent research[3,5] has demonstrated that autonomic and neuroglycopenic symptoms occur at similar glycemic thresholds, and that patients experience neuroglycopenic symptoms as frequently as other symptoms.

- The earliest signs of neuroglycopenia include a slowing down in performance and difficulty concentrating and reading.
- Subjectively, patients feel as if it takes more effort to perform routine tasks that are usually done easily.

   C As the blood glucose level drops further and neuroglycopenia progresses, the onset of the following symptoms occurs: frank mental confusion and disorientation, slurred or rambling speech, irrational or unusual behaviors, and extreme fatigue and lethargy.

- If the blood glucose level continues to fall, unconsciousness and seizures can occur.
- Neuroglycopenia is typically the cause of accidents and physical injuries that occur during hypoglycemic episodes.

   D Teach all patients that changes in their ability to do routine tasks can be a sign that blood glucose levels are too low. Being alert for such changes is especially important for patients with reduced autonomic symptoms who are more likely to experience neuroglycopenic symptoms as the first sign of impending hypoglycemia.

   E Instruct patients to treat themselves as soon as possible when neuroglycopenic symptoms occur. Failure to do so can cause patients to become so neuroglycopenic that they do not recognize that their blood glucose level is low.

   F Neuroglycopenia during hypoglycemia can severely compromise decision-making and self-treatment behavior; it is common for patients to resist attempts by others to give them carbohydrates or to even become belligerent when others try to persuade them to drink or eat.

   G Neuroglycopenia can also cause a number of changes in patients' emotional states and social behavior.[13]

- Some of the most common emotional changes, most of which are negative (eg, irritability and anxiety), are listed in Table 14.3. In children, these emotional changes may result in crying, argumentativeness, and misbehavior.[14]
- Some patients may also display positive emotional changes, such as inappropriate giddiness or euphoria.

H The effects of hypoglycemia on emotions can be a source of significant distress to patients, who often are not aware that such effects are common and who may be too embarrassed to talk to healthcare professionals about their behavior. Emotional changes are also a source of distress for family members and significant others because they have to contend with sudden negative shifts in their loved one's mood.

TABLE 14.3. CHANGES IN EMOTIONS AND SOCIAL BEHAVIOR ASSOCIATED WITH HYPOGLYCEMIA

Negative Moods	• Anxiety • Nervousness • Tension • Irritation	• Frustration • Anger • Sadness • Pessimism
Positive Moods	• Giddiness • Euphoria • Disinhibition	
Behaviors	• Arguing • Crying • Resisting treatment • Aggressive acts • Inappropriate social/sexual behaviors	

6 Symptoms of hypoglycemia can differ across individual patients and individual hypoglycemic episodes.

   A Hypoglycemic symptomatology tends to be idiosyncratic[3]; the most reliable warning symptoms for one patient may not be representative symptoms for others.

B It is important for patients to learn to identify their own most reliable symptoms.

- This identification process can be done systematically using a symptom diary like the one shown in Figure 14.1. Patients record their symptoms whenever they measure their blood glucose and then review the data to identify symptoms that occur reliably with hypoglycemia.

- A symptom diary also can be used to help patients with reduced hypoglycemia awareness (eg, loss of personally familiar symptoms) identify current reliable symptoms of hypoglycemia that they may not be aware of, such as neuroglycopenic symptoms.

C Individual patients also differ greatly in their ability to recognize and interpret symptoms accurately.[3] This variability among patients may be due to differences in physiological responses to hypoglycemia, as well as differences in psychological factors such as a tendency to attend to somatic cues.

D The type and magnitude of symptoms also can differ for a given individual from one hypoglycemic episode to the next.

- One reason why hypoglycemia episodes may vary within the same individual is because of delayed or reduced autonomic symptoms following a recent low blood glucose event.[12]

- Because neuroglycopenic symptoms do *not* appear to be affected, instruct patients to monitor themselves carefully for changes in their ability to perform routine tasks following a low blood glucose level.

E Foods and medications may influence autonomic symptoms.

- In some studies,[15] caffeine consumption has been found to increase autonomic symptoms.

- Alcohol consumption can diminish awareness of hypoglycemic symptoms and impede glycemic recovery by interfering with hepatic glucose production (gluconeogenesis).

- Some medications, such as propranolol, also can mask early warning autonomic symptoms.

Figure 14.1. Symptom Diary

Date	Time	Symptoms/Cues	Blood Glucose		Missed Cues	Causes of Hypoglycemia
			Estimate	Actual		

Instructions: (1) Fill in date and time. (2) Scan your body for symptoms. Also consider other blood glucose cues such as changes in your food, insulin, and exercise. Write down all of your symptoms and cues. (3) Based on your symptoms and cues, estimate your current blood glucose. Record this number in the "Estimate" column. (4) Measure and record your actual blood glucose. (5) If your actual blood glucose is <70 mg/dl, but your estimated blood glucose was >70 mg/dl, go back and scan your body for symptoms. List any symptoms you notice in the "Missed Cues" column. (6) Finally, if your blood glucose is <70 mg/dl, think about what might have caused it. For example, have you eaten less food, exercised more, or taken more insulin in the recent past?

CAUSES OF HYPOGLYCEMIA

1 Certain regimen factors and self-treatment behaviors can increase the risk of hypoglycemia.

A All hypoglycemic episodes are caused by excess blood glucose lowering medications (insulin, sulfonylureas or meglitinides) relative to food intake and caloric use.

- The first step in determining what is causing frequent hypoglycemia is a careful examination of the patient's insulin regimen. Insulin excess and hypoglycemia are more likely to occur at those times of the day when insulin action is peaking.

B Hypoglycemia is also more likely when no food has been eaten for several hours or when physical activity increases significantly.

- Many diabetes self-management behaviors related to food intake and physical activity can cause excess in hypoglycemic medication (insulin, sulfonylureas or meglitinides) thereby increasing the risk of hypoglycemia. Some of these behaviors are shown in Table 14.4.
- Alcohol consumption without food intake may result in hypoglycemia.

TABLE 14.4. DIABETES SELF-MANAGEMENT BEHAVIORS THAT INCREASE THE RISK OF HYPOGLYCEMIA

Insulin	• Frequent insulin adjustments • Irregular timing of insulin dosages • Failure to decrease insulin when eating less • Inaccurate preparation of insulin dose
Food	• Skipping meals/snacks • Delaying meals/snacks • Irregular timing of meals • Irregular carbohydrate content • Not carrying carbohydrate source
Physical Activity	• Failure to eat additional carbohydrates • High degree of variability in daily/weekly activity schedule • Failure to recognize significant increases in caloric demand

C More than 50% of all episodes of severe hypoglycemia occur during the night.

- Because patients may not awake by early warning symptoms with nocturnal hypoglycemia, the risk of severe episodes is greatly increased, especially in patients with deficient counterregulation. For patients with adequate counterregulation, it is not uncommon to sleep through episodes of nocturnal hypoglycemia.

- The most common symptom to awaken patients is sweating, although this symptom is absent in patients with diurnal hypoglycemic awareness. Partners may be awakened by the patient's moaning and thrashing if sweating is not present.

- Nocturnal hypoglycemia is often caused by exercise during the previous day or failure to eat a bedtime snack. A bedtime snack should always be eaten if the bedtime blood glucose level is <120 mg/dL.

TABLE 14.5. CALORIC DEMANDS FOR DIFFERENT PHYSICAL[16] ACTIVITIES

Very Low	Low	Moderate	High
•Bathing	• Auto repair	• Ballroom dancing	• Backpacking
•Driving	• Bowling	• Biking (12-14 mph)	• Basketball
•Eating	• Childcare (feeding/	• Canoeing	• Biking (>15mph)
•Mowing lawn	bathing)	• Carrying groceries	• Carrying heavy
(riding mower)	• Cooking	• Cleaning gutters	loads
•Playing board	• Croquet	• Digging garden	• Chopping wood
games/cards	• Darts	• Fencing	• Cross-country
•Playing musical	• Dusting	• Golf (carry clubs)	skiing
instruments	• Fishing	• Hanging storm	• Football
•Reading	• Hunting	windows	• Handball
•Sewing	• Laundry	• Hiking	• Hauling debris
•Sitting	• Leisurely biking	• Horseback riding	• Hockey (field or ice)
•Talking on phone	(4 mph)	• Mowing lawn	• Jogging
•Typing	• Making bed	(power push mower)	• Jumping rope
•Watching TV	• Miniature golf	• Outside carpentry	• Masonry work
•Working at desk	• Plumbing	• Painting	• Mowing (non-
	• Refinishing	• Planting	motorized mower)
	furniture	• Playing games with	• Playing "running"
	• Sexual activity	children (dodge	games with children
	• Shopping	ball, hopscotch)	• Racquetball
	• Standing	• Pushups/situps	• Sawing wood
	• Strolling	• Scrubbing floors/walls	• Scuba diving
	• Sweeping	• Skating/skateboarding	• Shoveling dirt/snow
	• Trimming shrubs/	• Softball	• Soccer
	trees	• Vacuuming	• Swimming
	• Watering garden	• Volleyball	• Tennis
	• Workshop	• Washing/waxing car	
	carpentry		
	• Yoga, stretching		

D Several factors contribute to nocturnal hypoglycemia:

- Predinner injections of intermediate-acting insulin (NPH, lente) may peak in action during the night and cause relative hyperinsulinemia in the predawn hours.

- Insulin requirements also appear to decrease between midnight and 3 AM, compared with insulin requirements at dawn.

- Additional contributors to nocturnal hypoglycemia include failure to eat a snack before bedtime and strenuous physical activity during the day.

E Significant increases in physical activity, combined with failure to increase carbohydrate consumption and/or reduce the insulin dose, are one of the most common causes of both diurnal and nocturnal hypoglycemia.

- Teach patients that *any* increase in physical activity can cause low blood glucose levels, even if they are not formally exercising (Different physical activities that have low, moderate, and high caloric demand are shown in Table 14.5.).

- Patients may not understand that activities such as shoveling snow are just as demanding as jogging and require the same adjustments in diabetes self-management (eg, eating extra carbohydrate).

F By increasing glucose requirements and utilization by muscle tissues, very intense physical activity can have both an immediate and a prolonged effect of lowering blood glucose levels (Table 14.6).

- Because of the depletion and need to replenish muscle glycogen stores, more carbohydrate may be required to raise blood glucose levels after prolonged strenuous exercise.

- Blood glucose levels may be lower or become hypoglycemic for as long as 12 to 24 hours after exercise, which often causes nocturnal hypoglycemia in patients who exercise during the day.

2 Other factors can increase the risk of hypoglycemia.

A Reproductive hormonal changes in women can affect blood glucose levels.

- The incidence of hypoglycemia increases significantly during the first trimester of pregnancy due to fetal demand for glucose and increased sensitivity to insulin. Frequent vomiting can also increase the risk of hypoglycemia.

- The risk and incidence of hypoglycemia decreases as pregnancy progresses, as increased levels of placental hormones result in an increase in peripheral insulin resistance (see Chapter 18, Pregnancy, for more information).

- The incidence of hypoglycemia increases significantly during the postpartum period due to increased insulin sensitivity and, if breast feeding, increased glucose use.
- During menses, a rapid decline in progesterone level and other physiological changes can cause a decrease in insulin requirements, thus increasing the risk of hypoglycemia.
- Women using intensive treatment programs frequently report higher blood glucose levels just prior to menses, followed by a lowering of blood glucose levels after the start of menstrual flow.

TABLE 14.6. IMMEDIATE AND PROLONGED EFFECTS OF INTENSE PHYSICAL ACTIVITY ON LOWERING BLOOD GLUCOSE LEVELS

Causes of Immediate Effects	• Increased glucose utilization by muscle tissue • Accelerated insulin absorption • Increased plasma insulin that inhibits normal glycogenolysis by the liver during exercise • Increased glucose utilization combined with decreased glucose production
Cause of Delayed or Prolonged Effects	• Depletion of glycogen stores in muscles and the liver that need to be replenished with glucose, possibly mediated by an increase in glucose carrier molecules on the surface of muscle cells

B The delayed absorption of carbohydrates and delayed gastric emptying caused by gastroparesis can cause hypoglycemia.

C Insulin sensitivity can affect blood glucose levels.

- Leaner patients tend to be more sensitive to insulin and have reduced insulin requirements.
- Physically fit patients also are more sensitive to insulin than those who have a more sedentary lifestyle.

PREVENTION OF HYPOGLYCEMIA

1   The most powerful tool for preventing hypoglycemia is diabetes patient education.

   A   Because the majority of hypoglycemic episodes are caused by overinsulinization, patients' knowledge about their diabetes treatment programs and the causes of hypoglycemia should be carefully assessed.

   B   Even well-educated and experienced patients may have misunderstandings or inadequate knowledge about hypoglycemia. For example, many patients do not know that high-fat foods have a delayed and depressed glycemic effect. Thus, eating a high-fat, low-carbohydrate meal after insulin injections or boluses can lead to hypoglycemia.

   C   Because knowledge does not always influence behavior, patients' self-management habits also need to be assessed.

2   Until recently, frequent hypoglycemia was often regarded as a sign of good glycemic control, and many patients continue to hold this belief.

   A   We now know that frequent episodes of mild hypoglycemia greatly increase the risk of an episode of severe hypoglycemia.

   B   Hypoglycemic episodes also have little or no effect on metabolic control, which is determined by the frequency of hyperglycemia.

   •   Hemoglobin A_{1c} values of 7.0% or less may be the result of wide high-low blood glucose fluctuations, which further emphasizes the importance of blood glucose record review.

3   Avoidance of nearly all hypoglycemic episodes is the ideal. However, it is especially important to prevent nocturnal hypoglycemia because patients cannot rely on being awakened by early warning symptoms. Guidelines for preventing nocturnal hypoglycemia are provided in Table 14.7.

TREATMENT OF HYPOGLYCEMIA

1   All blood glucose levels less than 70 mg/dL (3.9 mmol/L) need to be treated immediately, regardless of whether symptoms are present. Treatment guidelines are relatively straightforward.

   A   Eat or drink 10 to 15 grams of carbohydrate, which should raise the blood glucose level 30 to 45 mg/dL (1.7 to 2.5 mmol/L). Different foods and drinks that supply this amount of carbohydrate are listed in Table 14.8.

TABLE 14.7. GUIDELINES FOR PREVENTING NOCTURNAL HYPOGLYCEMIA

- Do not skip presleep snacks.
- Measure presleep blood glucose levels regularly.
- If the bedtime blood glucose level is 120 mg/dL (6.7 mmol/L) or lower, increase the carbohydrate and protein content of the snack.
- If daytime physical activity was increased, eat additional carbohydrate and protein at the night snack.
- Move the predinner NPH or lente to pre-sleep rather than decreasing the predinner dose, which can lead to fasting hyperglycemia. Use of ultralente instead of NPH or lente may also be effective.
- Measure 3 AM blood glucose levels at least once a week or more frequently if recurrent nocturnal hypoglycemia is a problem.
- Measure 3 AM blood glucose levels when daytime physical activity or food consumption was atypical and when insulin doses are being adjusted.

TABLE 14.8. CARBOHYDRATE SOURCES (15 TO 20 GRAMS) FOR TREATING HYPOGLYCEMIA

Source	Quantity
Glucose tablets	3 to 4
Lifesavers® candies	8 to 10
Brach's® hard candies	8 to 10
Raisins	2 tablespoons
Nondiet soft drinks	4 to 6 oz
Fruit juice	4 to 6 oz
Milk (no fat or low fat)	8 oz

- Carbohydrates are used to treat hypoglycemia so that blood glucose levels rise quickly. Drinks/food that are high in fat content take longer to raise blood glucose levels.

B If blood glucose levels are less than 50 mg/dL (2.8 mmol/L), 20 to 30 grams of carbohydrate may be needed.

C If possible, test blood glucose before beginning treatment. If pretreatment testing is not possible and symptoms are present, proceed with the treatment.

D Test blood glucose 15 to 20 minutes after initiating treatment. If the blood glucose level is still low, repeat the treatment even if symptoms have disappeared.

E If the patient will not be eating a meal within the next 1 to 2 hours, immediate treatment can be followed by eating additional food that contains some protein (eg, low-fat milk, peanut butter, or cheese and crackers). This combination of nutrients may keep blood glucose levels from falling back into the hypoglycemic range.

F Following very mild episodes of hypoglycemia, patients usually can resume normal activity fairly soon after treatment. With more significant hypoglycemia, recovery of mental and motor function lags behind glycemic recovery. Therefore, patients need to wait at least 30 minutes before resuming normal activities after hypoglycemic episodes in which the blood glucose was lower than 50 mg/dL (2.7 mmol/L).

G Following hypoglycemic episodes in which the blood glucose was lower than 40 mg/dL (2.2 mmol/L), mental and motor function may not return to normal for 1 or more hours. Advise patients not to engage in any potentially risky activities (eg, driving) during this period.

H Blood glucose levels between 70 and 120 mg/dL (3.5 to 6.6 mmol/L) with symptoms can be treated with 5 to 10 grams of carbohydrate.

2 The following patient guidelines are recommended for self-treatment of hypoglycemia.

A Do not keep eating after the initial treatment; wait 15 to 20 minutes, then test blood glucose to determine whether further treatment is needed.

B Do not keep eating until symptoms disappear.

C Avoid using high-fat foods for treatment because fat delays absorption so these foods will not raise blood glucose levels quickly enough (Table 14.9).

D Always carry some type of fast-acting carbohydrate.
- Keep something at your bedside to treat nocturnal hypoglycemia.

E Always wear diabetes identification.

F Overtreatment will cause posttreatment hyperglycemia.
- Overtreating hypoglycemia is relatively common and can be attributed to both physiological and psychological factors. Patients may eat until autonomic symptoms abate completely, rather than consuming the recommended amount of carbohydrate and waiting to see if symptoms subside or blood glucose increases.

Table 14.9. Foods with High Fat Content That are Poor Choices for Treating Hypoglycemia

- Ice cream
- Doughnuts
- Candy bars
- Meat

- Pies, cakes
- Cheese
- Nuts
- Cookie dough

- Pizza
- French fries
- Milkshakes
- Potato chips

- Other patients overtreat because of the fear of losing control due to neuroglycopenia. This fear is especially common in patients who live alone, care for small children, or have experienced a traumatic episode of severe hypoglycemia in the past.
- Using rapid-acting, commercially available, portion-controlled glucose products may help patients avoid overtreatment.

3 Appropriate treatment of hypoglycemia is also determined by such complicated psychological processes as decision-making and judgment.[17]
   A These processes can be compromised by diminished cognitive ability and inaccurate risk appraisal, either due to neuroglycopenia or inaccurate beliefs about hypoglycemia.
   B Once patients know that their blood glucose level is low, they make several decisions based on the following questions:
   - Treat immediately or wait?
   - What to eat and how much?
   - Stop current activity or continue?
   C Deciding to delay treatment is relatively common and often leads to severe hypoglycemia.
   - Reasons for delaying treatment include the desire to finish a task and embarrassment about eating when others are not.
   - Some patients may even deny they are becoming hypoglycemic because it is a reminder of their diabetes or perceived as an indication that they have made some mistake in diabetes management.
   D It is important to assess patients' attitudes and beliefs about hypoglycemia. Some patients believe there is no reason to treat low blood glucose levels unless they are below 50 mg/dL (2.8 mmol/L) or until they feel symptoms.
   - Many patients believe that their ability to function is not affected until blood glucose levels fall very low, which often is not the case.

Research shows that measurable deficits in mental and motor task performance occur at blood glucose levels of 65 mg/dL (3.5 mmol/L).

4 Treatment of hypoglycemia often must be done by family members or significant others.

A The hypoglycemic type 1 patient often has to be treated by others because of the effect of neuroglycopenia on judgment and behavior.

- Teach family members and significant others how to cope with episodes of severe hypoglycemia and what to expect in terms of the patient's behavior (eg, stupor or possible resistance). Some family members report that it is helpful to use favorite foods to coax the hypoglycemic patient to eat.

- Coworkers, friends, and teachers also need to know how to respond to symptoms of hypoglycemia, which can be a problem if individuals do not want to reveal their diabetes to others.

B The following basic guidelines are recommended for treating severe hypoglycemia.

- Patients who are able to swallow without risk of aspiration may be coaxed into drinking juice or a soft drink. If this is not possible, place some glucose gel, honey, syrup, or jelly inside the patient's cheek.

- Patients who are unable to swallow without risk of aspiration can be given glucagon by subcutaneous or intramuscular injection. *Glucagon* is a hormone secreted by the pancreatic alpha cells that stimulates hepatic glucose production and thereby raises blood glucose levels, usually about 20 to 30 mg/dL.

- Teach patients to keep glucagon in their homes at all times, and family members need to know how to administer it. Glucagon kits can be obtained by prescription and filled syringes can be stored in the refrigerator for one month.

- Glucagon can be injected subcutaneously or intramuscularly. Recommended doses are 1 mg for adults and older children, 0.5 mg for children < 5 years old, and 0.25 mg for infants.

- The glycemic effect of glucagon is quite short-lived, so as soon as the patient is able to swallow, carbohydrate liquid (eg, juice, soft drink, lowfat milk) should be administered to maintain normoglycemia (see Chapter 10, Pharmachologic Therapies, for more information on glucagon).

- Immediate treatment needs to be followed by a small snack containing carbohydrate and protein to keep blood glucose levels from falling before the next meal.

- Frequent blood glucose monitoring is needed over the next several hours to detect blood glucose levels that are falling again and to detect hyperglycemia due to overtreatment.
- Instruct patients to notify their healthcare professional following episodes of severe hypoglycemia.

C If episodes of severe hypoglycemia become frequent or recurrent, it is often helpful for the patient and team members to discuss how best to cope with these episodes. This discussion should only be attempted when the patient is not hypoglycemic.

PSYCHOSOCIAL IMPACT

1 Patients may develop emotional distress and fear of hypoglycemia after experiencing mild or severe hypoglycemia episodes.

A Negative moods, social embarrassment, and potential danger associated with hypoglycemia can clearly cause emotional distress for patients. Results from the DCCT[18] showed that the occurrence of severe hypoglycemia alone was not necessarily related to emotional distress, but recurrent episodes appeared to have a negative impact on quality of life.

B Patients may also develop significant anxiety about hypoglycemia and go to extreme measures to avoid its occurrence. The Hypoglycemia Fear Survey[19] is an assessment tool used to measure the extent to which patients worry about hypoglycemia and engage in behaviors to avoid hypoglycemia and its negative consequences. Patient groups at high risk for excessive fear of hypoglycemia are identified in Table 14.10.

TABLE 14.10. PATIENT GROUPS AT HIGH RISK FOR EXCESSIVE FEAR OF HYPOGLYCEMIA

Patient Characteristics

- Have just begun taking blood glucose lowering medication
- Have little or no experience in coping effectively with episodes of hypoglycemia
- Have frequent and/or recurrent episodes of hypoglycemia
- Have experienced emotionally traumatic episodes of hypoglycemia
- Tend to be overly anxious
- Have ineffective coping skills
- Have visual impairment or other physical disabilities

C High levels of fear can contribute to inappropriate diabetes management, such as keeping blood glucose levels above the target range to avoid hypoglycemic episodes, or phobic avoidance of certain situations such as being alone or driving.

- Conversely, low levels of fear can also contribute to inappropriate or high-risk behaviors, such as delaying treatment in response to symptoms.
- Assess the possible psychological sequelae of hypoglycemia on a routine basis, especially after a patient experiences an episode of severe hypoglycemia.

2 There are numerous aspects of hypoglycemia that contribute to conflicts between patients and significant others.

A The emotional changes associated with hypoglycemia (tension, irritation, and pessimistic thinking) can lead patients to become argumentative with others.

B When hypoglycemia is frequent or recurrent, patients may feel as if others blame them, so they become defensive and resentful; these behaviors can increase the likelihood of resisting treatment.

- Similarly, family members can become angry and resentful if they believe their loved one is not exerting enough effort to prevent hypoglycemia or behaving in ways that increase the risk.
- Spouses of patients who experience frequent, severe hypoglycemia report increased rates of marital conflict about diabetes-related issues, including the prevention and treatment of hypoglycemia.[20]

C In some families, power struggles occur over the management of hypoglycemia; these struggles may reflect other areas of unresolved conflict. The educator can offer to refer these couples or families for counseling.

3 Family members and significant others may experience similar emotional distress and fear of hypoglycemia similar to that of patients with diabetes.

A Family members also can develop significant fear of hypoglycemia, especially if they have experienced episodes associated with very frightening or traumatic consequences for their loved one.

- Spouses of patients who have experienced frequent, severe hypoglycemia show very high levels of fear compared with spouses of patients who have experienced only mild episodes.[20]

- Parents of children with type 1 diabetes report very high levels of fear in general, but especially if their child has been unconscious or had a seizure while hypoglycemic.[21]

B If nocturnal hypoglycemia has been a problem, family members may even develop sleep disorders such as insomnia or restless sleep if they feel they must remain vigilant during the night to recognize symptoms.[20]

ASSESSMENT AND INTERVENTION

1 Assessment of knowledge about hypoglycemia and individual risk factors is essential for developing effective educational and intervention plans.

A Hypoglycemia risk, treatment, and prevention are determined by many different factors, both general and specific for each patient, that may change over time. Therefore, education and intervention must be ongoing, individually tailored, and reassessed regularly to reflect changing patient needs.

B The frequency and severity of hypoglycemic episodes can change over the course of diabetes due to a variety of factors:

- Changes in diabetes treatment
- Physiological changes (eg, insulin sensitivity, hormonal counter-regulation)
- Changes in symptoms
- Lifestyle and schedule changes

C Objectively assess knowledge about hypoglycemia whenever possible. Patients often are reluctant to ask questions or admit that they do not understand the information they receive. Knowledge assessment can be done verbally, and written instruments also are available, such as the Hypoglycemia Knowledge Questionnaire.[22]

D In addition to basic knowledge, assess the patient's (or parents' if the patient is a child) personal habits and routine behaviors for treating and preventing hypoglycemia.

- It is important to identify beliefs about hypoglycemia and its treatment. Sample questions that can be used to identify personal risk factors and beliefs about hypoglycemia are listed in Table 14.10.

FIGURE 14.10. SAMPLE QUESTIONS TO DETERMINE PATIENT RISK FACTORS AND BELIEFS ABOUT HYPOGLYCEMIA

To what extent do you:	Not At All		Somewhat		A Great Deal
1 Always carry some type of food or drink with sugar?	1	2	3	4	5
2 Skip meals?	1	2	3	4	5
3 Skip snacks?	1	2	3	4	5
4 Worry about hypoglycemia?	1	2	3	4	5
5 Try to keep your BG levels below 100 mg/dL?	1	2	3	4	5
6 Delay eating when trying to finish a task?	1	2	3	4	5
7 Think having low BG is a sign of good control?	1	2	3	4	5
8 Eat extra food when you're going to be more active?	1	2	3	4	5
9 Recognize low BG symptoms?	1	2	3	4	5
10 Eat as little as possible to avoid gaining weight?	1	2	3	4	5
11 Increase your insulin whenever your blood glucose is too high?	1	2	3	4	5
12 Wait until you feel strong symptoms to treat a low BG?	1	2	3	4	5
13 Only treat very low BG levels (between 40 and 50 mg/dL)?	1	2	3	4	5
14 Believe you can function fine when your BG is below 50 mg/dL?	1	2	3	4	5

- Include possible emotional and social barriers to hypoglycemia management and treatment in the assessment. For example, adolescents often dislike having to eat a morning snack during school because it makes them feel different from their peers. Young women who are overly concerned about weight gain may be at increased risk of hypoglycemia due to low carbohydrate intake, even when blood glucose levels are low (see Chapter 6, Psychological Disorders, for more information).

E   Some aspects of hypoglycemia management can be assessed directly. For example, patients can be asked to show the educator their diabetes identification and the emergency glucose they are carrying.

F Symptoms and the ability to recognize low blood glucose levels should be assessed on a regular basis. Changes in symptoms (eg, loss of autonomic symptoms) and decreased ability to tell when blood glucose is low require additional education and intervention.

G At each routine visit, ask patients if any hypoglycemic episodes have occurred since their last appointment. If so, a structured interview can be given to evaluate the following factors. This type of structured evaluation is especially important after episodes of severe hypoglycemia to help identify specific risk factors and problem areas for individual patients.
- Date, time, and location of the hypoglycemic episode
- Severity of the episode
- Possible causes of the episode
- Degree of symptomatology and ability to recognize the need for treatment
- Ability to self-treat and/or respond to attempts by others to provide treatment
- Decisions made about when and how to treat
- Barriers to treatment (eg, no available food/drink)
- Type and amount of food eaten
- Negative consequences of the episode (eg, distress, accidents, or embarrassment)

H After severe, distressing, or traumatic episodes of hypoglycemia, patients need to be assessed for possible negative psychosocial sequelae. Objective measures of distress, such as the Hypoglycemia Fear Survey,[19] can be used. This assessment can also be accomplished by asking patients questions such as the following about the negative emotional and social effects of their hypoglycemic episode:
- How upsetting was the episode for you?
- How worried are you about another episode like that happening again?
- Have you changed your diabetes management to avoid another episode?
- Did the episode cause any problems between you and other people?

2 The core intervention for hypoglycemia management and treatment is effective education, although behavioral interventions may be needed when patients have a solid knowledge and understanding of hypoglycemia, yet continue to have problems.

A Goal setting and contracting can be used by patients to make specific behavioral changes.

B Teaching patients problem-solving techniques also can be effective for dealing with barriers to hypoglycemia management.

C When reduced hypoglycemic awareness is a problem, patients can use a diary to improve their ability to recognize and avoid hypoglycemia (Figure 14.2). Using a diary provides important benefits:

- Increased awareness of hypoglycemic symptoms and other predictors of low blood glucose levels
- Objective assessment of symptoms that are reliable signs of low blood glucose levels
- Objective assessment of how accurately low blood glucose is recognized
- Means of identifying patterns in hypoglycemic episodes (eg, causes, time of day)

D When frequent and/or severe hypoglycemic episodes continue in spite of medical, educational, and behavioral interventions, patients need referral to a mental health specialist who has experience working with diabetes-related psychosocial issues (see Chapter 6, Psychological Disorders, for more information).

- Patients who remain rather unconcerned or refuse to change their behavior, even after potentially dangerous episodes, also need referral for a psychological assessment.
- Referrals for counseling or psychotherapy also are appropriate when patients are experiencing emotional problems due to hypoglycemia, such as anxiety, phobias, or marital conflict.

E Currently, one psychoeducational intervention, Blood Glucose Awareness Training (BGAT)[23] has been demonstrated empirically to improve ability to recognize low blood glucose levels, reduce the frequency of low blood glucose levels, and reduce the incidence of severe hypoglycemia without jeopardizing diabetes control.

- BGAT involves eight weekly sessions using a manual with eight chapters (one per week) that provides training in recognizing hypoglycemic symptoms and predicting low blood glucose levels due to changes in insulin, food, and physical activity.
- Each chapter also provides exercises (eg, symptom diary) to be done during the rest of the week to increase awareness of hypoglycemia.

KEY EDUCATIONAL CONSIDERATIONS

1   Provide patients with type 1 diabetes basic information about hypoglycemia at diagnosis. This initial education includes
    A   An explanation of hypoglycemia and its causes
    B   A description of hypoglycemic symptoms
    C   Guidelines for treatment
    D   Preventive measures

2   At diagnosis, patients and their families are attempting to assimilate new information and are likely to process only a fraction of what they are taught.
    A   For this reason, give patients written materials such as handouts and articles about hypoglycemia for later review.
    B   Ask newly-diagnosed patients and their families to call back soon after the first hypoglycemic episode occurs to determine how they managed the episode and to receive further education.

3   Teach patients and their families that hypoglycemic symptoms are idiosyncratic, and that patients need to learn to recognize how they feel when their blood glucose is low.
    A   They need to know that hypoglycemic symptoms can sometimes be difficult to recognize and distinguish from other types of symptoms (eg, nervousness, sweating due to exertion).
    B   Describe the emotional and behavioral changes that can occur with hypoglycemia as biologically based and a normal manifestation of hypoglycemia.

4   In spite of the initial information overload, patients' families need to be taught immediately how to administer glucagon when severe hypoglycemia occurs. This information must be repeated and reinforced on subsequent visits because families who have not had to use glucagon may forget how to use it, forget where they have placed it, or fail to check the expiration date.

5   Initial education about hypoglycemia provides an opportunity to instill treatment habits such as using commercially-packaged glucose tablets and consuming carbohydrates immediately when blood glucose is low.

6 Patients with type 2 diabetes who are taking blood glucose-lowering medication also need to be taught about hypoglycemia, even though they appear to be at less risk for severe hypoglycemia due to a maintenance of the integrity of hormonal counterregulation.

- Patients who are changing from oral medications to insulin may have considerable fears and concerns about hypoglycemia and need to be taught to monitor themselves for warning symptoms, especially at those times of the day when they are at most risk (eg, just before lunch). These patients may also need to increase the frequency of self blood glucose monitoring.
- Many type 2 patients are not adequately educated about hypoglycemia when they begin taking blood glucose-lowering medications, and are not aware of the risks that hypoglycemia can impose. Knowledge about hypoglycemia, including warning symptoms, needs to be assessed even in patients who have been taking medication for a long period of time.
- Hypoglycemia due to oral medications is treated by carbohydrate consumption, following the guidelines prescribed for patients with type 1 diabetes. However, glucagon is not appropriate for type 2 diabetes because it stimulates insulin secretion.
- Sulfonylurea-induced hypoglycemia can be quite prolonged and can recur. For this reason, hospitalization may be necessary.

7 Education about hypoglycemia is an ongoing process.

A After diagnosis and initial education, the next important step in the learning process occurs when patients experience their first episode of hypoglycemia. Every hypoglycemic episode can be an opportunity for increasing knowledge.

B Use of the structured interview procedure can help teach patients about diabetes management behaviors that lead to lower blood glucose levels, their symptoms, and treatment decisions that increase the risk of severe episodes.

C Evaluation of specific episodes also provides an opportunity to give patients positive feedback when they have used their knowledge and judgment to avoid more severe problems with hypoglycemia.

8 Ask patients and their families to describe their concerns about hypoglycemia; their input provides focus and direction for the educational efforts. Because areas of concern differ greatly across different patient groups and developmental stages, educational priorities are based on the personal needs of individual patients.

A Parents of infants with type 1 diabetes may justifiably worry about the negative long-term effects of hypoglycemia on their child's intellectual abilities; provide this group with more intensive diabetes education aimed at prevention.

B The lifestyle changes and attitudes of adolescent patients often place them at increased risk of hypoglycemia. For example, adolescents will try alcohol and periodically skip meals or eat inappropriate foods. Adolescents need to be reminded frequently about the effects of alcohol and drug use, increased exercise, dietary indiscretion, and other risky behaviors on blood glucose levels.

9 Patients and their families need to be instructed about the risks of hypoglycemia and driving.

A These risks include automobile accidents and injury, as well as being mistakenly arrested for driving while intoxicated, which can happen when an individual is not wearing diabetes identification.

B At each visit, ask patients if they keep some kind of emergency carbohydrate in their car and, if so, what kind of food/drink they carry. They can also be asked to show their:
- Diabetes Identification
- Emergency carbohydrate they carry at all times in their purse pocket.

C Assess patients' beliefs about driving and hypoglycemia.
- Ask how low they believe their blood glucose needs to be before they will not drive.
- Many patients believe that they can continue to drive safely with blood glucose levels quite low.
- Patients should be instructed not to drive when their blood glucose is < 70 mg/dL because they may have motor impairments they do not recognize and because their blood glucose can quickly become lower while they are driving.

D Teach patients about the importance of checking their blood glucose before driving. This is especially important for patients who have previously experienced problems with hypoglycemia while driving or who have hypoglycemia unawareness.

SELF-REVIEW QUESTIONS

1 Define the different levels of hypoglycemia.

2 List ten symptoms associated with hypoglycemia and name the physiological basis for each of the symptoms.

3 State three reasons why hypoglycemic symptoms can vary across individual patients and different episodes.

4 Explain what reduced hypoglycemic awareness is and what causes it.

5 Describe emotional and behavioral changes that can occur with hypoglycemia.

6 List three of the most common causes of hypoglycemia.

7 Describe the reason prolonged, vigorous exercises have a delayed effect on blood glucose levels.

8 Describe the guidelines for treating a patient with a BG between 50 and 70 mg/dL (2.8 to 3.9 mmol/L). With a BG lower than 50 mg/dL.

9 Name three foods that are not as effective for treating hypoglycemia and explain why these foods are inappropriate choices.

10 Describe two beliefs about hypoglycemia that can lead patients to risky treatment behaviors such as delaying treatment.

11 Describe fear of hypoglycemia and the types of patients who are most likely to exhibit it.

12 Name three possible effects that hypoglycemia can have on family members and significant others.

CASE STUDY 1

LE is a 23-year-old female who has had type 1 diabetes for 12 years. Her metabolic control was fair during her adolescent and college years. LE currently is working full-time and living in an apartment with a roommate. For the last year, her glycemic control has been improving with regular insulin and NPH injections before breakfast and before dinner. She measures her BG before each insulin injection and sometimes before lunch. Because her fasting BG levels have been high, she has recently increased her predinner NPH. For weight control, LE jogs 3 miles after dinner several times each week and she only eats a bedtime snack if she feels hungry. At a routine office visit, LE reports that she is having two or three episodes of nocturnal hypoglycemia per week. In addition, she had many BG measurements during the day that were less than 50 mg/dL (2.8mmol/L) and she felt no symptoms at all. LE also reports that during one recent episode, her roommate had to force jelly into her mouth to treat her.

QUESTIONS FOR DISCUSSION

1 What clinical and behavioral factors increase LE's risk of hypoglycemia?

2 What steps can be taken by LE and her diabetes care team to reduce the frequency of LE's nocturnal hypoglycemic episodes without jeopardizing her improved metabolic control?

DISCUSSION

1 Several factors are contributing to LE's increased hypoglycemic risk:

A Increase in predinner NPH dose

B Failure to decrease predinner NPH dose before postdinner vigorous exercise

C Failure to eat regular bedtime snacks and larger snacks after evening exercise

D Failure to test bedtime BG levels

E Reduction in hypoglycemic symptoms due to deficient and/or delayed hormonal counterregulation

2 Ask LE to identify her concerns regarding hypoglycemia. Problem-solve with her about strategies to reduce nocturnal hypoglycemia. She can also make these behavioral goals.

3 Strategies she might identify are

A Consistently eat a bedtime snack. Check BG levels before eating the snack and make appropriate increases in the size of the snack depending on physical activity and BG level.

B If nocturnal hypoglycemia continues despite these interventions, LE could move her predinner NPH to bedtime and her predinner regular insulin could be adjusted. She also could switch to a regimen of ultra-lente twice a day, with preprandial regular insulin. The effect of insulin regimen changes should be assessed after a few days, with additional dose changes implemented, if necessary. Frequent contact with the healthcare provider is critical while insulin adjustments are being made.

C   Because of her reduced hypoglycemia awareness, LE could do more frequent blood glucose monitoring, and keep a blood glucose awareness diary. She should be taught to measure her blood glucose before driving or engaging in any other potentially risky activities.

D   Provide LE with a prescription for glucagon. LE can teach her roommate how to use it, and place it where her roommate can easily find it.

CASE STUDY 2

MJ is a 66-year-old man who is overweight and was diagnosed with type 2 diabetes 4 years ago. His blood glucose has been poorly controlled using a meal plan and exercise program, so glyburide each morning before breakfast was added. MJ was instructed that it was critical that he eat breakfast soon after taking his medication. He said that this would be no problem, describing himself as an old-fashioned, meat and potatoes man who always has a hearty breakfast. When MJ returned to the clinic for his 3-month checkup, his blood glucose records showed that most of his fasting and predinner levels were in a normal range. However, MJ reported that his medication was causing unpleasant side effects. He described feeling shaky, dizzy, and nauseous during the mid- to late-morning hours. While these symptoms seemed to eventually subside on their own, MJ found them to be quite aversive and disruptive to his work. He indicated that he wanted to stop taking the medication and attempt again to control his blood glucose levels with a meal plan and exercise.

QUESTIONS FOR DISCUSSION

1   What is the likely cause of MJ's unpleasant symptoms?
2   What can be done to help MJ continue to take his oral medications?
3   What dietary factors would you want to assess as possible contributors to MJ's problem?

DISCUSSION

1   Although it seems almost certain that MJ is experiencing midmorning hypoglycemia, this suspicion should be confirmed with daily midmorning BG measurements and additional measurements when symptoms occur.

2 Because MJ appears to be confused by his symptoms, additional education is needed about:

A Causes, warning symptoms, and treatment of hypoglycemia

B Importance of carrying carbohydrate at all times, including having food or drink at the office and in the car for quick treatment

3 MJ's meal pattern, especially breakfast foods, needs careful evaluation.

A He may eat a large breakfast that consists of high-fat, low-carbohydrate foods such as eggs, bacon, and milk. Consequently, his blood glucose levels may not be very high when his regular insulin peaks midmorning, causing him to become hypoglycemic.

B MJ should be given further nutritional education. Point out that by reducing fatty foods and increasing his carbohydrate intake at breakfast he may prevent hypoglycemia.

C Another of his options is to eat a midmorning snack on a routine basis.

4 If MJ continues to have problems with hypoglycemia in spite of these interventions, his morning dose of glyburide may need to be decreased, or he may need to switch to an oral agent that does not increase the risk for low blood glucose levels.

REFERENCES

1 The Diabetes Control and Complications Trial Research Group. The effect of intensive treatment of diabetes on the development and progression of long-term complications in insulin-dependent diabetes mellitus. N Engl J Med 1993; 329:977-86.

2 Cryer PE. Hypoglycemia: the limiting factor in the management of IDDM. Diabetes 1994;43:1378-89.

3 Cox DJ, Gonder-Frederick L, Antoun B, Cryer PE, Clarke WL. Perceived symptoms in the recognition of hypoglycemia. Diabetes Care 1993;6:519-27.

4 Santiago JV, Clarke WL, Shah SD, Cryer PE. Epinephrine, norepinephrine, glucagon and growth hormone release in association with physiological decrements in the plasma glucose concentration in normal and diabetic man. J Clin Endocrinol Metab 1980;51:877-83.

5 Clarke WL, Gonder-Frederick LA, Richards E, Cryer PE. Multifactorial origin of hypoglycemic symptom unawareness in IDDM: association with defective glucose counterregulation and better glycemic control. Diabetes 1991;40: 680-85.

6 Clarke WL, Cox DJ, Gonder-Frederick LA, Julian D, Schlundt D, Polonsky W. Reduced awareness of hypoglycemia in adults with IDDM. A prospective study of hypoglycemic frequency and associated symptoms. Diabetes Care 1995;18:517-22.

7 Amiel SA, Sherwin RS, Simonson DC, Tamborlane WV. Effect of intensive insulin therapy on glycemic thresholds for counterregulatory hormone release. Diabetes 1988;37:901-07.

8   Amiel SA, Tamborlane WV, Simonson DC, Sherwin RS. Defective glucose counter-regulation after strict glycemic control of insulin-dependent diabetes mellitus. N Engl J Med 1987;316:1376-83.

9   Cryer PE. Iatrogenic hypoglycemia as a cause of hypoglycemia-associated autonomic failure in IDDM. A vicious cycle. Diabetes 1992;41:255-60.

10   Cranston I, Lomas J, Maran A, Mac-Donald I, Amiel SA. Restoration of hypoglycaemia awareness in patients with long-duration insulin-dependent diabetes. Lancet 1994;344:283-87.

11   Fanelli CG, Epifano L, Rambotti AM, et al. Meticulous prevention of hypoglycemia normalizes the glycemia thresholds and magnitude of most neuroendocrine responses to, symptoms of, and cognitive function during hypoglycemia in intensively treated patients with short-term IDDM. Diabetes 1993;42:1683-89.

12   Heller SR, Cryer PE. Reduced neuroendocrine and symptomatic responses to subsequent hypoglycemia after 1 episode of hypoglycemia in nondiabetic humans. Diabetes 1991;40:223-26.

13   Gonder-Frederick LA, Cox DJ, Bobbitt SA, Pennebaker JW. Mood changes associated with blood glucose fluctuations in insulin-dependent diabetes mellitus. Health Psychol 1989;8:45-59.

14   McCrimmon RJ, Gold AE, Deary IJ, Kelnar CJ, Frier BM. Symptoms of hypoglycemia in children with IDDM. Diabetes Care 1995;18:858-61.

15   Kerr D, Sherwin RS, Pavalkis F, et al. Effect of caffeine on the recognition of and responses to hypoglycemia in humans. Ann Intern Med 1993;119:799-804.

16   Ainsworth BE, Haskell WL, Leon AS, et al. Compendium of physical activities: classification of energy costs of human physical activities. Med Sci Sports Exerc 1993;25:71-80.

17   Gonder-Frederick L, Cox D, Kovatchev B, Schlundt D, Clarke W. A biopsychobehavioral model of risk of severe hypoglycemia. Diabetes Care 1997; 20:661-69.

18   The Diabetes Control and Complications Trial Research Group. Influence of intensive diabetes treatment on quality-of-life outcomes in the diabetes control and complications trial. Diabetes Care 1996;19:195-203.

19   Irvine A, Cox D, Gonder-Frederick L. The fear of hypoglycemia scale. In: Bradley C, ed. Handbook of psychology and diabetes. Switzerland: Hardwood Academic Publishers, 1994:133-55.

20   Gonder-Frederick L, Cox D, Kovatchev B, Julian D, Clarke W. The psychosocial impact of severe hypoglycemic episodes on spouses of patients with IDDM. Diabetes Care 1997;20:1543-46.

21   Clarke WL, Gonder-Frederick LA, Miller S, Richardson T, Snyder A. Maternal fear of hypoglycemia in their children with insulin-dependent diabetes mellitus. J Pediatr Endocrinol Metab 1998;11:189-194.

22   Drass JA, Feldman RH. Knowledge about hypoglycemia in young women with type I diabetes and their supportive others. Diabetes Educ 1996;22:34-38.

23   Cox D, Gonder-Frederick L, Polonsky W, Schlundt D, Julian D, Clarke W. A multicenter evaluation of blood glucose awareness training—II. Diabetes Care 1995;18:523-28.

SUGGESTED READINGS

Cox DJ, Gonder-Frederick L, Clarke WL. Helping patients reduce severe hypoglycemia. In: Anderson BJ, Rubin RR, eds. Practical psychology for diabetes clinicians. Alexandria, Va: American Diabetes Association, 1996:93-102.

Cryer, PE. Hypoglycemia: pathophysiology, diagnosis and treatment. New York: Oxford University Press, 1997.

Gonder-Frederick L, Clarke WL, Cox DJ. The emotional, social, and behavioral implications of insulin-induced hypoglycemia. Semin Clini Neuropsychiatry 1997;2:57-65.

Gonder-Frederick L, Cox DJ, Clarke WL. Helping patients understand and recognize hypoglycemia. In: Anderson BJ, Rubin RR, eds. Practical psychology for diabetes clinicians. Alexandria, Va: American Diabetes Association, 1996:83-92.

Santiago JV, Levandoski LA, Bubb J. Definitions, causes, and risk factors for hypoglycemia in insulin-dependent diabetes. In: Bardin CW, ed. Current therapies in endocrinology and metabolism. Philadelphia: BC Decker, 1991:354-59.

Santiago JV, Levandoski LA, Bubb J. Hypoglycemia in patients with type I diabetes. In: Lebovitz HE, ed. Therapy for diabetes mellitus and related disorders. Alexandria, Va: American Diabetes Association, 1991:161-69.

OTHER RESOURCES

Blood Glucose Awareness Training was developed at the University of Virginia and is currently being used throughout the United States, Canada and Europe. Information about BGAT can be obtained by writing: The BGAT Institute, 555 Gillums Ridge Road, Charlottesville, VA 22901.

Illness and Surgery

15

Elaine Boswell, MSN, RN, CS, CDE
Vanderbilt Diabetes Research and Training Center
Nashville, Tennessee

Janie Lipps, MSN, RN, CS, CDE
Vanderbilt Diabetes Research and Training Center
Nashville, Tennessee

Introduction

1 This chapter will address the knowledge and skills needed by healthcare professionals and patients to manage diabetes during illness and surgery.

2 Illness can cause problems when managing diabetes. During times of illness, the body releases stress hormones that oppose the action of insulin and contribute to hyperglycemia and the formation and accumulation of ketones. If appropriate action is not taken, dehydration and ketosis or hyperglycemic hyperosmolar nonketotic syndrome (HHNS) can result, requiring hospitalization.

3 Surgery conditions can impact diabetes control. Persons with diabetes may require usual surgical interventions as well as surgery for associated complications such as coronary artery disease, peripheral vascular disease, neuropathic ulcers, kidney disease, and proliferative retinopathy.

   A Patients' usual treatment programs are affected when surgery is performed; typical adjustments involve medical nutrition therapy, medications, and mobility.

   B Surgery can place persons with diabetes at risk for infections if their blood glucose is not well controlled.

   C The perioperative management of persons with type 1 and type 2 diabetes can differ.

4 An understanding of normal physiology is necessary to provide adequate support to the person with diabetes who is experiencing an illness or undergoing a surgical procedure. Special care is needed to achieve and maintain euglycemia, maintain fluid and electrolyte balance, provide adequate nutrition, and prevent further complications.

Objectives

Upon completion of this chapter, the learner will be able to

1 Describe the physiological effects of illness and surgery on blood glucose levels, ketone levels, and fluid and electrolyte balance.

2 Describe specific guidelines that healthcare professionals can follow when managing the care of patients with intercurrent illnesses.

3 Identify sick-day situations that require evaluation and possible treatment in an office, emergency room, or hospital setting.

4 Identify assessment information needed preoperatively.

5 Describe methods of insulin/glucose management for the surgical patient.

6 Explain the importance of euglycemia during the perioperative period.

7 Explain postoperative concerns.

Physiologic Effects of Illness and Surgery on Blood Glucose Levels, Ketone Levels, and Fluid/Electrolyte Balance

1 Metabolic homeostasis is maintained by the balance of the anabolic hormone insulin and the major catabolic hormones of glucagon, catecholamines, cortisol, and growth hormone. Physiological stress caused by intercurrent illnesses, surgery, infection, injury, emotional trauma, or medications can disrupt homeostasis.

2 During illness and surgery, there is an increase in the secretion of counterregulatory hormones, including cortisol, catecholamines (epinephrine and norepinephrine), growth hormone, and glucagon.[1,2]

   A Catecholamines cause an increase in heart rate, which increases blood pressure and dilates the bronchi to maximize the amount of oxygen that is supplied to the body tissues. Blood is diverted from the vulnerable surface of the body to the core to supply the vital organs with essential oxygen.

   B Epinephrine decreases the uptake of glucose by the muscle tissue and inhibits the release of endogenous insulin.

3 In type 1 diabetes, counterregulatory hormones cause the following metabolic changes: glycogenolysis, gluconeogenesis, lipolysis, and ketogenesis.[3,4]

   A Counterregulatory hormones contribute to the release of glucose from the liver and oppose the action of insulin.

   B Catecholamines cause glycogen that is stored in the liver to break down into glucose (glycogenolysis) and be released into the bloodstream.

   C The adrenal cortex secretes cortisol, which causes the liver to create additional glucose (gluconeogenesis) from amino acids (alanine), glycerol, and lactate. Uptake of the glucose by the muscle tissue is inhibited by cortisol.

   D These responses all raise the blood glucose level.

4 With hyperglycemia, urine flow is increased due to osmotic diuresis; fluid requirements also increase.

    A Signs and symptoms resulting from increased urine flow can include muscle weakness and fatigue related to loss of sodium, potassium, and phosphorus.

    B Signs and symptoms related to increased fluid requirements include polydipsia and dry mouth.

    C If hyperglycemia persists, dehydration can occur. Vomiting and diarrhea can be warning signs of dehydration. Adequate insulin replacement must be given to avoid diabetic ketoacidosis (DKA).

5 Ketogenesis and lipolysis are caused by inadequate nutrition states and insufficient insulin. Ketonuria and/or ketonemia are clinical manifestations of lipolysis and ketogenesis.

    A Signs and symptoms of ketosis include nausea and anorexia. If ketosis goes untreated, acidosis can result.

    B Warning signals of ketoacidosis include fruity acidic breath, abdominal pain, and/or rapid, labored breathing/Kussmaul's respiration (see Chapter 13, Hyperglycemia for more information on DKA).

6 In type 2 diabetes, hyperglycemic hyperosmolar nonketotic syndrome (HHNS) can occur as a manifestation of severe metabolic decompensation. Although DKA and HHNS are often discussed as distinct entities, they may overlap in a spectrum of decompensation.

    A HHNS is differentiated from DKA by the absence of significant ketosis. In HHNS, volume depletion results but ketogenesis usually is suppressed secondary to some residual insulin secretion.

    B HHNS is characterized by severe hyperglycemia and hyperosmolarity.[5,6]

    C HHNS is seen most often in the elderly, who have poor fluid intake or a diminished thirst mechanism.[7,8]

    D If undetected, lethargy, impaired mental status, or coma may result.[9]

    E Recommendations for prevention and early treatment are similar to those for diabetic ketoacidosis.

GUIDELINES FOR SICK-DAY MANAGEMENT

1 Increase the frequency of blood glucose and ketone monitoring during suspected or acute illness.

    A The signs and symptoms of a developing acute illness can be preceded by elevated blood glucose levels and ketone levels.

B More frequent monitoring is indicated when the person experiences unusual physical symptoms such as malaise, anorexia, and nausea, or when blood glucose levels rise. These symptoms may disappear or may develop into an identifiable illness.

C The frequency of blood glucose monitoring may need to be increased to every 2 to 4 hours while glucose levels are elevated and/or until symptoms subside. Urine ketone levels also need to be tested every 4 hours until negative results are obtained. Monitoring is performed at times when decisions regarding the insulin dose are needed.

D Instruct patients to record their monitoring results in order to more readily provide this information to the healthcare professional over the telephone, if needed.

2 Continue and possibly increase medication during illness.

    A Insulin or oral agents are still needed during illness even when the patient is unable to eat. Omission of insulin is a common cause of ketosis.

- Continue the routine dose of intermediate- or long-acting insulin (NPH, lente, ultralente).
- The full dose of daily insulin usually is required.
- Individuals using continuous subcutaneous insulin infusion (CSII) pumps should continue their basal insulin. The pump should not be removed unless an adequate amount of insulin is administered via injections.

    B Supplemental doses of rapid-acting insulin (lispro) and short-acting insulin (regular) also may be required for continuously rising or persistently elevated blood glucose levels, large ketones, or persistent ketones. Teach patients to call the healthcare professional for instructions on taking extra insulin if they have not previously been given an insulin algorithm for sick days.

- Rapid-acting or short-acting insulins may be given every 1 to 4 hours.
- The doses of rapid- and short-acting insulin depend on the severity of the illness. During most illnesses, 10% of the total daily dose can be given safely as a supplemental dose of rapid- or fast-acting insulin. If the blood glucose level is higher than 300 mg/dL (16.7 mmol/L) with large ketones, 20% of the routine dose may be given as a supplement.

- In the rare event that hypoglycemia exists, the rapid- or short-acting insulin doses can be decreased while maintaining the usual intermediate- or long-acting insulin doses. Hypoglycemia may occur with nausea and vomiting of short duration without systemic involvement such as fever.

C Over-the-counter and prescription medications may contribute to hyperglycemia or hypoglycemia (see Chapter 10, Pharmacologic Therapies for more information).

D Labels on over-the-counter products used to treat cold symptoms often advise against use by persons with diabetes. There are two approaches regarding the use of over-the-counter medications to treat cold symptoms in persons with diabetes.

- Use of antihistamines/decongestants and cough medicines is acceptable if patients are performing blood glucose monitoring at least every 4 hours and using their insulin algorithm and/or calling the healthcare professional when blood glucose levels are elevated. Insulin dose adjustments can be made for hyperglycemia.

- Teach patients to use sugar-free antihistamines/decongestants and cough medicines to avoid consuming additional simple sugars that could elevate blood glucose levels.[10]

3 Maintain adequate hydration because of the risk of dehydration from decreased fluid intake, polyuria, and evaporative losses from fever, vomiting, and diarrhea.

A Instruct patients to drink at least 8 ounces (240 mL) of calorie-free fluids every hour while they are awake. Examples of calorie-free liquids include diet soft drinks, water, broth, and sugar-free Kool-Aid®. Because caffeine acts as a diuretic, the fluids consumed should be caffeine-free. Sports drinks, bouillon, consommé, and canned clear soups provide sodium and electrolytes as well as fluids.

B If the patient is unable to tolerate fluids by mouth, antiemetics or intravenous fluids may be required.

4 Substitute clear liquids if patients are unable to tolerate solid foods at meal times because of nausea or anorexia.

A If the blood glucose level is higher than 250 to 300 mg/dL (13.9 to 16.7 mmol/L), the usual amount of carbohydrate is not needed.

B To prevent ketosis, obligatory daily requirements are 150 grams of carbohydrate per day.[11]

C With intestinal viruses, if the blood glucose level is less than 180 mg/dL (10 mmol/L) prior to a meal, teach patients to consume more easily tolerated foods or beverages equivalent to the usual carbohydrate content of their meal plan. Many people regain their appetite when blood glucose levels return to less than 180 mg/dL (10 mmol/L).

D When using carbohydrate counting for diabetes meal planning, nutrition labels are helpful to determine the carbohydrate value of foods.

E The ADA exchange guidelines can also be used by the healthcare professional to calculate carbohydrates for patients (See Chapter 8, Nutrition, for more information).

F For those who are nauseated, vomiting, or unable to tolerate a large volume of fluids, a "sipping diet"[12] consisting of approximately 15 grams of carbohydrate such as Gatorade® (or similar sports drink) taken every 1 to 2 hours can be effective.

G The foods and beverages shown in Table 15.1 contain approximately 15 grams of carbohydrate and are appropriate for sick-day use. Clear liquids can be taken when nausea is present.

5 Teach patients when to call to their healthcare provider.

A Some patients hesitate to telephone the healthcare team because they are concerned that their call might be a bother. Encourage patients to call anytime when questions and problems arise.

B Instruct patients to call a healthcare professional *immediately* if any of the conditions in Table 15.2 develop.

Sick-Day Situations That Require Examination and Possible Treatment by a Healthcare Professional

1 The healthcare professional can determine whether telephone management is possible or if an assessment and evaluation in the clinic or emergency room is indicated.

2 Teach patients the signs and symptoms listed in Table 15.3 since they indicate a need for examination, treatment, and possible hospital care.

TABLE 15.1. FOODS THAT CONTAIN 15 GRAMS OF CARBOHYDRATE

- ½ cup apple juice
- ½ cup regular soft drink (not diet, caffeine-free)
- ¾ of a double-stick Popsicle®
- 5 Lifesavers®
- 1 slice dry toast
- ½ cup cooked cereal
- 6 saltines
- 1 cup broth-based soup
- ⅓ cup frozen yogurt
- 1 cup Gatorade® (replaces electrolytes)
- ½ cup regular ice cream
- ¼ cup sherbet
- ¼ cup regular pudding
- ½ cup regular gelatin/Jell-O®
- 1 cup nonfat, sugar-free yogurt (not frozen)
- Milkshake (⅓ cup lowfat milk and ¼ cup ice cream)

TABLE 15.2. CONDITIONS THAT REQUIRE IMMEDIATE CONTACT WITH A HEALTHCARE PROFESSIONAL

- Vomiting more than once
- Diarrhea more than five times or for longer than 24 hours
- Difficulty breathing
- Blood glucose levels higher than 300 mg/dL (16.7 mmol/L) on two consecutive measurements, that are unresponsive to increased insulin
- Moderate or large urine ketones

TABLE 15.3. SIGNS AND SYMPTOMS THAT REQUIRE ATTENTION/ TREATMENT BY A HEALTHCARE PROFESSIONAL

- Persistent vomiting or an inability to tolerate fluids by mouth
- Persistent diarrhea and progressive weakness
- Difficulty breathing, rapid and labored respirations
- Moderate or large ketones that do not improve after 12 to 24 hours of treatment
- Change in mental status

Perioperative Treatment for Patients With Diabetes

1   Prevention of hypoglycemia, excessive hyperglycemia, lipolysis, protein catabolism, and electrolyte disturbance are the goals of therapy during the perioperative periods.

   A   Hyperglycemia has been associated with problems such as decreased effectiveness of leukocytes, increased risk of platelet aggregation, and increased rigidity of the red blood cell, which results in decreased circulation through the small vessels and deprivation of oxygen and nutrients.

   B   Ketosis and ketoacidosis may ensue with persistent hyperglycemia, leading to a drop in pH concentration. Patients with type 1 diabetes undergoing surgery are more prone to developing acidosis even with moderate hyperglycemia.[11]

   C   All patients with glucose intolerance are susceptible to electrolyte abnormalities and volume depletion from osmotic diuresis.

   D   Unrecognized and untreated hypoglycemia may endanger the life of the surgical patient. Because hypoglycemia in the anesthetized patient can be difficult to identify, frequent perioperative blood glucose monitoring is imperative.

2   Theoretically, enhanced healing depends on establishing or reestablishing homeostasis. Normal glucose levels are essential for the normal protein synthesis that is required for wound healing.[13] For maximum healing the blood glucose level should be maintained between 125 mg/dL (6.9 mmol/L) and 200 mg/dL (11.1 mmol/L).[14]

General Preoperative Assessment and Preparation for Surgery

1   Preoperative care includes thorough history and physical examination.

2   Include the following information on the admission history:

   A   Date of diabetes diagnosis

   B   Medications, including type, manufacturer, and dosage of insulin and/or oral agents

   C   Over-the-counter medications

   D   Allergies

   E   Previous episodes of ketoacidosis, HHNS, and severe hypoglycemia

F Assessment of metabolic control using home blood glucose records and HbA₁c if available

G Current weight and maximum weight

H Previous hospital admissions for surgery and other illnesses

I Any current signs and symptoms

J For women, the last menstrual period and childbearing history

3 Diagnostic laboratory data should be reviewed prior to admission for surgery with special consideration given to electrolyte balance and blood count.

A An elevated HbA₁c may indicate that the patient has been in poor control, is dehydrated, and may have a greater risk for ketoacidosis. A glycosylated albumin (fructosamine) or glycosylated serum protein test may help determine the most recent level of glucose control.

B Just prior to surgery, a complete blood count and electrolyte profile should be performed to assess for any metabolic derangements. Patients who have been hyperglycemic may be dehydrated. Patients with diabetic neuropathy may need monitoring to avoid fluid overload and hyperkalemia. An elevated white blood cell count (WBC) may indicate an underlying infection that would impede post-operative recovery.

4 Special considerations need to be given to the patient's cardiovascular, cerebrovascular, peripheral vascular, respiratory, neurological, and renal systems.

A Certain cardiovascular assessments and considerations are necessary.

- A thorough assessment is performed of any past cardiac problems and any cardiovascular symptoms. Cardiac problems are the leading cause of death in persons with diabetes. The presence of carotid bruits or transient ischemia attacks (TIAs) prior to surgery may indicate cerebrovascular disease. Metabolic and hemodynamic stresses may compromise the cardiovascular system and lead to myocardial infarction, congestive heart failure, cerebral vascular accidents, or acute renal failure. Anesthesia agents can depress heart muscle function and may induce rhythm disturbances. Several events during surgery can place additional stress on the myocardium: bleeding may result in hypovolemia, hypotension, tachycardia, or bradycardia; volume overload, fever, and shivering all may put additional stress on the myocardium. Patients with diabetes are also at risk for developing postoperative myocardial ischemia.[11]

- Preoperative and postoperative electrocardiograms should be obtained as well as measurements of cardiovascular enzyme activity, when indicated.
- Blood pressure needs to be carefully monitored; antihypertensive medications should be reinstituted promptly after surgery.
- It is important that a patient with a history of congestive heart failure (CHF) be assessed for pulmonary and peripheral edema. Caution is needed to prevent overhydration and hypokalemia. The patient with CHF and hypertension may be at risk for hypokalemia due to previous diuretic therapy.

B Certain neurological assessments and considerations are necessary.
- If the patient has had recent TIAs, a neurological evaluation may be indicated.
- The presence of some manifestations of neuropathy may affect recovery from the operation. Orthostatic hypotension, neurogenic bladder, hyperesthesia or hypoesthesia, and gastroparesis are some manifestations of diabetic neuropathies. Physical assessment needed to identify these problems includes lying and standing blood pressure readings, reflex and pinprick assessment of the feet, and determination of residual urine, if indicated.

C Certain renal assessments and considerations are necessary.
- The presence of renal disease may alter the types and amounts of fluid infused and medication dosages. As part of the general assessment to guide diabetes management, measurement of urine protein and creatinine clearance may be indicated if the patient's diabetes has been diagnosed for more than 5 years and the tests have not been performed recently. If there is inadequate time to perform a 12- or 24-hour urine collection for a quantitative evaluation, random dipstick for proteinuria may be used for screening. A serum creatinine should be included in the electrolyte screen.
- Arteriography procedures using dye need to be undertaken with caution in the patient with renal disease. The use of low osmolar dyes may be indicated; adequate hydration is essential, and a nephrology consult may be warranted.
- Amphotericin B and aminoglycosides are extremely nephrotoxic and extreme caution should be used in administering these agents.

Perioperative Concerns for Patients with Type 1 Diabetes

1   Several protocols for insulin management of the surgical patient with diabetes are available and effective. Ideally, a diabetologist or endocrinologist will be consulted for insulin and fluid management. In all insulin protocols, however, the usual insulin dosage is altered for the day of surgery and adequate glucose is supplied.

A   A glucose and insulin infusion regimen is an option for providing optimal glucose control during surgery and the immediate postoperative period.

- Rapid- or short-acting insulin is mixed in a normal saline solution and infused intravenously using an infusion pump. An initial rate of 0.5 to 1.0 units per hour may be used. Published protocols report insulin requirements of .5u to 5u/hour. Beginning a dose at the low range is a safe way to start. Dose adjustments may be made frequently based on blood glucose monitoring.

- Most protocols use a 5% or 10% glucose solution in a separate bag from the insulin solution. The glucose solution is administered in a piggyback fashion with the insulin solution. This method allows the insulin dose to be adjusted as needed while also allowing adjustment of the glucose infusion.

- Hourly capillary blood glucose measurements are used to determine the dose of insulin based on an algorithm.[14]

B   Insulin is usually given subcutaneously with brief surgical procedures when the patient will be able to eat lunch.

- Subcutaneous rapid-acting insulin may be given with a 5% or 10% glucose intravenous solution to maintain the target glucose levels. Numerous methods have been used to calculate the dosage, from unit per kilogram to present total daily dose. The rate of insulin given usually varies from 0.5 to 5.0 units per hour.[11]

- Another approach is to withhold the morning rapid- or short-acting insulin and give one half to all of the morning intermediate-acting insulin. This method can lead to unpredictable glycemic excursions due to the variable absorption times of intermediate-acting insulin and the decreased peripheral perfusion during surgical procedures. However, if coverage is provided for basal insulin needs during a brief surgical procedure; rapid- or short-acting insulin can be given as needed based on bedside glucose monitoring.

2 Sufficient glucose to prevent hypoglycemia and to provide the basal energy requirement is administered during surgery in the insulinopenic patient. Rates between 50 to 150 mL/h of 5% dextrose can be used.[14]

3 Electrolytes may be given as needed and added to the glucose solution.[14]

4 Persons who must be on fluid restrictions due to renal failure or heart failure may receive 50% glucose solution and a smaller volume of fluid using a central venous line.[14]

5 Surgery or tests that require the patient to have nothing by mouth (NPO) should be scheduled early in the morning whenever possible to prevent long periods of fasting. If the test or procedure is scheduled mid-to-late morning or in the afternoon, intravenous fluids and insulin should be initiated on the morning of the procedure to prevent hyperglycemia and hypoglycemia. Frequent blood glucose monitoring is needed to provide the information to make treatment decisions.

6 Frequent blood glucose and urine ketone monitoring are necessary to evaluate the adequacy of the insulin dose and calorie replacement.
   A Urine ketone accumulation should be monitored every 4 to 6 hours, or anytime the blood glucose level is greater than 240 mg/dL (13.3 mmol/L).
   B The ease of obtaining and testing capillary samples using a reflectance meter makes frequent blood glucose testing feasible with less expense. At minimum, blood glucose levels need to be checked preoperatively and postoperatively and before insulin administration. If the patient is receiving intravenous insulin, it is essential to monitor the blood glucose every hour. Intraoperative blood glucose levels should be checked every 30 to 60 minutes.

PERIOPERATIVE CONCERNS FOR PERSONS WITH TYPE 2 DIABETES

1 Type 2 patients who undergo surgery may be using insulin to manage their diabetes.
   A These patients may respond metabolically like type 1 patients so the treatment is the same.

B The main determinants for therapy in type 2 patients are the magnitude of the procedure and the metabolic state of the patient on the day of surgery.[14]

2 Patients whose diabetes is well controlled with medical nutrition therapy (MNT) or MNT-plus-oral antidiabetes agents do not require specific therapy. Patients with fasting blood glucose levels lower than 140 mg/dL (7.8 mmol/L) treated with an oral agent can be given their medication and started on a glucose infusion the morning of surgery; however, it is sometimes suggested to stop the oral agent the evening before surgery. Discontinue the longer-acting chlorpropamide 48 to 72 hours prior to the surgical procedure. Discontinue metformin 48 hours before and after surgery.

3 Type 2 patients who are poorly controlled on oral agents will need insulin during their perioperative period using the same regimens as type 1 patients.[14] Aggressive treatment of hyperglycemia can prevent HHNS.

POSTOPERATIVE CARE

1 Impaired wound healing can occur when the blood glucose level is greater than 200 mg/dL (11.1 mmol/L).[11]

    A The wound needs to be observed carefully for any signs of inflammatory changes or drainage, and alterations in the patient's temperature noted. Meticulous wound care is essential to prevent infection.

    B Maintaining and improving circulation to promote wound healing is particularly important for the person with diabetes who may have peripheral vascular disease.

2 Continue monitoring of blood glucose and electrolytes in the postoperative period. Hypoglycemia is a particular concern because the blood glucose level and insulin dose may decrease dramatically as the stress of surgery declines or as an infection is treated.

3 Postoperative nutritional management consists of two phases. Involvement of a registered dietitian will help to ensure a successful transition through these phases and reinitiation of medication that are essential for a successful outcome.

    A The first phase of nutritional management is the initial catabolic phase that extends from the period just before surgery into the period immediately following the operation. The second phase is the transition time during which the patient moves from NPO status to the usual meal plan.

    B During the reintroduction of foods such as clear liquids, it is preferable to continue a low-maintenance dose of intravenous or subcutaneous rapid- or short-acting insulin along with fluids to maintain target blood glucose levels.

    C Returning to the usual meal plan as soon as possible will promote healing and reestablish homeostasis. Adequate carbohydrate is needed daily to prevent ketosis due to starvation. Solid foods can be started as soon as tolerated.

4 Once food tolerance is established, the intravenous insulin infusion is stopped and a new treatment program is planned, considering such elements as infection, pain, steroids, or total parenteral nutrition (TPN). For patients treated with oral agents, the usual dose may be given with supplements of rapid- or short-acting insulin. For insulin-treated patients, a combination of intermediate- and rapid- or short-acting insulin may be given. When using only rapid- or short-acting insulin, care must be taken not to leave insulinopenic patients without basal insulin.

5 It is very important to note that subcutaneous insulin needs to be given at least 30 minutes prior to the discontinuation of any intravenous insulin infusion to prevent hyperglycemia.

6 Capillary blood glucose monitoring is needed a minimum of 4 times per day, usually before meals and at bedtime to determine the effectiveness of the therapy.

7 Pain can cause the release of counterregulatory hormones that can increase the blood glucose level. Adequate pain management will help relieve this response. Because pain medication can make the patient drowsy, frequent assessment is necessary to recognize hypoglycemia. Hyperglycemia may heighten the perception of pain in older adults.

8 Peripheral neuropathy and peripheral vascular disease increase the risk of ulcerations. Careful monitoring of pressure areas and ambulation as soon as possible will help reduce the risk of these postoperative complications.

9 Written instructions are mandatory for postsurgical home care, with instructions for insulin, other medications, meal planning, physical activity, and wound care, if applicable.

Emergency Surgery

1 In situations that require emergency surgery, diabetes management will depend upon the metabolic condition of the patient. Surgical emergencies, particularly if there is underlying infection, can cause rapid metabolic decompensation, with dehydration and hyperglycemia, and ultimately ketoacidosis in the patient with type 1 diabetes. If the patient is in early or established DKA, the first priority is metabolic management.

2 If the patient is without severe metabolic disturbance, the initial diabetes management can involve intravenous insulin infusion. If the patient is dehydrated, normal saline if used for fluid replacement.[15]

Surgery in Children

1 Few published guidelines exist for the surgical management of diabetes in children. In general, adult regimens have been adapted for use.[15]

2 Caution needs to be taken in calculating fluid and insulin requirements. Consult a pediatric endocrinologist, if available.

Key Educational Considerations

1 Sick-day management is a survival skill and should be taught at an appropriate level to all patients with diabetes.
   A Sick-day instruction and reinforcement are a priority before a hospital discharge; before starting day care, school, or college; before the flu season; when administering the flu vaccine; and before overnight travel away from home.
   B Learning is reinforced and retained when it is applied immediately. Because sick-day guidelines usually are taught when patients are healthy, evaluation needs to include assessing the patient's immediate and long-term recall of knowledge about sick-day management.
   C Give patients written instructions as reinforcement, keeping the guidelines as simple as possible.

- If appropriate, ask the patient if it will help to copy the guidelines or highlight notes on a provided handout to enhance retention and personalize the written instruction.
- Ask the patient where the guidelines will be posted or placed for easy access when needed.
- Suggest that the patient pack a sick-day box with supplies and non-perishable items that can be stored for use during illness. Acknowledge that the patient may not be accustomed to keeping glucose-containing products such a Jell-O,® regular soft drinks, or regular sports drinks at home. Review the rationale for keeping these items on hand for sick days and if the patient is willing to prepare this kit. Ask about the site for storage or placement.

D Evaluate patient's actual skills during and following an intercurrent illness.

- During telephone contact and/or clinic visits on sick days, ask the patient to describe action taken during illness and assess results.
- Ask the patient to describe how the sick-day plan worked and identify what changes are needed to make the plan work better.
- During follow-up visits, props and simulations can be used for reinforcement and to assist the patient in recalling sick-day guidelines. For example, props such as rapid- or short-acting insulin vials, blood glucose and ketone testing materials, and an 8-ounce plastic glass can be used to emphasize sick-day care. Simulations such as telephone call role-playing, review of blood glucose records and actions to take may help to evaluate patient recall.

E During an illness, many patients experience malaise, fatigue, and sleepiness, making self-care more difficult. Therefore, family members or significant others need to be familiar with sick-day guidelines and know where sick-day supplies and instructions are kept. Discuss a plan for their role and participation prior to an illness. They also need to know when to call a healthcare professional.

2 The preoperative assessment may provide insight into the educational needs of the patient and significant other(s). Assessing the patient's knowledge will help provide direction for preoperative and postoperative diabetes teaching. Include family members or significant others in the preoperative teaching, so they understand the postoperative recovery care needed.

A Explain to the patient how the insulin dose will be administered and adjusted during surgery. Many patients are fearful of giving others the decision-making responsibility for insulin adjustment.

B Explain the need for dextrose in the intravenous solution. Many patients know that dextrose raises the blood glucose level and they are concerned that an error may be made.

C Explain to patients with type 2 diabetes who are treated with oral agents that they may need insulin just for the time before, during, and immediately after surgery. Many patients are concerned that insulin therapy may permanently replace their previous treatment.

D Prepare the patient for frequent capillary blood glucose and urine ketone testing. Blood glucose levels may be checked every 1 to 2 hours.

3 Provide written discharge instructions for any medications, including insulin (if applicable), meal plan, physical activity, and surgical and medical follow-up. Work with the significant other(s) to plan menus for the first few days at home. Prior to discharge, provide updated information about medical nutritional therapy.

SELF-REVIEW QUESTIONS

1 Describe the physiologic effects of illness and surgery on blood glucose levels, ketone levels, and fluid and electrolyte balance.

2 Discuss specific guidelines that healthcare professionals may use when managing an intercurrent illnesses.

3 List situations that require examination and possible treatment in an office, emergency room, or hospital setting during an illness.

4 Describe the effects of surgery on the cardiovascular system.

5 State the reason why the prevention of hyperglycemia is important to the surgical patient with diabetes.

6 List methods to prevent hyperglycemia in the surgical patient.

7 Describe what should be included in preoperative management.

8 List two alternatives for insulin therapy intraoperatively and immediately postoperatively. Discuss advantages and disadvantages of these alternatives.

9 List four potential postoperative problems that may be more common in the person with diabetes.

10 State which oral agent should be discontinued at least 48 hours prior to surgery.

Case Study 1

RS is a 32-year-old sales representative who was diagnosed with type 1 diabetes 1 year ago. He manages his diabetes with multiple daily injections of insulin consisting of long- and rapid-acting insulin before breakfast, rapid-acting insulin before lunch, and long- and rapid-acting insulin before dinner. He monitors his blood glucose 4 times per day, counts carbohydrates, and strives for consistency. RS has been instructed on the recognition and treatment of hypoglycemia, ketone testing, and sick-day management. He returns to the clinic for follow-up once every 2 to 3 months.

This morning RS calls you to report that he is feeling nauseated. He states that his blood glucose level before breakfast was 233 mg/dL, he administered his usual dose of insulin using his insulin algorithm, and then was only able to drink one small glass of apple juice before becoming nauseated. It is now noon and he is still nauseated and does not feel like eating lunch or going to the office. RS reports that he vaguely recalls being instructed on sick-day management, but he is unsure what he should do because this is his first episode of being sick since his diagnosis.

Questions for Discussion

1. What additional assessment data would you obtain at this point?
2. What instruction and/or advice might be given?

Discussion

1. Gather information to determine if the patient's condition is stable.
   A. Assess whether the patient has been vomiting or experiencing diarrhea, how often, and for how many hours.
   B. Listen for symptoms of respiratory distress and ask whether the patient has had difficulty breathing.
   C. RS reported no vomiting, diarrhea, or respiratory distress.

2. Once acute distress is ruled out, recent blood glucose and urine ketone results are needed. Although diabetic ketoacidosis usually develops over hours, hyperglycemia and ketosis could be present yet unknown if self-monitoring of blood glucose and ketone testing is not performed or if testing is performed incorrectly.

A RS had not tested his blood glucose since before breakfast and had not checked for ketones. He was asked to obtain blood glucose and urine ketone measurements.

B Depending on the circumstances, the healthcare professional may wait for the patient to report the testing results or ask the patient to call back immediately with the results.

C RS reported a blood glucose value of 363 mg/dL (20.2 mmol/L) and a small amount of ketones.

3 Assess fluid and food intake.

A Fluid intake was assessed and RS reported that he had been sipping on a diet soft drink during the morning because of thirst; because of nausea he had consumed only a total of approximately 8 ounces.

B He reported eating no solid foods.

C The concept of avoiding dehydration by consuming adequate fluids was explained.

D Because his blood glucose was 363 mg/dL, he agreed to have bouillon (a source of sodium and fluid) and a diet soft drink for lunch – both items were on hand and choices he likes. He also agreed to drink 8 ounces of calorie-free, caffeine-free fluids hourly during the afternoon and evening, drinking in sips if necessary.

4 Reinforce the rationale for not omitting insulin doses.

A RS was given reassurance that administering his morning dose of insulin was appropriate.

B He then was instructed to use his insulin algorithm and administer his pre-lunch dose of rapid-acting insulin immediately after the telephone conversation.

5 Review plan of care and when to call.

A RS was instructed to retest his blood glucose and urine ketone levels in 3 hours, pre-supper (7 PM), and at bedtime.

B He was reminded to call if his blood glucose values were higher than 300mg/dL (16.7 mmol/L) and if he had moderate or large ketones.

C RS was encouraged to telephone the clinic immediately if vomiting occurred more than once, if he experienced more than five episodes or diarrhea, or he had difficulty breathing.

CASE STUDY 2

CB is a 42-year-old female who was diagnosed with type 1 diabetes at age 17 years. She is being admitted for an elective cholecystectomy with general anesthesia. CB is hypertensive and being treated with ACE inhibitors. She also has background diabetic retinopathy and proteinuria.

CB monitors her blood glucose 3 to 4 times per day and injects 15 units of ultralente with 6 units of lispro before breakfast, 4 units of lispro before lunch, 8 units of lispro before dinner, and 15 units of ultralente at bedtime .

In a team meeting the day before CB's admission for surgery, the resident suggests the following plan:

1   <150 mg/dL (8.3 mmol/L) = no insulin
2   151 to 200 mg/dL (8.4 to 11.1 mmol/L) = 4 units
3   201 to 250 mg/dL (11.2 to 13.9 mmol/L) = 6 units
4   251 to 350 mg/dL (14.0 to 19.4 mmol/L) = 8 units
5   CB will be advised to take her usual ultralente dose on the morning of surgery.
6   Capillary blood glucose readings are ordered every 4 hours and she will be given lispro insulin using a sliding scale.

QUESTIONS FOR DISCUSSION

1   What problems do you see with the resident's plan?
2   What other options can be considered?
3   What pre- and post-operative teaching needs can you identify for CB and her family?

DISCUSSION

1   Use of an insulin/glucose infusion would be optimal.
  A   Use of an intermediate- or long-acting insulin prior to a lengthy surgical procedure could lead to difficulties with hypoglycemia or hyperglycemia.
  B   Subcutaneous insulin is not given during surgery due to unpredictable absorption from changes in body temperature, varying blood volumes, and anesthesia. Subcutaneous insulin pump use is discontinued during surgery when the insulin/glucose infusion method is used. The basal rate of the pump or the intermediate- or long-acting insulin should be

given 1 to 2 hours before discontinuing intravenous insulin. Rapid- or short-acting insulin given intravenously has a very short half-life.

C   Intravenous fluids will be discontinued after CB is able to tolerate food.

D   A patient with proteinuria may tolerate only small amounts of intravenous fluid. When necessary to meet the caloric needs of a patient with end-stage renal disease during surgery, a more concentrated dextrose solution may be used.

2   Blood glucose monitoring should be increased during the perioperative period.

A   Blood glucose monitoring should be done every 30 to 60 minutes during surgery and until CB awakens from the anesthesia.

B   Blood glucose monitoring should be done every 1 to 2 hours as long as CB receives intravenous insulin.

3   The ACE inhibitor could be given after surgery when CB fully awakens.

4   Both CB and her family have educational needs.

A   Preoperative teaching should include information about the frequency of glucose monitoring, the surgical procedure, and postoperative care.

B   CB will be discharged as soon as possible from the hospital with written instruction. Discharge instructions to CB and her family include wound care, assessment of her wound for infection, frequency of monitoring, safety issues related to the use of pain medication, when to call for assistance, and when to return for follow-up. When using narcotics, family members will need to ascertain that the patient has followed her diabetes self-care plan (eg, taken correct insulin dose, has eaten), and monitor her glucose for hypoglycemia.

REFERENCES

1   Rosenbloom AL, Hanas R. Diabetic ketoacidosis (DKA): treatment guidelines. Clin Pediatr 1996;35:261-66.

2   Schade DS, Eaton RP. Pathogenesis of diabetic ketoacidosis: a reappraisal. Diabetes Care 1979;2:296-306.

3   Alberti KG. Role of glucagon and other hormones in development of diabetic ketoacidosis. Lancet 1975;1:1307-11.

4   Keller U, Schnell H, Girard J, Stauffacher W. Effect of physiological elevation of plasma growth hormone levels on ketone body kinetics and lipolysis in normal and acutely insulin-deficient men. Diabetologia 1984;26:103-8.

5   Genuth S. Diabetic ketoacidosis and hyperosmolar hyperglycemic nonketotic syndrome in adults. In: Lebovitz HE, DeFronzo RA, Genuth S, Kreisberg RA, Pfeifer MA, Tamborlane WV, eds. Therapy for diabetes mellitus and related disorders. 2nd ed. Alexandria, Va: American Diabetes Association, 1994:65-76.

6   American Diabetes Association. Hospital admission guidelines for diabetes mellitus. Diabetes Care 1998;21(suppl 1):S77.

7   Ennis ED, Kreisberg RA. Diabetic ketoacidosis and the hyperglycemic hyperosmolar syndrome. In: LeRoith D, Taylor SI, Olesky JM, eds. Diabetes mellitus: a fundamental and clinical text. Philadelphia: Lippincott-Raven Publishers, 1996:276-86.

8   Matz R. Hyperosmolar nonacidotic diabetes (HNAD). In: Porte D Jr, Sherwin RS, eds. Ellenberg & Rifkin's diabetes mellitus. 5th ed. Stamford, Conn: Appleton & Lange, 1997:845-60.

9   Minaker KL. What diabetologists should know about elderly patients. Diabetes Care 1990; 13(suppl 2):34-46.

10 Campbell RK. Treating the common cold without sugar. Diabetes Professional 1988; (summer):16-18.

11 Gaare-Porcari JM, O'Sullivan-Maillet JM. Care for persons with diabetes during surgery. In: Powers MA, ed. Handbook of diabetes medical nutrition therapy. Gaithersburg, Md. Aspen Publishers, 1996:601-15.

12 Kulkarni K. Adjusting nutrition therapy for special situations. In: Powers MA, ed. Handbook of diabetes medical nutrition therapy. Gaithersburg, Md: Aspen Publishers, 1996:453-55.

13 Palmisano J. Surgery and diabetes. In: Kahn R, Weir G, eds. Joslin's diabetes mellitus. 13th ed. Philadelphia: Lea & Febiger, 1994:955-61.

14 Arauz-Pacheco C, Raskin P. Surgery and anesthesia. In: Lebovitz H, ed. Therapy for diabetes mellitus and related disorders. Alexandria, Va: American Diabetes Association, 1994:157-63.

15 Alberti KGMM. Diabetes and surgery. In: Rifkin H, Porte D Jr, eds. Ellenberg & Rifkin's diabetes mellitus: theory and practice. 4th ed. New York: Elsevier, 1990:626-33.

Suggested Readings

Kaufman FR, Dergan S, Roe TF, Costin G. Perioperative management with prolonged intravenous insulin infusion versus subcutaneous insulin in children with type 1 diabetes mellitus. J Diabetes Complications 1996;10:6-11.

Ley B, Goodman D. Sick-day management: preparing for the expected. Diabetes Spectrum 1991;4:173-76.

Lorber DM. Surgical management of the patient with diabetes. Pract Diabetology 1996;15(2):2-4.

White NH, Henry DN. Special issues in diabetes mellitus. In: Haire-Joshu D, ed. Management of diabetes mellitus: perspectives of care across the life span. 2nd ed. St. Louis: Mosby, 1997:378-84.

Skin, Foot, and Dental Care

16

Jessie H. Ahroni, PhD, ARNP, CDE
Veterans Affairs Puget Sound Health Care System
Seattle, Washington

Cheryl Hunt, RN, MSEd, CDE
Health Education and Resources
Alexandria, Virginia

INTRODUCTION

This chapter on skin, foot, and dental care deals with issues of having diabetes and its effect on the skin and its integrity. Emphasis has been placed on the foot because of the devastating personal, social, and financial impact neuropathy and skin breakdown can have on the person with diabetes. Understanding the effect of diabetes on the health of the skin, oral mucosa and teeth is also important as we work with patients with diabetes.

1 Skin, the largest organ of the human body, provides an important defense against infection when it is intact and healthy.

2 Hyperglycemia affects the condition of the skin by contributing to dry skin, rashes, boils, and increased growth of certain bacterial colonies. People with diabetes tend to have a higher risk of lower-extremity and group β-streptococcal infections than people without diabetes.[1]

3 Hyperglycemia in combination with vascular insufficiency; neuropathy; dry, cracked skin; and/or excoriations caused by pressure or blunt force trauma provide avenues for the sequelae of tissue breakdown, infection, and amputation.[2,3]

4 Controlling blood glucose levels, maintaining adequate nutrition and hydration, and caring for the skin can reduce the risk of infection in people with diabetes.

5 Lower-extremity complications of diabetes mellitus are serious personal, medical, social, and economic concerns.

    A The pathophysiological factors that lead to diabetic foot complications are peripheral sensory neuropathy, peripheral vascular disease, trauma, skin ulceration, faulty wound healing, infection, and gangrene.

    B These complications are costly, but beyond the financial concerns are the inevitable social and psychological distresses to patients and their families.

    C Despite many major advances in healthcare delivery over the last decade, foot problems continue to exact a heavy toll on the quality of life of people with diabetes.[4-8]

6 Amputation is one of the most feared and disabling consequences of long-term diabetes.

   A Certain ethnic groups may be at risk for diabetes-related lower-extremity amputations.

   - Amputation rates based on hospital discharges are generally higher for African Americans than for Caucasians after adjusting for age.[9]

   - For Native Americans living on the Gila River Indian Reservation, the incidence of amputations was 24.1 per 1000 patients years compared with 6.5 per 1000 patients years for the general US diabetic population.[10]

   - Others[11] have reported estimated age-adjusted diabetic amputation rates to be higher in African Americans than in Hispanics or non-Hispanic whites, although Hispanics had a higher proportion of amputations associated with diabetes than African Americans.

   - Population-based data seldom contain the information necessary to control for the potential confounding effects of socioeconomic status and access to health care. Selby and Zhang[12] found that African Americans did not have an increased risk for diabetes-related amputation when access to medical care was comparable.

   B The prognosis of people with diabetes who have undergone an amputation is poor.

   - In one study,[13] 2-year survival after a diabetes-related amputation was 50%. Five-year mortality following amputation ranged from 39% to 68%. The chance of a new or second leg amputation within one year of the first amputation has been estimated at 9% to 20%.

   - Within 5 years of an initial amputation, 28% to 41% of surviving amputees with diabetes have undergone a second leg amputation.[14]

   C Survivors of amputation report a lower quality of life and often are not successfully rehabilitated into the community.[15]

7 Among people with diabetes, periodontal disease occurs with such frequency and severity that it has been labeled the sixth complication of diabetes mellitus.[16]

8 Oral hygiene, regular dental care, and improved metabolic control in people with either type 1 or type 2 diabetes reduces the risk of periodontal disease.

OBJECTIVES

Upon completion of this chapter, the learner will be able to

1   State the relationship between metabolic control and healthy skin.
2   List two elements of effective skin care.
3   Identify the risk associated with loss of metabolic control when infection occurs in people with diabetes.
4   Identify the effects of neuropathy on the autonomic, sensory, and motor functions of the foot.
5   Identify the signs of peripheral vascular disease in the lower extremities of people with diabetes.
6   List the basic elements of a diabetic foot screening examination.
7   Explain the findings of a foot examination that would cause a person with diabetes to be classified as high-risk.
8   Describe treatment plans for a person with high-risk feet or a foot ulcer.
9   List guidelines for teaching foot care to both low- and high-risk individuals.
10 State the relationship between metabolic control and overall dental health.
11 Identify the factors that contribute to periodontal disease in people with diabetes.
12 List two effective dental care practices.

DIABETES AND SKIN DISEASE

1   Dry skin may occur more frequently in people with diabetes.

   A   Hyperglycemia resulting in polyuria may be a cause of dehydration and subsequent dry skin.

   B   *Anhidrosis*, which is defined as an autonomic neuropathic condition of diabetes in which little or no perspiration is produced in the feet and legs, may lead to drying and cracking of the skin.

   C   Elevated blood glucose levels and impaired circulation increase the risk of infection and present a situation of serious concern if either of the previous two circumstances are present.

2   People with diabetes demonstrate an increased risk for skin infection caused by staphylococci, β-hemolytic streptococci, and fungus.

3   Common infections of the skin that have a probable relationship to diabetes are

   A   Cutaneous infections: furunculosis and carbuncles

B Candida: affecting areas of the genitalia, upper thighs, and under the breast

C Cellulitis and/or lower-extremity vascular ulcers[17]

4 Infections usually increase the blood glucose level and, consequently, the patient's insulin requirements.

5 Maintaining metabolic control is important for both preventing and treating skin problems.

6 Cleanliness, adequate nutrition with appropriate consumption of fluids, and avoiding trauma to the skin are important components of care that help to maintain skin integrity and prevent infection. In addition using a mild soap, warm (not hot) water, moisturizing lotion (not oil-based and without alcohol), and sunscreen help to maintain healthy skin.

LOWER-EXTREMITY COMPLICATIONS

1 Lower-extremity complications are a significant cause of hospitalization, disability, morbidity, and mortality among patients with diabetes mellitus. Improvements in the prevention of diabetes-related foot ulceration and amputation are needed to avoid their considerable medical, social, and economic costs.

    A In a 1986 cost-of-illness study[18] assessing economic costs of type 2 diabetes in the US, chronic skin ulcers alone were estimated to account for $250 million in healthcare expenditures.

    B Approximately $500 million was spent in the US in 1988 for the care of diabetic patients with foot problems.[18]

    C A more recent economic study[19] in Sweden estimated the 1995 value cost per patient in US dollars for diabetes-related foot complications:
- For patients with ischemia who healed, the estimated cost was $26,700 US dollars.
- For patients without ischemia who healed, the estimated cost was $16,100 US dollars.
- For patients who healed with an amputation, the corresponding costs were $43,100 after a minor (below ankle) amputation and $63,100 after a major (above ankle) amputation.

    D The number of hospital discharges listing an amputation and diabetes in the National Hospital Discharge Survey[20] was 54 000 in 1990.

This number underestimates the problem because diabetes is not listed on the discharge record for 40% of all hospitalizations of people with diabetes.[21]

2 Lower-extremity complications of diabetes result from a combination of contributing causes rather than from a single cause. The pathophysiologic factors that lead to diabetic foot complications are peripheral neuropathy, peripheral vascular disease, trauma, skin ulceration, faulty wound healing, infection, and gangrene.

NEUROPATHY

1 Sensory, autonomic, and motor neuropathies> act synergistically to cause diabetic foot complications.

2 Peripheral sensory polyneuropathy is a major pathophysiologic risk factor for foot ulceration and amputation.
   A About 50% of people with diabetes of 15 years duration have peripheral sensory neuropathy.[21] Loss of protective sensation allows trauma to go undetected by the patient.
   B The earliest and most severe damage due to diffuse somatic bilateral distal symmetrical polyneuropathy occurs at the most distal enervated sites so that loss of protective sensation appears in a "stocking glove" pattern.
   C Bilateral distal symmetrical polyneuropathy usually affects the toes and feet first, although sensorimotor functions of the fingers and hands may also be impaired.
   D A quick and easy way to identify feet without protective sensation is to evaluate the ability of the patient to perceive the pressure of a 5.07 monofilament applied to vulnerable areas on the plantar surface and top of the feet (Figure 16.1).
      • A 5.07 monofilament delivers 10 grams of linear pressure when it bends into a "C" shape. Inability to perceive the monofilament at any site is evidence of neuropathy.[22]
      • Educators and providers who wish to use this tool should obtain instructions and practice under supervision before incorporating this test into their practice.
      • This procedure should be demonstrated first in an area of intact sensation, such as the arm.

- The examiner should then use the modified, two-alternative, forced-choice method[22] to test the most common sites of potential ulceration: the toe tips, metatarsal heads, and heels.
  — When the plastic wire bends to a "C" shape, 10 grams of pressure are being applied to the site being tested.
  — Neuropathy is diagnosed if the 5.07 monofilament cannot be perceived at any site on either foot.
  — The 5.07 monofilament is the best tool for discriminating between those with protective sensation and those without it.[22]

FIGURE 16.1. USING A MONOFILAMENT TO IDENTIFY FEET WITHOUT PROTECTIVE SENSATION

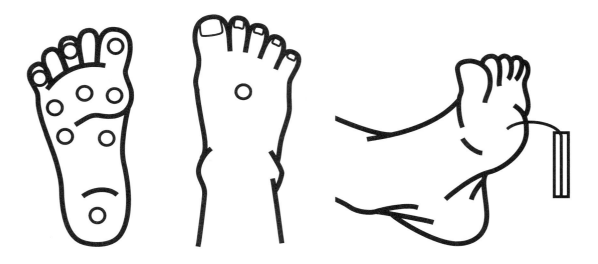

Suggested sites to test on each foot
The monofilament delivers 10 grams of pressure when it bends in a "C" shape.

4 Autonomic neuropathy causes changes in the nerves that control blood flow, skin hydration, and possibly bone composition of the foot.[23]
  A The lack of adequate skin hydration leads to dry skin, which can result in cracking and fissures of the skin of the foot.
  - Dry, cracked skin can be a portal for the microorganisms that cause infection.
  - Areas of callus are particularly prone to dryness.

B There may be changes in blood flow that result in vasodilation and shunting of blood away from the capillary bed.[24]

- Autonomic neuropathy may impair the ability of diabetic feet to mount an inflammatory response to trauma and infection.
- This impairment can contribute to skin ischemia and faulty wound healing, and an impaired ability to fight infection.[25]

C Some experts[23] propose that vasodilation and shunting of blood flow may cause bone demineralization and osteolysis that contribute to changes in the shape of the foot. Charcot's foot is an extreme example of such changes.

- In the acute stage of Charcot's foot, the foot becomes warm, swollen, and erythematous; this condition may be difficult to differentiate from infection.
- Although patients with Charcot's foot changes generally have severe neuropathy, they also may experience pain or tenderness. Because of relative insensitivity, however, many patients continue to walk, creating stress fractures and further disruption of the joint architecture.
- Although changes similar to Charcot's may occur in the forefoot, midfoot, or hindfoot, the most common presentation is collapse of the longitudinal arch. Diabetes educators should refer all patients suspected of having an acute Charcot's foot or a sudden change in foot shape for further orthopedic evaluation.
- Aggressive treatment in the early stage focuses on stabilizing the foot in a functional position, usually with a total contact cast. Without this treatment, the foot may develop a "rocker bottom" configuration or other bony prominence on the plantar surface that is prone to ulceration.[26] Once the Charcot foot has stabilized, protective shoes to accommodate changes in foot shape may be needed to prevent ulceration.

5 Motor neuropathy leads to muscle atrophy that results in weakness and changes in foot shape (Figure 16.2).

A The diabetic foot may take on a pes cavus shape, with a high arch and prominent metatarsal heads. The fat pad that normally protects the metatarsal heads at the ball of the foot becomes displaced.

B Weak intrinsic muscles allow flexors to predominate causing the toes to become deformed in a hammer or claw shape. Such abnormalities lead to irregular weight bearing and areas of high plantar pressure.

Figure 16.2. How Neuropathy Causes Changes in Foot Shape

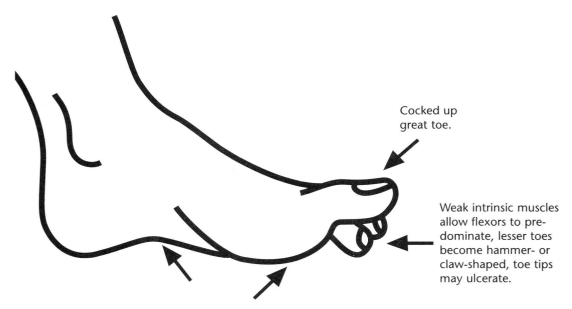

Cocked up great toe.

Weak intrinsic muscles allow flexors to predominate, lesser toes become hammer- or claw-shaped, toe tips may ulcerate.

The diabetic foot may take on a pes cavus shape, with a high arch and prominent metatarsal heads. The fat pad that normally protects the ball of the foot (metatarsal heads) is displaced. Higher plantar pressures result.

C There may also be subtle changes in posture and gait that cause changes in weight bearing and plantar pressure.[27]

D Assessment revealing muscle atrophy and/or changes in foot shape necessitates further orthopedic evaluation and shoes constructed to accommodate foot changes to alleviate pressure points.

PERIPHERAL VASCULAR DISEASE

1 Inadequate blood supply to the lower limbs deprives the tissues of oxygen and nutrients and impairs the removal of waste products.

    A Ischemia primarily results from atherosclerosis, which occurs early in the course of diabetes, progresses rapidly, and is associated with other risk factors such as aging, male gender, dyslipidemia, hypertension, smoking, obesity, a sedentary lifestyle, hyperglycemia, and hyperinsulinemia.[28] Thrombi from infection or blood clots can also cause ischemic changes.

B People with diabetes are more likely to have vascular disease below the knee. The estimated prevalence of arteriosclerosis obliterans, which totally occludes a vessel, is 15% after a 10-year duration of diabetes and 45% after 20 years.[29]

2 Symptoms of peripheral vascular disease include intermittent claudication, cold feet, and pain at rest that is relieved by dependency.

3 Vascular bypass surgery or angioplasty may enhance blood flow and improve the wound-healing process. However, arteriosclerosis is present not only in the larger vessels treated by these methods but also in the tiny vessels that supply the skin. These smaller vessels are not amenable to surgical interventions.

4 The single most important treatment for peripheral vascular disease is smoking cessation.[30] Self-management education should include risks faced by patients with diabetes who smoke, smoking cessation strategies, alternative nicotine devices, and referrals to aid in stopping.

5 Edema, whether from local infection or systemic causes, can adversely affect skin texture, cutaneous circulation, and wound healing.[31]

A Compression hose which can be obtained from a well-stocked drug store or pharmacy are useful. The patient's legs should be carefully measured as described on the packaging and the stockings fitted so as not to restrict arterial flow.

B Elevating the extremity above the heart may control dependent edema, but diuretics may be required for some patients. When arterial flow is severely compromised, patients may not be able to tolerate leg elevation, and may even need to sit with the feet dependent to facilitate blood flow to the feet.

TRAUMA

1 A 1990 study[3] of 80 amputations revealed that in 69 of the cases, the initial precipitating event was preventable minor trauma leading to skin ulceration. Common types of trauma include poorly fitting shoes, ingrown toenails, wrinkled stockings, foreign objects in the shoe, walking barefoot or sock footed, and inappropriate care of toenails, corns, and calluses.

A Chemical trauma results when caustic substances such as over-the-counter corn and callus removers destroy fragile tissue.

B Thermal injuries such as hot foot soaks, hot water bottles, heating pads, or walking on hot sand and pavement can cause severe burns to the insensitive and vascularly compromised foot.

- In a diabetic foot affected by autonomic neuropathy, the foot may become continually vasodilated.
- Applying heat to a diabetic foot increases metabolic demands.
- Tissue damage may occur when the vascular system is unable to meet the increased metabolic demands or unable to further vasodilate or sweat to release heat because of autonomic neuropathy.
- Most skin ulcers are caused by minor, repetitive pressure with each step (eg, walking on a bony, plantar prominence in a shoe with insufficient insole and sole cushioning) rather than a single episode of identifiable trauma.[32]

C Most amputations resulting from trauma can be prevented through patient education and effective self-care including properly fitting footwear. Elements of properly fitted shoes include

- Toe box that extends ½ inch beyond end of toes
- Toe box that leaves ¼ inch on each side
- Heel compartment that does not permit rubbing
- Metatarsal heads fitting in the widest part of the shoe
- Shoes with a soft and absorbent liner
- Lower heels, approximately 1 to 1½ inches
- Evaluation of shoe fit by performing a foot tracing and comparing it to the shoe in addition to examining the foot for pressure areas

---

ULCERATION

1 A foot ulceration is a full-thickness skin defect below the malleoli and penetrating to the subcutaneous tissue but not involving joint spaces, tendon, or bone.[33]

2 Any wound on the foot of a person with diabetes is a cause for serious concern.

A Diabetic foot ulceration need not result in infection or amputation. Proper wound management can heal many foot ulcers, and most amputations are preventable.

B There is disagreement on the details of foot ulcer management for patients with diabetes; however, there is substantial agreement on the major principles[34] of such care:
- Optimizing glycemic control
- Controlling sepsis
- Debriding necrotic tissues
- Applying dressings
- Treating local edema
- Bed rest or limited ambulation
- Utilizing protective footwear for the short- and long-term to redistribute weight, thus relieving pressure
- Providing foot care self-management education

INFECTION

1 The presence of purulence (pus), significant erythema, increased local warmth, tenderness, induration, fluctuance, or drainage indicates infection. If a diabetic foot lesion is infected, appropriate oral or parenteral antimicrobial therapy is prescribed after cultures are obtained, preferably by deep-tissue curettage.[35]

2 Acute or sub-acute infection (of less than 30 days duration) without systemic symptoms, gangrene, or osteomyelitis can effectively be treated using a single oral antibiotic for 2 weeks, with frequent follow-up and daily wound care.

A Gram-positive aerobic organisms, particularly staphylococci and streptococci, cause most foot infections in diabetes.

B Initial antibiotic therapy must cover these organisms and can be extended according to culture results or lack of clinical response.[35]

3 Patients with fever, leukocytosis, severe hyperglycemia, acidosis, hypotension, extensive cellulitis, lymphangitis, deep space infections, gangrene, crepitus, gas in the tissues, evidence of osteomyelitis, or failure of previous courses of therapy need to be admitted to the hospital for parenteral antibiotics and surgical drainage if necessary.[35] Patients who cannot perform or obtain needed outpatient care are also candidates for hospitalization.

GANGRENE

1 *Gangrene* is a nonspecific term for tissue death. Microthrombi that develop as a result of infection, arteriosclerosis, or other decreased blood flow, vasculitis, or increased platelet aggregation cause a complete blockage of the delivery of oxygen and nutrients to the tissue, resulting in tissue death or necrosis.

2 Dry gangrene is associated with ischemia.

   A When the gangrenous portion is sharply demarcated and affects only a small area, it may be left untreated but closely observed. In some cases, the affected part, usually a toe tip, will mummify and auto-amputate.

   B A wet or moist gangrenous area this is a sign that the process of tissue death is progressive or that infection may be involved. Because of the complete blockage of blood flow to the necrotic area, surgical intervention is usually required.

IDENTIFYING THE FOOT AT RISK

1 Identification of the at-risk foot can be done through screening of people who are asymptomatic. Screening allows classification regarding their likelihood of having a particular disease or outcome.

   A The screening itself, either a test, procedure, or examination, does not diagnose but simply identifies those who are at high risk.

   B Current published guidelines for establishing who is at risk for foot complications are not evidence-based.

2 Two commonly used risk stratification systems are the American Diabetes Association (ADA) Clinical Practice Recommendations[36] and the Hansen's Disease Center[37] (HDC) risk categories. Although these are the two main foot-risk stratification tools in the literature, neither of them can be considered a true screening procedure for the at-risk foot since both tools include patients with a history of foot ulcers or amputations and are therefore not truly asymptomatic.

   A The ADA Clinical Practice Recommendations describe two levels of risk for diabetic foot complications. These guidelines also outline the essentials of foot care for people with diabetes. The ADA provides no evidence in their recommendations for the inclusion or exclusion of any of these factors.

- High risk includes any of the following characteristics: neuropathy, vascular disease, structural deformities, abnormal gait, skin or nail deformities, a history of ulcers, poor understanding of, or inadequate self-care.
- Low risk includes none of the high-risk characteristics.

B The HDC recommends a four-level risk categorization scheme. The categories range from Category 0 (low risk) to Category 3 (high risk). The authors[37] cite unspecified personal experiences at the Hansen's Disease Center as evidence of the effectiveness of this risk-categorization.

- Category 0—no loss of protective sensation; very low risk of foot complications
- Category 1—loss of protective sensation; no weakness, deformity, callus, preulcer, or history of ulceration; intermediate, low-grade risk of foot complications
- Category 2—loss of protective sensation and any weakness, deformity, callus, or preulcer, but no history of ulceration; intermediate, high-grade risk of foot complications
- Category 3—history of plantar ulceration or ischemic index less than 0.45; high risk of foot complications

3 Risk factors for predicting foot ulceration were identified in a study[38] at the Veterans Affairs Puget Sound Health Care System, Seattle Division, using a stepwise logistic regression model.

A The following five risk factors were identified (statistical significance ranged from $P=.0001$ to $P=.0114$):

- Sensory neuropathy (inability to perceive a 5.07 monofilament)
- History of amputation
- Absent toe vibration (128-cycle tuning fork)
- Insulin treatment
- History of ulceration

B When none of the five variables are present, the probability of foot ulceration is .05%. When all five variables are present, the probability of foot ulceration is 68% and the likelihood ratio is 11.18 times (The likelihood ratio summarizes the odds of foot ulceration after a positive screening test).

4 Risk factors for predicting amputation were identified in the Seattle study.[38]

A The following five risk factors were identified (statistical significance ranged from $P=.0004$ to $P=.0237$):

- History of foot ulceration or amputation
- Charcot's foot
- Diabetes duration greater than 10 years
- Hammer or claw toes
- Self-reported nephropathy

B When none of the five variables are present, the probability of an amputation is .05%. When all five variables are present, the probability of an amputation is 84% and the likelihood ratio is 164[14] times (The likelihood ratio summarizes the odds of amputation after a positive screening test).

5 The presence of three of the multivariate criteria for predicting foot ulceration (history of ulceration, history of amputation, and insulin treatment), and possibly all five of the criteria for amputation can be detected through patient assessment. Those who have had a foot ulceration or amputation can automatically be categorized as high risk; no further screening questions or examinations are necessary to make this determination.

FOOT EXAMINATION

1 A powerful way to teach the importance of foot care is to demonstrate it through a careful foot examination at least once a year and asking about foot problems at every visit. A standardized assessment form that lists the specific screening activities that need to be done, the interventions recommended, and foot-risk categories can be used to document the examination. By taking advantage of this time the educator can emphasize the importance of this self-care activity and use the opportunity for individualized instruction.

2 A foot-risk screening includes assessing changes in the feet since the last visit. Areas to address include a history of peripheral vascular disease, intermittent claudication, symptoms of neuropathy, and a history of foot ulceration or amputation.

3 Record the presence or absence of a current foot ulceration. If an ulceration is present, refer the patient to a provider with expertise in foot care or a wound care clinic for ongoing care.

4 A vision assessment using a handheld or wall-mounted Snellen chart can help determine whether patients can see their feet well enough to perform an accurate visual inspection.

   A A foot inspection includes the tops, bottoms, and sides of each foot and between the toes. Ask the patient to demonstrate the ability to reach the feet for foot care and manual inspection.

   B Vision that is regarded as mildly to moderately impaired is probably inadequate for performing a reliable foot inspection.

   C If vision is poor, a manual inspection may substitute for the visual inspection. If poor vision or impaired mobility makes it difficult for the patient to reach the feet, a mirror, magnifying glass, or magnifying mirror may be used; a family member or other caregiver may need to assist with daily foot inspection (see Chapter 21, Eye Disease and Adaptive Education for Visually Impaired Persons).

5 In the clinical setting, sensory examination with a 5.07 monofilament is the single most practical measure for detecting neuropathy.[39]

6 Daily visual or manual foot inspection is recommended for patients with neuropathy.

   A Foot inspection consists of a brief examination for color, skin integrity, and toenail length in good light, such as when drying off after a shower or bath or when putting on socks.

   B Although patients without neuropathy are likely to be able to perceive injuries to their feet, daily foot inspection is a good habit to develop to promote early problem recognition and intervention.

7 The probability of vascular disease can be determined from knowledge of the patient's age, history of vascular disease, venous filling time, and examination of the lower-extremity pulses by palpation.[40] Segmental Doppler blood pressures and calculation of the ankle-arm index (AAI) need not be performed to determine risk for diabetic foot complications.

   A Palpation of the dorsalis pedis (DP) and posterior tibialis (PT) pulses should be performed and recorded as either present or absent.

   B The AAI should be determined in patients without palpable pulses or those otherwise suspected of having vascular disease of the lower extremities.

   C Venous filling time is easily determined.

- After identifying a prominent pedal vein, the examiner assists the patient in elevating the legs to 45° for 1 minute.
- The patient is then asked to sit up and hang the legs over the side of the examining table.
- The time (sec) until the veins bulge above the skin level is recorded.
- The time to reappearance of the veins can be recorded or results can be classified as normal (≤20 sec) or abnormal (≥20 sec).

D Those patients with ischemia who would benefit from vascular bypass surgery or angioplasty should be referred to appropriate health care providers.

8 Structural deformities are identified during the physical examination and the presence or absence of prominent metatarsal heads, hammer or claw toes, Charcot's foot deformity (collapse of the foot arch), bony prominences (exostosis), Hallux valgus (bunion), or hallus limitus (also called hallux rigidus, stiff great toe joint with limited range of motion), and corns and calluses are recorded.

A This is an ideal time to inspect the shoes and socks worn by the patient and to offer personalized information about footwear.
- Point out the need for shoes with cushioned insoles and soles.
- If claw or hammer toes are present, advise the patient to wear shoes with plenty of toe room (eg, in-depth or custom-made footwear).
- People with severe foot deformities need custom footwear available by prescription from foot care specialists: pedorthotist, orthotists, or podiatrists.

B Corns and calloused areas are signs of increased pressure.
- Excess keratin may be gently filed or buffed with an emery board or pumice stone.
- Over-the-counter corn and callus removers may cause burns or ulcers. Extremely thick corns or calluses need to be treated by a foot care specialist.

9 Skin abnormalities are also evaluated during the assessment. These may include excessive dryness and macerated, intertrigous areas indicating severe tinea pedis (athlete's foot fungus). Nail deformities such as fungal dystrophy (thickened and deformed toenails) or ingrown toenails should also be recorded.

A Dry skin can be treated with daily emollients or moisturizers.

- The best time to apply these agents is after a bath or shower. Emollients and moisturizers should not be applied between the toes.
- Soaking the feet is not routinely recommended for people with diabetes.

B Tinea pedis and toenail fungal infections can be treated with increased attention to drying between the toes and over-the-counter antifungal agents. Some patients find that loosely lacing pieces of lamb's wool between the toes helps prevent maceration and fungal infections. Fungal infections that are severe or persistent should be brought to the attention of a medical provider.

C Cut or file toenails straight across the contour of the toe, being sure that all sharp edges are filed smoothly.

- If the patient does not see well or has difficulty reaching the feet, a family member, nurse, or podiatrist should help with nail care.
- Patients with extremely thick toenails or ingrown toenails should be referred to a foot care specialist for treatment.

10 At the end of the examination, a foot risk category is determined and reviewed with the patient. A plan should be made for foot care education and at least annual foot exams (for low-risk patients). High-risk patients require more frequent foot exams and more detailed personalized education emphasizing daily inspection, protective footwear, and the need to report foot problems promptly.

IMPLICATIONS

1 Appropriate diabetes education and preventive care can reduce the risk of foot complications in susceptible patients.

A Meticulous foot care and proper patient education has been reported[41] to reduce the amputation rate associated with diabetes by 50%.

B Teaching patients and healthcare professionals ways to reduce risk factors and prevent limb loss due to foot disease is an important strategy in diabetes management and cost reduction.

C Predicting which patients are at the greatest risk could lead to more efficient use of resources.

2 Because present knowledge regarding the prevention and management of diabetic foot disease is not widely applied in practice, rates of foot ulcers and major amputations in the US remain high.[42]

3 For people without established end-stage complications of diabetes, better control of blood glucose levels has been shown to reduce the development of neuropathy and slow its progression.[43]

    A A fundamental principle in the strategy of prevention is that more cases are likely to emerge from a large number of people exposed to a low risk than a small number of people exposed to a high risk.

    B This principle suggests that significantly improving the glycemic control of the entire population of people with diabetes, thus lowering the incidence of risk factors and other complications, is likely to be more effective in preventing foot ulceration and amputation than focusing efforts only on members of the population already at high risk.

DIABETES AND DENTAL CARE

1 *Periodontal disease*, an inflammatory process that affects the supporting tissues of the teeth, may be accelerated in people with diabetes that is poorly controlled or of long duration.[44-46]

    A Periodontal disease is the most prevalent oral complication of diabetes.

    B Factors responsible for or contributing to the development of periodontal disease are
- Basement membrane thickening
- Possible changes in vasculature
- Changes in the microflora of periodontal tissues
- Collagen metabolism
- Leukocyte function and other aspects of the host response[44,47]

    C Because periodontal disease is often asymptomatic, people may have a false sense of dental health.[47]

2 Caries in the crown of a tooth seems to occur with greater frequency in adults with poorly controlled diabetes.[44] Hyperglycemia may contribute to elevated salivary glucose levels, which increase the risk of developing periodontal disease and dental caries.

3 Oral infections other than dental caries or periodontal disease are often more severe in people with poorly controlled diabetes than those with well-controlled diabetes or those who don't have diabetes.[44]

4 Insulin doses may need to be adjusted depending upon the degree of periodontal health.

A Infection may increase insulin requirements.

B Controlling infection and maintaining oral health may reduce insulin requirements.

5 Dental care and metabolic control contribute to the prevention of dental caries and periodontal disease.[44,47]

  A Bacterial plaque must be kept at a minimum.
  - Instruct patients to routinely brush and floss teeth.
  - Professional removal of plaque should be done periodically in association with regular dental exams.
  - The use of baking soda with hydrogen peroxide has been identified as being helpful in the eradication of subgingival microflora.

  B During routine medical visits, people with diabetes need to be assessed for signs of redness, foul odor, swelling, bleeding, loose teeth, or pain; offer appropriate referral if these periodontal symptoms develop. Instruct patients to see a dentist every six months, and more frequently if periodontal disease exists.

KEY EDUCATIONAL CONSIDERATIONS

1 Inform people with diabetes who have obvious signs of dry skin or compromised skin integrity about the risk of infection and further deterioration of the skin.

2 Emphasize the importance of metabolic control, cleanliness, moisturization, skin assessment, and reporting of problem areas to people with diabetes.

3 Advise patients to avoid trauma to the skin, especially the feet and legs. Use of properly fitting shoes and socks, protective sporting equipment when exercising, and general caution during routine daily activities can help reduce the risk of trauma to the skin.

4 Teach people with diabetes to
  A Bathe or cleanse skin with warm water and mild soap.
  B Avoid overexposure to water or cleansing products because these may strip the skin of its normal protective oils.
  C Pat skin dry with a soft, fluffy towel rather than rubbing it with the towel.

D Teach patients to thoroughly dry the skin between skin folds and toes. Powders or cornstarch may be applied to keep moist areas dry. Dry skin may be moistened with lanolin or hand lotion, but should not be used excessively.

E Emphasize the importance of a balanced nutritional plan with appropriate liquid consumption.

5 Approach issues of foot, skin, and dental care in a nonjudgmental way, maintaining sensitivity to individual and cultural differences.

A Many people with diabetes are fearful of the prospect of amputation. Present accurate information that will reinforce the importance of self-care to lower risks while reducing unrealistic fears.

B Apprehension associated with dental examinations and treatment can be reduced by explaining what to expect and by reinforcing the positive outcomes of dental care.

6 Before teaching foot care skills, the educator needs to assess the patient's present knowledge, behaviors, beliefs, and abilities.

A Ask "What are you doing now to care for your feet?"

B The challenge for the educator is to provide information tailored to the individual patient's risk level and current foot care practices.

C Homelessness or blindness represent situations for which the educator must adapt instructions to meet these patients' special needs.

7 Patients need to be given practical and realistic information about foot care that is presented in positives—"dos" rather than "don'ts." Give reasons why foot care is important and the purpose of recommendations.

8 It is helpful for patients to have some written guidelines about foot care to take home.

A Give patients only one handout at each visit to emphasize an important foot care concept. These might be:
- A reminder poster to hang on the back of the bathroom door, including a large-print or low-literacy version with graphics
- Reprints of articles written for the lay population

B To help personalize the information, the educator can highlight sections of the article that emphasize key principles and cross out information that is not applicable. Provide materials that are appropriate for the patient's language and literacy level.

9 Teach patients with diabetes the basic principles of foot care. Patients with neuropathy, vascular disease, or a history of foot ulceration or amputation should periodically be assessed for foot care practices and provided with personalized foot care education.

10 For high-risk patients, review the principles of foot care at every visit; for low-risk patients, an annual assessment and review is probably sufficient. Encourage patients to remove their shoes and socks at every healthcare visit, even if they are not asked to do so.

11 Teach and review the following principles of foot care:
  A Look at your feet and interdigital areas daily (eg, whenever putting on or taking off socks). A magnifying glass, mirror, or magnifying mirror may be helpful in examining the top, bottom, and sides of your feet for color and skin integrity.
  - Have the patient perform a return demonstration after explaining and demonstrating a foot inspection. Point out areas that need special attention.
  - If the patient is unable to do a demonstration, a family member or other care provider can perform the inspection.
  B Inspect shoes daily by feeling the inside of the shoe for torn or loose linings, cracks, pebbles, nails, or other loose objects and irregularities that may irritate the skin. Get in the habit of shaking out your shoes before putting them on.
  - Soft leather or canvas shoes that have cushioned insoles and fit well at the time of purchase offer the best protection.
  - Changing shoes during the day can limit repetitive local pressure.
  - Avoid going barefoot or sock footed. Wear footwear at the pool or beach. Use sunscreen to avoid burns.
  C Wash and dry the feet thoroughly, especially between the toes.
  - Use a thin layer of lamb's wool to separate toes that overlap or touch each other and to prevent maceration.
  - Caution patients to avoid hot-water burns by checking the bath or shower temperature with the forearm, elbow, or a bath thermometer.
  - Avoid routine foot soaks.

D Moisturize dry skin (except between the toes) with an emollient such as lanolin or hand lotion. Hand lotions containing alcohol are not suitable as the alcohol may contribute to drying or cracking of the skin.

E Cut toenails straight across and file the sharp corners to match the contour of the toe, making sure that all sharp edges are filed smooth. If the patient does not see well or has difficulty reaching the feet, this self-care task can be done by a family member, nurse, or podiatrist.

F Avoid self-treatment of corns, calluses, or ingrown toenails.
- Using chemicals, sharp instruments, or razor blades to treat these problems can lead to ulceration or infection.
- Flaky fungal debris can be loosened and removed with a soft nail brush during regular bathing.
- A patient or family member may gently buff corns or calluses with a pumice stone while the skin is damp; emollient lotion or creme should then be applied to keep the corn or callus soft.

G Wear well-fitting, soft cotton or wool socks. Avoid using hot water bottles, heating pads, or microwave foot warmers as they can cause burns.

H Seek prompt medical attention for any problems (eg, cuts, blisters, calluses, any wounds that do not heal, or signs of infection such as redness, swelling, pus, drainage, or fever). Treat fungal infections promptly with antifungal cream, spray, or powder; change footwear periodically to keep the area between the toes clean and dry.

12 Stress the importance of preventing dental complications through routine dental examinations, effective brushing and flossing, and keeping blood glucose levels near normal.

13 Advise persons taking sulfonylureas or insulin, to schedule dental appointments about 1 hour after a meal to reduce the chances of hypoglycemia. When anesthesia is to be used, inform patients that the best outcome may be facilitated by having the dentist or oral surgeon collaborate with their doctor or nurse practitioner.

14 Nutritional modification and appropriate instruction may be necessary for preventing and/or treating periodontal disease. Instruction may focus on a balanced medical nutrition plan; use of sugars; important vitamins and minerals; and changes to accommodate treatments or impaired ability to chew foods.

15 Be prepared to recommend dentists or local dental clinics for people who have not established a program of routine dental care.

SELF-REVIEW QUESTIONS

1 What steps should be included in every diabetic foot risk screening examination?

2 Describe changes in the appearance of the foot due to autonomic, motor, and sensory neuropathies.

3 List the signs of peripheral vascular disease.

4 Describe the indications of a high-risk diabetic foot.

5 What is the best indicator of peripheral sensory neuropathy?

6 Describe the best preventive measures for dental problems in people with diabetes.

7 State why products for the skin containing alcohol should be avoided.

CASE STUDY 1

JF is an elderly gentleman who has had type 2 diabetes for 12 years is referred to you for foot care education. He does not have a history of peripheral vascular disease, retinopathy, nephropathy, foot ulceration, or amputation. He is insensate to the 5.07 monofilament at several sites on each foot. He has thin, bony feet with a high arch, prominent metatarsal heads, clawed toes, and dry skin. JF is wearing well-worn loafers with no insoles and a thin leather sole. He says he doesn't get overly concerned about his feet and tends to only look at them when toweling off after a shower.

QUESTIONS FOR DISCUSSION

1 How would you classify JF's risk for foot ulceration?

2 What aspects of foot care education are important to emphasize for someone at this risk level?

Discussion

1   This patient has neuropathy and is at high risk for foot ulceration or amputation.

2   Before teaching foot care skills, the educator needs to assess JF's present knowledge, behaviors, beliefs, and abilities.

3   It is essential to assess if JF's can see functionally and reach his feet before teaching is begun.
   A   Wearing loafers may be a sign that he is unable to bend over to tie shoes.
   B   Wearing shirt styles that are easier to put on (eg, pullover versus button), may be a clue to possible neuropathy of the hands.

4   Explain to JF that you are concerned that his casual inspection is no longer adequate because his feet are now insensate. Recommend that he closely examine his feet daily and use a mirror if necessary.
   A   Good opportunities to examine the feet are while drying the feet after bathing, when putting on socks, when getting ready for bed, or when applying emollients to dry skin.
   B   Remind him to not put the emollient between his toes. However, he should still examine the areas between the toes.
   C   If JF is unable to inspect his feet daily, ask about other family members or caregivers who might be able to assist in performing this inspection.

5   JF's current shoes are not ideal diabetic footwear because of their lack of support, both inside and outside.
   A   If he has or can obtain financial resources, athletic shoes with a cushioned sole/insole and a rounded toe box will offer protection.
   B   Shoes with Velcro® straps may be easier for him to fasten than those with shoelaces. If this type of shoe is not available commercially, a pedorthotist can make this alteration in the shoes.
   C   Medicare may offer coverage for therapeutic shoes, inserts, and shoe modifications for certain people with diabetes. Information and claim forms can be obtained from the Department of Health and Human Services.

CASE STUDY 2

A 20-year-old female (SA) with type 1 diabetes diagnosed 5 years ago has been referred to you for diabetes education. She is afraid of the complications of diabetes, especially amputation, and intends to do everything possible to prevent these. She does not have any complications of diabetes at this time and can perceive the 5.07 monofilament at all sites tested on each foot. SA's feet are shaped normally and she is wearing high-quality athletic shoes.

QUESTIONS FOR DISCUSSION

1   How would you classify SA's risk for foot ulceration?
2   What aspects of foot care education are important for someone at this risk level?

DISCUSSION

1   SA does not have neuropathy, a history of foot ulceration or amputation, or other complications of diabetes or foot deformities. She currently has a low risk of foot complications.

2   Before teaching foot care skills, the educator needs to assess the SA's present knowledge, behaviors, beliefs, and abilities.

3   Although SA has sensation on all parts of her feet, daily foot inspection is a good habit to develop.
   A   Briefly looking at the feet in good light after bathing or before putting on socks is all that is necessary for foot inspection at this time.
   B   If SA discovers any foot problems or abnormalities, she should promptly report these to her healthcare provider.

4   Reassure SA that at the present time her risk of foot complications is low. Even if she were to get a foot ulcer, it would probably heal easily.

5   Emphasize that she should continue wearing good shoes with cushioned soles/insoles and have an annual foot exam with testing for neuropathy. Stress the importance of keeping her blood glucose near normal to also help prevent foot problems from developing.

6   Point out the additional risks of smoking for people with diabetes.

Case Study 3

TL is a 63-year-old female with a history of type 2 diabetes for 8 years. She has tried a variety of oral medications to control her blood glucose, with little success. TL's blood glucose levels remain elevated in the range of 220 mg/dL to 280 mg/dL for no obvious reason. Today you notice that her gums are unusually red and you detect a foul breath odor as she speaks to you. Further questioning reveals that TL has recently had to alter her eating habits to soft foods because her mouth has been so tender and her gums bleed so easily. TL tells you she fears the dentist and she has not seen one in the past 4 years.

Questions for Discussion

1   How could infection in the gingiva affect TL's blood glucose?
2   What are age-appropriate concerns related to TL's oral health?
3   What are aspects of personal oral hygiene important to discuss with TL?
4   Who are possible professional referrals you can offer to TL?

Discussion

1   Periodontal disease may be responsible for TL's persistently elevated blood glucose levels that have failed to respond to pharmacologic therapy. In addition, elevated blood glucose levels increase the risk for periodontal disease.

2   Teach TL about the various aspects of oral hygiene and how dental problems such as periodontal disease can affect blood glucose levels.

3   She should be given referrals to appropriate dental health professionals (a dentist, periodontist, or oral surgeon) to treat her oral health problems while she continues to work with her diabetes care team to lower her blood glucose levels.

4   Given the relationship between her age, current state of dental health, and glycemic control, the following outcomes should be considered:
    A   Impact of loss of teeth, soreness, and/or infection in the oral cavity
    B   Influence of normal changes in taste and smell on her willingness to use a meal plan as part of her diabetes care

REFERENCES

1 Boyko EJ, Lipsky BA. Infection and diabetes. In: National Diabetes Data Group, eds. Diabetes in America. 2nd ed. Bethesda, Md: National Institutes of Health, 1995; NIH publication no. 95-1468:485-500.

2 Reeves WG, Wilson RM. Infection, immunity, and diabetes. In: Alberti KGMM, DeFronzo RA, Keen H, Zimmet P, eds. International textbook of diabetes mellitus. New York: John Wiley & Sons, 1992:1165-71.

3 Pecoraro RE, Reiber GE, Burgess EM. Pathways to diabetic limb amputation. Basis for prevention. Diabetes Care 1990;13:513-21.

4 Ahroni JH, Boyko EJ, Davignon DR, Pecoraro RE. The health and functional status of veterans with diabetes. Diabetes Care 1994;17:318-21.

5 Bild DE, Selby JV, Sinnock P, Browner WS, Braveman P, Showstack JA. Lower extremity amputation in people with diabetes: epidemiology and prevention. Diabetes Care 1989;12:24-31.

6 Boulton AJM, Connor H. The diabetic foot 1988. Diabetic Med 1988;5:796-98.

7 Levin ME, O Neal FW. The diabetic foot. St. Louis: CV Mosby, 1988.

8 Most RS, Sinnock P. The epidemiology of lower extremity amputations in diabetic individuals. Diabetes Care 1983;6:87-91.

9 Centers for Disease Control and Prevention. Diabetes surveillance 1993. Atlanta: US Department of Health and Human Services, Public Health Service, 1993.

10 Nelson RG, Gohdes DM, Everhart JE, et al. Lower extremity amputations in NIDDM: 12-year follow-up study in Pima Indians. Diabetes Care 1988;11:8-16.

11 Lavery LA, Ashry HR, vanHoutum W, Pugh JA, Harkless LB, Basu S. Variation in the incidence and proportion of diabetes-related amputations in minorities. Diabetes Care 1996;19:48-52.

12 Selby JV, Zhang D. Risk factors for lower extremity amputation in persons with diabetes. Diabetes Care 1995;18:509-16.

13 Deerochanawong C, Home PD, Alberti KGMM. A survey of lower limb amputation in diabetic patients. Diabetic Med 1992;9:942-46.

14 Reiber GE, Boyko EJ, Smith DG. Lower extremity foot ulcers and amputations in diabetes. In: National Diabetes Data Group, eds. Diabetes in America. 2nd ed. Bethesda, Md: National Institutes of Health, 1995; NIH publication no. 95-1468:409-28.

15 Pell JP, Donnan PT, Fowkes FG, Ruckley CV. Quality of life following lower limb amputation for peripheral arterial disease. Eur J Vasc Surg 1993;7:448-51.

16 Loe H. Periodontal disease. The sixth complication of diabetes mellitus. Diabetes Care 1993;16:329-34.

17 American Diabetes Association. Detection and treatment of complications. In: Medical management of non-insulin-dependent (type II) diabetes. 3rd ed. Alexandria, Va: American Diabetes Association, 1994:66-86.

18 Reiber GE. Diabetic foot care. Financial implications and practice guidelines. Diabetes Care 1992;15(suppl 1):29-31.

19 Apelqvist J, Ragnarson-Tennvall G, Larsson J, Persson U. Long-term costs for foot ulcers in diabetic patients in a multidisciplinary setting. Foot Ankle Int 1995;16:388-94.

20 Ford ES, Wetterhall SF. The validity of diabetes on hospital discharge diagnoses. Diabetes 1991;40(suppl 1):449A.

21 Franklin GM, Kahn LB, Baxter J, Marshall JA, Hamman RF. Sensory neuropathy in non-insulin dependent diabetes mellitus. The San Luis Valley Diabetes Study. Am J Epidemiol 1990;131:633-43.

22 Holewski JJ, Stess RM, Graf PM, Grunfeld C. Aesthesiometry: quantification of cutaneous pressure sensation in diabetic peripheral neuropathy. J Rehabil Res Dev 1988;25(2):1-10.

23 Young MJ, Adams JE, Marshall A, Selby PL, Boulton AJM. Osteopenia, neurological dysfunction and the development of Charcot neuroarthropathy. Diabetes Care 1995;18:34-38.

24 Edmonds ME, Roberts VC, Watkins PJ. Blood flow in the diabetic neuropathic foot. Diabetologia 1982;22:9-15.

25 Flynn MD, Tooke JE. Aetiology of diabetic foot ulceration: a role for the microcirculation? Diabetic Med 1992;9:320-29.

26 Sanders LJ, Frykberg RG. Diabetic neuropathic osteoarthropathy: the Charcot foot. In: Frykberg RG, ed. The high risk foot in diabetes mellitus. New York: Churchill-Livingston, 1991:197-338.

27 Lippmann HI, Perotto A, Farrar R. The neuropathic foot of the diabetic. Bull New York Acad Med 1976;52:1159-78.

28 Reiber GE. Who is at risk of limb loss and what to do about it? J Rehabil Res Dev 1994;31:357-62.

29 Palumbo PH, Melton LJ. Peripheral vascular disease and diabetes. In: National Diabetes Data Group, eds. Diabetes in America. 2nd ed. Bethesda, Md: National Institutes of Health, 1995: NIH publication no. 95-1468:401-08.

30 Bell DS. Lower limb problems in diabetic patients: What are the causes? What are the remedies? Postgrad Med 1991;89: 237-40, 243-44.

31 Pecoraro R. The nonhealing diabetic ulcer: a major cause for limb loss. In: Barbul A, Caldwell MD, Eaglestein WH, et al, eds. Clinical and experimental approaches to dermal and epidermal repair: normal and chronic wounds. New York: Wiley-Liss, 1991:27-43.

32 Brand PW. Repetitive stress in the development of diabetic foot ulcers. In: Levin ME, O'Neal LW, eds. The diabetic foot. St. Louis: CV Mosby, 1988:83-90.

33 Pecoraro RE, Ahroni JH, Boyko EJ, Stensel VL. Chronology and determinants of tissue repair in diabetic lower extremity ulcers. Diabetes 1991;40:1305-13.

34 Ahroni JH. The care of lower extremity lesions in patients with diabetes. Nurse Pract Forum 1991;2:188-92.

35 Lipsky BA, Pecoraro RE, Larson SA, Hanley ME, Ahroni JH. Outpatient management of uncomplicated lower-extremity infections in diabetic patients. Arch Intern Med 1990;150:790-97.

36 American Diabetes Association. Position statement. Foot care in patients with diabetes mellitus. Diabetes Care 1998;21 (suppl 1):S54-55.

37 Duffy JC, Patout CA, Jr. Management of the insensitive foot in diabetes: lessons learned from Hansen's disease. Mil Med 1990;155:575-79.

38 Ahroni JH. The evaluation and development of diabetic foot risk stratification tools. Dissertation Abstracts International. 0453 (University Microfilms No. 9804430).

39 McNeely MJ, Boyko EJ, Ahroni JH, et al. The independent contributions of diabetic neuropathy and vasculopathy in foot ulceration. How great are the risks? Diabetes Care 1995;18:216-19.

40 Boyko EJ, Ahroni JH, Davignon D, Stensel V, Prigeon RL, Smith DG. Diagnostic utility of the history and physical examination for peripheral vascular disease among patients with diabetes mellitus. J Clin Epidemiol 1997;50:659-68.

41 Edmonds ME, Blundell MP, Morris ME, Thomas EM, Cotton LT, Watkins PJ. Improved survival of the diabetic foot: the role of a specialized foot clinic. Quarterly J Med 1986;60:763-71.

42 Fylling CP. Wound healing: an update. Comprehensive wound management for prevention of amputation. Conclusions. Diabetes Spectrum 1992;5:358-59.

43 The Diabetes Control and Complications Trial Research Group. The effect of intensive treatment of diabetes on the development and progression of long-term complications in insulin-dependent diabetes mellitus. N Engl J Med 1993;329:977-86.

44 Loe H, Genco RJ. Oral complications in diabetes. In: National Diabetes Data Group, eds. Diabetes in America. 2nd ed. Bethesda, Md: National Institutes of Health, 1995;NIH publication no. 95-1468:501-06.

45 Sznajder N, Carraro JJ, Rugna S, Sereday M. Periodontal findings in diabetic and non-diabetic patients. J Clin Periodont 1978;49:445-48.

46 Hugoson A, Thorstennson H, Falk H, Kuylenstierna J. Periodontal conditions in insulin-dependent diabetics. J Clin Periodont 1989;16:215-23.

47 Hallmon W, Measley BL. Implications of diabetes mellitus and periodontal disease. Diabetes Educ 1992;18:310-15.

SUGGESTED READINGS

Ahroni JH. Teaching foot care creatively and successfully. Diabetes Educ 1993;19:320-25.

Betschart JM, Betschart JE. Periodontal disease and diabetes mellitus. Diabetes Spectrum 1997;2:112-18.

Centers for Disease Control and Prevention. The prevention and treatment of complications of diabetes mellitus: a guide for primary care practitioners. Atlanta, Ga: US Department of Health and Human Services, 1991; DHHS publication no. 93-3464.

Holdren RD, Patton LL. Oral conditions associated with diabetes mellitus. Diabetes Spectrum 1993;6:11-17.

Haas LB. Lower extremity amputations: strategies for prevention. Diabetes Spectrum 1995;8:206-31.

"Feet Can Last a Lifetime" patient and professional materials available from the National Diabetes Information Clearing House (301-654-3327) or at http://www.niddk.gov under health information.

DIABETES AND THE LIFE CYCLE

DIABETES AND THE LIFE CYCLE

Childhood and Adolescence 17

Jean Betschart MSN, MN, CPNP, CDE
Department of Endocrinology Diabetes and Metabolism
Children's Hospital of Pittsburgh
Pittsburgh, Pennsylvania

INTRODUCTION

1   The impact of diabetes is unique for each developmental stage.

2   Diabetes can profoundly affect the normal physical, cognitive, and emotional developmental stages of childhood and adolescence. Likewise, each developmental stage has implications for diabetes management and care.

3   The unrelenting demands of diabetes management also affect families and their social network and may disrupt the developmental tasks of the child within the family.

4   Understanding the unique considerations of diabetes management in children and adolescents, the impact of diabetes on normal development, the effect of the diagnosis on parents, and the dynamic nature of managing diabetes in youth can help health professionals provide appropriate support, flexible care, and age-specific education.

OBJECTIVES

Upon completion of this chapter, the learner will be able to

1   State the major developmental concerns about diabetes in infants and toddlers, preschool/school-age children, and preadolescents/adolescents.

2   Explain how the care, management, and education of children and adolescents with diabetes are different from that of adults, focusing on meal planning, insulin therapy, blood glucose monitoring, and exercise.

3   Describe the parental burden of managing a child's diabetes and the benefit of social networks and support.

4   Describe the acute and chronic complications of diabetes in childhood.

5   Identify age-appropriate educational materials and considerations for each age group.

INCIDENCE

1   Type 1 diabetes occurs in children and adolescents at a rate of 13.8 to 16.9 per 100,000 for Caucasian American children and from 3.3 to 11.8 per 100,000 for African American children.[1] Approximately 100 000

children and adolescents under the age of 19 years have diabetes.[2] The worldwide prevalence and incidence of type 1 diabetes varies from one geographic location to another, with the highest incidence being in the Scandinavian countries of Sweden, Finland, and Norway, and lowest incidence in Japan. Evidence[3] suggests that the incidence of type 1 diabetes is increasing globally.

2 Approximately 95% of new onset diabetes in children and adolescents is type 1. Nontype 1 diabetes in children, once believed to be a disease of predominantly obese adults, is on the increase in the pediatric population.[4]

A The incidence of type 1 diabetes increases with age and peaks in at puberty.

B Seasonal variations have also been reported, with diabetes being diagnosed more frequently in the winter than in the summer months.[3]

3 The remaining cases are either nontype 1 diabetes in youth, which includes maturity onset diabetes in youth (MODY), atypical diabetes, secondary diabetes, or gestational diabetes.

A Recent progress in further defining genetic typing and the ability to easily identify islet cell antibodies (ICA) will allow a more accurate definition of the subtypes of nontype 1 diabetes.

B There has been an acute rise in the prevalence and incidence of nontype 1 diabetes in children in the United States.[4] Children at greatest risk for nontype 1 diabetes are those of African American, Jamaican, Native American, and Mexican American heritage.[5]

C The presentation, onset of symptoms, and clinical course of nontype 1 diabetes should be carefully followed to further classify subtypes. As one subtype, MODY, should be suspected in any youth with new-onset diabetes who presents with physical characteristics such as obesity, acanthosis nigricans, and/or hypertension. MODY is characterized by impaired insulin secretion with minimal or no defects in insulin action. MODY can now be further defined into three or more genotypes, which are inherited in an autosomal dominant pattern.[6]

4 Diagnostic criteria for children and adolescents are generally the same as those for adults (see Chapter 7, Pathophysiology of the Diabetes Disease State).

TABLE 17.1. POSSIBLE COMPLICATIONS OF DIABETES IN CHILDHOOD AND ADOLESCENCE

Acute Complications	• Hypoglycemia (especially unrecognized in young children) • Ketoacidosis • Vaginal yeast infections/thrush • Cellulitis due to infection/injury (rare)
Chronic Complications*	• Hypertension • Nephropathy • Neuropathy • Retinopathy • Eating disorders • Depression • Cognitive deficits
Other Complications	• Lipohypertrophy and lipoatrophy at injection sites • Mauriac syndrome (rare; characterized by insulin insufficiency, growth and pubertal delay) • Necrobiosis lipoidica diabeticorum (rare)

*not usually seen before puberty

GUIDELINES FOR THERAPY FOR CHILDREN AND ADOLESCENTS

1   General goals of therapy for children or adolescents with diabetes include

   A   Achieve normal growth and development

   B   Optimal glycemic control

   C   Minimal acute or chronic complications (Table 17.1)

   D   Positive psychosocial adjustment to diabetes

2   There are unique considerations for using insulin therapy with children and adolescents.

   A   Adequate growth and appropriate pubertal development are important indices of insulin sufficiency. Children with type 1 diabetes have normal onset of puberty and normal sexual maturation; however, diminished height gain after diagnosis has been reported.[7] When insulin insufficiency occurs during childhood and adolescence, normal growth and development may be delayed. Poor growth or weight gain should be evaluated to be sure that it is not a result of other medical or psychosocial problems.

- Mauriac syndrome, a diabetes-related growth disorder, is characterized by delayed linear growth, delayed sexual maturation, hepatomegaly, and among other findings.[8] Although rarely seen today in its severe form, mild variations are seen in children and adolescents with poorly controlled diabetes.

- Height and weight need to be carefully plotted at 3- to 4-month intervals on a standard growth chart. If height and weight fall below the child's normal growth percentile, the child should be evaluated for glycemic control, insulin sufficiency, nutritional adequacy, or the presence of other endocrine disorders or disease.

B Therapy endeavors to balance the fluctuating food intake, insulin requirements, and exercise levels that are characteristic of the growing and developing child. Making frequent adjustments in insulin dosages to account for daily differences in activity and food is usually necessary.

- It is important to be able to adjust insulin to avoid hypoglycemia and hyperglycemia.

- Commercially prepared premixed insulins generally do not allow for the flexibility of daily dosage adjustment based on blood glucose values and exercise levels, which are especially variable in children. However, they may be useful for some adolescents who are unable or unwilling to regularly adjust insulin doses or have difficulty accurately mixing insulin.

- Young children may require dose adjustments in increments of one half unit.

C Approximately 70% of children and adolescents with diabetes move into a remission phase (or "honeymoon" phase), requiring decreased insulin dosages.[9] This phase can be highly variable in duration, ranging approximately from two weeks to two years after diagnosis.

- Recent evidence suggests that beta cell preservation may be enhanced by provision of basal insulin. Therefore, maintaining tight glycemic control without frequent or severe hypoglycemia during remission by providing round the clock basal insulin may be desirable.[10-12]

D Most children require approximately 1 unit of insulin per kg of body weight per day (other than during remission).[8] A range of 0.5 to 1.5 units/kg/day is acceptable and allows for individual differences based on age, activity, eating habits, and metabolic requirements.

E School-age children are frequently capable of giving themselves insulin injections with supervision. When determining the ability of a child to perform self-care skills, it is important to identify readiness and individual considerations (locus of control, maturity, and family factors) rather than define specific age ranges for task performance.

- Broad differences have been identified among children and adolescents in their ability to master and take responsibility for self-care tasks.

- Parental involvement and/or supervision appears to enhance self-care behaviors and glycemic control.[13,14]

- Diabetes self-management education programs for children can be effective for facilitating greater responsibility for self care.[15]

F Usual injection sites for young children are the legs, arms, and the upper/outer quadrant of the buttocks.

- School-age children and adolescents can be encouraged to use the abdomen on a regular basis. However, abdominal injections may not be advisable in children with little subcutaneous abdominal fat or in very young children. For these children, the abdomen is usually the least-favored site.

- Rotating sites in a consistent manner (eg, arms in the morning, legs in the evening) may help provide a consistent rate of absorption.

- It is not yet clear whether the findings from adult studies about insulin absorption are applicable to children.[16]

- Using 30-gauge (short) needles may provide more comfortable injections for the very young or the very lean.

- Avoiding even mildly hypertrophied sites is recommended to enhance insulin absorption.

3 The principles of medical nutrition therapy for children and adolescents differ from those for adults because children usually do not require weight reduction, and children need to focus on consuming sufficient calories and protein for growth and pubertal development.

A The specific goals of medical nutritional therapy for children are shown in Table 17.2.

B Nutritional recommendations for children and adolescents are based on a nutrition assessment.

- The distribution of calories from fat and carbohydrate can vary and can be individualized based on the nutrition assessment and treatment program.[17]

TABLE 17.2. SPECIFIC GOALS OF MEDICAL NUTRITION THERAPY FOR CHILDREN

- Maintaining normal growth, weight, and sexual development
- Preventing obesity, excessive glycemic excursions, hypoglycemia, and hyperlipidemia
- Controlling blood pressure
- Preventing future complications of diabetes

- The benefits and risks of reducing protein intake in children without nephropathy have not been established.

C Meal plans must be individualized to meet individual food preferences, cultural influences, family eating patterns and schedules, age, weight, activity level and insulin action peaks.

- Most children over the age of 6 years require three meals per day plus snacks in midafternoon and at bedtime.
- Children under the age of 6 years or children who must go more than 4 or 5 hours between breakfast and lunch usually require a midmorning snack.
- When older children and adolescents dislike having to eat during schooltime, insulin dosages can usually be adjusted to make snacks at school unnecessary.
- Unless the child or adolescent is over his or her ideal body weight, the usual caloric guidelines for healthy children are followed. For example, it is not uncommon for a normal-weight, very active adolescent boy with diabetes to require between 3500 and 4500 calories per day. Carbohydrate counting principles are the same for children as adults and can allow greater flexibility and alternatives in a child's meal plan.
- Meals and snacks are timed to correspond with the peak action of the injected insulin. For this reason, it is generally recommended that children and teens try to not deviate from their normal schedules by more than 1 hour. In the summer, for example, the daily schedule can be started later if the child wants to sleep later.
- Children and teens who sleep very late in the morning may awaken hypoglycemic because it has been a long time since they have eaten, or hyperglycemic due to insulin insufficiency. A reasonable

rule of thumb might be to always have breakfast by 9 AM. A child who wants to sleep later can take the scheduled insulin, eat breakfast, and then go back to bed.

4 Although exercise may not always result in better glycemic control in every child with diabetes, physical activity is encouraged to promote cardiovascular fitness and long-term weight control and to enhance social interaction and self-esteem through team play.[18]

    A Physically fit adolescents with diabetes have greater insulin sensitivity.[19]

    B Physical training in young children with a short duration of diabetes may improve glycemic control when their HbA_{1c} is high. However, changes in HbA_{1c} appear to be independent of changes in fitness.[20]

    C Additional carbohydrate with protein or fat may be eaten before exercising. Typical preactivity snacks might be a peanut butter sandwich or cheese and crackers with skim or lowfat milk or juice. Adolescents may prefer to use drinks such as various sport drinks or fruit juice before, during, and after sports because of the difficulty of exercising with a full stomach.

    D School personnel, especially gym teachers and coaches, need to be informed that children and adolescents with diabetes require a snack before and/or sometimes during strenuous exercise. They must also be prepared to identify and treat hypoglycemia with a form of readily available glucose.

    E Because of the prolonged hypoglycemic effect of exercise, parents are frequently concerned about the possibility of their child developing hypoglycemia during the night. To replenish glycogen stores depleted during high-intensity exercise, a child or adolescent with diabetes may require additional food at bedtime and at 3 or 4 AM. Bedtime monitoring may help identify children who are at risk for nocturnal hypoglycemia[21] (see Chapter 9, Exercise, for additional information about exercise and hypoglycemia).

5 Monitoring of blood glucose and urine ketone levels must be done regularly to enable parents and children to interpret any symptoms and make the necessary adjustments in insulin doses.

    A In general, the recommended frequency for blood glucose monitoring for children is before each meal and bedtime snack, with additional tests performed if the child has symptoms of hypoglycemia, hyperglycemia, ketosis, or illness. For those trying to maintain tight glycemic control, 3 or 4 AM monitoring may be recommended on a weekly basis.

B Testing blood glucose levels before lunch may be necessary for children and adolescents on multiple daily injections and those who change insulin doses based on glycemic patterns. The child and school personnel may need assistance in finding a safe and comfortable way for the child to perform these required self-management tasks.

C The general recommendation regarding urine ketone testing for children and adolescents is once daily in the morning, when blood glucose levels exceed 240 mg/dL (13.3 mmol/L), and when illness occurs.

D Ketones may be present in the urine following hypoglycemia.
- Persistent small amounts of urine ketones found in the morning may be indicative of nocturnal hypoglycemia.
- To verify nocturnal hypoglycemia, parents may be asked to test their child's blood glucose level between 1 and 4 AM.

E There has been no consensus on adapting glycemic goals for pediatric use.
- Goals must be individualized with each family based on age, ability to recognize hypoglycemia, self-management capabilities, and history of severe hypoglycemic episodes or seizures.
- Target ranges for blood glucose levels of children and adolescents vary depending on the judgement of the provider or health care team and the individual goals set with the child and his/her parents.
- Guidelines for target levels can range from 80 to 120 mg/dL (4.4 to 6.7 mmol/L) at fasting and from 80 to 180 mg/dL (4.4 to 9.9 mmol/L) at other times of the day.
- Permissible levels for children under 6 years of age may range from 90 to 130 mg/dL (4.9 to 7.1 mmol/L) at fasting and from 90 to 200 mg/dL (4.9 to 11.1 mmol/L) at other times.[22]

F Blood glucose monitoring results are also used to help parents determine food types and quantities for balancing activities and food intake or providing a bedtime snack to avoid nocturnal hypoglycemia.

6 Providing appropriate family education and support is essential.

A Optimally, all family members of the child or adolescent with diabetes (including grandparents, babysitters, and other caregivers when possible) are educated regarding diabetes management.

B The educational process needs to be an open-ended, ongoing experience between the child, family, friends, and the diabetes team.[23]

C Developing effective stress management/coping skills and problem-solving skills is considered as important to successful therapy as insulin administration, meal planning, blood glucose monitoring, and exercise[24] (see Chapter 5, Behavior Change, for information about coping skills).

D Recognize and encourage individual efforts to create more effective coping strategies which support self-care and problem solving should be recognized and encouraged.[23]

IMPACT ON THE FAMILY

1 The role of the parent varies greatly depending on the child's age and ability to perform self-care activities.

2 Daily adjustment of insulin, food, monitoring, and exercise are part of successful diabetes self-management. These tasks are either assumed or supervised by a parent or caretaker.

3 These demands of daily diabetes management can be quite stressful to parents and cause worry, anxiety, and family disruption. In some instances, both the child and the family respond by developing dysfunctional methods of coping.[25,26]

4 Children with diabetes who come from families with minimal support, lower socioeconomic status, or a chaotic home environment may be at greater risk for acute and chronic complications.

5 The educator can help provide parents with the guidance and support needed by teaching extended family members, encouraging, counseling, closely reviewing blood glucose monitoring results, and enhancing family support networks.

6 Many families who have a child with diabetes have health insurance. However, these families still incur larger out-of-pocket healthcare expenses than families who do not have a member with diabetes. Families coping with diabetes may have additional financial burdens.[27]

Issues of Childhood and Adolescent Development

1 A number of developmental factors must be considered in the care of the infant and toddler (birth to 2 years) with diabetes.

A Normal growth and development for infants and toddlers progresses rapidly and predictably, from large muscle developmental tasks to fine motor skills.

• Infants may require significant amounts of sleep, and toddlers usually need daily naps.

• Parents and caretakers can be taught ways to fit naps into the child's schedule at times that do not interfere with meals or snacks.

• Regular scheduled nighttime feedings are important for avoiding hypoglycemia in infants and the very young.

B In normal development, differentiation and "hatching" begin at around 4 to 5 months of age; tentative experimentation with separation-individuation begins at around 6 months; and early practicing of crawling begins at around 9 months.

• Infants 10 to 12 months of age practice walking and manual skills and have been described by Mahler as having "a love affair with the world."[28]

• As toddlers approach 2 years of age, they begin to separate and individuate, testing their separateness by saying no and behaving in an oppositional manner. Most parents know this stage as the "terrible twos." Providing choices at this age can give the toddler with diabetes some control, but the choices need to be framed in such a way that the child is not allowed to make important decisions. For example, asking "Which finger shall we choose?" works better than asking "Do you want to do your blood test now?"

C Infants usually nurse or eat predictably.

• A 3- to 4-hour flexible feeding schedule is effective for maintaining a steady blood glucose level.

• In order to prevent hypoglycemia, infants older than 4 months of age may be given additional cereal along with their bottle at feedings prior to the peak effect of insulin.

• Balancing food with insulin and activity to prevent hypoglycemia can be challenging, particularly because of the sporadic and spontaneous nature of physical activity in infants.

D Appetite may become erratic in toddlers when rapid growth begins to subside. Food and feedings can become problematic for parents and caretakers of a picky toddler.

- Toddlers usually eat three meals and three snacks daily, but additional snacks may be required.
- The normal sporadic eating habits of toddlers can be worrisome for parents who try to balance food with insulin and activity.
- Normal activity in toddlers is sporadic and spontaneous, interspersed with sudden bursts of whole body movement.
- To prevent hypoglycemia, activity needs to be balanced with intake of extra food or beverages such as milk or juice.
- If a toddler will not eat, offer favorite foods and substitute alternative choices of carbohydrate-containing beverages (eg, milk, juice). Avoid becoming a short-order cook for a demanding toddler.
- Although there is limited research on the use of lispro insulin (Humalog) in children, clinical observations suggest that giving this insulin analog to children with or after a meal or snack after parents observe how much and what foods are consumed can be effective. Currently, however, rapid-acting insulin has not been approved by the FDA for use in children.

E Infants and young children may become dehydrated quickly because they have a large percentage of body surface area and are unable to retain large volumes of fluids taken by mouth.

- Dehydration can take place rapidly in any child when illness occurs; this effect is enhanced in the infant or toddler with diabetes.
- The potential for rapid dehydration makes infants and young children with diabetes especially vulnerable when illness, vomiting, or diarrhea occurs. Instruct parents to notify their diabetes care team or physician whenever a young child is ill and carefully monitor the child's blood glucose and urine ketone levels.
- Intravenous hydration may be necessary if vomiting does not subside and/or the child shows signs of dehydration, urinary ketones, ketoacidosis, or hypoglycemia (see Chapter 15, Illness and Surgery, for information about diabetes management during illness).

F Infants and toddlers are developmentally unable to effectively communicate symptoms of hypoglycemia and must rely on the observations of caretakers for recognition and treatment.

- Signs of hypoglycemia in an infant may be pallor, listlessness, crying, clammy skin, irritability, sleepiness, hunger, restless sleep and/or shakiness.
- Toddlers may also exhibit uncoordinated gait, stumbling, or inactivity.

G Onset of diabetes early in life is associated with impaired cognitive functions (eg, abstract and visual reasoning) or attention deficits. The reason for cognitive differences in those with diabetes is not yet clear. However, the differences may be due to undetected hypoglycemia or a seizure resulting from hypoglycemia.[29,30]

- Consensus has not been reached regarding treatment guidelines for hypoglycemia in young children. However, it is generally agreed that glucose levels in young children need to be as tightly controlled as possible without risking severe or frequent hypoglycemia.
- Multiple-dose insulin therapy does not appear to increase the incidence of profound hypoglycemia as long as psychosocial support and active education are provided.[31] The number of injections is not necessarily related to the tightness of glycemic control.

H A basal insulin such as a split-dose of NPH insulin given morning and evening may be effective for balancing frequent feedings and providing a steady-state level of insulin.[22]

I Recommended carbohydrate intake for the treatment of hypoglycemia in the infant is shown in Table 17.3.

TABLE 17.3. RECOMMENDED CARBOHYDRATE INTAKE FOR TREATING HYPOGLYCEMIA IN INFANTS

Carbohydrate, g	Source	Quantity
5 to 10	Karo syrup	1 to 2 teaspoons
15	Undiluted baby fruit juice or glucose water	4 oz
15 to 30	Cake decorator frosting or commercially prepared glucose gels	1 small tube

* Honey should be avoided in infants for treatment due to association with infantile botulism.

J Parents of infants and toddlers must rely on frequent blood glucose monitoring to distinguish normal infant and toddler behaviors from symptoms of hypoglycemia because infants and toddlers are often defiant, demanding, sleepy, or cranky as part of their normal development. Test results help parents make daily management decisions.

K Blood for glucose monitoring can be obtained from the child's fingers, big toes, and external, lateral aspect of the heel.

L The burden of responsibility for constant care can be quite difficult for parents and caretakers of children with diabetes. Supportive extended family, friends, or babysitters may be needed to offer relief by sharing in the care of these children.

M Blood glucose readings in young children can be erratic, at best. Parents may need additional support during this difficult period from members of the diabetes treatment team who have experience in pediatric diabetes.

2 Developmental considerations of the preschool-age child (3 to 5 years) include many of the concerns pertinent to the toddler in addition to specific developmental issues of the preschool child.

    A Physical growth slows after the toddler stage but is still relatively rapid. Fine motor skills continue to develop in the preschool child and cognitive language develops rapidly as children learn to play and enjoy stories.

        • Children of this age engage in magical thinking; they may believe that if they think or wish something they can cause it to happen.[32] For example, when Susan was admitted to the hospital with diabetes, her 4-year-old brother, who earlier that day had shouted angrily that he wished she would go away, later revealed that he thought he had caused Susan's diabetes to happen.

        • Separation-individuation issues continue during this stage as children learn to define themselves as being separate from their parents.

    B Preschool children are concerned about the intactness of their bodies.

        • Fear of intrusive procedures is characteristic of this age, and children may act out their anxieties at the times when insulin injections and blood testing are done.

        • Preschool-age children have a difficult time understanding the need for insulin injections and blood tests, particularly if they are feeling well.

        • The use of bandaids is helpful to the preschool child, as they help to address concerns about body integrity.

    C The advantages and use of play therapy have been well recognized.[33-35] Children establish a balance between their inner life and reality by continually exploring and testing through their play.

- Guided play, or play therapy, provides a forum and vehicle for children to express their concerns and provides a mechanism for emotional release by helping the child learn to deal with these issues through creative expression.
- Giving a child a "safe" syringe, family and health professional dolls, meter supplies, and other diabetes paraphernalia will provide an opportunity for supervised play.
- Children may choose one of the dolls to have diabetes and will play out their personal life issues and concerns about having diabetes through doll or puppet play.

D Normal eating patterns for preschool age children are often unpredictable.

- This variability in eating is not considered harmful but rather normal from a developmental point of view. For example, children may want to eat only bananas and peanut butter for days at a time, then they will switch to grilled cheese and apples.
- Increased appetites tend to precede growth spurts and, food intake is usually balanced over a period of weeks.
- This erratic eating makes glucose control difficult for this age group because parents worry about hypoglycemia when their children will not eat.
- Parents can allow the child some control over eating by providing reasonable choices without allowing the child to control eating situations. By giving young children limited choices, parents may avoid a battle of wills.

E Undetected hypoglycemia is a risk in the preschool years.

- Frequent blood glucose testing helps in the management decision-making process.
- Many preschool-age children are able to identify symptoms of hypoglycemia and can alert adults.

F Infants, toddlers, and preschool-age children are especially vulnerable to elevated blood glucose values and ketonuria when acute infections of childhood occur (eg, otitis media, vomiting illnesses, or the common cold). Conversely, hypoglycemia can also result.

- Wide excursions in blood glucose levels are common and can be frustrating and frightening for parents.
- Dehydration and diabetic ketoacidosis (DKA) can develop rapidly.

- Intravenous therapy may be necessary either to prevent further dehydration and treat ketoacidosis, or to acutely provide glucose to treat hypoglycemia if the child is unable to eat or drink.

G Educating the staff in preschool or daycare centers is critical for the management of acute and chronic diabetes-related problems. Recognition, detection, and treatment of hypoglycemia are essential. The number of day care centers able and willing to accommodate blood glucose monitoring and other procedures is increasing as a result of the Americans with Disabilities Act.

3 The school-age child (6 to 10 years) is better coordinated physically, has a vivid fantasy life, speaks fluently, has a conscience, and is able to share and cooperate. This is the age of concrete reasoning, and repetition compulsion is played out in games and skills.

A Although the school-age child has increasing need for independence, the power and protection of the parent is very important to the child's feeling of well-being.

B In terms of diabetes management, the parent's role is to perform diabetes care tasks while moving the child toward independence through supervision, encouragement, and support.

- At times the child may be willing and able to perform blood glucose monitoring, prepare his or her own snacks, and administer insulin. At other times, the parent will need to perform the test or administer insulin. Parent-child sharing of these responsibilities is essential during the school-age years.[13]

- Parents of the school-age child with diabetes may be more understandably protective than other parents. This attitude can make it difficult for the child with diabetes to attain the same level of independence as a nondiabetic child of the same age.

- Diabetes management planning for special events and activities is important to promote independence and minimize differences. By planning ahead, most children can safely participate in all childhood activities.

C One of the greatest drives of school-age children is to avoid failure. They acquire strategies to keep from feeling different from peers. Monitoring, eating special snacks, taking injections, and fear of peers witnessing symptoms of hypoglycemia can alter diabetes self-care routines and ultimately affect self-esteem.

- Helping the child to fit diabetes management into normal routines both at home and at school can minimize these differences. A teacher, for example, can implement a snack break for all children in the classroom.

D Because school-age children spend a large portion of their day in school, it is reasonable to expect school personnel to become informed about diabetes care. School districts and personnel are obligated to provide an individualized plan to accommodate a child's special healthcare needs.

- Certain federal laws address these issues. The Education for All Handicapped Children Act of 1975, commonly referred to as Public Law No. 94-142, is a federal mandate that entitles all physically, developmentally, emotionally, and other health-impaired children to free, appropriate public education.
- The other law, Section 504, is a more general civil rights law that makes it illegal for any agency or organization that receives federal funds to discriminate in any way against qualified people with disabilities.[36]

E Beginning each school year with a conference involving the child with diabetes, parents, and school personnel is an effective way to establish a plan of care, communication, and a means of addressing important issues and concerns.

- The administration of glucagon in schools is highly variable, depending on state laws. When a physician's order is provided, the school must designate a person to administer glucagon to a hypoglycemic child with diabetes just as they are required to give epinephrine to an acutely allergic child who sustains a bee sting.
- Parents need to provide basic information about diabetes, the causes of hypoglycemia, the specific requirements of their child's daily management plan, and their child's usual signs and symptoms. This information is used to develop a plan of care that satisfies the needs of the child, parents, and school policies. This written plan includes who will administer the care and the location of the treatment supplies.
- When scheduling changes occur in the daily school routine (eg, field trips or parties) the school needs to notify parents prior to the event so that appropriate care can be administered.

- A review of meal plan basics provides school personnel with a general awareness of what the child eats. Providing a plan to enable the child to manage parties and snacks in school is also beneficial.

F Children with diabetes can have feelings of sadness, anxiety, friendlessness, and isolation.[25] Support groups, individual counseling, or diabetes camps can be useful for assisting the child in resolving these feelings. Determining the child's individual coping skills, supporting adaptive strategies, and providing interventions should be initiated early.[23]

ISSUES OF ADOLESCENT DEVELOPMENT

1 There are large differences between the three stages of adolescence. These stages are early adolescence or preadolescence (12 years), middle adolescence (13 to 15 years), and late adolescence (16 to 18 years).

A At no other time of life do environment and heredity produce such a variance in individual development. Broad differences normally occur in emotional, social, and physical development.

- In girls, the onset of breast budding and the growth of pubic hair occur at an average age of 10 to 11 years; in boys, the growth of pubic hair and the enlargement of testicles occur at an average age of 12 to 16 years.
- Changes in size, weight, body proportions, muscular development, strength, coordination, and skill are seen at this age. These changes may occur slowly or rapidly.
- The age of onset of pubescent growth is determined by genetic familial factors but can also be affected by culture, economy, nutrition, health, and habitat. Poor glycemic control can delay the onset of puberty.

B Puberty is characterized by the onset of hormonal activity, which is under the influence of the central nervous system, especially the hypothalamus and pituitary gland. The major effects of puberty are the increased production of adrenocortical and gonadal hormones and the production of mature ova and spermatozoa.

- Metabolic control, as represented by increasing glycosylated hemoglobin levels, deteriorates during adolescence despite significantly higher insulin doses.[37,38]

- It has been suggested that the hormonal changes of puberty cause a state of relative insulin resistance as a result of declining peripheral insulin action and changing counterregulatory hormonal responses.[39] However, the etiology of the insulin resistance associated with puberty is not fully understood and is likely multifactorial.

C Certain important characteristics mark the normal period of early adolescence.
- The child becomes acutely aware of body image.
- Dependent versus independent struggles begin between parent and child.
- There may be great vacillation between childlike and adult behaviors.
- There is less social involvement with family and more with peers.
- Parental criticism becomes difficult to accept.
- Turmoil and conflict within the parent-child relationship may begin.

D Certain important characteristics are typical of the normal period of middle adolescence.
- Peer group allegiance develops.
- Greater experimentation and risk taking occurs.
- Physical and social activity increases.
- Sexual relationships emerge and are important.
- Formal operational thinking begins with the beginning of abstract reasoning.
- Teens and parents often struggle and experience conflict in their relationship.

E Certain important characteristics are part of the normal period of late adolescence.
- Cognitive abilities and abstract morals develop.
- The peer group loses its primary importance.
- There is increasing separation from the family unit.
- Teens become future oriented.
- Conscience is able to stand without support or validity from others.

F Diabetes affects normal adolescent development.
- Identity and self-image concerns can revolve around diabetes concerns such as the appearance of the injection site or self-identification as "a diabetic."
- Normal independence issues may be thwarted as a result of parental protectiveness or the teen's failure to assume responsibility for self-care.

- Physical growth and development have a strong impact on a teen's self-image.[40,41] Adolescents with diabetes can become particularly concerned about their growth and sexual maturation even though they usually display normal growth patterns and normal onset and progression of pubertal development.
- Attitudes of experimentation and rebellion and risk-taking behaviors normally associated with adolescence can revolve around diabetes issues such as taking insulin regularly, monitoring, and the quality and quantity of food consumption.

G It is essential for educators to be aware of and address issues of substance abuse (tobacco use, alcohol consumption, drug use) and sexual practices and attitudes in their assessment of adolescent diabetes management.

- Risk taking and lack of health promoting behaviors is widespread, especially among adolescents.
- Family dynamics, family health beliefs, communication style, and support networks all affect adolescents' ability to do what is necessary to manage diabetes.
- Adolescent females with diabetes must be taught the importance of planning pregnancy and meticulously using contraception. Their instruction should include a frank dialogue about the potential fetal/ maternal health risks of an unplanned pregnancy in a woman with diabetes.
- Discuss sexual issues in a relaxed, comfortable manner. Comfort in discussing sexual topics comes with practice and a sense of control over the subject matter. The comfort level of the educator is communicated to the patient and sets the tone for the discussions.
- Begin sex education in the preteen ages so that it becomes a routine part of diabetes assessment and education.
- The use of unbiased, gender-neutral language is important when assessing sexual orientation, practice, frequency, use of contraceptives, and consistency of contraceptive practices.
- Point out that abstinence is the only 100% effective contraceptive method for preventing pregnancy, STDs, and AIDS. Emphasize the importance of using condoms at all times to prevent STDs and AIDS.
- Include the female's partner, whenever possible, as part of the contraception and other education process. It is important to ask for the date of last intercourse and whether the woman or couple wants to have a baby.[42]

H The privilege of driving is an adult responsibility. Health professionals and parents of teens who are approaching the age to drive should begin discussions with the teen about the responsibility of safety when driving. Guidelines for safety include:
- responsible diabetes self-care
- desire or motivation to consider the safety of self and others
- self-monitoring before driving
- testing blood glucose at two hour intervals while driving
- carrying appropriate supplies
- wearing a medical ID
- never driving if there are signs of hypoglycemia

2 Several important conditions in children and adolescents may be associated with poor glycemic control and/or health outcomes.

   A Biologically, the adolescent's earlier and greater epinephrine responses to moderate drops in blood glucose concentrations, combined with heightened insulin resistance, may contribute to some of the lability in metabolic control.

   B A chaotic home environment, chronic family stress or parental over or under involvement can contribute to poorer metabolic control for children and adolescents as a result of increased epinephrine responses to physical or psychological neglect or abuse, or to the frank omission of insulin.

   C Knowledge and cognitive maturity levels are important elements of diabetes self-management. Occasionally, developmental delay or learning disabilities may hamper understanding of diabetes care.

   D Emotional disturbance can cause disequilibrium and precipitate frequent episodes of ketoacidosis. Insulin insufficiency may occur in response to physical or emotional stress, resulting in overproduction of counterregulatory hormones.
- Early adolescent girls who are extraordinarily sensitive to emotional stress are most likely to demonstrate recurrent DKA.[22]
- Repeated episodes of DKA warrant investigation, as DKA can be deliberately induced to displace family tensions. Family patterns of interaction may reveal family enmeshment, rigidity, poor communication and overprotectiveness.[43]
- Treatment may include family counseling and aggressive insulin therapy when illness, stress, or ketones appear.

E Adolescents frequently develop DKA because they fail to take their insulin.

- Insulin doses can be missed when parents are not involved in an adolescent's diabetes management.[44]
- Adolescent females may decide to skip injections for the purpose of weight control, which is a variant of an eating disorder.

F Diabetes and the regimen may provide the right conditions for those who are at risk of developing an eating disorder because of the focus on food and discipline required.

- Educators need to be aware of the possibility of pathologic eating behaviors, particularly among adolescent and young adult females (see Chapter 6, Psychological Disorders, for more information about eating disorders in people with diabetes).

KEY EDUCATIONAL CONSIDERATIONS

1 Parents, friends, neighbors, caretakers, babysitters, and any other support persons can either help or hinder a child's adjustment to diabetes and self-care. For this reason, it is important to be consistent and provide the same information to all who are involved with the child.

2 When working with children and adolescents, learning materials, content, and expectations need to be age-appropriate, and the teaching approach and schedule matched to the age and attention span of the individual child.

A Educating the preschool child is often limited to spontaneously occurring opportunities that revolve around diabetes management and questions asked by the child.

- Young children often do well when provided with simple choices such as "Do you want raisins or a banana?"
- The need for insulin injections and fingersticks can be explained in terms of "keeping you healthy."
- Preschool and school-age children process what they have learned primarily through play. Doll play or puppet play are valuable teaching/learning methods for children of this age.
- An essential topic for the young children is hypoglycemia: identifying the symptoms, knowing that treatment involves consuming juice or food, and recognizing the need to tell an adult about any symptom of hypoglycemia. Discussing how the child felt before each hypo-

glycemic episode can help a child recognize the symptoms the next time. Many young children are able to identify the symptoms of hypoglycemia and tell an adult about what they are experiencing.

- Parents often are concerned that they may not recognize an episode of hypoglycemia. They are likely to benefit from reading a detailed description of the symptoms of hypoglycemia and/or seeing a video about hypoglycemia.

B The school-age child needs to be assessed individually for learning readiness, which can be highly variable in this age group. School-age children are able to learn most effectively when the information about diabetes is presented in an interesting and fun way. They also have the ability to learn concrete survival skills quite well.

- Games, puzzles, and videos are effective educational tools.
- The school-age child also learns well through play.

C Most health professionals agree that learning educational content is not the most difficult task for the adolescent with diabetes but rather assuming responsibility for self-management.

- Adolescents learn best when the educational content is pertinent to adolescent issues. Topics of particular concern to adolescents are diabetes and sexuality (including contraception), alcohol and tobacco use, drugs, diabetes identification, driving issues, and special concerns such as party advice, managing diabetes and sports, prom-night management, career information, and travel.
- Educational materials can include books and videos, but discussion groups among peers are often most effective.

D Educators can use a number of strategies for dealing with teens with diabetes.

- Enhance self-esteem by promoting feelings of normalcy. The behavior of teens frequently matches their self-image.
- Develop a primary relationship with teens and a collaborative one with parents.
- Provide honest communication and don't minimize feelings.
- Listen to what is being said as well as what is not being said. Negative feelings exist before negative acts.
- Solve problems together and negotiate treatment strategies.
- Enlist the assistance of a supportive person (boyfriend, girlfriend, sibling).
- Candidly discuss perceptions of barriers.

- Provide ongoing positive reinforcement.
- Convey enjoyment in working with adolescents.

E Diabetes camps provide an excellent setting for facilitating formal and informal learning. Children and adolescents learn from each other in an environment where they share the common thread of having diabetes. They can relate to each other in terms of similar feelings, concerns, and experiences from living with diabetes; no one feels different because of the diabetes.

F Support groups also promote learning and are most effective when structured around an activity that is fun.

G Factors that contribute to impaired self-care are family dynamics (including the family's health belief model), communication style, emotional tone, and inappropriate expectations of children and adolescents.

H It is important for both children and adolescents that blood glucose results be treated as information only and not as bad or good numbers. Less judgmental expressions for blood glucose readings should be used, such as "in range" or "out of range." The same is true for the commonly used word, *cheating* to describe making food choices outside of the meal plan. This word is judgmental, meaning to defraud or deceive, and may create more anger, guilt, and acting-out behaviors.

SELF-REVIEW QUESTIONS

1 Describe three characteristics for each of the following developmental stages: infancy and toddlerhood; preschool-age; school-age; and early, middle, and late adolescence.

2 Explain the potential impact of diabetes on each developmental stage.

3 Describe the burden of care and potential stress that falls on parents and caretakers; list two possible sources of support.

4 List three conditions that may be associated with poor glycemic control or health outcomes.

5 State two educational considerations regarding learning styles and abilities for each of the following age groups: preschool, school-age, and adolescent.

CASE STUDY 1

HP is a 21-year-old single mother whose 11-month-old son (BP) has just been hospitalized and diagnosed with type 1 diabetes. The mother is a high-school graduate currently employed part-time as a waitress and working a 4 PM to midnight shift. HP is having financial problems. Her sister, who has four children of her own, has agreed to watch BP on the nights his mother works.

BP's doctor has prescribed two injections of NPH per day, which BP receives before breakfast and dinner. Regular insulin was tried and discontinued at this time because of hypoglycemia. BP is still being bottle-fed and receives a bottle before bedtime. The dietitian and HP have developed a 1200-calorie meal plan with three meals and three snacks per day.

QUESTIONS FOR DISCUSSION

1 What are the primary management and social issues?

2 What are potential educational strategies?

3 What interventions could be implemented immediately, and which can be planned for a later time?

DISCUSSION

1 One of the main concerns for this single mother is finding the support and resources needed to adequately care for her child. One approach might be to ask if the mother needs additional support and who could provide it. Or the diabetes educator could explore relationships with other people besides the sister, such as neighbors and friends, and include them in the educational process.

2 Include all individuals in HP's support network in the diabetes education process from the beginning so they are fully aware of the seriousness of her needs.

3 Discuss with the sister her willingness and assess her ability to learn to give insulin injections, do monitoring, and so forth.

4 Social service workers might be able to assist with community resources and explore financial considerations such as expansion of Social Security benefits for this mother.

5 HP also will most likely need a great deal of support, close follow-up and a positive relationship with her son's healthcare providers. Ongoing evaluation of her level of stress and coping should provide indications for the direction of follow-up care.

6 The infant should not be weaned from the bottle during the period of diagnosis and hospitalization, although this is an appropriate goal to work toward after BP is settled at home. Because hospitalization is a traumatic experience for a very young child, the stress should not be compounded by weaning him at this time from an obvious comfort.

7 Home healthcare nurses might be consulted to look in on and assist this young mother in her efforts to provide a regular schedule and care for her child.

Case Study 2

JJ is a 15-year-old male who was diagnosed with type 1 diabetes 8 years ago. As a child his blood glucose was reasonably well controlled and had no hospital admissions. Over the past year, JJ has been admitted to the hospital three times for DKA and once for severe hypoglycemia. His HbA$_{1c}$ concentration has risen over the past 2 years from 10.3% to 14.8% (normal = 5.5% to 7.4%). He has been frank about admitting to not testing his blood glucose level. JJ also states that he occasionally forgets to take his insulin, especially the second injection of the day. He lives at home with both parents and two younger siblings, does average work in school, and has a girlfriend. He has become very oppositional at home and argues frequently with his parents.

Questions for Discussion

1 What are the primary goals of therapy for this young man?

2 What educational approaches might be effective?

3 What concerns described above are typical adolescent behaviors from a developmental perspective?

DISCUSSION

1   The main goals of therapy are (1) to prevent the recurrent DKA, (2) prevent severe hypoglycemia, and (3) decrease JJ's HbA$_{1c}$ concentration.

2   Critical to achieving these goals is JJ taking his prescribed doses of insulin and eating regularly.

3   Exploring JJ's goals and the reasons for not taking his insulin might reveal insights that can help JJ to address and problem-solve about his difficulties.

   A   JJ needs to understand the positive and negative consequences of his decisions and goals, focusing on the present.

   B   If JJ is out with friends and is either too embarrassed to take his insulin or has not had the foresight to bring it, these issues can be addressed. He may be a candidate for a premixed insulin at the evening meal, using an insulin pen. This may be more portable and convenient, increasing the likelihood of taking his second injection.

   C   If JJ agrees, his friends, including his girlfriend, can be asked to support these efforts and be invited to attend education classes.

   D   Asking parents to observe JJ taking his insulin can reinforce the importance of this request.

4   JJ also probably needs an updated educational review because he was at a developmentally younger age when he last received diabetes education.

5   JJ might contract with the educator for small behavior changes that are achievable and mutually agreeable, and maintain frequent contact to monitor progress.

6   One motivating factor for JJ may be the potential inability to obtain a drivers license. He may be motivated by the understanding that the adult responsibility of driving is based on safety issues for himself and others on the road. Demonstrating responsibility and safety in his diabetes self-care is a sign that he is ready to take on the adult responsibility of driving.

7   JJ can be assisted in the problem-solving process using hypothetical adolescent situations. One strategy might be to remove the parents from the center of the conflict and communicate directly with JJ without eliminating parental involvement.

8   A referral for counseling, peer support groups, or camp might also be beneficial as JJ passes through a very difficult period of development.

9   Developmental concerns include declining glycemic control due to the insulin resistance of the hormones of puberty and the accompanying characteristics of middle adolescence. In particular, JJ is most likely striving for greater independence, and is increasingly busy with his girlfriend and social agenda. He is showing experimentation and and risk-taking behaviors. In addition, he is having increasing conflict with his parents. These are typical developmental characteristics of middle adolescence, all of which can affect glycemic control.

REFERENCES

1   Tull ES, Roseman JM. Diabetes in African Americans. In: Diabetes in America. 2nd ed. Bethesda, Md: National Institute of Diabetes and Digestive and Kidney Diseases, 1995;613-25.

2   US Department of Health and Human Services. Diabetes Statistics. Bethesda, Md: National Institutes of Health, 1995; NIH publication no. 96-3926.

3   LaPorte RE, Matsushima M, Chang YF. Prevalence and incidence of insulin-dependent diabetes. In: Diabetes in America.

4   LaPorte RE, Matsushima M, Chang YF. Diabetes in America. 2nd ed. Bethesda, Md: National Institute of Diabetes and Digestive and Kidney Diseases, 1995;37-45.

5   Pinhas-Hamiel O, Dolan LM, Daniels SR, et al. Increased incidence of non-insulin dependent diabetes mellitus among adolescents. J Pediatr 1996;128:608-15.

6   Tull ES, Jordan OW, Simon L, Laws M et al. Incidence of childhood-onset IDDM in black African-heritage populations in the Caribbean. Diabetes Care 1997; 20:309-10.

7   Rewers M, Hamman RF. Risk factors for non-insulin dependent diabetes. Diabetes in America, 2nd ed, Bethesda, Md: National Institute of Diabetes and Digestive and Kidney Diseases, 1995; 170-202.

8   Salerno M, Argenziano A, Di Maio S, et al. Pubertal growth, sexual maturation and final height in children with IDDM. Diabetes Care 1997;20:721-24.

9   Drash A. Management of the child with diabetes mellitus: clinical course, therapeutic strategies, and monitoring techniques. In: Lifshitz F, ed. Pediatric endocrinology, a clinical guide. 2nd ed. New York: Marcel Dekker, 1990:681-700.

10 Becker D. Complications of insulin-dependent diabetes mellitus in childhood and adolescence. In: Lifshitz F, ed. Pediatric endocrinology, a clinical guide. 2nd ed. New York: Marcel Dekker, 1990:701-18.

11 Shah SC, Malone JI, Simpson NE. A randomized trial of intensive insulin therapy in newly diagnosed insulin-dependent diabetes mellitus. N Engl J Med 1989;320:550-54.

12 Atkinson MA, Maclaren NK, Luchetta R. Insulitis and diabetes in NOD mice reduced by prophylactic insulin therapy. Diabetes 1990;39:933-37.

13 Zhang ZJ, Davidson L, Eisenbarth G, Weiner HL. Suppression of diabetes in nonobese diabetic mice by oral administration of porcine insulin. Proc Natl Acad Sci USA 1991;88:10252-6.

14 Follansbee D. Assuming responsibility for diabetes management: what age? what price? Diabetes Educ 1989;15:347-53.

15 Wysocki T, Meinhold PA, Abrams KC, et al. Parental and professional estimates of self-care independence of children and adolescents with IDDM. Diabetes Care 1992;15:43-52.

16 McNabb WL, Quinn MT, Murphy DM, Thorp FK, Cook S. Increasing children's responsibility for diabetes self-care: the In Control study. Diabetes Educ 1994;20:121-24.

17 Becker D. Management of insulin dependent diabetes mellitus in children and adolescents. Curr Opinion Pediatr 1991;3:710-23.

18 American Diabetes Association. Position statement. Nutrition recommendations and principles for people with diabetes mellitus. Diabetes Care 1998;21(suppl 1):S32-35.

19 American Diabetes Association. Position statement. Diabetes mellitus and exercise. Diabetes Care 1998;21(suppl 1):S40-44.

20 Arslanian S, Nixon PA, Becker D, Drash AL. Impact of physical fitness and glycemic control on in vivo insulin action in adolescents with IDDM. Diabetes Care 1990;13:9-15.

21 Campaign BN, Lampman RM. Exercise in the clinical management of diabetes. Champaign, Il: Human Kinetics Publishing, 1994:62.

22 Porter PA, Keating B, Byrne G, Jones TW. Incidence and predictive criteria of nocturnal hypoglycemia in young children with insulin dependent diabetes mellitus. J Pediatr 1997;130:366-72.

23 Drash A. Clinical care of the diabetic child. Chicago: Year Book Medical Publishers, 1987:16.

24 Boland EA, Grey M. Coping strategies of school-age children with diabetes mellitus. Diabetes Educ 1996;22:592-97.

25 Drash A, Becker DJ. Behavioral issues in patients with diabetes mellitus with special emphasis on the child and adolescent. In: Rifkin H, Porte D Jr, eds. Ellenberg and Rifkin's diabetes mellitus theory and practice. 4th ed. New York: Elsevier Publishing, 1990:922-33.

26 Kovacs M, Feinberg T. Coping with juvenile onset diabetes mellitus. In: Singer JE, Baum A, eds. Handbook of medical psychology. Vol 2. Hilldale, NJ: Lawrence Erlbaum Associates, 1982;165-212.

27 Almeida CM. Grief among parents of children with diabetes. Diabetes Educ 1995;21:530-32.

28 Songer TJ, LaPorte R, Lave JR, Dorman JS, Becker DJ. Health insurance and the financial impact of IDDM in families with a child with IDDM. Diabetes Care 1997;20:577-84.

29 Mahler M, Pine F, Bergman A. The psychological birth of the human infant. New York: Basic Books, 1975.

30 Ryan C, Vega A, Drash A. Cognitive deficits in adolescents who developed diabetes early in life. Pediatrics 1985;75:921-27.

31 Rovet J, Alvarez M. Attentional functioning in children and adolescents with IDDM. Diabetes Care 1997;20:803-10.

32 Nordfeldt S, Ludvigsson J. Severe hypoglycemia in children with IDDM. Diabetes Care 1997;20:497-503.

33 Fraiberg S. The magic years. New York: Charles Scribner's Sons, 1959.

34 Rogerson C. Play therapy in childhood. New York: Oxford University Press, 1939.

35 Pothier P. Resolving conflict through play fantasy. J Psychiatr Nurs 1967;5:141-47.

36 Marcus S. Therapeutic puppetry. In: Philpott AR, ed. Puppets and therapy. New York: Plays Inc, 1977.

37 94-142 and 504: numbers that add up to educational rights for children with disabilities. Washington, DC: Children's Defense Fund, 1989.

38 Daneman D, Wolfson D, Becker DH, Drash AL. Factors affecting glycosylated hemoglobin values in children with insulin-dependent diabetes mellitus. J Pediatr 1981;99:847-53.

39 Blethen S, Sargeant DT, Whitlow MG, Santiago JV. Effect of pubertal stage and recent blood glucose control on plasma somatomedian C in children with insulin-dependent diabetes mellitus. Diabetes 1981;30:868-72.

40 Amiel SA, Sherwin RS, Simonson DC, Lauritano AA, Tamborlane WV. Impaired insulin action in puberty: A contributing factor to poor glycemic control in adolescents with diabetes. N Engl J Med 1986;315:215-19.

41 Committee on Adolescence/Group for the Advancement of Psychiatry. Normal adolescence: its dynamics and impact. New York: Charles Scribner's Sons, 1968.

42 Blos P. On adolescence: a psychoanalytic interpretation. New York: Free Press of Blencoe, 1962.

43 Betschart J. Oral contraception and adolescent women with insulin-dependent diabetes mellitus: risks, benefits and implications for practice. Diabetes Educ 1996;22:374-78.

44 Anderson BJ, Auslander WC. Research on diabetes management and the family: a critique. Diabetes Care 1980;3:696-702.

45 Golden MP, Herrold AJ, Orr DP. An approach to prevention of recurrent diabetic ketoacidosis in the pediatric population. J Pediatr 1985;107:195-200.

EDUCATIONAL MATERIALS FOR CHILDREN, ADOLESCENTS, AND PARENTS

Betschart J. A magic ride in Foozbah Land [Book and audiotape]. Minneapolis, Minn: Chronimed, 1995.

Betschart J. Thom S. In-control: a guide for teens with diabetes. Minneapolis, Minn: Chronimed, 1995.

Betschart J. It's time to learn about diabetes. Minneapolis, Minn: Chronimed, 1995.

Betschart J. It's time to learn about diabetes [Video]. Minneapolis, Minn: Chronimed, 1993.

Brackenridge B. Diabetes 101: a pure and simple guide for people who use insulin. Minneapolis, Minn: Chronimed, 1993.

Brackenridge B, Rubin R. Sweet kids: How to balance diabetes control and good decision making with family peace. Alexandria, Va: American Diabetes Association, 1996.

Childs B. Caring for children with diabetes. Alexandria, Va: American Diabetes Association, 1990.

Diabetes: one part of me. Boston: Joslin Diabetes Center, 1986.

Giordano B, Giordano J. Diabetes drama. Denver: The Children's Hospital, 1993.

Hayes J. Necessary toughness. Alexandria, Va: American Diabetes Association, 1990.

Martin A. The babysitter's club: the truth about Stacey. New York: Scholastic Inc, 1986.

Martin A. The babysitter's club: Stacey's emergency. New York: Scholastic Inc, 1991.

Miller J. Grilled cheese at four o'clock in the morning. Alexandria, Va: American Diabetes Association, 1988.

Moynihan P, Balik B, Eliason S, Haig B. Diabetes youth curriculum: a toolbox for educators. Minneapolis, Minn: International Diabetes Center, 1988.

Moynihan P, Haig B. Whole parent, whole child. Minneapolis, Minn: Chronimed Publishing, 1989.

Siminerio L, Betschart J. Raising a child with diabetes. Alexandria, Va: American Diabetes Association, 1995.

Wysocki T. The ten keys to helping your child grow up with diabetes. Alexandria, Va: American Diabetes Association, 1997.

SUGGESTED READINGS

Anthony E, Benedek T, eds. Parenthood: its psychology and psychopathology. Boston: Little, Brown, 1972.

Chase P. Understanding insulin dependent diabetes. 8th ed. Denver: Children's Diabetes Foundation, 1995.

Daneman D. Childhood, adolescence, and diabetes: a delicate developmental balance. Diabetes Spectrum 1989;2(4):225-43.

Giordano BP, Petrila AT, Mamien CR, et al. Transferring responsibility for diabetes self-care from parent to child. Pediatr Health Care 1992;6(Sep-Oct):5.

Holzmeister LA. Medical nutrition therapy for children and adolescents with type 1 diabetes mellitus. Diabetes Spectrum 1997;10:268-75.

Kleinberg S. Educating the chronically ill child. Rockville, Md: Aspen Publishers, 1982.

Lorenz R, Wysocki T. The family and childhood diabetes. Diabetes Spectrum 1991;4(5):261-92.

Petrillo M. Emotional care of hospitalized children. Philadelphia: JB Lippincott, 1980.

Pond JS, Peters ML, Pannell DL, Rogers CS. Psychosocial challenges for children with insulin-dependent diabetes mellitus. Diabetes Educ 1995;21:297-99.

Vandagriff J, Marrero D, Ingersoll GM, Fineberg NS. Parents of children with diabetes: what are they worried about? Diabetes Educ 1992;18:299-302.

DIABETES AND LIFE CYCLE

Pregnancy: Preconception to Postpartum

18

Donna Jornsay, BSN, RN, CPNP, CDE
North Shore University Hospital
Great Neck, New York

INTRODUCTION

1   Diabetes mellitus is one of the most commonly encountered complications of pregnancy, affecting more than 150 000 pregnancies in the United States annually.[1]

2   The outlook for pregnant women with diabetes and their children has improved dramatically over the last 25 years due to improvements in diabetes care such as the use of self-monitoring of blood glucose and intensive insulin therapy to normalize maternal metabolism throughout the gestation period, better fetal monitoring, and advances in neonatal intensive care.

3   The perinatal mortality rate of infants of women with diabetes has decreased dramatically from 25% of live births in the 1960s to a near normal 2% of live births in the 1980s.[2]

4   Despite these recent advances in care, women with diabetes and their infants remain at greater risk for a number of complications, most notably congenital malformations, which account for 40% to 50% of the perinatal deaths in these infants. To prevent these anomalies, euglycemia must begin in the preconception period and continue throughout the period of organogenesis.

5   The diabetogenic state of pregnancy leads to the diagnosis of gestational diabetes in 2% to 15% of all pregnant women.
    A   The fetal risks and infant morbidity are related to the severity of the maternal hyperglycemia and consequent fetal hyperinsulinism.
    B   To prevent these short- and long-term metabolic and growth complications, glycemic control must be maintained throughout pregnancy through provision of multidisciplinary team care and targeted self-management education.

6   Topics that are addressed in this chapter include the metabolism of normal pregnancy and the alterations that occur in maternal diabetes, potential maternal and neonatal complications, the essentials of preconception counseling and care, and diabetes management and patient education for pregestational and gestational diabetes.

OBJECTIVES

Upon completion of this chapter, the learner will be able to

1 Identify how gestational diabetes differs from type 1 or type 2 diabetes that existed prior to pregnancy.

2 Identify risk factors associated with a poor outcome in a pregnancy complicated by diabetes.

3 Describe normal maternal metabolism during pregnancy.

4 List neonatal complications.

5 Explain the relationship between preconception glucose control and the incidence of congenital anomalies and spontaneous abortions.

6 State potential maternal complications for the patient with pregestational diabetes.

7 State blood glucose guidelines for pregnancy.

8 Describe two important topics to discuss with patients during preconception counseling.

9 Identify strategies to achieve blood glucose levels.

10 Identify specific patient education needed for self-management during pregnancy.

11 Define the screening guidelines for gestational diabetes.

12 Describe postpartum care and education for women with pregestational and gestational diabetes.

DEFINITION OF DIABETES IN PREGNANCY

1 The types of diabetes that occur during pregnancy can be divided into two groups.

   A The first group consists of women with preexisting diabetes, either type 1 diabetes or type 2 prior to pregnancy (pregestational).

   B The second group consists of women who develop *gestational diabetes,* which is defined as carbohydrate intolerance of variable severity with the onset or first recognition during pregnancy.[3-6] This group may actually include women who have had previously undiagnosed type 2 diabetes but who are first diagnosed during pregnancy. The risks for complications in this latter group are greater than for the woman with gestational diabetes only, and may include women who present at diagnosis with evidence of existing diabetes complications.

2 Approximately 0.2% to 0.3%[7] of all pregnancies occur in women with insulin-treated diabetes diagnosed prior to pregnancy. Another 2% of all

women in the United States of childbearing age have undiagnosed type 2 diabetes mellitus. In Australia, 4.3% to 15% of pregnant women were found to have gestational diabetes when tested during the second half of pregnancy depending on their country of origin.[8] These prevalence statistics support earlier data showing a significant variance in the rate of gestational diabetes among various racial and ethnic groups.[9,10]

CLASSIFICATION SYSTEMS FOR PREGNANCY COMPLICATED BY DIABETES

1 Various classification systems have been developed to identify risk factors in patients who are pregnant and have diabetes.

2 The White classification system[11] was for many years the most widely applied system for assessing the risk factors of pregnancy complicated by diabetes.

    A White[11] observed that the age of onset of maternal diabetes, duration, and the presence of vascular complications all had an important impact on the outcome of pregnancy.

    B In terms of outcome measures, problems with the White classification include omission of any mention of glycemic control and guidelines regarding insulin treatment for gestational diabetes. For these reasons, many diabetes and pregnancy programs rely on narrative descriptions of women with both preexisting and gestational diabetes to more closely predict maternal and neonatal outcomes.

3 Pederson et al[12] offered another classification system for poor pregnancy outcomes. They noted five prognostically bad signs of pregnancy associated with unfavorable outcomes: ketoacidosis, pyelonephritis, pregnancy-induced hypertension, poor clinic attendance, and self-neglect.

4 Both White's Classifications[11] and Pederson's prognostically bad signs[12,13] have been used to identify patients at risk for poor pregnancy outcomes.

5 Buchanan and Coustan[14] offer another classification system which takes into account glycemia, the presence of diabetic vascular complications, and the type of diabetes (Table 18.1) These factors appear to be more important predictors of perinatal outcome than either the age at onset or the duration of maternal diabetes.

Table 18.1. Classification of Diabetes During Pregnancy

Pregestational Diabetes	Risks
Type of maternal diabetes	
Type 1	• Ketoacidosis
Type 2	• Obesity, hypertension
Metabolic control and timing	
Early pregnancy	• Birth defects, spontaneous abortions
Later pregnancy	• Hyperinsulinemia, overgrowth, stillbirth, polycythemia, RDS
Maternal vascular complications	
Retinopathy	• Worsening during pregnancy
Nephropathy	• Edema, hypertension, intrauterine growth retardation
Atherosclerosis	• Maternal death
Gestational Diabetes	
Fetal risks	• Hyperinsulinemia and macrosomia, possibility of stillbirth
Maternal risks	• Hypertensive disorders in pregnancy, diabetes following pregnancy
Metabolic control	
Fasting glucose <105 mg/dL (Class A$_1$)	
Fasting glucose (≥105 mg/dL (Class A$_2$)	

Source: Adapted from Buchanan and Coustan.[14]

Normal Metabolism

1 An understanding of the metabolic changes that occur in a nondiabetic pregnancy is necessary to be able to normalize metabolism for the best possible outcome in a diabetic pregnancy.

   A The fetus depends upon the mother for an uninterrupted supply of fuel. To meet fetal needs, the following maternal adaptations occur:[15] Increased tissue glycogen storage and peripheral glucose utilization, enhanced hepatic glucose production

   • A shift toward production of free fatty acids and ketones

- Pancreatic cell hypertrophy with resultant increased insulin response to glucose
- Decreased maternal alanine (gluconeogenetic amino acid) leading to hypoglycemia and lower fasting blood glucose levels than in the nongravid state

B There is a passive diffusion of glucose across the placenta.

C Hyperemesis and food intolerance may occur.

D The early months of a nondiabetic pregnancy can be described as a period of maternal anabolism during which maternal fat storage takes place.

2 The metabolic changes related to pregnancy increase progressively during the second and third trimesters. The changes occur in both the fasting and fed states.

A The fasting state of pregnancy is characterized by a more rapid diversion to fat metabolism (accelerated starvation).[16] This results in an increased risk for diabetic ketoacidosis (DKA) and fasting ketosis.

- Whenever food is withheld, concentrations of free fatty acids and ketones reach higher levels in pregnant women than in nongravid women, again increasing the risk for DKA.
- Plasma glucose levels and amino acids are markedly lower in pregnant women during a fasting state, increasing the risk for severe hypoglycemia. This is especially true in the first half of pregnancy.

B Food ingestion results in higher and more prolonged plasma glucose concentrations in pregnant women compared with nongravid women.[17] This more sustained, postprandial hyperglycemia enhances transplacental delivery of glucose to the fetus and promotes growth of the fetus. (Maternal insulin and glucagon do not cross the placenta.)

3 During late pregnancy, a woman's basal insulin levels are higher than nongravid levels, and food ingestion results in a two- to threefold increase in insulin secretion.[17]

A The cause of this state of progressive insulin resistance is related to the increasing levels of human placental lactogen (HPL), prolactin, and free and bound cortisol.

B Insulin resistance may be responsible for the diabetogenic effect of pregnancy and the risk for gestational diabetes (GDM).

NEONATAL COMPLICATIONS

1 There are increased rates of neonatal complications in pregnancies complicated by diabetes. These complication rates can be correlated to the level of glycemia.

   A Complications can result from high glucose levels during the first trimester (ie, congenital malformations and spontaneous abortions). These are generally seen in women with preexisting type 1 or type 2 diabetes.

   B Metabolic complications can be seen secondary to maternal hyperglycemia in the second and third trimester after the fetal pancreas has begun to function. These include neonatal hyperglycemia, macrosomia, increased childhood rates of obesity and impaired glucose tolerance, stillbirth, respiratory distress syndrome (RDS), hyperbilirubinemia, hypocalcemia, and polycythemia. These complications are seen in women with preexisting type 1 or type 2 diabetes, as well as in infants of women with GDM.

2 First trimester hyperglycemia can result in a number of complications including congenital malformations and spontaneous abortions.

   A Congenital malformations often develop before the woman knows she is pregnant; fetal organogenesis occurs during the first 8 weeks of gestation.[18]

   • The incidence of congenital malformations is 6% to 13% in pregnancies complicated by preexisting diabetes where glycemic control is not established prior to conception. This rate of congenital malformations is two to three times greater than the 2% to 3% rate for the general population.[19-21]

   • Studies of maternal glycosylated hemoglobin levels at the end of the first trimester as an index of glycemia during organogenesis generally reveal an anomaly risk of 2% to 5% in women with diabetes who have normal to moderately elevated glycosylated hemoglobin levels.[21-23]

   • Infants of mothers diagnosed early in pregnancy, thereby suggesting previously impaired glucose tolerance, and in whom there is an elevation of the glycosylated hemoglobin values are potentially at risk for malformations and/or spontaneous abortions as well as neonatal complications.

- When glycosylated hemoglobin levels are markedly elevated at the end of the first trimester, the malformation rate rises substantially, reaching as high as 20% to 40% in some studies.[22-24]

- The association between glycemic control and birth defects prompted several studies of preconception management in women with diabetes. Fuhrmann et al[25,26] Steel et al,[27] and Kitzmiller et al[28] have reported a virtual elimination of excess anomalies in studies designed to achieve very good glycemic control prior to conception. The results of these studies suggest that it may be possible to eliminate the high rate of congenital malformations by achieving a normalized glycosylated hemoglobin value prior to conception. Therefore, planned pregnancies are extremely important for women with diabetes.

- The types of birth defects that occur in infants of women with poorly controlled diabetes during organogenesis are varied but most often involve the cardiovascular, central nervous, and skeletal systems (see Table 18.2).

- Congenital heart defects are the most common birth defect seen in infants of mothers with type 1 diabetes, occurring in 4% of all diabetic pregnancies.[18] Transposition of the great vessels, ventricular septal defects, and coarctation of the aorta are other common cardiac defects.

- The birth defects in the infants of women with diabetes are commonly multiple, more severe, and more often fatal than those in the general population.

B Spontaneous abortion rates have also been found to correlate with first trimester glycosylated hemoglobin values. These rates have been reported to be as high as 30% to 60%, depending on the degree of hyperglycemia at the time of conception (Figure 18.1).[29] In the Diabetes and Early Pregnancy Project (DIEP)[13] and a study by Greene et al,[23] the frequency of spontaneous abortions was similar to the frequency expected in nondiabetic pregnancies when first trimester glycosylated hemoglobin levels were in the normal to moderately elevated ranges. Once the glycosylated hemoglobin value was three standard deviations above the norm, the risk for spontaneous abortion increased more and more steeply as the levels of glycohemoglobin got further from normal.

Table 18.2. Congenital Malformations in Infants of Diabetic Mothers (Type 1 Diabetes)

Anomaly	Gestational Age After Last Menstrual Period
Sacral Agenesis (Caudal regression)	5 weeks
Spina bifida, hydrocephalus, or other CNS defect	6 weeks
Anencephalus	6 weeks
Heart anomalies	
Transposition of great vessels	7 weeks
Ventricular septal defect	8 weeks
Atrial septal defect	8 weeks
Anal/rectal atresia	8 weeks
Renal anomalies	
Agenesis	7 weeks
Cystic kidney	7 weeks
Ureter duplex	7 weeks
Situs Inversus	6 weeks

Source: Reprinted with permission from Mills et al.[18]

Figure 18.1. Major Malformations and Spontaneous Abortions According to First Trimester HbA1c

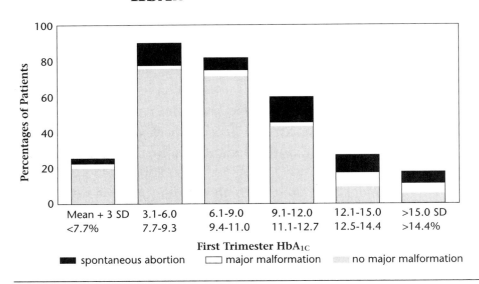

Source: Adapted from: Jovanovic L.[29]

3 Second- and third-trimester hyperglycemia results in increased neonatal metabolic complications.

  A *Hypoglycemia* in the neonate, the most common metabolic complication, is defined as plasma glucose values less than 35 mg/dL (1.92 mmol/L) in term infants and less than 25 mg/dL (1.37 mmol/L) in preterm infants.[30]

- When blood glucose levels are elevated during pregnancy, the fetus receives larger amounts of glucose, amino acids, and fatty fuels than are required for normal growth and development. The increased delivery of these nutrients stimulates fetal growth and maturation of normally immature pancreatic beta cells in the fetus.

- At delivery, when the maternal blood supply is eliminated, the fetus continues to produce excess amounts of insulin that may result in neonatal hypoglycemia.

- The peak incidence of neonatal hypoglycemia is 6 to 12 hours after birth; but if severe it can persist for several days or more.

  B *Macrosomia* (abnormally large body size) in the neonate is generally defined as a weight of 4000 grams or greater.[31] It should be noted that there is no widely agreed upon weight definition. Any evaluation of fetal weight must be considered in the context of gestational age.

- A fetus with a gestational age of 32 weeks and an estimated fetal weight of 3800 grams or ≥90% for gestational age is nonetheless considered large for gestational age (LGA) and also has an increased perinatal morbidity similar to a fetus with macrosomia. LGA is the most common clinical definition of macrosomia.

- In the general population, macrosomia occurs in 10% of all pregnancies, and a fetus with a weight of 4500 grams occurs in only 1% of all pregnancies. In pregnancies complicated by diabetes, the incidence of macrosomia is between 20% and 32%, making macrosomia the most common complication of diabetes during pregnancy.

- Macrosomia occurs in pregnancies with preexisting diabetes as well as gestational diabetes. Macrosomia decreases dramatically in gestational diabetes when insulin therapy and glucose monitoring are instituted.[32]

- Macrosomic and LGA fetuses have increased demands for oxygen. When the demands for oxygen exceed the supply, asphyxia results. This reaction may account for the increased death rate in macrosomic fetuses in the late third trimester. Thus, close follow-up and fetal surveillance are needed.

- The development of macrosomia in late pregnancy is highly correlated with maternal glycemia as explained by the Pederson hypothesis.[19]
- The hypothesis states that maternal hyperglycemia leads to fetal hyperglycemia, which in turn stimulates the fetal pancreas to produce excessive amounts of insulin (a growth factor for fetal tissue).
- Fetal macrosomia is evidenced by the enlargement of the abdominal and chest circumference compared with the head circumference. Increased skin fold thickness and a fetal fat line are specific to infants of mothers with poor glucose control and can be seen on ultrasound. In two separate studies,[33,34] ultrasonographic evidence of these fetal morbidities confirmed poor glucose control and was associated with a glycosylated hemoglobin of 6.3% or greater (normal = 4.4% to 6.4%).
- Most of the perinatal morbidity associated with pregnancies complicated by diabetes result from the traumatic delivery of a macrosomic infant. Macrosomia is a risk factor for shoulder dystocia, which can lead to birth trauma such as Erb's palsy. A Cesarean Section is judicious when the estimated fetal weight is in excess of 4500 grams.[35]

C Increased rates of obesity, hypertension, glucose intolerance, and diabetes have been identified in the offspring of women with diabetes during pregnancy.[36-39] Near normal blood glucose levels throughout pregnancy have been associated with lowered perinatal mortality, decreased prevalence of macrosomia, and improved delivery and maternal postpartum outcomes. At this time, however, there is little evidence regarding the long-term benefits for the offspring.

D Stillbirth is a complication of a diabetic pregnancy that can be dramatically reduced when glycemic control is maintained throughout pregnancy and delivery and sophisticated fetal monitoring tests are employed. The precise cause of stillbirths in pregnancies complicated by diabetes is still not known.

E Respiratory distress syndrome now is an infrequent complication of a diabetic pregnancy.
- In the past, obstetricians commonly induced preterm delivery which often resulted in RDS because the infant's lungs were not fully mature.
- Because of blood glucose monitoring and new approaches to care resulting in improved glycemic control, sophisticated fetal monitoring, and the ability to document fetal lung maturity, most

babies can now be delivered close to term (38 to 40 weeks), thereby eliminating the problems of preterm delivery.

F Hypocalcemia, hyperbilirubinemia, and polycythemia occur more frequently in infants of mothers with less-than-optimal glucose control during the third trimester of pregnancy. These problems are infrequent in babies whose mothers maintained glycemic control and who were delivered at term (37 to 40 weeks gestation). The pathogenesis of hypocalcemia is not well understood. Polycythemia is related to increased levels of erythropoietin (which correlate directly with maternal insulin levels), and hyperbilirubinemia results from the breakdown of the excess red blood cells that are needed during pregnancy.

PRECONCEPTION COUNSELING AND CARE

1 Preconception care in the US remains the exception rather than the rule, despite the fact that clinical trials over the last decade have demonstrated its effectiveness in reducing the incidence of malformations.

A In Copenhagen between 1982 and 1986, 76% of women with diabetes sought care prior to conception.[40]

B In contrast, in the California Diabetes and Pregnancy Program (CDAPP), only 7% of women sought preconception care between 1982 and 1986.[41]

C In Maine between 1987 and 1990, 34% of eligible women sought care prior to conception.[42]

D In Singapore, 29% of patients were diagnosed to have pregestational diabetes after their 6-week postpartum oral glucose tolerance test. Of these, only 5% presented for preconception care in a subsequent pregnancy.

2 The economics of preconception care were examined in two separate studies.[43,44] In the first study by Elixhauser et al,[43] the costs of preconception care for women with established diabetes were $1721 per enrolled patient, and the benefit-cost ratio was 1.87. In other words, for every dollar spent on preconception care, $1.87 was gained. A second study by Scheffler and colleagues[44] examined actual hospital charges and lengths of stay, comparing women from the CDAPP who enrolled prior to 8 weeks gestation versus after 8 weeks gestation. A savings of $7253 for each enrolled patient was realized, and the benefit-cost ratio for the program was between $5 and $6. This suggests that for every dollar spent on preconception care, $5 to $6 was recovered in direct medical costs.

3 Preconception care for women with preexisting diabetes ideally begins 3 to 6 months prior to conception to allow sufficient time to evaluate the mother's health status and to normalize or maximize glycemic control, thereby offering the best chance for the unborn child.

4 Two percent of women of childbearing age have unrecognized type 2 diabetes.

   A Women of childbearing age who have risk factors for diabetes need to be tested before they attempt conception.

   B Provide counseling for women with diabetes of childbearing age about the potential risks of an unplanned pregnancy. Appropriate contraception also needs to be emphasized and offered.

   C Women with type 2 diabetes need to make the transition from oral antidiabetes agents to insulin before conception. The safety of all currently available oral agents has not been established in pregnancy and may lead to prolonged neonatal hypoglycemia,[45] and are therefore not recommended.

5 Neonatal and maternal problems may develop if blood glucose control is not maintained prior to and throughout gestation, and if skilled obstetrical care is not available. For this reason, team management by an endocrinologist, obstetrician/perinatologist, nurse educator, dietitian, and social worker is highly desirable. In addition, women with diabetes who have complications require special attention by the appropriate medical subspecialist.

6 Topics that are important to discuss with each patient and her significant other include fertility, spontaneous abortion rates, incidence of congenital anomalies, incidence of diabetes in offspring, and the effects of pregnancy on existing complications.

   A The discussion of risks needs to be done with sensitivity to the distress that it may cause. Offer realistic but positive messages. Discuss psychosocial concerns and offer support as an integral part of care and education.

   B The increased financial burden of a pregnancy with diabetes also needs to be discussed (eg, testing and fetal surveillance, diabetes supplies, and the potential for lost time from work).

   C The following information is helpful for discussing these issues with patients:

- There is no evidence to suggest that women with diabetes are less fertile than nondiabetic women.
- The risk of spontaneous abortion in women with diabetes appears to be no greater than the risk for nondiabetic women when glycemic control is good to fair.[13,23] Spontaneous abortion rates increased dramatically in these studies when glycosylated hemoglobin levels were markedly elevated.
- Results from one long-term follow-up study[46] indicated a net cumulative risk of 2% for type 1 diabetes in children born to mothers with type 1 diabetes. In contrast, the prevalence of type 1 diabetes in the offspring of type 1 fathers is reported to be 6%.[46] The risk for offspring of mothers with type 2 diabetes is not precisely known but is related to ethnic origin and the presence or absence of obesity. The empiric risk for offspring to develop diabetes or some form of glucose intolerance is 33%.[47] Frequently, diabetes or impaired glucose tolerance of the offspring is not manifested until adulthood.
- An essential preconception consideration is achieving optimal diabetes control prior to and throughout early pregnancy.
- With normal or near-normal glycosylated hemoglobin levels in early pregnancy the risk of birth defects is reduced to a level similar to that in the general population. However, a perfectly healthy baby cannot be guaranteed because the risk in the general population is still 2% to 3%.[19-21,25]
- Women with markedly elevated glycosylated hemoglobin levels, need to be informed that they may be at higher risk for an infant with a congenital malformation and that the risk may be as high as 20% to 40%. While this is difficult for patients to hear, it is important for them to know.
- When counseling about birth defects, offer maternal serum alpha-fetoprotein screening for neural tube defects and ultrasonographic evaluation for central nervous system, heart, renal, and skeletal anomalies. It must be emphasized that none of these tests is 100% sensitive for detecting fetal malformations.

7 The following preconception protocol is recommended prior to discontinuing contraception.

    A A thorough assessment is needed to detect any vascular complications, including a dilated retinal examination, a 24-hour urine collection for creatinine, creatinine clearance, and microalbumin, thyroid function tests, and an EKG. Any detected complications needs evaluation by the appropriate subspecialist as indicated on an individual basis.

B Discontinue oral agent if applicable.

C Provide dietary counseling because the meal plan may no longer be appropriate for current needs. The dietary intake of calcium, iron, and folic acid are particularly important. Provide information about the use of alternative sweeteners during pregnancy.

D Assess diabetes self-management skills.

- Observe self-monitoring of blood glucose to assess technique and accuracy, and to make sure that the meter is accurate.
- Observe insulin dose and administration technique.
- Provide education about hypoglycemia to the patient and her significant other including the administration of glucagon.

E Achieve glycosylated hemoglobin levels within or close to the normal range and acceptable mean blood glucose levels. Ideally, the glucose levels will mimic those of a nondiabetic pregnancy where fasting glucose values are 60-90 and 1-hour postmeal values never exceed 140 mg/dL. The glycosylated hemoglobin value should be within two standard deviations of the mean for the nondiabetic range prior to conception.

F Start folic acid supplements.

G Continue contraception until glucose goals are attained.

- Patients may have already discontinued contraception by the time they present for preconception care. Reinforce the importance of maintaining contraception until normal or near normal glucose values have been achieved.
- Basal body temperatures at this time are helpful to maximize the opportunity for conception and to accurately date conception.

H Obtain a serum pregnancy test if menses does not occur within 15 to 18 days following ovulation.

8 Women with diabetic retinopathy as well as the other vascular complications of diabetes present additional concerns.

A Counsel women who have diabetic retinopathy about the effect of pregnancy on their eyes. All women with type 1 diabetes for 5 years or more, or type 2 diabetes at diagnosis, require a thorough dilated ophthalmologic evaluation.[49] This may necessitate preconception fluorescein angiography as dye studies are generally contraindicated during pregnancy. These evaluations need to be completed prior to counseling if possible, and certainly prior to attempting conception. Laser therapy, if indicated, also needs to be completed prior to conception.

B The severity of retinopathy is related to the duration of diabetes,[49] the level of glycemia,[50] the patient's age at diagnosis,[49] the presence of proteinuria, and higher diastolic blood pressures.

- The Kroc study[51] demonstrated that retinopathy progresses when diabetes control is rapidly achieved. It is therefore advisable to normalize blood glucose levels in the presence of retinopathy over a period of 6 to 9 months.[52] Women with retinopathy need close ophthalmologic follow-up prior to conception.

- Rosenn et al[53] found that pregnancy-induced or preexisting chronic hypertension was the most important risk factor associated with progression of retinopathy in pregnancy.

C Pregnancy per se is an independent risk factor that accelerates retinopathy. Pregnancy is associated with a marked elevation in placental lactogen and other hormones that cause vascular changes and may in fact accelerate retinopathy.

D Nonproliferative (background) retinopathy does not generally threaten vision and is not considered a contraindication to pregnancy (see Chapter 21, Eye Disease and Adaptive Diabetes Education for Visually Impaired Persons). When a woman has background retinopathy at the start of her pregnancy, there is a 16% to 50% risk of progression during the pregnancy (Table 18.3).[53-57] In most situations, background retinopathy that occurs during pregnancy regresses after delivery.[55]

E Earlier data[55] showed that women with proliferative eye disease who had photocoagulation prior to pregnancy encountered a low risk (~5%) of significant disease progression during gestation. Rosenn et al,[53] however, reported risk of progression as high as 63% for women with proliferative retinopathy.

- Women with untreated proliferative retinopathy have the greatest risk of progression,[55] and pregnancy is contraindicated until they receive laser photocoagulation to stabilize their eye disease.

- Because retinopathy is known to regress postpartum, the need for photocoagulation during pregnancy continues to be controversial. Most centers treat patients with significant neovascularization rather than risk retinal hemorrhage.

- The mode of delivery is an important consideration as ophthalmologists warn women with proliferative retinopathy to avoid the

Valsalva maneuver. Many obstetricians recommend a cesarean delivery or a vacuum extracted vaginal delivery to avoid pushing during a vaginal delivery.

TABLE 18.3. PROGRESSION OF DIABETIC RETINOPATHY IN PREGNANCY STRATIFIED BY INITIAL RETINAL FINDINGS

Author, Year	No. of Pregnancies	No. (%) with Progression Given the Initial Findings		
		None	Background	Proliferative
Horvar et al, 1980	160	13/118 (11)	11/35 (31)	1/7 (14)
Moloney and Drury, 1982	53	8/20 (40)	15/30 (50)	1/3 (33)
Dibble et al, 1982	55	0/23 (0)	3/19 (16)	7/13 (54)
Ohrt, 1984	100	4/50 (8)	15/48 (31)	1/2 (50)
Rosenn et al, 1992	154	18/78 (23)	28/68 (41)	5/8 (63)

Source: Adapted from Jovanovic-Peterson et al.[48]

---

9 Diabetic nephropathy is the complication of diabetes most likely to affect pregnancy outcomes.[56-61] In two studies,[59,60] 61% and 27%, respectively, of women with nephropathy were undiagnosed until they were examined during pregnancy (see Chapter 23, Nephropathy, for more information).

   A It is recommended that a thorough evaluation of renal function be part of routine preconception care for all women with type 1 diabetes of greater than 5 years duration or at diagnosis with type 2 diabetes. This evaluation includes a 24-hour urine collection for creatinine, creatinine clearance, and microalbumin performed in a reference laboratory because of technical problems encountered with the albumin assay. Established nephropathy is staged and counseling provided about the potential risks to both maternal and fetal well-being.

   B Because the use of ACE inhibitors is contraindicated during pregnancy, Kitzmiller et al[60] and others have recommended methyldopa as a first-line agent for hypertension control. Prazosin or clonidine can be added if additional therapy is necessary in early pregnancy; diltiazem can be added at the end of the first trimester. Blood pressure control often worsens as pregnancy progresses.

C Preeclampsia is the most frequent, serious complication of maternal nephropathy. Combs et al[64] found that the rate of preeclampsia in women with diabetes depended on the initial level of proteinuria. Preeclampsia occurred in 7% of women with proteinuria of <190 mg/day, 31% with proteinuria of 190 to 499 mg/day, and 38% with proteinuria of >500 mg/day. This increased risk of preeclampsia with proteinuria >190 mg/day persisted after controlling glycemia, parity, and diabetes complications.

D In general, the chances for a successful outcome are good for women with diabetic nephropathy. Studies[58-65] have shown that the perinatal survival rate in this group has been between 89% and 100% (Table 18.4). However, the course of pregnancy is not necessarily easy.

- There are increased risks for pregnancy-induced hypertension and/or a progression of already existing hypertension, intrauterine growth retardation resulting in small-for-gestational-age infants, preterm deliveries secondary to fetal distress, and a tenfold increase in the incidence of stillbirth over women with diabetes but without nephropathy.[58-62]

- Preterm delivery and stillbirth are most likely related to the fact that women with diabetes, hypertension, and chronic proteinuria have a high frequency of atherotic lesions in the uterine arteries that compromise the oxygenation of the fetus.

E Studies[58,60,66] over the last decade have addressed the long-debated question of what effect pregnancy has on the natural history of renal disease. Conclusions from these studies indicate that renal function deteriorates after pregnancy in women with overt nephropathy, but the rate of deterioration is not different (10 mL/min/y decrease in creatinine clearance) than would be expected without pregnancy.

- A later study by Miodovnik and colleagues[65] demonstrated that pregnancy in women with diabetes does not increase the risk for the subsequent development of diabetic nephropathy. Results from this study also supported the findings from the earlier studies that pregnancy does not accelerate the progression of renal disease in women who already have nephropathy.

- It is important to counsel women with nephropathy and their partners that diabetic nephropathy worsens over time and women with this condition must consider the possibility of a future complicated by dialysis or renal transplantation.

TABLE 18.4. DIABETIC NEPHROPATHY, PERINATAL SURVIVAL, AND CONGENITAL MALFORMATIONS IN FOUR SERIES OVER 15 YEARS

	Kitzmiller (1981) Boston	Grenfell (1986) London	Reece (1988) New Haven	Pierce (1992) California
Years of study	1975-1978	1974-1984	1975-1984	1986-1990
Infants	27	23	31	39
*Fetal deaths**	2	0	2	1
Neonatal deaths	1	0	0	0
Perinatal survival	88.9%	100%	93.5%	97.4%
Major anomalies	3 (11.1%)	1 (4.3%)	3 (9.7%)	3 (7.7%)

*Elective and spontaneous abortions excluded.
Source: Adapted from Kitzmiller JL, Combs CA.[64]

10 Significant coronary artery disease is two to four times more common in patients with overt diabetic nephropathy than in those without nephropathy. Prior to conception, it is recommended that women with overt nephropathy be given a comprehensive physical examination with a thorough history, and an electrocardiogram.

    A Manske et al[68] found virtually no significant coronary disease among people with diabetes and end-stage renal disease as long as their age was less than 45 years, their duration of diabetes was less than 25 years, and there were no ST-T wave changes in the electrocardiogram. In the presence of any of these risk factors, exercise tolerance testing is needed.

    B Pregnant women with diabetes and coronary artery disease have a maternal mortality rate of 25% to 50% based on limited data.[69] These women along with their partners must be advised of the considerable risk of pregnancy.[69]

11 Diabetic neuropathy with severe gastroparesis may lead to significant nausea, vomiting, hypoglycemia or hyperglycemia, and problems with maternal and, indirectly, fetal nutrition. Metoclopramide can be used for women with symptoms of gastroparesis to improve comfort, nutritional status, and glucose control; symptoms of diarrhea are safely treated with loperamide during pregnancy.[69]

CARE AND EDUCATION DURING PREGNANCY

1   Care and education are focused on achieving and maintaining excellent blood glucose levels to maximize chances for a positive outcome. Glucose metabolism in a normal pregnancy provides the reference point for glycemic control.

    A   Lower fasting and preprandial blood glucose levels are normal during the second and third trimesters of pregnancy.

    B   Because of the greater tendency for maternal ketosis during fasting and the possible adverse effects of ketones on the fetus, periods of fasting during pregnancy need to be avoided to help prevent ketonemia.[70,71]

    C   Because of the increased resistance to insulin during the latter half of pregnancy, increasing doses of short-acting insulin with meals often are necessary. In addition, larger amounts of intermediate- or long-acting insulins or increased basal rates are needed to maintain insulin levels overnight. It is not unusual for a woman's insulin requirement to increase two- to threefold during the course of pregnancy.

2   No general consensus exists regarding optimal dietary guidelines for women with diabetes. Because no evidence exists to indicate otherwise, it is generally assumed that nutritional guidelines for pregnant women with type 1 and type 2 diabetes are similar to recommendations for pregnant women who do not have diabetes. Caloric requirements increase in the latter half of pregnancy.

    A   Goals of meal planning during pregnancy are to provide adequate nutrition throughout pregnancy for the baby and mother, to assist in appropriate gestational weight gain that is neither subnormal nor excessive, and to minimize blood glucose excursions.

    B   The recommended dietary allowances were revised in 1989[72] and are presented in Table 18.5. Of particular concern during pregnancy are protein, calcium, iron, folate, and calories.

       • Pregnant women require an additional 10 g/day of protein to support the metabolic changes in the mother and the growth of the fetus.

       • Pregnant women require 1200 mg/day of calcium to calcify fetal bones and teeth. This need is most dramatic in the third trimester.

       • The iron requirement increases substantially in pregnancy. There is no increased need in the first trimester, but the need doubles in the second and third trimester for a total of 30 mg/day.

Table 18.5. Selected Recommended Dietary Allowances for Women 25 to 50 Years Old

	Pregnant 1980	Nonpregnant 1989	Nonpregnant 1989
Protein (g)	74	60	50
Average kcal*	2300	2500	2200
Vitamin C (mg)	80	70	60
Vitamin B6 (mg)	2.6	2.2	1.6
Folate (µg)	800	400	180
Calcium (mg)	1200	1200	800
Magnesium (mg)	450	320	280
Iron (mg)	30-60	30	15
Zinc (mg)	20	15	12

*Additional calories are needed during the second and third trimesters only.
Source: Reprinted with permission from Jovanovic-Peterson et al.[29]

- Folate requirements more than double during pregnancy from 180 to 400 ug/day. Because folate supplementation has been associated with a decrease in neural tube defects, folate supplementation is recommended when contraception is stopped.
C The 1990 National Academy of Science[73] has established recommended ranges for total weight gain for pregnant women based on prepregnancy body mass index (BMI) (Table 18.6).

Table 18.6. Recommended Ranges of Total Weight Gain for Pregnant Women

Weight-for-Height Category	Recommended Total Weight Gain
Low (BMI <19.8)	28-40 lb (12.5 - 18 kg)
Normal (BMI 19.8 - 26)	25-35 lb (11.5 -16 kg)
High (BMI 26-29)	15-25 lb (7 - 11.5 kg)
Obese (BMI >29)	>15 lb (6 kg)

*BMI = weight (kg)/height (m)^2 x 100

- Weight gain by women who give birth to healthy infants is highly variable. Obese women have significantly heavier babies independent of weight gain. It is generally recommended that obese women gain a minimum equivalent to the products of conception, 15 lb (6.8 kg), although lower weight gains are often compatible with optimal birth weight.[74]

- Recommended weight gain is approximately 1 lb/week[74] (0.3 to 0.7 kg) during the second or third trimester; overweight women can gain at half that rate. Gains of less than 2 lb/month (0.9 kg month) or more than 6.5 lb/month (3 kg/month) for normal weight women warrant further evaluation.

D Adequate calories are needed to provide for weight gain in underweight and normal weight women and for weight maintenance or minimum weight gain in obese women. Weight loss is contraindicated.

- There are no universal recommendations for determining calories required during pregnancy (see Chapter 8, Nutrition, for more information). One method that can be used is to determine caloric requirements based on prepregnancy weight and add an additional 100 to 300 calories per day for the last two trimesters.[75,76] Using this method, the American Diabetes Association[29] prepared the recommendations shown in Table 18.7. A preferred method is to take a detailed diet history, prepare an individualized meal plan, follow up with food records, and monitor weight gain.

- Every attempt should be made to avoid ketonemia either from ketoacidosis or accelerated starvation ketosis in all pregnant women.[71]

- Monitoring blood glucose levels, urine ketones, appetite, and weight gain can guide the registered dietitian in developing an appropriate individualized meal plan and in making adjustments to the meal plan throughout the pregnancy.[76]

E Insulin can be matched to food intake, but maintaining consistency of times and amounts of food eaten is essential. Frequent smaller meals and snacks are often helpful. A snack at bedtime is important to prevent overnight starvation ketonuria and/or ketonemia.

F High-intensity sweeteners, in general, can be consumed during pregnancy.

- Saccharin can cross the placenta to the fetus, although there is no evidence that this sweetener is harmful to the fetus. However, avoiding excessive use of saccharin during pregnancy would seem prudent.[77]

- Aspartame is safe for use during pregnancy except for women with phenylketonuria.[77] Reproduction studies[77] in laboratory animals show that consumption of aspartame at intake levels of at least three times the 99th percentile poses no risk to the mother or fetus.
- Although acesulfame K crosses the placenta, reproduction studies[77] show no adverse effect; it can be used safely during pregnancy.

G Morning sickness can present a challenge. The following recommendations may be helpful:
- Suggest trying dry crackers or toast before rising.
- Small frequent meals help some women minimize nausea.
- Avoid caffeine and foods that are spicy or have a high fat content.
- Drink fluids between meals rather than with meals.
- Some women find it beneficial to take their prenatal vitamins before bedtime.
- Hypoglycemia aggravates morning sickness. Instruct patients to check blood glucose levels when nausea appears at unpredictable times and to always carry treatment for potential reactions.
- If vomiting occurs after taking the premeal short-acting insulin dose, administration of 0.15 mg of glucagon subcutaneously increases blood glucose 30 to 40 mg/dL and can help prevent hypoglycemia until the vomiting wanes. This increase in glucose level generally lasts 1 to 2 hours so the glucagon dose may need to be repeated until the peak short-acting insulin action has subsided. Advise any woman with continued vomiting to contact her healthcare team.[78,79]

3 Exercise can have a beneficial effect on blood glucose levels as well as overall well-being during pregnancy.

A Pregnancy generally is not a time for a woman who was previously sedentary to initiate strenuous activity. However, walking is possible for most women; a 15- to 20-minute walk can lower blood glucose by 20 to 40 mg/dL.

B Active women can continue to do similar activity during pregnancy but need to limit exercise periods to less than 30 minutes to help prevent hypoglycemia. Caution about becoming dehydrated, overheated, tachycardiac (heart rate >140 bpm), or dyspneic.

C As with exercise for any person with diabetes, planning, adjustments, and education for safety (eg, always carry additional food in case of hypoglycemia) are needed.

4 The glycemic goals of pregnancy are to achieve the blood glucose levels for that in a pregnant woman without diabetes. The most widely recommended glucose thresholds for early pregnancy are those of Kitzmiller et al:[28] fasting values of 60 to 100 mg/dL (3.3 to 5.6 mmol/L) and 1-hour postprandial blood glucose ranges of 100 to 140 mg/dL (5.6 to 7.8 mmol/L). The frequency of birth defects in patients who attained these goals in the preconception period and in early pregnancy was comparable to the frequency in a nondiabetic population (approximately 2%). The American Diabetes Association[29] recommends the maternal glucose goals shown in Table 18.8.

    A When defining glycemic goals during pregnancy, it is important to recognize that these targets are not always attainable. In Kitzmiller's successful preconception study,[28] 90% of the patient population achieved mean blood glucose levels of 104 to 160 mg/dL (5.8 to 8.9 mmol/L) during organogenesis, which was substantially higher than the recommended goals. Even with these blood glucose ranges there was no excess of congenital anomalies.

    B Discussing and establishing glucose goals with the woman and her partner is one of the most important aspects of both preconception and prenatal care. They need to understand the costs, benefits, barriers, and strategies of glycemic control in order to determine safe and realistic goals. If a woman has impaired glucose counterregulation or hypoglycemia unawareness, preprandial blood glucose levels under 100 mg/dL (3.3 to 5.6 mmol/L) may not be safe. Hypoglycemia has not been found to be teratogenic in human studies,[21,27,28] although animal studies suggest otherwise.[80]

    C Neonatal complications other than congenital malformations are associated with the level of glycemia throughout pregnancy. The fetal pancreas begins to function at approximately 13 weeks gestation. Elevations of glucose beyond this point stimulate fetal hyperinsulinism[13] which accelerates fetal growth beyond normal (macrosomia). Neonatal hypoglycemia, hyperbilirubinemia, and hypocalcemia have all been associated with maternal hyperglycemia.

    D Several authors[81,82] have reported lowered rates of macrosomia, neonatal hypoglycemia, and cesarean deliveries when glucose values were monitored postprandially rather than preprandially.

5 Many patterns of insulin administration can be used to achieve the desired ranges of glycemia.

TABLE 18.8. BLOOD GLUCOSE GOALS IN DIABETIC PREGNANCY

Fasting	60-90 mg/dL (3.3-5.0 mmol/L)
Premeal	60-105 mg/dL (3.3-5.8 mmol/L)
1 h postprandial	100-120 mg/dL (5.5-6.7 mmol/L)
2 h-6 h	60-120 mg/dL (3.3-6.7 mmol/L)

Source: Adapted with permission from Jovanovic-Peterson et al.[29]

A Because only human insulin with its faster absorption is used during pregnancy, the vast majority of women with diabetes will require three injections to achieve glucose goals: intermediate- and short-acting insulin in the morning, short-acting insulin predinner, and intermediate-acting insulin at bedtime. Intermediate-acting insulin before dinner is not advised because of the increased risk of overnight hypoglycemia during pregnancy.

B Other women may achieve their goals with short-acting insulin prior to meals and intermediate-acting insulin at bedtime.

C Still others will benefit from continuous subcutaneous insulin infusion (CSII) therapy, which can be particularly helpful during pregnancy.[83] CSII lowers the amount of circulating basal insulin, thereby decreasing the incidence of premeal hypoglycemia while efficiently controlling the more dramatic rise in postprandial glucose common during pregnancy. Frequent and severe hypoglycemia is an indication for pump therapy.

- Pregnant women using insulin pumps require extensive education to avoid complications that could arise from any interruption in insulin delivery. In the third trimester there is an increased risk of DKA. Marcus and colleagues[84] recommended using 0.2 u/kg of NPH or lente insulin at bedtime in addition to the usual basal rate in order to reduce the incidence of DKA to <0.5% during pregnancy.

- Insulin pump therapy is best initiated before conception, but successful therapy can and should be started at any point if glycemic control is suboptimal.

D Keeping activity and timing and content of meals as constant as possible will help as the patient learns her own glucose patterns. As she becomes more knowledgeable and the glucose patterns normalize, greater flexibility is possible and the insulin dosage can be varied to keep up with her changing insulin requirements.

E Insulin requirements are estimated based on current weight, gestational age, blood glucose monitoring results, and caloric intake. Generally, 0.6 u/kg/day total daily dose during preconception, increasing to 0.7 at 6 weeks gestation, 0.8 at 16 weeks gestation, 0.9 at 26 weeks gestation, and 1.0 at 36 weeks gestation are recommended.[85] Women who are >150% of desirable body weight may need 1.5 to 2.0 u/kg secondary to insulin resistance due to obesity.

E Adjustments need to be made cautiously in the first trimester because of the significant incidence of hypoglycemia.

- Kimmerle and colleagues[86] reported a rate as high as 41%; 84% of these episodes occurred before 20 weeks gestation and 77% occurred during sleep. Women with a previous history of severe hypoglycemia were at particular risk. Diamond et al[87] suggested that impaired counterregulatory responses in women with type 1 diabetes may be responsible for this increased rate.

- Provide education to all patients regarding hypoglycemia prevention and treatment, including instructing family members in the use of glucagon.

6 Diabetes control is monitored through blood glucose levels, urinary ketone measurements, and glycosylated hemoglobin concentrations. In addition, some centers have successfully measured glycosylated serum protein levels to evaluate short-term glycemic control.[88]

A Self blood glucose monitoring is needed before each meal and before the bedtime snack. Additionally, postprandial measurements are used to evaluate the effectiveness of short-acting insulin, and 3 AM levels are helpful to detect asymptomatic hypoglycemia or evaluate unexplained fasting hyperglycemia.

- Verifiable data are preferred to document blood glucose results. Pregnant patients are no different than nonpregnant patients in their abilities to fabricate data. Along with the use of memory meters, detailed record keeping is useful to help patients identify their glucose patterns.

B Urine monitoring for ketones in the first morning urine specimen is needed daily, any time the blood glucose level exceeds 200 mg/dL (10.0 mol/L), during illness, or when the patient is unable to eat as a result of nausea and/or vomiting. The glucose value at which a woman will spill ketones is lower during pregnancy, and therefore the risk of DKA is greater. Urine measurements for ketones are needed because of the increased tendency toward fat catabolism during pregnancy. Ketones cross the placenta if the patient has ketonemia and may be potentially harmful to the fetus.

- The presence of ketonuria with normal or low blood glucose levels is suggestive of starvation ketonuria and usually indicates inadequate food intake.
- The presence of ketonuria in the face of mildly elevated blood glucose levels may indicate incipient ketoacidosis.
- The main cause of ketoacidosis is infection.
- Ketoacidosis in pregnancy is associated with a high perinatal mortality rate.
- ß-sympathomimetic therapy such as ritodrine or terbutaline used to treat premature labor has been reported to cause deterioration of blood glucose control and ketosis in pregnant diabetic women.[89] These agents should not be the first line of therapy for women with diabetes; if they are used, blood glucose levels must be carefully monitored.
- Ketoacidosis has been reported in pregnancy with normal glucose values.

C Glycosylated hemoglobin measurements may be obtained monthly. Ideally, patients' levels will be in the mid-normal range throughout pregnancy. Relatively mild elevations of glycohemoglobin have been associated with increased fetal morbidity.[33]

7 Hospitalization may be indicated whenever a woman with diabetes who has not been using intensive management prior to conception becomes pregnant. Other indications for hospitalization include a lack of self-management skills, nausea and vomiting that prevent adequate caloric intake, deterioration of blood glucose control that is unresolved with close telephone contact, hyperglycemia with moderate or large ketonuria, nonadherence, and any obstetric complication such as preeclampsia or premature labor.[90]

Monitoring of the Fetus During Pregnancy

1 Fetal ultrasonography in the first or early second trimester allows confirmation of gestational age and helps to verify the absence of any malformations. A fetal echocardiogram in midpregnancy is used to screen for

congenital heart defects. Serial ultrasounds thereafter are used to assess fetal growth, measure the amniotic fluid volume, and evaluate the state of the placenta (Table 18.9).

2   A blood test to screen maternal serum alpha-fetoprotein (MSAFP) levels provides additional information when trying to identify the fetus at risk for a neural tube defect. In women with diabetes, the incidence of neural tube defects is 20 per 1000, which is 10- to 20-times greater than in the general population.[91] Thus, all women with diabetes need referral for targeted ultrasound regardless of their MSAFP test result.

   A   Neural tube defects develop from defective closure of the neural tube during embryogenesis, which results in anencephaly, encephalocele, and all variants of spina bifida.

   B   The MSAFP test should be offered between 15 and 18 weeks of gestation (Table 18.9). An elevated result identifies a fetus that may have a neural tube defect or other abnormality.

   • There are many conditions that can falsely raise this test result including diabetes, inaccurate dates, or multiple gestations.

   • Advise patients that the MSAFP is a screening test to identify fetuses that require a closer look and is not diagnostic in and of itself.

   • Patients with positive results may be advised to have a further evaluation with ultrasound and/or amniocentesis.

3   Fetal movement recording is an accurate, reliable, and inexpensive way for the pregnant women to assess her baby's overall health. Fetal kick counting, as it is popularly called, is advisable for all pregnant women with diabetes beginning in the early third trimester.

   A   One method is to keep track of fetal movements over a 12-hour period. If fewer than 10 movements are observed during the 12-hour period, or if it takes progressively longer before the 10 movements are identified, the woman should notify her obstetrician immediately. In many cases, further evaluation of fetal status is indicated.[92]

   B   Another method is to count fetal movement for several 30-minute or 1-hour periods each day. The patient may be asked to keep written records of fetal movement (Figure 18.2).

Table 18.9. Fetal Testing Timeline for Women With Preexisting Diabetes

	Tests	Number of Weeks Into the Pregnancy
First Trimester	Early ultrasound to date the pregnancy	8 weeks
Second Trimester	Alpha-fetoprotein test	15 to 18 weeks
	Comprehensive ultrasound Fetal echocardiogram	18 to 22 weeks 20 to 22 weeks
Third Trimester	Kick counting	26 weeks
	Nonstress test	If there are complications, twice a week starting at 28 weeks. If there are no complications, twice a week starting at 32 to 34 weeks.
	Biophysical profile	28 to 32 weeks to begin
	Fetal echocardiogram	32 to 33 weeks if needed
	Amniocentesis to test lung maturity	If birth is induced before 39 weeks

Source: Adapted with permission from Jornsay DL. Diabetes Self-Manage 1996;13(3):40.

4 The nonstress test (NST) is a safe, noninvasive assessment of the overall health of the fetus. Two transducers are placed on the mother's abdomen; one records the fetal heart rate while the other detects uterine contractions. The fetal heart rate should increase with activity and/or stimulation. This is called a reactive test.

   A In some centers, nonstress tests are performed weekly from the gestational age of 32 to 34 weeks, then twice weekly from 36 weeks until delivery (Table 18.9). If a nonstress test is abnormal or nonreactive, a contraction stress test or a biophysical profile may be ordered.

   B Earlier and more frequent testing may be necessary for patients who have vascular disease.

5 Weekly contraction stress tests are used by some centers to assess fetal well-being beginning at 32 to 34 weeks. The contraction stress test (CST) is a record of the fetal heart rate response to mild uterine contractions, which are induced by intravenous pitocin or by nipple stimulation.

A If late decelerations of the fetal heart rate occur following more than 50% of the uterine contractions, the test is considered positive.

B A positive CST may indicate fetal distress and the need for delivery.

6 A biophysical profile is another test to discriminate between fetuses that are well adapted to their intrauterine environment and those in danger of fetal demise (Table 18.9).

A A *biophysical profile* involves the evaluation of five parameters. Ultrasound is used to assess four components: fetal breathing, fetal body movement, fetal muscle tone, and amniotic fluid volume. Fetal heart-rate activity is evaluated by means of a nonstress test. Two points are given for the normal observation of each of these five parameters. The lowest score is 0 and the highest score is 10. A score of 8 to 10 is desirable; scores lower than 6 generally warrant further evaluation.

B A biophysical profile sometimes is performed when a NST is nonreactive or a CST is positive.

7 If an amniocentesis is performed, it is used to assess fetal lung maturity (Table 18.9). Amniocentesis may be part of the protocol when induction of labor or elective Cesarean Section is planned prior to 39 weeks.

8 Many pregnancies can safely progress to term as long as fetal health does not appear to be compromised and no maternal complications (such as preeclampsia) are present.

DIABETES CARE DURING LABOR AND DELIVERY

1 The goals of managing diabetes during labor are to provide adequate carbohydrate intake to meet maternal energy requirements and to maintain maternal euglycemia.

A Glucose is administered 2.0 to 2.5 mg/kg/min by continuous intravenous infusion to meet maternal energy requirements and thus to prevent ketosis.[93] This dosage corresponds to approximately 5 to 10 g/hour in lean individuals.

B Maternal blood glucose values are measured every 1 to 2 hours, and short-acting insulin is administered by multiple subcutaneous doses or by continuous intravenous infusion as necessary to maintain euglycemia,. Maternal euglycemia may help prevent undue stimulation of fetal insulin secretion prior to delivery to prevent neonatal hypoglycemia.[92]

FIGURE 18.2. FETAL MOVEMENT RECORD[92]

Reprinted with permission: Hollister Incorporated, Libertyville, Illinois, ©1988

- CSII has been used successfully during labor and delivery.
- Regardless of the method, the key to successful intrapartum management is to monitor blood glucose levels frequently and administer insulin and glucose as necessary.

POSTPARTUM PERIOD

1 The postpartum period is characterized by an immediate decrease in insulin requirements.

   A In general, insulin requirements are recalculated at 0.6 u/kg current weight for nonlactating women and 0.4 u/kg current weight for lactating women.

   B Occasionally little or no insulin is required during the first 24 to 48 hours following delivery.

   C No reduction in insulin requirements may indicate an underlying infection such as endometritis or a urinary tract infection.

2 Many issues surround the patient in the postpartum period. The role of the educator is to continue to offer support and information during this period of adjustment.

   A She needs to learn to balance her own self-care needs with the needs of her infant. Assess for postpartum depression or other psychosocial needs related to diabetes or the demands of motherhood.

   B The risk of hypoglycemia is very significant in the first few weeks postpartum. Review hypoglycemia knowledge and skills with the new mother and her partner, including the need to first care for herself then her baby when hypoglycemic.

   C Provide close follow-up of diabetes control to reestablish her baseline insulin requirement.

   D Offer referral to a registered dietitian concerning weight reduction and/or prevention of hypoglycemia while breast-feeding.

   E Offer referral for counseling or other support if the outcome was not positive.

Lactation

1 Provide support and education for women who desire to breast-feed.

   A In most situations, breast-feeding mothers require less insulin because of the calories expended with nursing. Lactating women have reported drops in glucose of 50 to 100 mg/dL over a 30-minute nursing session.

   B All lactating women with diabetes need information about the prevention and prompt recognition and treatment of hypoglycemia.

2 Approximately the same meal plan as that of the third trimester of pregnancy is appropriate during lactation. The bedtime snack may need to be adjusted and the intermediate-acting insulin may be given at bedtime, because of the significant risk for hypoglycemia following nighttime breast-feeding.

3 Oral antidiabetes agents cannot be used while lactating. Other medications may also affect breast milk.

4 Women with type 2 diabetes whose glucose values are not maintained with medical nutrition therapy alone will need to continue to take insulin throughout lactation.

Contraception and Family Planning

1 The use of contraception in *all* women with diabetes or a prior history of GDM cannot be emphasized strongly enough. This is the only way to ensure that preconception care can be provided.

2 Barrier methods of contraception create mechanical and/or chemical barriers to fertilization.

   A Barrier methods include diaphragms, male condoms, spermicidal foam, jelly or foam, cervical caps and female condoms.

   B Although these methods pose no health risks to women with diabetes, they are user-dependent, require correct application or insertion before intercourse, and have a high failure rate of 12% to 28%[94,95] in the first year because of improper use. With experience and motivation, these failure rates may be reduced to levels of 2% to 6%.[94,95]

3 Oral contraceptives remain the most popular form of birth control despite controversy over potential side effects.

    A The main reasons for their popularity are their failure rate of generally less than 1% and ease of use.

    B Low-dose formulations are preferred and are recommended only for patients without vascular complications or additional risk factors such as smoking or a strong family history of myocardial disease.[96]

4 An intrauterine device (IUD) is the most effective nonhormonal device.[94]

    A It should only be offered to women who have a low risk of sexually transmitted diseases because any infection might place the patient with diabetes at risk for sepsis and ketoacidosis.

    B Patient education includes the early signs of sexually transmitted diseases, such as increased and abnormal vaginal discharge, dyspareunia, heavy, painful menses, lower abdominal pain, and fever.[97] Teach patients to seek prompt health care attention if any of these occur.

5 Depoprovera® and Norplant® are long-acting progestins that provide highly effective pregnancy prevention.

    A Depoprovera® is administered intramuscularly every 3 months and works by inhibiting ovulation.

    B Norplant® is a long-acting, reversible, silicone/rubber-covered, hormonal implant that offers 5-year protection and 99% effectiveness.[96] Norplant® works by inhibiting ovulation, thickening cervical mucus, and changing the uterine lining.

    C The high efficiency and long period of action of Depoprovera® and Norplant® make them attractive options for women with diabetes or previous gestational diabetes mellitus (GDM), especially women with a history of poor medication-taking.[94] Unfortunately, these long-acting progestins have not been studied in women with diseases.

6 Permanent sterilization, including tubal ligation and vasectomy, may be considered by the patient or her partner when they desire no more children.

GESTATIONAL DIABETES

1 *Gestational diabetes mellitus* is the most common medical complication of pregnancy, occurring in 1% to 15% of patients depending on the population described and the criteria used for diagnosis.[97]

A GDM is defined as carbohydrate intolerance of variable severity with onset or first recognition during pregnancy.[3-6] This definition applies regardless of whether insulin was instituted during pregnancy or the condition persisted following pregnancy. The definition does not exclude the possibility that unrecognized glucose intolerance may have antedated the pregnancy.

B GDM is usually detected between 24 and 28 weeks gestation when the insulin resistance of pregnancy becomes marked.

2 GDM has implications for both the mother and her offspring. Women with undetected or untreated GDM have an increased risk for perinatal morbidity and mortality, and are at high risk for the development of overt type 2 diabetes later in life.

A A 6.4% perinatal mortality rate has been observed in pregnancies complicated by untreated GDM in women over 25 years of age compared with a 1.5% rate in pregnant women with normal glucose tolerance.[65]

B Today, in patients with appropriately treated GDM, the likelihood of intrauterine death is not significantly higher than in the general population.[98]

C GDM also is associated with many of the same fetal and neonatal morbidities observed in patients with pregestational diabetes, including macrosomia, shoulder dystocia, hypoglycemia, hypocalcemia, polycythemia, and hyperbilirubinemia.[99,100]

D The rates for these neonatal complications are dependent upon the quality of glycemic control throughout gestation.

- Macrosomia is the most common of these perinatal concerns and is observed two to three times more often than in women with normal glucose tolerance.[6]
- GDM, with its onset in late pregnancy, is not associated with an increased incidence of birth defects. However, preexisting diabetes diagnosed for the first time during pregnancy as GDM, may result in a higher risk of birth defects.[6]

E Studies suggest that the long-range implications for offspring of women with GDM may include an increased risk of obesity in adolescence[37-39] and impaired glucose tolerance and diabetes later in life.

- The prevalence of type 2 diabetes has been reported as high as 45% by age 20 to 24 in the offspring of mothers with gestational diabetes during pregnancy.[37]

- Rizzo and associates,[101] found that poorer maternal metabolic control was associated with the child's poorer performance on standard measures of psychomotor development at ages 6 and 9.

F Many studies[82,102,103] have documented an increased maternal risk for preeclampsia, polyhydramnios, and operative delivery in pregnancies complicated by GDM.

- The added maternal implication of GDM is also a high risk for the development of overt type 2 diabetes mellitus later in life.[104,105]
- Elevated fasting plasma glucose levels, increased maternal age, obesity, a diagnosis of gestational diabetes prior to 24 weeks, and the need for insulin therapy during pregnancy all correlate with an increased risk for abnormal glucose tolerance in the immediate postpartum period or within the first postpartum year.[105,106] Kjos and associates[106] have shown the rate of postpartum glucose intolerance to be as high as 10% in women 5 to 8 weeks postpartum.
- Coustan and associates[107] studied former gestational diabetic women and found diabetes or impaired glucose tolerance (IGT) in 6% of women with GDM tested at 0 to 2 years, 13% at 3 to 4 years, 15% at 5 to 6 years, and 30% at 7 to 10 years postpartum.
- Peters and colleagues[108] found that episodes of insulin resistance due to additional pregnancies increased the rate for developing type 2 diabetes independent of pregnancy-associated weight gain.

3 There are various considerations regarding screening for gestational diabetes mellitus.

A Considerable international debate has ensued regarding the recommendation that all pregnant women be screened for glucose intolerance. Initially this recommendation was made by the Second International Workshop[4] on gestational diabetes because clinical risk factors such as previous birth of a large baby, maternal obesity, glycosuria, or family history of diabetes have been shown to be poor predictors of GDM[109-111]; and GDM is generally asymptomatic.

B Current recommendations by the Expert Committee on the Diagnosis and Classification of Diabetes Mellitus, working under the sponsorship of the American Diabetes Association[112] are that universal screening may not be necessary in women who meet *all* of the following criteria:

- <25 years of age
- Normal body weight
- No first degree relatives with diabetes mellitus

- Not of an ethnic group at increased risk for type 2 diabetes mellitus. These groups include Latinos, Native Americans, Asians, Africans and African Americans, Pacific Islanders, indigenous Australians, and anyone from the Indian subcontinent.[112] It is felt that screening may not be cost-effective in these women, who have no increased risk.

- Universal screening is still recommended in women who are in a high-risk group (ie, those with any of the risk factors listed above).

C Screening for GDM is recommended between the 24th and 28th week of gestation if a woman has not been identified as having glucose intolerance before the 24th week of gestation.[4,6]

D Any woman who presents with a history suggestive of prior or current glucose intolerance, who is markedly obese, or who has a strong family history of type 2 diabetes or glucosuria should be screened immediately.

E A fasting plasma glucose measurement of 126 mg/dL (7.8 mmol/L) or a random plasma glucose measurement of 200 mg/dL (11.1 mmol/L) outside the context of a formal glucose challenge suggests diabetes and warrants immediate further investigation.[6,112]

F The screening test, or glucose challenge test (GCT) as it is frequently called, involves obtaining a venous plasma glucose measurement 1 hour after consuming 50 g of oral glucose without regard to the time of the last meal or the time of day.

- Whatever assay method is used must have good precision, as defined by a coefficient of variation <3.5%. Capillary glucose meters do not have sufficient precision and accuracy for establishing the diagnosis of GDM.[6]

- A value of 140 mg/dL (7.8 mmol/L) or greater is a positive screening test,[4,6] as established by the Second, Third, and Fourth International Workshop-Conferences on GDM, and requires further evaluation with an OGTT (see Table 18.10).

- It should be noted that 10% of all women with GDM had screening test values between 130 mg/dL and 139 mg/dL.[110] However, if screening values were lowered to this range, it would result in an increase in glucose tolerance testing from 14% to 23%, and an increase in attendant costs.[74]

G An alternative to the two-step screening process offered above has been recommended by the Fourth International Workshop-Conference. This one-step process eliminates the glucose screen and immediately goes to the diagnostic glucose tolerance test. It utilizes a

75 g GTT based on WHO criteria rather than the 100 g GTT which has traditionally been used in this country.

TABLE 18.10. SCREENING/TESTING FOR GDM

Who	When	Type of Test	Results
All women with risk factors	24 to 28 weeks	50 g 1-hour GCT vs 75 g 2-hour OGTT	+ GCT result ≥140 mg/dL (7.8 mmol/L); GDM if 100 g meets revised Carpenter and Coustan criteria[115]
Women who have a positive screen	24 to 28 weeks	100 g 3-hour OGTT	+ Diagnosis if meets Carpenter and Coustan criteria[115]
Women who have a clinical history/normal screen	32 to 34 weeks	Repeat 1-hour GCT or OGTT	Repeating screen is based upon clinical judgment
Women diagnosed with GDM	6 to 8 weeks postpartum	75 g 2-hour OGTT	Classify according to National Diabetes Data Group[116]

GCT=glucose challenge test, OGTT=oral glucose tolerance test.

H Women with risk factors for glucose intolerance and an abnormal screen but a normal 3-hour OGTT might be candidates for a repeat 3-hour OGTT at 32 weeks. This is especially true for women with one abnormal value on the OGTT. Jornsay and colleagues[113] recommend the following criteria for retesting:
- Positive screen at 24 to 28 weeks and one abnormal OGTT value
- Maternal age >35 years
- Maternal obesity (> 120% desirable body weight)
- Current glucosuria
- Ultrasound evidence of fetal compromise, (ie, polyhydramnios, macrosomia, or accelerated abdominal circumference growth)
- Current betamimetic or glucosteroid therapy

I If the glucose screen is >185 mg/dL, a 3-hour OGTT is contraindicated, and the patient needs treatment for diabetes.[114]

4 There are various considerations regarding making the diagnosis of gestational diabetes mellitus. The 100 g OGTT values diagnostic for GDM have been those recommended by the National Diabetes Data Group

(NDDG).[116] These values were derived from the work of O'Sullivan and Mahan.[111] More recent work by Carpenter and Coustan[115] challenged the NDDG criteria. Sacks and colleagues[117] conducted further investigations and discovered that the NDDG conversions were above the 95% confidence limits for all but the fasting sample, whereas the Carpenter and Coustan criteria were always within the 95% confidence intervals. Table 18.11 summarizes the various diagnostic criteria for GDM using the 100 g OGTT.[118] These lower values result in a higher prevalence of GDM.

A The diagnosis of GDM may now be based on the results of either the 100 g OGTT, according to the diagnostic criteria of Carpenter and Coustan[115] or the NDDG,[116] or a 75 g OGTT, based on the WHO criteria, depending on the risk characteristics of the local population.

- It is recommended that oral glucose tolerance testing be performed in the morning after an overnight fast of at least 8 hours but no greater than 14 hours. At least 3 days of unrestricted diet (150 g carbohydrate per day) and unrestricted activity need to precede the test.

- Women need to remain seated and not smoke during the test.

- A definitive diagnosis of GDM requires that two or more of the venous plasma glucose levels listed in Table 18.11 are met or exceeded.[6,118]

- It may be prudent to notify the patient's provider of the fasting blood glucose level before administration of the glucose load.

- A fasting level >126 mg/dL is sufficient to make the diagnosis and may make further glucose administration dangerous.[112]

- The glucose load is best tolerated when it is chilled and citrus rather than cola flavored. Women who are unable to tolerate glucola without vomiting, may attempt an alternative such as jelly beans.[119] However, these alternatives have not been as extensively evaluated as has glucola. The intravenous glucose tolerance test (IVGTT)[120] has been examined as an alternative method. Comparisons of the IVGTT and the OGTT and found a poor correlation between the two tests. The IVGTT is more expensive and cumbersome, and it is therefore unlikely that this will be extensively utilized as an alternative to the OGTT.[120]

5 Treatment of gestational diabetes consists of improving the metabolic abnormalities associated with GDM through meal planning and insulin therapy (if indicated), and providing close maternal and fetal surveillance.

TABLE 18.11. DIAGNOSTIC CRITERIA FOR GDM USING THE 100 G OGTT[111,115,116]

Time (h)	mg/dL	(mmol/L)
0	105	5.8
1	190	10.6
2	165	9.2
3	145	8.1

A Medical nutrition therapy is the foundation of GDM treatment. The goals and strategies for nutrition care are the same as during a pregestational diabetic pregnancy. Consultation and ongoing nutrition follow-up with a perinatal nutritionist is recommended to develop the meal plan based on the woman's prepregnancy body weight,[121] activity levels, food preferences, and daily schedule.

- The goal is to provide adequate calories and optimal nutrition for pregnancy without hyperglycemia or ketonemia.

- Frequent small meals with limited carbohydrates at breakfast often will return blood glucose levels to normal. Meal plans include three meals and two to four small snacks (see Chapter 8, Nutrition).

- While caloric restriction does improve glycemic control, it results in ketonuria and potential ketonemia.[122,123] It is, therefore, not generally recommended because of the potential effects on the fetus.

- The use of protein-rich foods helps blunt the effects of the carbohydrates on blood glucose. These foods also provide extra calories without increasing the carbohydrate content of meals.

- Blood glucose monitoring and food records help the patient learn the effects of foods on blood glucose levels.

- The ideal percentage and type of carbohydrate is controversial. A reasonable meal plan for GDM has between 45% and 65% of the carbohydrate, predominately complex and high fiber, at meals. When snacks are included, approximately 38% to 45% of the calories for the total day are from carbohydrate, 20% to 25% from protein, and 30% to 40% from fat. These new guidelines[124] provide greater flexibility in the amount of carbohydrate and fat.

- More important than percentages are the actual grams of carbohydrate. Breakfast meals generally require less than 30 grams of carbohydrate to prevent excessive elevations of postprandial blood glucose levels. Teach patients to eliminate concentrated sources of carbohydrates and to be aware that highly processed foods often produce higher postmeal glucose values.

B Exercise can be helpful in lowering postprandial glucose elevations. Women with GDM who have an active lifestyle may continue a program of moderate exercise[6] combined with frequent blood glucose monitoring and close follow-up.[125]

- While more studies are needed to determine the effects of cardiovascular fitness training on fetal outcome and the effects of such exercise on ketone production,[6] it is sensible that a program of moderate regular exercise, particularly after meals, will have a beneficial effect on the blood glucose levels.

C The Third International Workshop Conference on GDM[6] noted that "self-monitoring of capillary blood glucose has been useful in allowing the woman to participate in her own management," but its utility "in mild GDM not requiring insulin, although reasonable and logical, has not been formally proved."

- Evidence does exist, however, to support the role of glucose monitoring in GDM pregnancies. Wechter and associates[126] demonstrated a reduction in the incidence of macrosomia in infants of mothers with GDM to that seen in the normal population by utilizing nutrition therapy and home blood glucose monitoring. Insulin was used only if needed as determined by glucose results and clinical assessment. Significant reductions in macrosomia and LGA infants were found by using home monitoring to selectively determine who required insulin by Goldberg and colleagues.[32] Langer et al,[127] in a large, partially randomized study of women with GDM, showed that more intensive management (seven meter-verified glucose results versus four visually read glucose results) resulted in significant reductions in macrosomia, shoulder dystocia, stillbirths, and cesarean delivery as compared to the women in the conventionally treated (four visual results) group. More intensive glucose monitoring resulted in a higher percentage of patients taking insulin.[32]

- The controversies regarding the timing for blood glucose testing were quieted by de Veciana and associates[82] who in a prospective, randomized study found that fasting and 1-hour postprandial glucose monitoring resulted in improved glycemic control and significant decreases in neonatal hypoglycemia, birth weight, and percentage of LGA infants, shoulder dystocia, and cesarean deliveries when compared with preprandial glucose monitoring.

- Daily urine ketone accumulation is measured in the first voided morning specimen to determine if dietary carbohydrate and caloric intake are sufficient. Teach patients to monitor urine ketones if they have not eaten for more than 5 hours and any time the glucose level is in excess of 200 mg/dL.

  - Buchanan and colleagues[90] have suggested a management strategy which combines the use of a fetal ultrasound at 29 to 33 weeks and fasting glucose levels checked every 2 weeks to determine the need for insulin. While this approach may be helpful, it does not provide for any assessment of postmeal glucose values, which have been shown to more closely correlate with overall glycemic control than fasting values.[82] It is also more costly than glucose monitoring and does not give the patient the immediate feedback of the effects of meal planning on glycemia.

  - The goals of glycemic control are stated in Table 18.8.

D Insulin therapy is necessary to achieve euglycemia in 20% to 50% of women with GDM depending on the goals of glycemia. The major benefits derived from this therapy are reductions in perinatal morbidity, especially in the incidence of macrosomia in the newborn.[32,127-130]

- The initiation of insulin is now widely recommended when the fasting plasma glucose levels of <105 mg/dL (<5.8 mmol/L) and/or a 2-hour postprandial plasma glucose levels of <120 mg/dL (<6.7 mmol/L) are not consistently maintained with medical nutrition therapy.[6,131] Many centers, however, initiate insulin at fasting values of 90 mg/dL or above, or 1-hour postprandial values above 120 mg/dL, as this lowers the rate of macrosomia.[126,129]

- There is a relationship between the level of glycemia and neonatal weight.[126,127] Undertreatment results in macrosomia and overtreatment with insulin may result in small-for-gestational-age (SGA) infants. Langer et al[127] have reported that a mean blood glucose level consisting of both preprandial and postprandial values <87 mg/dL (4.8 mmol/L) increased the incidence 2.55-fold for the development of SGA infants.

- When insulin is required, human preparations are used because the insulin antibodies produced in response to animal insulins can cross the placenta.
- Oral antidiabetes agents are not recommended during pregnancy because they cross the placenta and may potentiate fetal hyperinsulinism.[45] Glyburide is the one oral agent which does not appear to cross the placenta and may have a future in the management of GDM.[132]
- At this time, prophylactic insulin treatment for patients whose glucose values are within normal limits is not recommended.[118]
- Insulin therapy can generally be initiated on an outpatient basis, provided glycemic control is not grossly compromised, the patient is able to give and cope with injections, and 24-hour access to health care is available.

E Fetal monitoring tests are an important part of the management of GDM. The tests utilized are the same as those described in the section on preexisting diabetes fetal monitoring (Table 18.9).

- The time in pregnancy to initiate these tests depends upon the practice in a given institution, whether the woman with GDM is taking exogenous insulin, whether her fetus demonstrates any abnormalities of growth, and whether the woman has any other factors complicating her pregnancy.
- Patients generally are permitted to begin labor spontaneously at term unless fetal health appears compromised. The goals of management for the woman with gestational diabetes in labor are the same as those previously outlined in the pregestational diabetes section.
- Blood glucose is periodically monitored during labor. Normal glucose levels can generally be maintained during labor without insulin.
- Insulin treatment can usually be discontinued in the immediate postpartum period. Women who then manifest nongravid diabetes can be treated as indicated.

6 The postpartum period demands special education and follow-up because of the high risk of subsequent diabetes in the mother.

A Following delivery, teach all women with GDM to request reevaluation for glucose intolerance. The American Diabetes Association[133] and the Second and Third International Workshop-Conferences on Gestational Diabetes[4,6] recommend that all women receive their initial evaluation (a 2-hour oral glucose tolerance test with 75 grams of glucose) at the first 6- to 8-week postpartum visit.

B Based on the result of this test, the woman is then categorized as having previous abnormality of glucose tolerance, impaired glucose tolerance, or diabetes mellitus in the nonpregnant adult (see Chapter 7, Pathophysiology of the Diabetes Disease State).

C Because the risk of subsequent diabetes is so high, oral glucose tolerance tests are done in some centers in the postpartum period and yearly thereafter.

D Patient education for prevention of future type 2 diabetes includes the importance of attaining and maintaining a reasonable body weight, receiving annual blood glucose testing, and contacting a member of the healthcare team if symptoms of hyperglycemia develop. The role of meal planning and exercise on glucose tolerance and weight loss and/or control cannot be stressed strongly enough.

E Low-dose oral contraceptives appear to be safe in women with prior GDM who demonstrate normal glucose tolerance in the postpartum period.[6] High-dose synthetic estrogen/progestin contraceptives are not recommended.

F Additionally, the use of other medications that may affect glucose metabolism adversely, such as thiazides, steroids, and ß-blockers, requires careful consideration.[6]

G The postpartum 75 g 2-hour OGTT may be affected by lactation; if abnormal, the patient needs reevaluation postlactation.

KEY EDUCATIONAL CONSIDERATIONS FOR WOMEN WITH PREEXISTING DIABETES

1 Information needed by patients in the pre- and/or early postconception period includes the effects of maternal diabetes on her baby. Explain that glucose and ketones cross the placenta, while insulin and glucagon do not. This concept is also quite helpful in helping women to understand the importance of waiting until glycemia is normalized before conceiving.

2 Explain that it is usual for the insulin dose to increase during pregnancy and that she may need a two- to threefold increase toward the end of pregnancy. Discuss with her that her insulin requirements will increase because the placenta produces hormones that act against insulin, not because her diabetes is more severe. Tell her explicitly that her diabetes is not getting worse.

3 Explain how it may be difficult to accomplish glycemic goals and that her numbers do not need to be perfect to have a normal glycohemoglobin value and a healthy baby. Be sure to make adjustments for the patient who has problems with hypoglycemia awareness.

4 Offer referral to a registered dietitian for nutritional counseling. It is important that the patient understand sick day rules because hyperemesis can be a problem in early pregnancy. It is also important that she understand the role of snacks in preventing ketonuria.

5 Assess her blood glucose monitoring technique periodically. Verify her meter's accuracy with a laboratory plasma glucose test done simultaneously with a capillary blood glucose reading. Ideally, the capillary value should be within 10% to 15% of the laboratory value.

6 Review the signs, symptoms, causes, treatment, and prevention of hypoglycemia with the patient, her partner or other family member. Instruct family members on glucagon administration. Recommended treatment may change from concentrated sources of carbohydrates (eg, orange juice) to milk. Advise her to carry food at all times and provide information on how to obtain diabetes identification.

7 Review injection sites and the differences in absorption times for different sites. Reassure her that it is fine to use her abdomen.

8 Ask the patient about her daily routine and create a schedule together with times for meals, snacks, testing, and insulin injections. If the patient does not follow a schedule, it is virtually impossible to successfully titrate her insulin dosage to keep up with the changing requirements of pregnancy.

9 Provide the patient with written parameters for when to contact you or another member of the healthcare team. Suggest that she or a family member notify you if any of the following occurs: a marked change in blood glucose levels, moderate or large ketonuria, vomiting, hypoglycemia requiring a glucagon injection or any severe episode, fever, vaginal bleeding, severe headache, blurred vision, a decrease in fetal movement (in the second half of pregnancy), uterine contractions, or other pregnancy complications.

10 Following the birth of her baby and months of intensive monitoring, it is common for the mother to lose interest in for her own self-management. Remind her that she worked hard to have a healthy infant and healthy babies need healthy mothers. Careful diabetes management will help ensure future successful pregnancies and reduce the risk for long-term diabetes complications such as retinopathy and/or nephropathy.

11 Work with the mother closely in the postpartum period to avoid maternal hypoglycemia, which can be a safety issue for her infant and/or herself.

KEY EDUCATIONAL CONSIDERATIONS FOR WOMEN WITH GESTATIONAL DIABETES

1 When educating women about gestational diabetes, it is important to recognize that they may be casual about following treatment guidelines because they feel well and are approaching the end of pregnancy.

   A When teaching the pathophysiology of GDM, describe the role of insulin action in the body to keep blood glucose levels in the normal range. Explain that in the second half of pregnancy the need for insulin increases because the placenta produces hormones that work against the insulin's ability to lower blood glucose levels. Discuss that 2% to 15% of all women develop GDM because they are unable to produce enough of the additional insulin needed during pregnancy, causing their blood glucose levels to become elevated. Reassure the patient that she did not do anything to cause this condition and that her infant will not have diabetes. Explain that GDM is easily treated with meal planning or a combination of meal planning and insulin injections. Reinforce that oral agents cannot be taken during pregnancy because they cross the placenta to the developing baby.

   B Review the results of her 3-hour OGTT and use it to explain glucose fluctuations.

2 Emphasize that it is important to diagnose and treat GDM because it has implications for both the mother and her baby.

   A The maternal implication is a higher incidence of type 2 diabetes later in life, although there are preventive steps she can take to lower her risk.

B The potential neonatal implications are macrosomia and other neonatal metabolic complications at birth, and a greater propensity toward obesity and diabetes later in life.

3 Review the basics of type 2 diabetes, explaining the relationship between food, endogenous insulin (also exogenous insulin if the patient requires insulin therapy), and activity. Provide referral to a registered dietitian. Emphasize the importance of eating all of the planned foods so that the baby receives adequate nutrition. (Some patients may eat less to lower their blood glucose levels and thus avoid insulin injections. This eating pattern may lead to starvation ketosis.)

4 Discuss the goals of glycemia and explain that there may be a need for insulin injections if her fasting and/or postprandial blood glucose levels do not respond to meal planning and exercise.

   A Reassure her that if she requires insulin, it will most likely be only for the duration of pregnancy.

   B Reassure her that exogenous insulin lowers her glucose and thereby decreases her baby's production of insulin. Insulin has only positive effects on the baby.

5 Teach self blood glucose monitoring and how to use the results. Capillary blood glucose monitoring helps document her glycemic response of foods and aids in insulin adjustments, if needed.

6 Teach all patients with GDM to test their first morning urine sample for ketones.

7 Be alert for patients who present with a second GDM pregnancy and are using an outdated meter or strips. Provide reeducation in all the necessary skills.

8 Provide written guidelines describing when to contact you or another member of the healthcare team. Suggest that she notify you if any of the following occurs: elevated blood glucose levels, hypoglycemia (if the patient requires insulin), moderate or large ketonuria, a decrease in fetal movement (in the second half of pregnancy), fever, vaginal bleeding, severe headache, blurred vision, uterine contractions, or other pregnancy complications.

9   Stress the importance of follow-up in the postpartum period for glucose intolerance. Advise her that she needs a 2-hour 75 g OGTT 6 to 8 weeks postpartum and to request if not offered.

SELF-REVIEW QUESTIONS

1   Describe the normal metabolic changes related to pregnancy during the latter half of gestation.

2   State reasons why it is important to achieve optimal diabetes control prior to conception.

3   List four potential neonatal complications that may occur in pregnancies complicated by diabetes mellitus

4   State why nonstress tests are routinely ordered in pregnant women with diabetes.

5   List three maternal complications associated with diabetes and pregnancy.

6   When and why should pregnant women with diabetes test their urine for ketones?

7   Describe elements of preconception counseling to include.

8   Define gestational diabetes.

9   Describe reasons women need to be screened for gestational diabetes between the 24th and 28th weeks of pregnancy.

10 List two methods that might be used to assess fetal status.

11 Describe areas to address with women who had gestational diabetes in the postpartum period.

12 Discuss contraceptive options for women with diabetes.

CASE STUDY 1

NC is a 29-year-old newly married woman with type 1 diabetes who presents to the Diabetes in Pregnancy Center for preconception counseling and care. NC was diagnosed with type 1 diabetes at age 10 years and has been in good health with the exception of one episode of DKA at age 12 years when she had the flu. She has never been pregnant and is using a diaphragm with spermicidal cream as her method of contraception. NC denies a history of diabetic nephropathy and claims that she is normotensive. Her history is significant for background retinopathy that was diagnosed 1 year ago.

At this initial visit, a physical examination was also performed. NC's blood pressure was 110/70 and her urine sample tested 1+ for protein on dipstick. Her blood glucose records during the previous 2 weeks were reviewed. She appeared to be in reasonably good diabetes control with fasting blood glucose values ranging from 80 to 130 mg/dL (4.4 to 7.2 mmol/L) and predinner values from 95 to 140 mg/dL (5.3 to 7.8 mmol/L). NC tests her blood glucose levels twice daily. She takes three-injections per day with short- and intermediate-acting insulin prior to breakfast, short-acting insulin prior to dinner, and intermediate-acting insulin prior to bedtime. NC did not bring her blood glucose meter with her during this initial visit.

QUESTIONS FOR DISCUSSION

1 What are appropriate laboratory tests for this patient?
2 What are potential topics that need to be addressed with her?
3 How would you involve her husband in the education?

DISCUSSION

1 Baseline renal function studies including a 24-hour urine for creatinine clearance, quantitative protein, and microalbumin are needed. A urinalysis to rule out a urinary tract infection which might have caused the 1+ proteinuria is also needed.

2 A glycosylated hemoglobin is needed to assess overall glycemic control, as well as a rubella titer to assess her immune status. If NC is nonimmune, an inoculation could be administered during this preconception period. If thyroid function tests have not been performed in the last year, these should be done now.

3 In addition to these laboratory tests, referrals to a retinal specialist for a reassessment of her background retinopathy, and to the team dietitian to evaluate her nutritional intake and meal plan are needed. If she is interested, the dietitian can work with NC to initiate exercise.

4 Discuss blood glucose goals during preconception and pregnancy with NC and the purpose of blood glucose checks prior to each meal, 1 hour post-meal, and at bedtime. Weekly calls to the diabetes educator are needed so

that any necessary insulin and/or meal plan adjustments can be made. Assess NC's understanding and willingness to work towards these targets.

5 Counsel NC to continue her barrier method of contraception until she, her husband, and the healthcare team agree it is safe to discontinue (eg, when blood glucose levels are optimal and the glycosylated hemoglobin level is in the normal or near-normal range).

6 Discuss the topics of fertility, spontaneous abortion rate, incidence of diabetes mellitus in offspring, effects of pregnancy on existing vascular complications, and the incidence of congenital and answer any questions. Assess NC's emotional response throughout the discussion.

7 Ask NC how her husband has coped with her diabetes during their marriage and what he knows about pregnancy and diabetes. Invite NC to bring her husband to her next appointment and all future appointments so that he can learn about diabetes in pregnancy and how to administer glucagon.

8 Additionally, ask NC to bring her glucose meter so her technique and meter accuracy can be assessed.

CASE STUDY 2

RG is a 26-year-old G2P1000 (gravida, term, preterm, abortion, live), obese Hispanic woman who presents to the outpatient Diabetes in Pregnancy Center at 28 1/7 weeks of gestation. RG stated that she was referred to the center by her family practitioner because he thought that her expected baby was excessively large.

RG's past obstetric history was significant for GDM in her first pregnancy, 2 years earlier. That pregnancy resulted in the delivery of a 9 lb 12 oz (4.4 kg) stillborn son at 38+ weeks of gestation. RG's mother had type 2 diabetes, diagnosed at 40 years of age.

A 3-hour OGTT was done 3 days later. The following results were obtained:

Time (h)	Plasma Glucose mg/dL (mmol/L)
FBS	112 (6.2)
1	250 (13.9)
2	224 (12.4)
3	190 (10.6)

RG was diagnosed with GDM, although the possibility of previously undiagnosed type 2 diabetes could not be ruled out at this time, and started taking three injections per day of insulin because of her fasting glucose levels. She met with the dietitian and they developed a meal plan that included the ethnic foods RG prepares at her husband's request. In addition, RG learned how to monitor capillary blood glucose levels and urine ketone levels. Weekly nonstress tests were instituted at 34 weeks of gestation and RG was instructed to call immediately if she experienced any decrease in fetal movement. As a result of intensive diabetes care, education, self management, and careful fetal monitoring, RG successfully delivered a healthy, term 7 lb 11 oz infant.

Questions for Discussion

1 What other information would you like to have received about this patient?

2 What would you have done differently if she had presented at 6 weeks of gestation instead of at 28½ weeks?

3 What advice would you give RG about the long-term implications of GDM?

4 How can the educator show sensitivity to RG's cultural background?

Discussion

1 It would be important to find out if RG had received an OGTT following the delivery of her stillborn son to determine if she still had diabetes, had impaired glucose tolerance, or was normoglycemic when she was not pregnant. Ideally she would have been screened in early pregnancy because of her obstetric history. More information surrounding the stillbirth would have been helpful. The absence of obstetric complications suggest, but do

not prove, that the stillbirth was related to maternal diabetes. Therefore, RG should be asked the following questions: Was she preeclamptic? Was there a cord accident? Did she have a placental abruption?

A It is also important to assess her beliefs about why the stillbirth occurred as it will influence how she cares for herself and her current emotional status. In addition, knowing about her mother's experiences with diabetes and her self-care practices may provide important insights.

2 Screening early in pregnancy helps to identify those women who probably were glucose intolerant prior to conception. If RG had first presented for care at 6 weeks rather than at 28½ weeks of gestation, she should have been screened for diabetes immediately because she had several risk factors for GDM (obesity, family history of diabetes, and a history of a stillborn macrosomic infant). She may have remained hyperglycemic following her first pregnancy.

3 In the postpartum period, RG needs to be told that she is at a high risk for developing diabetes later in life. After she discontinues breast-feeding, she will need an OGTT. In addition prevention strategies such as weight loss, physical activity, and educational support need to be offered. Inform RG how to obtain annual blood glucose testing if her OGTT is normal and advise her to contact her provider if she develops any signs or symptoms of hyperglycemia.

4 Discuss contraception, including any personal, religious or culturally related concerns. Assess her use of alternative forms of birth control. Suggest that if RG desires any more children, she needs to be tested for diabetes before becoming pregnant. She also needs to understand that any subsequent pregnancies increase her risks for type 2 diabetes.

5 It is important to assess the influence of her culture on the care of her pregnancy and her diabetes.

A Ask, "Are there cultural or religious practices that affect how you care for yourself or your pregnancy?"

B It is also important to assess the use of alternative therapies (eg, herbs, vitamins) for pregnancy.

References

1   Freinkel N, Metzger BE, Potter JM. Pregnancy in diabetes. In: Ellenberg M, Rifkin H, eds. Diabetes mellitus: theory and practice. 3rd ed. New York: Medical Examination Publishing Co, 1983:689-714.

2   Weintrob N, Karp M, Hod M. Short- and long-range complications in offspring of diabetic mothers. J Diabetes Complications 1996;10:294-301.

3   National Diabetes Data Group. Classification and diagnosis of diabetes mellitus and other categories of glucose intolerance. Diabetes 1979;28:1039-57.

4   Freinkel N, Gabbe SG, Hadden DR, et al. Summary and recommendations of the Second International Workshop-Conference on Gestational Diabetes Mellitus. Diabetes 1985;34(suppl 2):123-26.

5   Freinkel N, Josimovich J, Conference Planning Committee. American Diabetes Association Workshop-Conference on Gestational Diabetes. Summary and recommendations. Diabetes Care 1980;3:499-501.

6   Metzger BE, Organizing Committee. Summary and recommendations of the Third International Workshop-Conference on Gestational Diabetes Mellitus. Diabetes 1991;40(suppl 2):197-201.

7   Connell FA, Vadheim C, Emmanuel I. Diabetes in pregnancy: a population-based study of incidence, referral for care, and perinatal mortality. Am J Obstet Gynecol 1985;151:598-603.

8   Beischer NA, Oats JN, Henry OA, Sheedy MT, Walstab JE. Incidence and severity of gestational diabetes mellitus according to country of birth in women living in Australia. Diabetes 1991;40(suppl 2):35-38.

9   Freinkel N. Gestational diabetes 1979: philosophical and practical aspects of a major public health problem. Diabetes Care 1980;3:399-401.

10 Dooley SL, Metzger BE, Cho NH. Gestational diabetes mellitus: influence of race on disease prevalence and perinatal outcome in a US population. Diabetes 1991;40(suppl 2):25-29.

11 White P. Pregnancy complicating diabetes. Am J Med 1949;7:609-16.

12 Pederson J, Perdersen LM, Andersen B. Assessors of fetal perinatal mortality in diabetic pregnancy: analysis of 1,332 pregnancies in the Copenhagen series, 1946-1972. Diabetes 1974;23:302-5.

13 Mills JL, Simpson JL, Driscoll SG, et al. Incidence of spontaneous abortion among normal women and insulin-dependent diabetic women whose pregnancies were identified within 21 days of conception. N Eng J Med 1988;319:1617-23.

14 Buchanan TA, Coustan DR. Diabetes mellitus. In: Burrows GN, Ferris TF, eds. Medical complications during pregnancy. 4th ed. Philadelphia: WB Saunders, 1994:29-61.

15 Metzger BE, Hare JW, Freinkel N. Carbohydrate metabolism in pregnancy. IX: Plasma levels of gluconeogenetic fuels during fasting in the rat. J Clin Endocrinol Metab 1971;33:869-72.

16 Metzger BE, Ravnikar V, Vilelsis RA, Freinkel N. "Accelerated starvation" and the skipped breakfast in late normal pregnancy. Lancet 1982;1:588-92.

17 Phelps RL, Metzger BE, Freinkel N. Carbohydrate metabolism in pregnancy. XVII. Diurnal profiles of plasma glucose, insulin, free fatty acids, triglycerides, cholesterol, and individual amino acids in late normal pregnancy. Am J Obstet Gynecol 1981;140:730-36.

18 Mills JL, Baker L, Goldman AS. Malformations in infants of diabetic mothers occur before the seventh gestational week: implications for treatment. Diabetes 1979;28:292-93.

19 Pederson J. The pregnant diabetic and her newborn infant. 2nd ed. Baltimore, Md: Williams & Wilkins, 1977:191-97.

20 Simpson JL, Elias S, Martin AO, et al. Diabetes in pregnancy. Northwestern University series (1977-1981): Prospective study of anomalies in offspring of mothers with diabetes mellitus. Am J Obstet Gynecol 1983;146:263-70.

21 Mills JL, Knopp RH, Simpson JL, et al. Lack of relation of increased malformation rates in infants of diabetic mothers to glycemic control during organogenesis. N Engl J Med 1988;318:671-76.

22 Miller E, Hare JW, Cloherty JP, et al. Elevated maternal hemoglobin A1c in early pregnancy and major congenital anomalies in infants of diabetic mothers. N Engl J Med 1981;304:1331-34.

23 Greene MF, Hare JW, Cloherty JP, et al. First-trimester hemoglobin A1 and risk for major malformation and spontaneous abortion in diabetic pregnancy. Teratology 1989;39:225-31.

24 Ylinen K, Aula P, Stenman UH, et al. Risk of minor and major fetal malformations in diabetics with high hemoglobin A1c values in early pregnancy. Br Med J 1984;289:345-46.

25 Fuhrmann K, Reiher H, Semmler K, et al. Prevention of congenital malformations in infants of insulin-dependent diabetic mothers. Diabetes Care 1983;6:219-23.

26 Fuhrmann K, Reiher H, Semmler K, Glockner E. The effect of intensified conventional insulin therapy before and during pregnancy on the malformation rate in offspring of diabetic mothers. Exp Clin Endocrinol 1984;83:173-77.

27 Steel JM, Johnstone FD, Hepburn DA, Smith AF. Can prepregnancy care of diabetic women reduce the risk of abnormal babies? Br Med J 1990;301:1070-74.

28 Kitzmiller JL, Gavin LA, Gin GD, et al. Preconception care of diabetes: Glycemic control prevents congenital anomalies. JAMA 1991;265:731-36.

29 Jovanovic-Peterson L, Abrams RS, Coustan DR, et al, eds. Medical management of pregnancy complicated by diabetes. Alexandria, Va: American Diabetes Association, 1995.

30 Cornblath M, Schwartz R. Disorders of carbohydrate metabolism in infancy. Philadelphia: WB Saunders, 1976.

31 Reece EA, Friedman AM, Copel J, Kleinman CS. Prenatal diagnosis and management of deviant fetal growth and congenital malformations.

32 Goldberg JD, Franklin B, Lasser D, et al. Gestational diabetes: impact of home glucose monitoring on neonatal birth weight. Am J Obstet Gynecol 1986;154:546-50.

33 Wyse LJ, Jones M, Mandel F. Relationship of glycosylated hemoglobin, fetal macrosomia, and birthweight macrosomia. Am J Perinatal 1994;11:260-62.

34 Morris MA, Grandis AS, Litton JC. Glycosylated hemoglobin concentration in early gestation associated with neonatal outcome. Am J Obstet Gynecol 1985;153:651-54.

35 Coustan DR. Delivery: timing, mode and management. In: Reece EA, Coustan DR, eds. Diabetes mellitus in pregnancy. New York: Churchill-Livingston, 1995:353-60.

36 Pettitt DJ, Baird HR, Aleck KA, Bennet PH, Knowler WC. Excessive obesity in offspring of Pima Indian women with diabetes during pregnancy. N Engl J Med 1983;308:242-45.

37 Pettitt DJ, Knowler WC, Bennett PH, Aleck KA, Baird HR. Obesity in offspring of diabetic Pima Indian women despite normal birth weight. Diabetes Care 1987;10:76-80.

38 Pettitt DJ, Baird HR, Aleck KA, Knowler WC. Diabetes mellitus in children following maternal diabetes during gestation. Diabetes 1982;31(suppl 2):66A.

39 Pettitt DJ, Bennett PH, Knowler WC, et al. Gestational diabetes mellitus and impaired glucose tolerance during pregnancy: long-term effects on obesity and glucose tolerance in the offspring. Diabetes 1985;34:119-22.

40 Damm P, Molsted-Pedersen L. Significant decrease in congenital malformations in the newborn infants of an unselected population of diabetic women. Am J Obstet Gynecol 1989;161:1163-67.

41 Cousins L. The California Diabetes and Pregnancy Programme: a statewide collaborative program for the preconception and prenatal care of diabetic women. Clin Obstet Gynecol 1991;5:443-59.

42 Willhoite MB, Bennert HW Jr, Palomaki GE, et al. The impact of preconception counseling on pregnancy outcomes. The experience of the Maine Diabetes and Pregnancy Program. Diabetes Care 1993;16:450-55.

43 Elixhauser A, Weschler JM, Kitzmiller JL, et al. Cost-benefit analysis of preconception care for women with established diabetes mellitus. Diabetes Care 1993;16:1146-57.

44 Scheffler RM, Feuchtbaum LB, Phibbs CS. Prevention: the cost-effectiveness of the California Diabetes and Pregnancy Program. Am J Public Health 1992;82:168-75.

45 Placquadio, K, Hollingsworth D, Murphy H. Effect of in-utero exposure to oral hypoglycaemic drugs. Lancet 1991; 338:866-69.

46 Warram JH, Krolewski AS, Kahn CR. Determinants of IDDM and perinatal mortality in children of diabetic mothers. Diabetes 1988;37:1328-34.

47 Kobberly J, Tallil H. Empirical risk figures for first degree relatives of non-insulin-dependent diabetics. In: Genetics of diabetes mellitus. Proceedings of the Serone Symposia. Vol 47. London: Academic Press, 1982:201.

48 Jovanovic-Peterson L, Peterson CM. Diabetic retinopathy. In: Reece EA, Coustan DR, eds. Diabetes mellitus in pregnancy. New York: Churchill-Livingston, 1995:303-14.

49 Klein R, Klein BE, Moss SE, et al. Retinopathy in young-onset diabetic patients. Diabetes Care 1985;8:311-15.

50 The Diabetes Control and Complication Trial Research Group. The effect of intensive treatment of diabetes on the development and progression of long-term complications in insulin-dependent diabetes mellitus. N Engl J Med 1993;329:977-86.

51 The Kroc Collaborative Study Group. Diabetic retinopathy after two years of intensified insulin treatment. Follow-up of the Kroc Collaborative Study. JAMA 1988;260:37-41.

52 Laatikainen I, Teramo K, Hieta-Heikurainen, et al. A controlled study of the influence of continuous subcutaneous insulin infusion treatment on diabetic retinopathy during pregnancy. J Intern Med 1987;221:367-76.

53 Rosenn B, Miodovnik M, Kranias G, et al. Progression of diabetic retinopathy in pregnancy: association with hypertension in pregnancy. Am J Obstet Gynecol 1992;166:1214-18.

54 Moloney JB, Drury MI. The effect of pregnancy on the natural course of diabetic retinopathy. Am J Ophthalmol 1982;93:745-56.

55 Dibble CM, Kochenour NK, Worley RJ, et al. Effect of pregnancy on diabetic retinopathy. Obstet Gynecol 1982;59:699-704.

56 Horvat M, Maclean H, Goldberg L, Crock GW. Diabetic retinopathy in pregnancy: a 12-year prospective survey. Br J Ophthalmol 1980;64:398-403.

57 Serup L. Influence of pregnancy on diabetic retinopathy. Acta Endocrinol 1986;277:122-24.

58 Reece EA, Coustan DR, Hayslett JP, et al. Diabetic nephropathy: pregnancy performance and fetomaternal outcome. Am J Obstet Gynecol 1988;159:56-66.

59 Jovanovic R, Jovanovic L. Obstetric management when normoglycemia is maintained in diabetic pregnant women with vascular compromise. Am J Obstet Gynecol 1984;149:617-23.

60 Reece EA, Winn HN, Hayslett JP, Coulehan JJ, Wan M, Hobbins JC. Does pregnancy alter the rate of progression of diabetic nephropathy? Am J Perinatal 1990;7:193-97.

61 Kitzmiller JL, Combs CA. Maternal and perinatal implications of diabetic nephropathy. Clin Perinatal 1993;20:561-70.

62 Combs CA, Rosenn B, Kitzmiller JL, et al. Early-pregnancy proteinuria in diabetes related to preeclampsia. Obstet Gynecol 1993;82:802-7.

63 Hou SH, Grossman SD, Madias NE. Pregnancy in women with renal disease and moderate renal insufficiency. Am J Med 1985;78:185-94.

64 Grenfell A, Brudenell JM, Doddridge MC, Watkins PJ. Pregnancy in diabetic women who have proteinuria. Q J Med 1986;59:379-86.

65 Miodovnik M, Rosenn BM, Khoury JC, Grigsby JL, Siddiqi TA. Does pregnancy increase the risk for development and progression of diabetic nephropathy? Am J Obstet Gynecol 1996;174:1180-91.

66 Kitzmiller JL, Brown ER, Phillippe M, et al. Diabetic nephropathy and perinatal outcome. Am J Obstet Gynecol 1981;141:741-51.

67 Kitzmiller JK. Diabetic nephropathy. In: Reece EA, Coustan DR, eds. Diabetes mellitus in pregnancy. New York: Churchill-Livingston, 1995:315-44.

68 Manske CL, Thomas W, Wang Y, Wilson RF. Screening diabetic transplant candidates for coronary artery disease: identification of a low risk subgroup. Kidney Int 1993;44:617-21.

69 Brown FM, Hare JW. Diabetic neuropathy and coronary heart disease. In: Reece EA, Coustan DR, eds. Diabetes mellitus in pregnancy. New York: Churchill-Livingston, 1995:345-51.

70 Churchill JA, Berendes HW. Intelligence of children whose mothers had acetonuria during pregnancy. In: Perinatal factors affecting human development. Pan American Health Organization scientific publication. Washington, DC: Pan American Health Organization, 1969;185:300.

71 Rizzo T, Metzger BE, Burns WJ, Burns K. Correlations between antepartum maternal metabolism and child intelligence. N Engl J Med 1991;325:911-16.

72 National Research Council. Recommended dietary allowances. Washington, DC: National Academy Press, 1990.

73 National Academy of Science. Nutrition during pregnancy. Washington, DC: National Academy Press, 1990.

74 Abrams BF, Laros Jr RK. Prepregnancy weight, weight gain, and birthweight. Am J Obstet Gynecol 1986;154:503-9.

75 National Research Council. Recommended dietary allowances. 10th ed. Washington, DC: National Academy Press, 1989.

76 Powers MA, Metzger BE, Freinkel N. Pregnancy and diabetes. In: Powers MA, ed. Handbook of diabetes nutritional management. Rockville, Md: Aspen Publishers, 1987:332-51.

77 American Dietetic Association. Position statement. Use of nutritive and non-nutritive sweeteners. J Am Diet Assoc 1993;93:816-21.

78 Jornsay DL. Managing morning sickness. In: Jovanovic-Peterson L, Abrams RS, Coustan DR, et al, eds. Medical management of pregnancy complicated by diabetes. Alexandria, Va: American Diabetes Association, 1995:39-44.

79 Jornsay DL. Managing morning sickness. Diabetes Self-Manage 1990;10(2):10-12.

80 Buchanan TA, Schemmer JK, Freinkel N. Embryotoxic effects of brief maternal insulin-hypoglycemia during organogenesis in the rat. J Clin Invest 1986;78:643-49.

81 Combs CA, Gunderson E, Kitzmiller JL, et al. Relationship of fetal macrosomia to maternal postprandial glucose control during pregnancy. Diabetes Care 1992;15:1251-57.

82 de Veciana M, Major CA, Morgan MA, et al. Postprandial versus preprandial blood glucose monitoring in women with gestational diabetes mellitus requiring insulin therapy. N Engl J Med 1995;333:1237-41.

83 Jornsay DL. Pregnancy and continuous insulin infusion therapy. Diabetes Spectrum 1998;11:26-32.

84 Marcus AO, Fernandez MP. Insulin pump therapy. Postgrad Med 1996:3.

85 Jovanovic L, Peterson CM. Optimal insulin delivery for the pregnant diabetic patient. Diabetes Care 1982;5(suppl 1):24-37.

86 Kimmerle R, Heinemann L, Delecki A, Berger M. Severe hypoglycemia incidence and predisposing factors in 85 pregnancies of type 1 diabetic women. Diabetes Care 1992;15:1034-37.

87 Diamond MP, Reece EA, Caprio S, et al. Impairment of counterregulatory hormone responses to hypoglycemia in pregnant women with insulin-dependent diabetes mellitus. Am J Obstet Gynecol 1992;166:70-77.

88 Nelson DM, Barrows HJ, Clapp DH, Ortman-Nabi J, Whitehurst RM. Glycosylated serum protein levels in diabetic and nondiabetic pregnant patients: an indicator of short-term glycemic control in the diabetic patient. Am J Obstet Gynecol 1985;151:1042-47.

89 Mordes D, Kreutner K, Metzger W, Colwell JA. Dangers of intravenous ritodrine in diabetic patients. JAMA 1982;248:973-75.

90 Buchanan TA, Unterman TG, Metzger BE. The medical management of diabetes in pregnancy. Clin Perinatal 1985;12:625-50.

91 Main DM, Mennuti MT. Neural tube defects: issues in prenatal diagnosis and counselling. Obstet Gynecol 1986;67:1-16.

92 Landon MB. Diabetes mellitus and other endocrine disorders. In: Gabble SG, Niebyl JR, Simpson JL, eds. Obstetrics: normal and problem pregnancies. New York: Churchill-Livingston, 1991:1097-136.

93 Jovanovic L, Peterson CM. Insulin and glucose requirements during the first stage of labor in insulin-dependent diabetic women. Am J Med 1983;75:607-12.

94 Kjos SL. Contraception in women with diabetes mellitus. Diabetes Spectrum 1993;6:80-86.

95 Trussell J, Hatcher RA, Cates W Jr, et al. Contraceptive failure in the United States: an update. Stud Fam Plan 1990;21:51-54.

96 Lipinski KA. Birth control choices. Diabetes Self-Manage 1991;8(3):6-16.

97 Metzger BE, Cho NH. Epidemiology and genetics. In: Reece EA, Coustan DR, eds. Diabetes mellitus in pregnancy. New York: Churchill-Livingston 1995:11-26.

98 Coustan DR. Gestational diabetes. In: National Diabetes Data Group, eds. Diabetes in America. 2nd ed. Bethesda, Md: National Institutes of Health, National Institute of Diabetes and Digestive and Kidney Diseases, 1995: 703-17.

99 Hod M, Rabinerson D, Peled Y. Gestational diabetes mellitus: is it a clinical entity? Diabetes Reviews 1995;3: 602-13.

100 Blank A, Grave GD, Metzger BE. Effects of gestational diabetes on perinatal morbidity reassessed. Report of the International Workshop on Adverse Perinatal Outcomes of Gestational Diabetes Mellitus. Diabetes Care 1995;18:127-29.

101 Rizzo TA, Dooley SL, Metzger BE, et al. Prenatal and perinatal influences on long-term psychomotor development in offspring of diabetic mothers. Am J Obstet Gynecol 1995;173:1753-58.

102 Magee MS, Walden CE, Benedetti TJ, Knopp RH. Influence of diagnostic criteria on the incidence of gestational diabetes and perinatal morbidity. JAMA 1993;269:609-15.

103 Sermer M, Naylor D, Gare DJ, et al. Impact of increasing carbohydrate intolerance on maternal-fetal outcomes in 3,637 women without gestational diabetes. Am J Obstet Gynecol 1995;173:146-56.

104 O'Sullivan JB. Long-term follow-up of gestational diabetes. In: Camerini-Davalos RA, Cole HS, eds. Early diabetes in early life. Third International Symposium. New York: Academic Press, 1975:503-18.

105 Metzger BE, Bybee DE, Freinkel N, et al. Gestational diabetes mellitus: correlations between the phenotypic and genotypic characteristics of the mother and abnormal glucose tolerance during the first year postpartum. Diabetes 1985; 34(suppl 2):111-15.

106 Kjos SL, Buchanan TA, Greenspoon JS, et al. Gestational diabetes mellitus: the prevalence of glucose intolerance and diabetes mellitus in the first two months postpartum. Obstet Gynecol 1990; 163:93-98.

107 Coustan DR, Carpenter MW, O'Sullivan PS, Carr SR. Gestational diabetes mellitus: predictors of subsequent disordered glucose metabolism. Am J Obstet Gynecol 1993;168:1139-45.

108 Peters RK, Kjos SL, Xiang A, Buchanan TA. Long-term diabetogenic effect of single pregnancy in women with previous gestational diabetes mellitus. Lancet 1996;347:227-30.

109 O'Sullivan JB, Mahan CM, Charles D, et al. Screening criteria for high-risk gestational diabetic patients. Am J Obstet Gynecol 1973;116:895-900.

110 Coustan DR, Nelson C, Carpenter MW, Carr SR, Rotondo L, Widness JA. Maternal age and screening for gestational diabetes: a population-based study. Obstet Gynecol 1989;73:557-61.

111 O'Sullivan JB, Mahan CM. Criteria for the oral glucose tolerance test in pregnancy. Diabetes 1964;13:278-85.

112 American Diabetes Association. Report of the Expert Committee on the Diagnosis and Classification of Diabetes Mellitus. Diabetes Care 1997;20:1183-97.

113 Jornsay DL, Smith-Levitin M, Petrikovsky B. Diabetes in pregnancy: how to manage? Neonatal Intensive Care 1997;10: 45-50.

114 Landy HJ, Gomez-Marin O, O'Sullivan MJ. Diagnosing gestational diabetes mellitus: use of a glucose screen without administering the glucose tolerance test. Obstet Gynecol 1996;87:395-400.

115 Carpenter MW, Coustan DR. Criteria for screening tests for gestational diabetes. Am J Obstet Gynecol 1982;144:768-73.

116 National Diabetes Data Group. Classification and diagnosis of diabetes mellitus and other categories of glucose intolerance. Diabetes 1979;28:1039-57.

117 Sacks DA, Abu-Fadil S, Greenspoon JS, Fotheringham N. Do the current standards for glucose tolerance testing for pregnancy represent a valid conversion of O'Sullivan's original criteria? Am J Obstet Gynecol 1989;161:638-41.

118 Carr DB, Gabbe S. Gestational diabetes: detection, management, and implications. Clin Diabetes 1998;16:4-11.

119 Boyd KL, Ross EK, Sherman SJ. Jelly beans as an alternative to a cola beverage containing fifty grams of glucose. Am J Obstet Gynecol 1995;173:1889-92.

120 Carpenter MW. Testing for gestational diabetes. In: Reece EA, Coustan DR, eds. Diabetes mellitus in pregnancy. New York: Churchill-Livingston, 1995:261-75.

121 King JC. New National Academy of Sciences guidelines for nutrition during pregnancy. Diabetes 1991;40(suppl 2):164.

122 Algert S, Shragg P, Hollingsworth DR. Moderate caloric restriction in obese women with gestational diabetes. Obstet Gynecol 1985;65:487-91.

123 Knopp RH, Magee MS, Raisys V, Bendetti T. Metabolic effects of hypocaloric diets in management of gestational diabetes. Diabetes 1991;40(suppl 2):165-71.

124 Gunderson EP. Intensive nutrition therapy for gestational diabetes. Diabetes Care 1997;20:221-26.

125 Durak EP, Jovanovic-Peterson L, Peterson CM. Physical and glycemic responses of women with gestational diabetes to a moderately intense exercise program. Diabetes Educ 1990;16:309-12.

126 Wechter DJ, Kaufmann RC, Amankwah KS, et al. Prevention of neonatal macrosomia in gestational diabetes by the use of intensive dietary therapy and home glucose monitoring. Am J Perinatal 1991;8:131-34.

127 Langer O, Rodriguez DA, Xenakis EMJ, et al. Intensified versus conventional management of gestational diabetes. Am J Obstet Gynecol 1994;170:1036-47.

128 Coustan DR, Imarah J. Prophylactic insulin treatment of gestational diabetes reduces the incidence of macrosomia, operative delivery, and birth trauma. Am J Obstet Gynecol 1984;150:836-42.

129 Drexel H, Bichler A, Sailer S, et al. Prevention of perinatal morbidity by tight metabolic control in gestational diabetes mellitus. Diabetes Care 1988;11:761-68.

130 Jovanovic-Peterson L, Peterson CM, Reed G, NICHD-DIEP. Maternal postprandial glucose levels predict birthweight. Am J Obstet Gynecol 1991;164:103-11.

131 American College of Obstetricians and Gynecologists. Diabetes and pregnancy. ACOG technical bulletin #200. Washington, DC: ACOG, 1994.

132 Langer O. Management of gestational diabetes. Clin Perinatal 1993;20:1-15.

133 American Diabetes Association. Gestational diabetes mellitus. Ann Intern Med 1986;105:461.

Suggested Reading

AADE Task Force on Diabetes and Pregnancy. Educational guidelines for pre-existing diabetes complicated by pregnancy. Diabetes Educ 1993;19:15-17.

California Diabetes and Pregnancy Program. Sweet Success: guidelines for care. Campbell, Calif: Education Program Associates, 1992.

Franz M, Cooper N, Mullen L, Birk PS, Hollander P. Gestational diabetes: guidelines for a safe pregnancy and a healthy baby. Minneapolis, Minn: Diabetes Center Inc, 1988.

Jornsay DL, Carlson M, Meyer SL. The best for you and your baby: Answers about gestational diabetes. Indianapolis, Ind: Boehringer Mannheim Corp, 1993.

Jovanovic L, Abrams RS, Coustan DR, et al, eds. Medical management of pregnancy complicated by diabetes. Alexandria Va: American Diabetes Association, 1995.

Kitzmiller JL, Gavin LA, Gin GD, et al. Managing diabetes and pregnancy. Curr Probl Obstet Gynecol Fertil 1988;11:113-67.

Kitzmiller JL, Gavin LA, Gin GD, et al. Preconception care of diabetes: glycemic control prevents congenital anomalies. JAMA 1991;265:731-36.

Metzger BE, Buchanan TA. Diabetes and birth defects. Diabetes Spectrum 1990;3:149-83.

Radak JT. Why worry about gestational diabetes? Diabetes Forecast 1996;49(3):46-47.

DIABETES AND THE LIFE CYCLE

Diabetes in the Elderly
19

Anne T. Nettles RN MS CDE
Healthcare Consultant
Minneapolis, Minnesota

Introduction

1   Diabetes mellitus has been underdiagnosed and undertreated in the United States, particularly among people in the oldest age groups.

2   Nearly 40% of those age 65 to 75 years may be affected by hyperglycemia. More individuals may be affected by hyperglycemia after the age of 75 years because of rising glucose intolerance.[1]

3   Because the classical symptoms of diabetes often are absent in the elderly, diagnosis is more often made when the long-term effects of poor glucose control result in a crisis. Harris, et al[2] estimate that the diagnosis is made an average of 6.5 years after the onset of the disease.

4   Because of the magnitude of underdiagnosis in this population, the American Diabetes Association, in cooperation with worldwide health organizations modified the recommendations for diagnosis in 1997. If the criteria are put into practice, elderly individuals will be diagnosed and treated sooner.

5   Diabetes educators need to understand the atypical manifestations of diabetes in the aged to properly educate and care for this age group.

Objectives

Upon completion of this chapter, the learner will be able to
1   Describe the pertinent effects of aging.
2   Identify the unique risks of poor glucose control in the elderly.
3   Explain adaptations in treatment approaches for older individuals.
4   List potential barriers and strategies for teaching the elderly about diabetes management.

Changes of Aging

1   Aging is more than a matter of just physiological changes. Psychosocial factors play a significant role in how aging is expressed. For example, a 75-year-old may be more robust than someone who is 65 years of age.

2 Many of the physiological changes of aging resemble those of diabetes and include impaired hormone regulation, decreased vision, elevated blood pressure, decreased glomerular filtration, bone loss, muscle wasting, and loss of skin tone.

3 The changes of aging are accelerated and compounded by having diabetes (Table 19.1).

4 Dementia, certain cognitive disorders, and memory have been shown to improve with glucose control.[3]

DIAGNOSIS AND TREATMENT

1 Undiagnosed and untreated diabetes is more common in the elderly. The prevalence of diabetes is higher among African Americans, Hispanics, Pima Indians, Micronesians, Scandinavians, and male Japanese.[4]

2 The same diagnostic criteria used for all adults are used for the elderly. Recent changes in diagnostic criteria are likely to reveal more older adults in need of treatment for diabetes.

3 Because consensus has not been established regarding target glucose levels for elderly patients, diabetes management should be individualized with attention to eliminating glycemic symptoms. Longevity and potential risks for long-term effects of poor glucose control also should be considered.

4 Uncontrolled diabetes causes symptoms and acute illnesses that, at the least, impair quality of life; some complications such as hyperglycemic hyperosmolar nonketotic syndrome (HHNS) may be fatal.[5]

5 The lifespan of people in the US is increasing (Table 19.2), therefore, people over age 65 years may live long enough to develop the long-term complications of poor glucose control.[6]

6 Educators must avoid assuming that an elderly patient has a short life expectancy (Table 19.2).

TABLE 19.1. AGING AND DISEASE OF THE ELDERLY THAT INFLUENCE DIABETES CARE

Ophthalmic
- Decreased acuity
- Slowed light/dark adaptation
- Decreased color perception
- Increased blinding diseases (senile cataracts, macular degeneration)

Cardiovascular
- Conduction defects
- Systolic hypertension
- Decreased cardiac output
- Increased vascular resistance
- Increase in cerebral vascular accidents
- Increase in myocardial infarction
- Peripheral vascular diseases

Gastrointestinal
- Decreased secretion, absorption, motility
- Changes in appetite

Dental
- Tooth loss
- Gum/periodontal disease

Musculoskeletal
- Arthritis, joint diseases
- Decreased muscle mass and strength
- Foot deformities

Neurological
- Slower learning, processing time
- Slower reactions
- Decreased taste, smell, and thirst
- Peripheral and autonomic neuropathies
- Increase in organic brain diseases

Renal
- Decreased glomerular filtration rate (GFR)

TABLE 19.2. LIFESPAN OF OLDER ADULTS IN THE UNITED STATES

Age, y	Additional Life Expectancy Mean, y
Males	
65	14.44
75	8.97
85	5.15
95	3.22
Females	
65	18.57
75	11.70
85	6.44
95	3.65

Source: Adapted from Manton and Stallard.[6]

MANAGEMENT ISSUES

1 Diabetes that is diagnosed in the elderly is primarily type 2 and related to impaired insulin release in all elderly persons and insulin resistance in obese elderly persons.[4,7]

2 Among obese people, modest weight loss and mildly increased activity can improve glucose control.[8]

MEAL PLANNING

1 Adequate nutrition is the primary goal of meal planning. Those who are dependent or have low functional ability should be assessed for risk of malnutrition.

2 Failure to thrive in older people is generally due to a combination of malnutrition, decreased physical function, depression, and cognitive impairment.[9] Elderly patients with diabetes are at additional risk because of high rates of depression.

3 Be alert for rapid weight loss or other coexisting problems in underweight older people and refer these individuals for diagnosis and treatment.

4 Meal planning for weight maintenance or weight gain includes the following considerations:

    A Preferences

    B Palatability

    C Food consistency

    D Lifelong eating habits

    E Purchasing and preparing food

    F Financial considerations

    G Cultural preferences and/or religious practices

5 The following weight reduction strategies are appropriate for older adults:

    A Use a gradual approach.

    B Incorporate and prioritize other restrictions such as sodium.

    C Provide adequate protein and calcium.

    D Reduce overall fat content.

EXERCISE

1 Exercise plans should be designed to accommodate the patient's activity preferences and assessment of functional capacity and coexisting cardiovascular diseases. Exercise has been shown to prevent and reverse some microvascular/muscle changes in older people.[8]

2 Physical limitations can be accommodated through such activities as stationary bicycling, swimming, water aerobics, walking, or chair exercises.

3 Exercising with others provides safety and opportunities for socialization.

4 As with younger people, education is needed about risks and benefits, hypoglycemia, and timing of exercise.

MEDICATIONS

1 Including a pharmacist in the diabetes management team can improve detection of redundant therapies, interactions with other diseases, drugs and food, and identify ways to simplify medication programs for those with comorbidities.

2 The ideal oral antidiabetes agent for elderly people is unknown given the number of new drugs and the lack of long-term experience administering these drugs to elderly patients. Diabetes specialists have conflicting recommendations. To date, however, most of the recently developed hypoglycemics have been used safely in elderly populations when carefully monitored and individualized.[4,10-17]

3 The risks associated with hypoglycemia due to an oral agent must be weighed against the risks associated with uncontrolled hyperglycemia and dehydration.

4 Key considerations for selection of oral antidiabetes agents include
   A Simplify regimens (eg, fewer pills less often).
   B Other drugs may interfere with effectiveness.
   C Comorbidities may create contraindications.
   D Side effects may complicate management of other existing diseases.
   E Costs may be prohibitive for some agents.
   F Effects on weight or lipids.

5 The appropriateness of all drug therapy should be assessed at each visit when patients have renal, liver, or cardiac impairment.

6 All oral antidiabetes agents should be started at the lowest possible doses to avoid toxicity.

7 Effective therapy requires that the patient takes medications as recommended. The following approaches may increase the likelihood of patients taking their medications in the prescribed manner:
   A Find ways to incorporate the medication schedule into daily routines.
   B Teach patients how to read their prescription labels carefully and thoroughly.
   C Devise or procure memory aides.[18]

8 Provide brief, easy-to-read written and verbal information about the specific oral agent that is being used. Inquire about side effects at each visit.

9 Assistive devices (eg, date/time pill boxes, counting or pill-splitting aids, and magnifiers) can be recommended to elderly patients to reduce errors and simplify medication taking.

10 Insulin should be started when maximum doses of single or combined oral agents fail to control glucose levels.

11 Physician and educator attitudes have been shown to be the most important factors in acceptance of insulin therapy. Discussing the benefits and potential challenges of insulin therapy may help patients make a decision about initiating insulin.[19]

12 Providing time for supervised practice can increase the ability of older people to accurately administer insulin, particularly if they have motor or visual problems.

13 Plan to observe the patient's insulin injection technique on a regular basis to detect a need for adaptive techniques, such as additional lighting, magnification, and premixed syringes. Home care and visiting nurses can assist with applying these techniques in the home.

14 Patients who require insulin may benefit from using lispro insulin because it may reduce the likelihood of hypoglycemia for those with irregular food intake or unpredictable digestion/absorption.[20]

15 Include family members who are involved in day-to-day care in all educational and clinical sessions. These caregivers often are elderly spouses for whom educational adaptation will also be needed.[21]

16 Establish goals for management by discussing with the patient existing diabetes complications, comorbidities, abilities, and willingness to carry out the treatment plan.[22]

GLUCOSE MONITORING

1 Blood glucose monitoring is recommended over urine testing as the latter is unreliable in older people. Monitoring frequency and method will depend on the stability and level of glucose control as well as self-testing skills.

2 Older people can learn to test as accurately as younger people.[23]

3 Determine whether problems exist with manual dexterity, vision, or memory of the procedure. Choose a meter that is best suited to the needs of each specific patient.

4 Adjust the dosing frequency based on the level and stability of glucose control as well as patient ability.

5 Incorporate urine ketone testing for those with type 1 diabetes and those with type 2 diabetes who are lean and take insulin.

SELF-MANAGEMENT EDUCATION

1 Older patients may not have had previous diabetes education. Therefore, it is important to evaluate their current level of knowledge about diabetes, correct existing misconceptions, and provide updated information.

2 Positive attitudes of educators can have a positive effect on patient behavior. Do not assume that mental or physical incompetence is part of normal aging.

3 Cultural or social barriers may exist between older people and the educator in part because of age differences. Create a comfortable, accepting environment to overcome these barriers.

4 Provide meaningful and practical information. Avoid jargon.

5 Assess the social and financial support available as well as the patient's expectations about the relationship with healthcare providers.

6 Because hyperglycemia impairs learning and retention,[3,24] instruction should be simplified and include significant others. Patients should be given written reinforcement and access to the educator for clarification especially when hyperglycemia is present.

7 When glucose is under control, assess residual mental changes using standardized instruments, such as the Mini Mental State, Short Portable Mental Status, or Neurobehavioral Cognitive Status Examination.[25]

8 The following approach can be effective for accommodating persistent sensory or neurological limitations:

   A Slow the pace of teaching; focus on one or two points and make the learning sessions brief.

   B Use printed materials that are easy to read; assess color vision (use red, orange, or yellow instead of green or blue if color blindness exists), and use fonts that are simple, bold, and large size.

   C Present audio information clearly; speak slowly, distinctly, augment spoken information with visual aids, avoid shouting, and prevent distracting noises or activity.

   D Include frequent practice opportunities, telephone follow-up, or home care for those with limited mobility.

   E Enhance memory by using cues such as calendars or pill boxes, repeating key learning points, and using familiar concrete examples.

9 Consider group education that includes coping skills. This approach may significantly improve glycemic control as well as enhance learning over time.[26]

PSYCHOSOCIAL ISSUES

1 Depression is common in people with diabetes (15% to 20%) but may be masked in elderly people by multiple physical symptoms and other mental changes associated with medications or the aging process.[27] Depression may be accompanied by alcohol abuse.

2 Inadequate income, isolation, loss of a spouse, or limited mobility can lead to inadequate self-care or a sense of hopelessness. Depression has been correlated with mortality in older people with diabetes.[28]

3 Assess for signs and symptoms of depression at each appointment. Because diagnosis may be difficult in the presence of dementia or cognitive impairment, refer patients to mental health professionals for evaluation when you suspect depression.

4 Advocate for assistance with transportation, shopping, social contact, or negotiation with healthcare systems when patients appear to need this type of support.[29]

HYPERGLYCEMIC HYPEROSMOLAR NONKETOTIC SYNDROME (HHNS)

1   HHNS is most often seen in the elderly or those with undertreated type 2 diabetes (see Chapter 13, Hyperglycemia, for more information).

2   Both patients and provider-related causes can increase the risk of HHNS:

    A   Patient causes include infection, polypharmacy, and inadequate food/liquid intake due to decreased thirst sensation or swallowing difficulties.

    A   Provider-related causes include reluctance to aggressively treat elderly people, and inadequate monitoring especially in settings where patients are dependent or during concurrent illness (see Chapter 15, Illness and Surgery, for more information).

HYPOGLYCEMIA

1   The elderly are at higher risk for medication-induced hypoglycemia due to the following conditions:

    A   Renal changes

    B   Slowed hormonal counterregulation

    C   Inadequate hydration

    D   Polypharmacy

    E   Inadequate or erratic food intake

    F   Slowed intestinal absorption

2   Hypoglycemia can result in fatal strokes or myocardial infarctions.

3   Review the common signs and symptoms of hypoglycemia regularly with patients and caregivers. Patients may attribute hypoglycemic symptoms to comorbidities, drug side effects, or normal aging.

4   Appropriate bedtime snacks for people on medication can prevent nocturnal hypoglycemia. Keeping a glucose source at the bedside may help prevent falls.

5   Avoid reliance on symptoms because they may be absent or confused with other disease symptoms. Blood glucose monitoring can be used to detect asymptomatic hypoglycemia.

6 Oral agents without hypoglycemic effects should be used when feasible.

7 Higher blood glucose targets may be appropriate for people with a history of severe hypoglycemia.

8 A "check-in" system can be helpful for those at high risk of developing hypoglycemia. Individuals who live alone can call a relative at a preappointed time; emergency pager devices also may be useful.

LONG-TERM COMPLICATIONS OF DIABETES

1 Elderly people have a higher incidence and accelerated development of long-term complications. Some complications (especially retinal and lower extremity) often are present at diagnosis.[30,31]

2 Amputation is twice as common in patients over age 65 years. Peripheral neuropathy and decreased vision can compromise self-detection of lower extremity problems (see Chapter 16, Foot, Skin and Dental Care, for more information).

A Stress the importance of frequent foot inspection, incorporating assistance from others (family, friends, and home health nurses) as needed.

B Create teaching opportunities by observing foot care and inspecting footwear during clinical visits.

C Assist patients to obtain footwear that accommodates the shape of their feet and specific sensation problems. Refer to a podiatrist or orthotic specialist as necessary.

3 Hypertension, a diabetes-related complication, contributes to stroke, renal failure, and myocardial infarction.

A Screen blood pressure regularly.

B Evaluate sodium intake and teach patients ways to decrease if appropriate.

C Alternative seasonings can be suggested for those with decreased taste sensation.

D It is important to advocate for early treatment.

E Monitor closely for drug side effects (eg, orthostatic hypotension, decreased cardiac output).

F Consider potential drug-drug interactions each time a new medication is started (see Chapter 10, Pharmacologic Therapies, for more information).

4 Myocardial infarction and cerebrovascular incidents are more prevalent in elderly persons with diabetes. In addition to the usual preventive care and education, the elderly patient has special needs that must be considered.

A Preventive strategies should be weighed against needed treatments for comorbidities and expected benefits.

B Stroke prevention efforts for the elderly are focused on glucose control, treating atrial fibrillation, and control of hypertension.[32]

C Routine EKGs should be given and patients should be monitored for the signs/symptoms of congestive heart failure to provide early detection and treatment of cardiac disease.[33]

5 Vision loss is more likely to occur in the elderly.

A Eye diseases, in general, are more common with aging. This fact, coupled with changes from diabetes, make older people more susceptible to vision loss.

B Limited vision can seriously impact self-care for diabetes.

C Glucose control affects the progression of retinopathy in the elderly.[34]

D Annual screening and treatment of retinopathy and maculopathy for older patients can save vision.[35]

E Emphasize the importance of annual screening because yearly eye exams are not ordered routinely.[36]

F Assess functional vision regularly and during educational sessions to determine its impact on self-monitoring, medication administration, and foot care.

6 Diabetic nephropathy coupled with the renal changes associated with aging and other causes of renal insufficiency (eg, arteriosclerosis, hypertension, congestive heart failure, drugs, infection, and cancer) can precipitate kidney failure.

A Routine screening for kidney disease is needed for early detection and treatment (see Chapter 23, Nephropathy, for more information).

B Warn patients about the dangers of nephrotoxic contrast media and selected drugs.

C Teach ways to prevent urinary tract infections and signs/symptoms for early treatment.

D Evaluate the need for a low-protein diet carefully when it is recommended.

7 The effect of dental diseases on eating and nutrition can be significant.
  A Assess whether mobility and financial difficulties are affecting preventive care.
  B Assess and facilitate oral hygiene and dental care.

CARE OF THE HOSPITALIZED ELDERLY

1 Elderly people are hospitalized more frequently than younger people. One third of those who are 75 years of age and have diabetes are hospitalized in the course of a year.[37,38]

2 Because 65% of elderly people who are hospitalized are undernourished at admission, the nutritional status of elderly patients should be carefully assessed on admission and follow-up provided as needed.[39]

3 The diagnosis of diabetes may not be included in the hospital records of patients with diabetes. Furthermore, undetected diabetes is common in hospital populations.[40]

4 Hospital-based diabetes educators have a unique opportunity to promote diagnosis and improved treatment of older people with diabetes.

5 Costs of hospitalization make up 40% of all costs of care for people with diabetes.[41] Earlier detection and treatment in the geriatric population may help reduce personal suffering and the healthcare costs.

NURSING FACILITIES

1 Dependent individuals with diabetes comprise 18.3% of residents in nursing care facilities.[42]

2 Priorities of care for residents with diabetes include
  A Personal/family priorities
  B Eliminating glycemic symptoms
  C Achieving/maintaining optimal daily functioning
  D Balancing treatment with overall prognosis

3 A team approach is possible for residents with diabetes because the involvement of nurses, dietitians, pharmacists, physicians, and therapists is mandated by regulations for long-term care facilities. The nature of this environment in terms of consistency and team care can result in optimal control of diabetes without unnecessary burden. Staff education is necessary and has been should to be effective.[43-45]

Key Educational Considerations

1 Assess elderly patients as individuals but anticipate special needs related to aging.

2 Determine the patient's priorities. Limit instruction to content that matches the older adult's specific diabetes-related goals.

3 Modify instruction so that key information is presented in easily read or heard messages.

4 Routinely teach at a slower pace, use memory aides and incorporate significant others and caregivers in instruction.

5 Evaluate learning often, especially when hyperglycemia is present.

6 Evaluate care recommendations with consideration for cost, accessibility, safety, support systems, and the effect on quality of life.

Case Study 1

FM is a 70-year-old Native American man who lives on the local reservation. He has been admitted to the hospital for hypoglycemia, and you have been asked to evaluate his treatment and educational needs. His HbA$_{1c}$ is 10%. Currently, FM is taking the following medications:
- Troglitazone 400 mg, glipizide 10 mg bid
- 70/30 insulin: 45 units before breakfast, 25 units at 6 PM
- Aspirin, 1 daily
- Lasix, 40 mg daily
- Vasotec, 5 mg daily
- Albuterol, 2 puffs 4 times daily

FM has had diabetes for 15 years and is followed at the reservation clinic several times a year. Due to poor eyesight he is not using his blood glucose meter to test his blood sugars.

QUESTIONS FOR DISCUSSION

1 What approach would you use for your first visit with this patient?
2 Are the patient's current medications appropriate for him?
3 What resource issues will need to be assessed?

DISCUSSION

1 To prepare for FM's first visit:

A Ask FM to bring a family member or friend with him.

B Ask FM to bring all of his medications and monitoring supplies.

C Make sure you have magnifiers and low-vision educational materials available for FM to use.

D Contact his provider to confirm his medications and get his most recent lab results.

E Determine if community health workers or home health care is available to him on the reservation.

2 The first visit will likely focus on assessing FM's ability to do self-care, the cause of his current episode of hypoglycemia, dietary intake and nutritional needs, identification of support systems, and influence of his cultural beliefs and practices on his self-care (eg, food preparation and choices, use of alternative therapies).

3 It is likely that FM's complex diabetes medication regimen can be simplified to assure accurate administration.

A Sulfonylureas are not indicated because FM is likely to have reduced insulin secretion at his age.

B Combination regimens with three or more drugs are not recommended.

- There are no studies that demonstrate a therapeutic advantage of adding a third drug to a treatment regimen.

- A simplified regimen is more likely to result in increased accuracy in dosing, administration and reduced costs. Therapy can be initiated with either insulin or an oral agent, but not both.

C If troglitazone is continued, FM will need to be monitored for liver dysfunction.

4 FM has visual problems that will have to be accommodated.

5 Develop a teaching plan with FM so that other educational and management issues can be addressed at future visits. This plan also can be used to report back to FM's case manager or provider as needed.

6 It is likely that FM will benefit from ongoing brief educational sessions. A significant other should be taught to help him with reinforcement or memory problems. Given the high incidence of diabetes in Native Americans, FM's family members or friends may personally benefit from receiving information about diabetes.

7 A community health worker or home health nurse can assist with instruction and evaluate his home environment.

Case Study 2

EK is an obese 76-year-old widow with type 2 diabetes. She is referred to you for instruction about blood glucose monitoring. EK lives alone in a high-rise apartment building in a large city. Her daughter lives nearby and drives her to medical appointments. Although she takes glyburide 5 mg twice daily, her blood glucose levels are consistently 300 mg/dL (16.7 mmol/L) when measured using the glucose meter in her provider's office. EK does not report symptoms of high or low blood sugar but is concerned about having to get up during the night to urinate as a result of her "water pill." Other medical problems that she reports are arthritis (which limits her activity), cataract surgery 2 years earlier, and a mild heart problem for which she takes digitalis.

Questions For Discussion

1 What difficulties might EK have doing blood glucose monitoring?

2 What might be the causes of her persistent hyperglycemia?

3 In addition to her concerns, what other areas might you identify in your educational plan?

DISCUSSION

1 In light of her previous cataract surgery, EK may have difficulty seeing adequately, and her manual dexterity may be affected by her arthritis.

2 She may benefit from (1) a meter with easy-to-use features, (2) being given supervised opportunities to practice using her meter, and (3) receiving brief written reminders on how to use the device. Demonstrate different meters that are available so she can understand her options in making a selection.

3 Until her blood glucose is in good control, EK may have difficulty learning and retaining information. Therefore, all verbal information should be reinforced with written forms as well. Her daughter can also be taught how to reinforce her mother's technique and recall, such as posting the procedure where she tests and making sure there is good lighting.

4 EK is at risk for dehydration because of her hyperglycemia and polyuria; getting up at night increases her risk of falling since her mobility is limited.

5 Her glyburide is at maximum dose and improved glycemic control may be better achieved with an oral agent that does not cause hypoglycemia.

6 Another possible cause of her hyperglycemia is infection. The upper respiratory tract is the most common site of infection in people with diabetes.

7 Information on meal planning, weight, blood pressure, recent HbA$_{1c}$, serum and urine creatinine, and EKG needs to be provided. Include a foot exam at every office visit, a referral to an ophthalmologist and emphasize regular eye care during educational sessions.

8 Financial and access issues must be discussed early so that appropriate resources can be provided.

9 Determine whether the hyperglycemia was caused by inadequate medication, dietary intake, or infection. Other issues to assess include activity level and other medications.

REFERENCES

1 Kenny SJ, Aubert RE, Geiss LS. Prevalence and incidence of non-insulin-dependent diabetes. In: National Diabetes Data Group, eds. Diabetes in America. 2nd ed. Bethesda, Md: National Institutes of Health, 1995; NIH publication no. 95-1468:49-54.

2 Harris MI, Klein R, Welborn TA, Knuiman MW. Onset of NIDDM occurs at least 4-7 yr before clinical diagnosis. Diabetes Care 1992;15:815-19.

3 Gradman TJ, Laws A, Thompson LW, Reaven GM. Verbal learning and/or memory improves with glycemic control in older subjects with non-insulin-dependent diabetes mellitus. J Am Geriatr Soc 1993;41:1305-12.

4 Meneilly GS, Tessier D. Diabetes in the elderly. Diabetic Med 1995;12:949-60.

5 Wachtel T, Silliman R, Lamberton P. Prognostic factors in the diabetic hyperosmolar state. J Am Geriatr Soc 1987; 35:737-41.

6 Manton KG, Stallard E. Cross-sectional estimates of active life expectancy for the US elderly and oldest-old populations. J Gerontal 1991;46: S170-82.

7 Sacks DB, McDonald JM. The pathogenesis of type II diabetes mellitus. A polygenic disease. Am J Clin Pathol 1996; 105:149-56.

8 Williamson JR, Hoffmann PL, Kohrt WM. Endurance exercise training decreases capillary basement membrane width in older nondiabetic and diabetic adults. J Appl Physiol 1996;80:747-53.

9 Markson EW. Functional, social, and psychological disability as causes of loss of weight and independence in older community-living people. Clin Geriatr Med 1997;13:639-52.

10 Bressler R, Johnson DG. Oral antidiabetic drug use in the elderly. Drugs Aging 1996;9:418-37.

11 Mooradian AD. Drug therapy of non-insulin dependent diabetes mellitus in the elderly. Drugs 1996;51:931-41.

12 Oki JC, Isley WL. Rethinking new and old diabetes drugs for type 2 disease. Practical Diabetol 1997;16(3):27-40.

13 Umeda F. Potential role of thiazolidinediones in older diabetic patients. Drugs Aging 1995;7:331-37.

14 White JR. Combination oral agent/insulin therapy in patients with type 2 diabetes mellitus. Clinical Diabetes 1997;152: 102-12

15 Shorr RI, Ray WA, Daugherty JR, Griffin MN. Incidence and risk factors for serious hypoglycemia in older persons using insulin or sulfonylureas. Arch Intern Med 1997;157:1681-1686

16 Gregorio F, Ambrosi F, Filipponi P, Manfrini S, Testa I. Is metformin safe enough for aging type 2 diabetic patients? Diabetes Metab 1996;22:43-50.

17 Jennings PE. Oral antihyperglycemics. Considerations in older patients with non-insulin-dependent diabetes mellitus. Drugs Aging 1997;10:323-31.

18 Wallsten SM, Sullivan RJ Jr, Hanlon JT, Blazer DG, Tyrey MJ, Westlund R. Medication-taking behaviors in the high- and low-functioning elderly: MacArthur field studies of successful aging. Ann Pharmaco Ther 1995;29:359-64.

19 Wolffenbuttel BH, Drossaert CH, Visser AP. Determinants of injecting insulin in elderly patients with type II diabetes mellitus. Patient Educ Couns 1993;22:117-25.

20 Hoogwerf BJ, Mehta A, Reddy S. Advances in the treatment of diabetes mellitus in the elderly. Development of insulin analogues. Drugs Aging 1996; 9:438-48.

21 Silliman RA, Bhatti S, Khan A, Dukes KA, Sullivan LM. The care of older persons with diabetes mellitus: families and primary care physicians. J Am Geriatr Soc 1996;44:1314-21.

22 Halter J. Geriatric patients. In: Lebovitz HE, ed. Therapy for diabetes mellitus and related disorders. Alexandria, Va: American Diabetes Association, 1991: 155-60.

23 Bernbaum M, Albert SG, McGinnis J, Brusca S, Mooradian AD. The reliability of self blood glucose monitoring in elderly diabetic patients. J Am Geriatr Soc 1994;42:779-81.

24 Meneilly GS, Cheung E, Tessier D, Yakura C, Tuokko H. The effect of improved glycemic control on cognitive functions in the elderly patient with diabetes. J Gerontol 1993;48:M117-21.

25 Chenitz WC, Stone JT, Salisbury SA. Clinical gerontological nursing. Philadelphia: WB Saunders, 1991.

26 Garcia R, Suarez R. Diabetes education in the elderly: a 5-year follow-up of an interactive approach. Patient Educ and Couns 1996;29:87-97.

27 Lustman PJ, Griffith LS, Clouse RE. Recognizing and managing depression in patients with diabetes. Anderson BA, Rubin RR, eds. In: Practical psychology for diabetes clinicians. Alexandria, Va: American Diabetes Association, 1996: 143-52.

28 Ganzini L, Smith DM, Fenn DS, Lee MA. Depression and mortality in medically ill older adults. J Am Geriatr. Soc 1997; 45:307-12.

29 Zrebiec JF. Caring for elderly patients with diabetes. Anderson B, Rubin R, eds. In: Practical psychology for diabetes clinicians. Alexandria, Va: American Diabetes Association, 1996:35-42.

30 Abraira C, Colwell J, Nuttall F, Sawin CT, Henderson W, Comstock JP. Cardiovascular events and correlates in the Veterans Affairs Diabetes Feasibility Trial. Arch Intern Med 1997;157:181-8.

31 Turner RC, Holman RR. Lessons from UK prospective diabetes study. Diabetes Res Clin Pract 1995;28:S151-57.

32 Kuusisto J, Mykkanen L, Pyorala K, Laakso M. Non-insulin-dependent diabetes and its metabolic control are important predictors of stroke in elderly subjects. Stroke 1994;25:1157-64.

33 Azzarelli A, Dini FL, Cristofani R, et al. NIDDM as unfavorable factor to the postinfarctual ventricular function in the elderly: echocardiography study. Coronary Artery Dis 1995;6:629-34.

34 Morisaki N, Watanabe S, Kobayashi J, Kanzaki T, Takahashi K, Yokote K. Diabetic control and progression of retinopathy in elderly patients: five year follow-up study. J Am Geriatr Soc 1994; 42:142-45.

35 Agardh E, Agardh CD, Hansson-Lundblad C, Cavallin-Sjoberg U. The importance of early diagnosis of treatable diabetic retinopathy for the four-year visual outcome in older-onset diabetes mellitus. Acta Ophthalomol Scand 1996;74:166-70.

36 Pagano G, Bargero G, Vuolo A, Bruno G. Prevalence and clinical features of known type 2 diabetes in the elderly: a population based study. Diabetic Med 1994; 11:475-79.

37 Aubert RE, Geiss LS, Ballard DJ, Cocanougher B, Herman WH. Diabetes-related hospitalization and hospital utilization. In: National Diabetes Data Group, eds. Diabetes in America. 2nd ed. Bethesda, Md: National Institutes of Health, 1995; NIH publication no. 95-1468:559.

38 Rosenthal MJ, Fajardo M, Gilmore S, Morley JE, Naliboff B. Hospitalization and mortality of diabetes in older adults. Diabetes Care 1998;21:231-35.

39 Sullivan D, Lipschitz D. Evaluating and treating nutritional problems in older patients. Clin Geriatr Med 1997;13: 753-68.

40 Levetan CS, Passaro M, Jablonski K, Kass M, Ratner RE. Unrecognized diabetes among hospitalized patients. Diabetes Care 1998;21:246-49.

41 Diabetes 1996 vital statistics. Alexandria, Va: American Diabetes Association, 1997:67.

42 Mayfield JA, Deb P, Potter DEB. Diabetes and long term care. In: National Diabetes Data Group, eds. Diabetes in America. 2nd ed. Bethesda, Md: National Institutes of Health, 1995; NIH publication no. 95-1468:571.

43 Tonino R. Diabetes education: what should health-care providers in long-term nursing care facilities know about diabetes? Diabetes Care 1990;13(suppl 2):55-59.

44 Wylie-Rosett J, Villeneuve M, Mazze R. Professional education in a long term care facility: program development in diabetes. Diabetes Care 1985;8:481-85.

45 Mooradian AD. Caring for the elderly nursing home patient with diabetes. Diabetes Spectrum 1992;5:318-22.

Suggested Readings

Amato L, Paolisso G, Cacciatore F, Ferrara N, Canonico S, Rengo F. Non-insulin-dependent diabetes mellitus is associated with a greater prevalence of depression in the elderly. Diabetes Metab 1996;22:314-18.

Atiea JA, Moses JL, Sinclair AJ. Neuropsychological function in older subjects with non-insulin-dependent diabetes mellitus. Diabetic Med 1995;12:679-85.

Belmin J, Valensi P. Diabetic neuropathy in elderly patients. What can be done? Drugs Aging 1996;8:416-29.

Bohannon NJ, Jack DB. Type II diabetes: tips for managing your older patients. Geriatrics 1996;51(3):28-35.

Deakins DA. Teaching elderly patients about diabetes. Am J Nurs 1994;94(4):38-42.

Gurwitz JH, Field TS, Glynn RJ, Manson JE, Avorn J, et al. Risk factors for non-insulin-dependent diabetes mellitus requiring treatment in the elderly. J Am Geriatr Soc 1994;42:1235-40.

Helkala EL, Niskanen L, Viinamaki H, Partanen J, Uusitupa M. Short-term and long-term memory in elderly patients with NIDDM. Diabetes Care 1995; 18:681-85.

Joergens V, Gruesser M. Three years' experience after national introduction of teaching programs for type II diabetic patients in Germany: how to train general practitioners. Patient Educ Couns 1995;26:195-202.

Leibson CL, Rocca WA, Hanson VA, Cha R, Kokmen E, O'Brien PC, et al. Risk of dementia among persons with diabetes mellitus: a population-based cohort study. Am J Epidemiol 1997;145:301-8.

Niskanen L, Rauramaa R, Miettinen H, Haffner SM, Mercuri M, Uusitupa M. Carotid artery intima-media thickness in elderly patients with NIDDM and in nondiabetic subjects. Stroke 1996;27:1986-92.

Paolisso G, Balbi V, Volpe C, Varricchio G, Gambardella A, Saccomanno F. Metabolic benefits deriving from chronic vitamin C supplementation in aged non-insulin dependent diabetics. J Am Coll of Nutr 1995;14:387-92.

COMPLICATIONS

COMPLICATIONS

Chronic Complications of Diabetes: An Overview   **20**

Michael A. Pfeifer, MD
East Carolina University
School of Medicine
Greenville, North Carolina

INTRODUCTION

1 Education concerning the reduction of modifiable risk factors for the chronic complications of diabetes is an essential component of diabetes self-management training. Although the influence of hyperglycemia has become part of standard diabetes self-management education, other risk factors have often received less attention.

2 Patients need information about risk factors that may increase chronic complications, however, in order to make informed decisions and fully participate in their own care.

3 The diabetes educator can play a key role in the prevention of chronic complications by providing information to patients about behaviors and nonpharmacologic options that may affect their development.

4 This chapter will enumerate both the modifiable and nonmodifiable risk factors of diabetes complications in order to provide both the background and a framework for the content incorporated in the complication-specific chapters, and to assist educators to present this information to patients in a meaningful way.

5 Chronic complications of diabetes were virtually unknown until 10 to 20 years after the discovery of insulin in 1921.

    A Descriptions of renal disease, neuropathy, and retinopathy did not appear until the 1930s and 1940s. At that time, it was not clear whether these complications (especially the microvascular abnormalities) were an integral part of diabetes mellitus or a consequence of poor blood glucose control.

    B Studies such as the Diabetes Control and Complications Trial (DCCT)[1] among individuals with type 1 diabetes and the Kumamoto study[2] among individuals with type 2 diabetes have demonstrated that these complications are not inevitable.

6 The chronic complications of diabetes significantly impact the cost of health care. Approximately 25% of the total Medicare budget is dedicated to the treatment of diabetes and its chronic complications. It has been estimated that by reducing or eliminating risk factors, 85% of the chronic complications could be delayed or the progression slowed. This would save the Medicare budget more than $17 billion annually.[3]

7 The pathogenesis of diabetes complications has been studied for the last 50 years. No single etiology explains all of the complications; rather, multiple etiologies exist that are specific to each.

   A Assuming that hyperglycemia plays a role in the etiology of all complications, there are also additional risk factors associated with each, resulting in complex, and perhaps independent, etiologies.

   B The etiology of complications is further confounded by the variation in risk factors among individuals. In some individuals, one or more risk factors may play a greater role than in other individuals.

   C Determining which risk factor carries the greatest possibility for the development of each complication, as well as the variation among individuals, has been an area of intense investigation.

8 Pathophysiologic mechanisms which are hypothesized to contribute to the development of specific complications include

   A Accumulation of intracellular sorbitol from the conversion of glucose to sorbitol (polyol pathway)

   B Autoimmunity

   C Tissue ischemia and hypoxia

   D Glycosylation of cellular proteins (advanced glycosylated endproducts [AGE])

   E Coagulation defects

   F Insulin resistance

OBJECTIVES

Upon completion of this chapter, the learner will be able to

1 State the modifiable risk factors for individuals with diabetes for cardiovascular disease, neuropathy, nephropathy, and retinopathy.

2 State the non-modifiable risk factors for persons with diabetes for cardiovascular disease, neuropathy, nephropathy, and retinopathy.

3 Describe the impact of hyperglycemia on the long-term complications of diabetes.

CARDIOVASCULAR COMPLICATIONS

1 Cardiovascular complications include coronary artery disease, myocardial infarction, peripheral vascular disease, and cerebral vascular disease (see Chapter 24, Macrovascular Complications, for more information).

2 Nonmodifiable risk factors include duration of diabetes, age, genetics, race, and gender.

   A A linear relationship appears to exist between the duration of diabetes and cardiovascular complications. This relationship may be more observable in individuals with type 1 diabetes, since the onset of type 2 diabetes is not easily established.

   B As in individuals without diabetes, there is a relationship between age and the prevalence of cardiovascular disease. The older the individual with diabetes, the greater the risk for cardiovascular complications.

   C Genetics play a role in the incidence of cardiovascular complications, although predictive genetic characteristics have not been fully elucidated.

   D African-American individuals with diabetes are at risk for macrovascular disease but have an overall lower prevalence rate of myocardial infarction (MI) than Caucasian individuals.[4] Mexican-American individuals appear to have an increased risk for peripheral vascular disease, but a lower prevalence of MI than Caucasian individuals.[5]

   E Premenopausal women without diabetes are at less risk than males without diabetes for cardiovascular events and complications. This gender-protective advantage does not exist for females with diabetes, who have an equal risk for cardiovascular events and complications as males with diabetes.[6]

3 Modifiable risk factors include hyperglycemia, hypertension, dyslipidemia, increased platelet adherence, smoking, diet, increased homocysteine level, obesity, increased insulin level, lack of exercise, and type A personality.

   A There is little evidence that treatment of hyperglycemia will result in a decrease in cardiovascular events or complications. The DCCT[1] data were suggestive (45% to 54% reduction) but did not reach statistical significance regarding this relationship. Nonetheless, improved glucose control will decrease total cholesterol levels, decrease LDL cholesterol, and decrease platelet adherence.

B Hypertension appears to play a major role in the development of cardiovascular complications in individuals with diabetes as well as individuals without diabetes.

- Hypertension is twice as common in African-American individuals than in Caucasion individuals with diabetes.[4]
- Hypertension prevalence increases with age among people with diabetes. A larger percentage of individuals with diabetes have hypertension than do age-comparable individuals without diabetes.
- An increase in vascular response to stimuli may play a role in hypertension in diabetes.
- Hyperinsulinemia, theoretically, might play a role by increasing the tubular reabsorption of sodium and thereby increasing blood volume.

C Dyslipidemia involves four major areas of concern for individuals with diabetes: decreased high density lipoprotein cholesterol level (HDL), increased low density lipoprotein (LDL) cholesterol level, increased triglyceride (TG) level, and increased lipoprotein(a) [Lp(a)] level.

D People with diabetes can have an increase in platelet adherence and aggregation that may lead to abnormalities in microcirculation and add to plaque formation. Improved metabolic control has been shown to decrease platelet adherence and aggregation.[7,8]

E The link between smoking and cardiovascular events and complications is well established in individuals with or without diabetes. The benefits of smoking cessation has been demonstrated in non-diabetic populations. There is no reason to believe that smoking cessation would not be beneficial for individuals with diabetes.

F Diets high in fat have been suggested to increase atherosclerosis via increased cholesterol levels. There is controversy, however, whether educational and nutritional efforts should be directed towards a very low-fat composition versus a low saturated fat/high monounsaturated fat composition.

G Homocystine is increased only in individuals with diabetes and vascular disease or retinopathy. Elevated homocystine levels may cause tears in the endothelium. No prospective studies have been conducted demonstrating that a decrease in homocystine level results in decreased cardiovascular events. Homocystine levels may be decreased by pharmacological doses of pyridoxine (vitamin B6), vitamin B12, and folic acid.

H Obesity, particularly central adiposity, has been linked to atherogenesis. However, no prospective, randomized clinical trial has shown that a decrease in adiposity will decrease cardiovascular events. Because increased adiposity is linked with hypertension, dyslipidemia, hyperinsulinemia, and hyperglycemia, it seems prudent that a decrease in adiposity would contribute to decreasing cardiovascular events.

I Increased insulin levels have been linked to both hypertension and atherosclerosis in cross-sectional data in non-diabetic populations,[7] leading to a suggestion that insulin resistance is associated with increased cardiovascular risks. However, no data indicating that insulin is atherogenic in humans are available.

J Lack of exercise is associated with cardiovascular events and complications. Routine exercise decreases blood pressure, often decreases blood glucose levels, is important for cardiac toning, and is useful as a way to cope with stress and as an adjunct to weight loss. There are few data that link the benefits of exercise to prolongation of life after myocardial infarction. Cross-sectional epidemiologic and anecdotal data suggest that a routine exercise program can help prevent cardiovascular events in patients who have not had a myocardial infarction.

K Individuals with a Type A (high strung) personality are at increased risk for cardiovascular events and their complications.[10] Psychological and behavioral therapies have been shown to decrease cardiovascular events in individuals without diabetes. This benefit is thought to be realized by individuals with diabetes as well.

4 Other risk factors include plasminogen activator inhibitor 1, Von Willebrand factor, fibrinogen, fibrinolysis, and microcirculation. All of these factors have been linked, in cross-sectional studies in animals, to increased cardiovascular events, suggesting they may also play a role in humans with diabetes. However, convincing prospective studies are lacking.

5 Characteristics not believed to be risk factors for cardiovascular complications.

A Controversy exists concerning whether the type of antidiabetes medication is a risk factor for cardiovascular complications.

B The type of diabetes does not appear to be a factor in the development of cardiovascular disease. However, cardiovascular events and complications occur with higher frequency in individuals with type 2 diabetes than in individuals with type 1 diabetes. Individuals with type 1 diabetes develop cardiovascular disease at a younger age.

C There is no known evidence of an autoimmune process causing cardiovascular complications in individuals with diabetes.

NEUROPATHY

1 Diabetic neuropathy includes distal symmetrical polyneuropathy, autonomic neuropathy, mononeuropathies, plexopathies, proximal motor neuropathy, and entrapment neuropathies (see Chapter 22, Neuropathy, for more information).

2 Nonmodifiable risk factors include duration of diabetes, age, genetics, race, height, and autoimmunity.

A There is a linear relationship between the duration of diabetes and the development of diabetic neuropathy; the longer one has diabetes, the greater the risk of developing diabetic neuropathy.

B Age also appears to be related in a linear fashion to the development of diabetic neuropathy; older age in a person with diabetes is associated with a greater likelihood that neuropathy will develop.

C Diabetic neuropathy is influenced by genetics; human leukocyte antigens (HLA) DR3 and DR4 have been linked to an increased incidence of this complication.[11]

D African Americans are more likely to develop diabetic neuropathy than Caucasians.[12,13]

E Taller individuals tend to have more diabetic neuropathy than shorter individuals, possibly due to the length of the nerve and the increased probability of abnormalities due to this length.[14]

F Autoimmunity involves the body's antibodies attacking itself in an unwanted assault, in this case, against the nerves. There is an increase in the level of autoantibodies to nerves in some individuals with diabetes and neuropathy.[15] It is not clear whether the autoantibodies are a response to damaged nerves or the autoantibodies cause the damage. Thus, it is not clear whether this is a primary etiology in the development of neuropathy. Once autoantibodies are formed, they hasten the progression of the diabetic neuropathy.

3 Modifiable risk factors include hyperglycemia, hypertension, dyslipidemia, abnormal microcirculation, and alcohol use.

A Hyperglycemia may play several roles in the development of diabetic neuropathy.

- Hyperglycemia may cause an increased incidence of glycosylated neural proteins and formation of advanced glycosylated endproducts (AGEs). Such alterations of the neural proteins may decrease nerve transport and affect protein function.

- Hyperglycemia can competitively inhibit the uptake of myoinositol by the nerve. Myoinositol is important for nerve membrane function and maintaining the Na-K-ATPase activity.

- Hyperglycemia can activate the polyol pathway, leading to increased concentration of sorbitol within the nerve. This, in turn, can cause swelling within the space between the nerve fibers (endoneuria) within the nerve sheath, which can damage the nerve and alter nerve function. In addition, activation of the polyol pathway may decrease nerve myoinositol through unknown mechanisms.

- Hyperglycemia can decrease nitric oxide synthethase activity, which, in turn, may decrease microcirculation to the nerve.

- Insulin deficiency may retard the conversion of the fatty acid linoleic acid to gamma-linoleic acid. This may cause a deviation in prostaglandin pathways, causing a decrease in the formation of arachidonic acid. This decrease in arachidonic acid alters the constituents of the nerve membrane.

B Hypertension,[12] particularly the diastolic level, is linked to the development of diabetic neuropathy. This finding is consistent in several correctional studies including the DCCT.[1] At least one study[16] has shown an increase in nerve conduction velocity when patients were placed on an angiotensin-converting enzyme (ACE) inhibitor.

C Hypercholesterolemia is associated with the development of diabetic neuropathy. However, no prospective studies have shown that a decrease in cholesterol levels will decrease the onset or slow the progression of diabetic neuropathy.

D The relationship between heavy alcohol ingestion and an increased incidence of neuropathy has been clearly demonstrated. Alcohol alone can cause nerve damage. Combining the effects of alcohol with the nerve damage due to diabetes may worsen the overall clinical picture.

4 Characteristics not believed to be risk factors for neuropathy.

   A There are no data to suggest that the type of antidiabetes medications predisposes patients to nor protects patients from, diabetic neuropathy.

   B Males were once thought to be at greater risk for developing diabetic neuropathy than females. However, considering that males are generally taller than females, it is felt that it is the height of the individual, not the gender, that predisposes individuals to develop diabetic neuropathy.

   C There is no evidence to suggest that specific diets may predispose patients to diabetic neuropathy. Conversely, a diet high in myoinositol has been shown to increase nerve conduction velocity.[17]

   D Neither increased nor decreased adiposity has been linked to the development of, or protection from, diabetic neuropathy.

   E Exercise does not seem to play a role in the development of, or protection from, diabetic neuropathy. Exercise may put the insensate foot at risk for traumatic injury resulting in diabetic foot ulcers.

   F There is no evidence to suggest a relationship between increased insulin levels and increased incidence of diabetic neuropathy.

   G Some studies[13,18] have indicated that there is a cross-sectional relationship between smoking and diabetic neuropathy; however, this relationship has not been universally found.

FOOT ULCERS

1 Foot ulcers develop primarily as a consequence of vascular disease, various types of neuropathies, foot deformities, or other factors affecting the health of the foot. Each of these causative factors has specific modifiable or nonmodifiable risk factors (see Chapter 16, Skin, Foot and Dental Care, for more information).

2 Peripheral vascular disease plays a major role in the development of foot ulcers.

3 Neuropathy plays an essential role in the development of diabetic foot ulcers.

   A An insensate foot puts the patient at increased risk for traumatic damage without an awareness of the injury. As a result, proper attention and care is often not sought in a timely manner.

    B Autonomic dysfunction of the sweat glands of the foot may cause the skin to become dry and cracked, and prone to ulceration.

    C Patients with diabetic neuropathy often have motor abnormalities which may predispose them to trauma secondary to an unsteady gait and falls secondary to lack of proprioception (awareness of where the foot is in space).

    D Neuropathy in the muscular part of the foot, leading to foot deformities and increased pressure points may predispose the foot to ulcers. The metatarsal heads, interdigital joints, and tips of toes particularly are at high risk for development of foot ulcers from neuropathic muscular changes.

4 Amputation rates are higher among African Americans,[4] Hispanics,[5] and Native Americans[19] than Caucasians.

5 Exercise may predispose the insensate foot to traumatic damage if it is done in an imprudent manner. Choosing activities that avoid repeated pounding to the feet (swimming, bicycling) may be more prudent than jogging.

6 Other risk factors include improperly fitting shoes and nail abnormalities, visual impairments, lack of self-management skills.

NEPHROPATHY

1 Diabetes is the most common cause of nephropathy. It is also, at present, the most costly complication of diabetes, due to the success of renal dialysis and kidney transplants. Early evidence of nephropathy is determined by the presence of albumin in urine. As the disease progresses the amount of albumin increases until end-stage renal disease is reached (see Chapter 23, Nephropathy, for more information).

2 Nonmodifiable risk factors include duration of diabetes, age, genetics, and race.

    A A relationship between duration of diabetes and end-stage renal disease is well established in individuals with type 1 diabetes but not in individuals with type 2 diabetes, partly because the onset of type 2 diabetes is seldom well documented.

- The natural history (clinical stages) of nephropathy is thought to be the same in type 1 and in type 2 diabetes.
- Generally, end-stage renal disease occurs between 10 to 25 years duration of diabetes. There is a decline in the prevalence of end-stage renal disease after 25 to 30 years duration, although the risk is not totally eliminated.

B A linear relationship exists between age and the development of diabetic nephropathy. The older the individual, the greater the risk of developing nephropathy.

C Certain human leukocyte antigen (HLA) types are associated with the development of diabetic nephropathy.[20]

D African Americans,[4] Hispanics,[5] and Native Americans[19] all have a greater prevalence of diabetic nephropathy than Caucasians with diabetes.

3 Modifiable risk factors include hypertension, dyslipidemia, hyperglycemia, diet, smoking, and frequent urinary tract infections.

A The effect of hypertension on the development of nephropathy in individuals with diabetes or without diabetes is well documented.
- There is some evidence that treatment with certain antihypertensive agents may reduce the incidence or slow the progression of nephropathy. In particular, ACE inhibitors decrease blood pressure (that is, reduce pressure going into the glomeruli) as well as reduce resistance within the glomeruli.
- In prospective trials[21], the ACE inhibitor captopril has been shown to increase the time to reach a doubling of the serum creatinine level, thus slowing the progression to end-stage renal disease.

B Cross-sectional studies[22] have linked hypercholesterolemia to the presence of diabetic nephropathy.
- In prospective trials[23], treatment with HMG-CoA reductase inhibitor antilipidemia agents ("statin" drugs such as pravastatin, lovastatin, atorvastatin, fluvastatin, simvastatin, cerivastatin) has been shown to decrease cholesterol levels and increase the time to doubling of the serum creatinine level compared with the placebo group.

C Hyperglycemia may play several roles in the development of diabetic nephropathy.
- Hyperglycemia can lead to glycosylation (increased amount of sugar molecules attaching to proteins) of glomerular proteins and the formation of advanced glycation end products (AGEs). The develop-

ment of AGEs results in protein structural changes which can alter protein function.

- Hyperglycemia can result in activation of the polyol pathway. Accumulation of sorbitol produced by increased activity of the polyol pathway has been demonstrated in the glomeruli. This may lead to a decrease in glomerular function and allow micro quantities of albumin to leak into the urine (microalbuminuria).

D There is little evidence that a high-protein diet results in the development of diabetic nephropathy or that a low-protein diet prevents the development of diabetic nephropathy. However, once diabetic nephropathy develops, the rate of progression of the nephropathy can be slowed by placing the patient on a low-protein diet.[24]

E Cross-sectional studies[25] have linked smoking to the presence of diabetic nephropathy. No prospective trials have been done.

F Frequent urinary tract infections predispose a patient to glomerulonephritis and papillary necrosis, thus worsening existing renal dysfunction.

4 Certain characteristics not believed to be risk factors.

A There is no evidence that the type of antidiabetes treatment protects or predisposes an individual to diabetic nephropathy. However, certain antidiabetes medications are contraindicated in renal disease because of the elimination profile of the drug.

B There is no evidence that gender protects or predisposes an individual to the development of diabetic nephropathy.

C Cross-sectional or prospective data are not available to document autoimmunity as a possible pathogenesis.

D Strenuous exercise can increase proteinuria but there is no evidence of long-term damaging effects provided the patient does not have clinical evidence of renal disease. There is no evidence that exercise helps slow the progression of diabetic nephropathy.

E There is no evidence that adiposity is either protective or predisposes a patient for diabetic nephropathy.

F There is no evidence that increased insulin levels are associated with the development of diabetic nephropathy.

RETINOPATHY

1 Diabetic retinopathy is the leading cause of blindness in the US and has been the focus of several large, multicenter, double-blind, randomized clinical trials. Diabetic retinopathy is described by the changes that occur in the retina, including microaneurysms, hard exudates, soft exudates, hemorrhages, and peripheral retinopathy (see Chapter 21, Eye Disease and Adaptive Diabetes Education for the Visually Impaired, for more information).

2 Nonmodifiable risk factors include duration of diabetes, age, genetics, and race.

    A Duration of diabetes is linked to the development of retinopathy in type 1 diabetes.[26] A similar relationship is believed to exist for type 2 diabetes, but is not as well understood.

        • There is seldom a need for laser therapy within the first 10 years duration of diabetes; laser therapy is most often needed between 10 and 22 years of duration of diabetes.

        • There is a small increase in the need for laser therapy after 22 years of duration of diabetes.

        • Some diabetic retinopathy is present in 90% of patients with diabetes by 20 years disease duration.

    B There is a linear relationship between age and prevalence of diabetic retinopathy.

    C Diabetic retinopathy is influenced by genetics; human leukocyte antigens (HLA) DR3 and DR4 predispose for the development of this complication more than other HLA types.[27]

    D African Americans and Hispanics[4,5] are more likely to develop diabetic retinopathy than Caucasians. Retinopathy has also been reported in many Native American tribes.[19]

3 Modifiable risk factors include hyperglycemia, hypertension, dyslipidemia, abnormal microcirculation, and smoking.

    A The development and progression of retinopathy correlates strongly with the degree of glycemic control.[1,2]

        • One mechanism may be hyperglycemia-activation of the polyol pathway in the pericytes. The pericytes are the first cells to become abnormal and "pericyte ghosts" are formed early in the development of diabetic retinopathy. As a result, leakage (hard exudates) of albumin occur within the retina. In addition outpouching of the capillary walls (microaneurysms) develop as a result of pericyte loss.

    B Hypertension clearly plays a role in the development of diabetic retinopathy. Current data[28] suggest that ACE inhibitors may be particularly effective in slowing the progression of diabetic retinopathy.

    C High cholesterol levels have been linked to the development of diabetic retinopathy in cross-sectional studies.[26] No prospective studies have been done.

    D Areas of microischemia and microinfarctions (soft exudates) produce areas of hypoxia. As a result, there is increased formation of new blood vessels. However, the vessels are not well supported because of the vitreous fluid. These vessels are often very fragile and susceptible to bleeding, resulting in hemorrhage.

    E Smoking has been linked to the development of retinopathy. Prospective randomized studies have not been performed.

4 Certain characteristics not believed to be risk factors

    A To date, there are no data concerning whether the type of antidiabetes treatment protects or predisposes individuals to diabetic retinopathy.

    B There are very few data concerning whether gender protects or predisposes an individual to the development of diabetic retinopathy.

    C The type of diabetes does not protect an individual from diabetic retinopathy; persons with all types of diabetes may develop retinopathy. However, the incidence of proliferative retinopathy is greater in type 1 than in type 2 diabetes.

    D Although the predisposing human leukocyte antigen (HLA) types may imply an autoimmune basis, no autoantibodies have been identified to date.

    E Diet does not appear to be protective nor predisposing to diabetic retinopathy.

    F Some studies[26] have demonstrated that increased adiposity is associated with the presence of retinopathy. However, this association has not been universally found.

    G There is no evidence that increased insulin levels influence the incidence of diabetic retinopathy.

    H Although exercise has many benefits, aerobic exercise may cause high intraocular pressure that may result in increased bleeding in the eye (see Chapter 9, Exercise, for more information).

Other Long-Term Concerns or Issues

Certain long-term problems are not complications of diabetes, but occur more frequently in people with diabetes and have significant impact upon quality of life for the patient and family.

1 Cataracts
   A Individuals with diabetes are more likely to develop cataracts than individuals without diabetes.
   B Increased polyol pathway activity, due to hyperglycemia, may contribute to lens opacity.
   C Improved blood glucose control is associated with decreased incidence of cataracts.
   D Routine annual eye exams (dilated) is the most effective preventative for vision loss from cataracts.

2 Glaucoma
   A Glaucoma is more common in individuals with diabetes than in individuals without diabetes.
   B There is a linear relationship between the incidence of glaucoma and age with the incidence increasing with age.
   C The duration of diabetes is related in a linear fashion to an increase in glaucoma.
   D The pathogenesis of the glaucoma in individuals with diabetes is poorly understood at this time.
   E Routine annual eye exams (dilated) is the most effective preventative for vision loss from glaucoma.

3 Depression
   A Depression is not a complication of diabetes but is often a consequence of the complications of diabetes or chronic illness.
   B Depression has a reported incidence of 30% to 70% in patients with diabetes, and may be as high as 75% in patients with more than one complication.[29]
   C Assessment for depression among patients with complications is an important role for diabetes educators at all phases in the course of the complication (see Chapter 4, Psychosocial Assessment, for more information).

KEY EDUCATIONAL CONSIDERATIONS

1   Certain modifiable risk factors (hyperglycemia, hypertension, hyperlipidemia, smoking) play a role in the development of most complications of diabetes.

2   Teach all patients about the benefits of improving blood glucose control since this intervention can be expected to reduce the risks for cardiovascular complications, neuropathy, nephropathy, retinopathy, and cataracts. It also favorably affects lipid levels and platelet adherence.

3   Hypertension is second only to hyperglycemia as a risk factor for the development and progression of diabetic complications. Inform patients that normalization of blood pressure can be expected to reduce the risks for cardiovascular complications, neuropathy, nephropathy, and retinopathy.

4   Treatment of hypertension using an angiotensin-converting enzyme (ACE) inhibitor may be particularly advantageous, unless contraindicated.

5   Medical nutrition therapy and exercise offer direct as well as indirect benefits in reducing the risk for certain complications.

6   Smoking cessation may be especially difficult for patients to accomplish. Assessment of readiness to quit, referral to smoking cessation programs or support groups, alternative nicotine delivery systems, or other cessation aids or medications can be offered at the appropriate time to assist patients in their efforts to quit.

7   Teaching patients behavioral strategies, goal-setting, and problem-solving skills can be useful as they choose and make changes that affect lifestyle-related risk factors.

REFERENCES

1   The DCCT Research Group. The effect of intensive treatment of diabetes on the development and progression of long-term complications in insulin-dependent diabetes mellitus. N Engl J Med 1993;329:977-86.

2   Ohkubo Y, Kishikawa H, Araki E, et al. Intensive insulin therapy prevents the progression of diabetic microvascular complications in Japanese patients with non-insulin-dependent diabetes mellitus: a randomized prospective 6-year study. Diab Res and Clin Pract 1995;28:113-17.

3   American Diabetes Association. Direct and indirect costs of diabetes in the United States in 1992. Alexandria, Va: 1993.

4   Tull ES, Roseman JM. Diabetes in African Americans. In: National Diabetes Data Group, eds. Diabetes in America. 2nd ed. Bethesda, Md: National Institute of Diabetes and Digestive and Kidney Diseases, 1995;613-30.

5   Stern MP, Mitchell BD. Diabetes in Hispanic Americans. In: National Diabetes Data Group, eds. Diabetes in America. 2nd ed. Bethesda, Md: National Institute of Diabetes and Digestive and Kidney Diseases, 1995;631-60.

6   Kuhn F, Rackley C. Coronary artery disease in women: risk factors, evaluation, treatment, and prevention. Arch Intern Med 1993;143:2626-36.

7   Home PD. Insulin resistance is not central to the burden of diabetes. Diabetes Metab Rev 1997;13:87-92.

8   Colwell JA. Pathophysiology of vascular disease in diabetes: effects of gliclazide. Am J Med 1991;90(6A):50S-54S.

9   Paffenberger RS Jr, Hyde RT, Wing AL, Hsieh CC. Physical activity, all-cause mortality and longevity of college alumni. N Engl J Med 1986;314:605-13.

10 Williams RB Jr, Haney TL, Lee KL, et al. Type A behavior, hostility, and coronary atherosclerosis. Psychosom Med 1980; 42:539-49.

11 Barzilay J, Warram JH, Rand LI, Pfeifer MA, Krolewski AS. Risk for cardiovascular autonomic neuropathy is associated with the HLA-DR3/4 phenotype in type I diabetes mellitus. Ann Intern Med 1992;116:544-49.

12 Harris M, Eastman R, Cowie C. Symptoms of sensory neuropathy in adults with NIDDM in the US population. Diabetes Care 1993;16:1446-52.

13 Sands ML, Shetterly SM, Franklin GM, Hamman RF. Incidence of distal symmetric sensory neuropathy in NIDDM. Diabetes Care 1997;20:322-29.

14 Gadia MT, Natori N, Ramos LB, Ayyar DR, Skyler JS, Sosenko JM. Influence of height on quantitative sensory, nerve-conduction, and clinical indices of diabetic peripheral neuropathy. Diabetes Care 1987;10:613-16.

15 Vinik AI, Milicevic Z, Pittenger GL. Beyond glycemia. Diabetes Care 1995;18:1037-41.

16 Reja A, Tesfaye S, Harris ND, Ward JD. Is ACE inhibition with lisinopril helpful in diabetic neuropathy? Diabetic Med 1995;12:307-9.

17 Mayer JH, Tomlinson DR. Prevention of defects of axonal transport and nerve conduction velocity by oral administration of myoinositol or an aldose reductase inhibitor in streptozotocin-diabetic rats. Diabetologia 1983;25:433-38.

18 Mitchell BD, Hawthorne BD, Hawthorne VM, Vinik AI. Cigarette smoking and neuropathy in diabetic patients. Diabetes Care 1990;13:434-37.

19 Gohdes D. Diabetes in North American Indians and Alaska Natives. In: National Diabetes Data Group, eds. Diabetes in America. 2nd ed. Bethesda, Md: National Institute of Diabetes and Digestive and Kidney Diseases, 1995;683-702.

20 Krolewski AS, Canessa M, Warram JH, et al. Predisposition to hypertension and susceptibility to renal disease in insulin dependent diabetes mellitus. N Eng J Med 1988;318:140-45.

21 The Microalbumin Captopril Study Group. Captopril reduces the risk of nephropathy in IDDM patients with microalbuminuria. Diabetologia 1996; 39:587-93.

22 Mulec H, Johnson S-A, Björck S. Relationship between serum cholesterol and diabetic nephropathy. Lancet 1990;335:1537-38.

23 Tonolo G, Ciccarese M, Brizzi P, et al. Reduction of albumin excretion rate in normotensive microalbuminuric type 2 diabetic patients during long-term simvastatin treatment. Diabetes Care 1997;20:1891-95.

24 Zeller K, Whittaker E, Sullivan L, Raskin P, Jacobson HR. Effect of restricting dietary protein on the progression of renal failure in patients with insulin-dependent diabetes mellitus. N Engl J Med 1991; 324:78-84.

25 Sawicki PT, Didjurgeit U, Mühlhauser I, Bender R, Heinemann L, Berger M. Smoking is associated with progression of diabetic nephropathy. Diabetes Care 1994;17:126-31.

26 Klein R, Klein BEK. Vision disorders in diabetes. In: National Diabetes Data Group, eds. Diabetes in America. 2nd ed. Bethesda, Md: National Institute of Diabetes and Digestive and Kidney Diseases, 1995;293-338.

27 Rand LI, Krolewski AS, Aiello LM, Warram JH, Baker RS, Maki T: Multiple factors in the prediction of risk of proliferative diabetic retinopathy. N Eng J Med 113:1433-38, 1985

28 Chaturvedi N, Sjolie AK, Stephenson JM, et al. Effect of lisinopril on progression of retinopathy in normotensive people with type 1 diabetes. The EUCLID study group. EURODIAB controlled trial of lisinopril in insulin-dependent diabetes mellitus. Lancet 1998;351:28-31.

29 Goodnick PJ, Henry JH, Buki VM. Treatment of depression in patients with diabetes mellitus. J Clin Psychiatry 1995;56(4)128-36.

SUGGESTED READINGS

Bloomgarden, ZT. Pathogenesis, treatment and complications of diabetes. Pract Diabetol 1992;11(3):18-22.

Boulton AJM. Pathogenesis of diabetic neuropathy. In: Marshall SM, Home PD, Alberti KGMM, Krall LP, eds. Diabetes Annual/8. New York: Elsevier Science Publishing: 1993:192-210.

Clark CM, Lee, DA. Prevention and treatment of the complications of diabetes mellitus. N Eng J Med 1995; 332:1210-17.

DCCT Research Group. Factors in development of diabetic neuropathy: baseline analysis of neuropathy in the feasibility phase of Diabetic Control and Complications Trial (DCCT). Diabetes 1988;37:476-81.

DeFronzo RA, Bonadonna RC, Ferrannini, E. Pathogenesis of NIDDM: A balanced overview. Diabetes Care 1992;15:318-68.

Dinsmoor RS. AGE's-Closing in on complications. Diabetes Self-Management 1997; 14(2):6-10.

Eastman RC, Javitt JC, Herman WH, Dasbach EJ, et al. Model of complications of NIDDM. I. Model contruction and assumptions. Diabetes Care 1997; 20:725-34.

Eastman RC, Javitt JC, Herman WH, Dasbach EJ, et al. Model of complications of NIDDM. II Analysis of the health benefits and cost-effectiveness of treating NIDDM with the goal of normoglycemia. Diabetes Care 1997; 20:735-44.

Eastman RC et al. Lessening the burden of diabetes: Intervention strategies. Diabetes Care 1993;16:1095-102.

Gelber DA, Pfeifer MA. Management of diabetic neuropathy. In: Marshall SM, Home PD, eds. Diabetes Annual/8. New York: Elsevier Science Publishing, 1994:349-63.

Graham C, Lasko-McCarthey, P. Exercise options for persons with diabetic complications. Diabetes Educ 1990;16:212-20.

Greene DA, Sima AAF, Pfeifer MA. Neuropathy. In: Mogensen CE, Standl E, eds. Prevention and treatment of diabetic late complications. Diabetes Forum Series; Excerpta Medica. Berlin: Walter DE Gruyter, 1989:93-149.

Greene DA, Pfeifer MA, Carroll PB. Diabetic neuropathy. In: Becker KL, ed. Principles and practice of endocrinology and metabolism. Philadelphia: JB Lippincott Company, 1990:1136-44.

Greene DA, Sima AAF, Pfeifer MA. Diabetic neuropathy. In: Rifkin H, Porte Jr D, eds. Diabetes mellitus. New York: Elsevier Science Publishing, 1990:710-55.

Greene DA, Sima AF, Feldman EL, Stevens MJ, Pfeifer MA. Diabetic neuropathy: screening and management. Contemp Int Med 1993;5(4):79-91.

Greene DA, Feldman EL, Stevens MJ, Sima AAF, Albers JW, Pfeifer MA. Diabetic neuropathy. In: Porte Jr D, Sherwin RS, eds. Ellenberg and Rifkin's diabetes mellitus. 5th ed. New York: Elsevier Science Publishing, 1997:1009-76.

Haire-Joshu, D. Smoking cessation, and the diabetes health care team. Diabetes Educ 1991; 17:54-64.

Klein, R. Hyperglycemia and microvascular and macrovascular disease in diabetes. Diabetes Care 1995; 18:258-68.

Kostraba, JN. Contribution of diabetes duration before puberty to development of microvascular complications in IDDM subjects. Diabetes Care 1989;12:686-93.

Lloyd CE, Matthews KA, Wing RA, Orchard TO. Psychosocial factors and complications of IDDM. Diabetes Care 1992; 15:166-72.

Low P. Panel Members of the American Academy of Neurology. Assessment: Clinical autonomic testing report of the therapeutics and technology assessment subcommittee of the American Academy of Neurology. Neurology 1996;46:873-80.

McLaughlin S. Nutritional considerations for other complications of diabetes. Diabetes Educ 1992; 18:527-29.

Orchard TJ. From diagnosis and classification to complications and therapy. Diabetes Care 1994; 17:326-38.

Pfeifer MA, Greene DA. Diabetic neuropathy. Current Concepts Booklet. The Upjohn Company, 1985.

Robertson C. Coping with chronic complications. RN 1989;52(9):34-41.

Rovner JF. Diabetes and the brain: A complex relationship. Diabetes Spectrum 1997; 10:23-70.

Ryan C. Magnificent seven. Diabetes Forecast 1994; 48(1):37-39.

Strowig S, Raskin, P. Glycemic control and diabetic complications. Diabetes Care 1992; 15:1126-1140.

Vinicor FA. Epidemiology of diabetes complications. Diabetes Spectrum 1992; 5(2): 86-122.

Walker EA, Wylie-Rosett J, Shamoon H, et al. Program development to prevent complications of diabetes: Assessment of barriers in an urban clinic. Diabetes Care 1995; 18:1291-93.

COMPLICATIONS

Eye Disease and Adaptive Diabetes Education for Visually Impaired Persons

21

Marla Bernbaum, MD
St. Louis University Health Sciences Center
Division of Endocrinology
St. Louis, Missouri

Tamara Stich, RN, MSN, CDE
St. Louis University Health Sciences Center
Division of Endocrinology
St. Louis, Missouri

INTRODUCTION

1   Diabetes is a leading cause of vision impairment in the United States. Diabetic retinopathy is the most prevalent ophthalmic disease among individuals with diabetes. However, persons with diabetes are also at increased risk for other eye conditions that may impact visual function. Persons with preexisting vision impairment due to other causes who develop diabetes also need self-management skills.

2   The extent of vision impairment and the individual's ability to adapt to the vision loss must be evaluated before undertaking adaptive education. The adaptive education and training needs of persons with preexisting eye disease due to other causes may differ from persons experiencing a new onset of diabetic retinopathy.

3   The diabetes educator can play a key role in referring patients with visual impairment to the proper rehabilitative and psychosocial services.

4   This chapter provides basic information and describes skills required for working with visually impaired patients with diabetes.

OBJECTIVES

Upon completion of this chapter, the learner will be able to

1   Describe the stages of diabetic retinopathy and appropriate treatment for each stage.
2   List three other ophthalmic conditions that may occur in people with diabetes.
3   Identify three factors for assessing function with vision loss.
4   Identify the appropriate time for referral and the general services that are available for individuals with diabetes and visual impairment.
5   List three ways to enhance interactions with individuals who are visually impaired.
6   Describe five ways to adapt diabetes self-management skills for the visually impaired patient.

Identifying and Treating Diabetic Eye Disease

1   Diabetes is the leading cause of blindness in the United States for persons between the ages of 20 and 74 years.[1-4] Diabetes accounts for 12% of legal blindness in the US.[2,3] Literature[1-4] suggests there are 8 000 to 23 000 new cases of legal blindness associated with diabetes annually. Rates for less severe levels of vision impairment have not been estimated.

   A   Persons with either type 1 or type 2 diabetes are susceptible to eye complications.

   B   Diabetic retinopathy, the most prevalent diabetic eye complication, is often detectable within 5 years of the diagnosis of diabetes.[2]

   - Since diabetes may not be detected in type 2 patients until years after the onset, up to 21% of patients may have retinopathy at the time of diagnosis.
   - Retinopathy is present in more than 90% of type 1 patients and 55% to 80% of type 2 patients after 15 years of diabetes.
   - Over 600 000 persons are in the stage of the disease at which vision is threatened (Table 21.1).

Table 21.1. Percentage of Persons with Diabetic Retinopathy 15 Years After Diagnosis of Diabetes[2]

Stage of Retinopathy	Type of Diabetes		
	Type 1	Type 2 Treated With Insulin	Type 2 Treated Without Insulin
Nonproliferative	97%	80%	55%
Proliferative	30%	10% to 15%	5%

   C   One half to two thirds of the approximately 30% of persons with diabetes who are on work disability have vision impairment.

   - The financial impact in terms of Social Security and disability benefits is estimated at $6,900 per person annually[1,5]
   - The cost of the recommended treatment is estimated at $2,000 per person–year of vision spared.
   - Blindness is 20 times more common among people with diabetes than with the general population.

D The development and progression of retinopathy correlates strongly with degree of glycemic control in addition to duration of diabetes.

- This relationship was demonstrated in the Diabetes Control and Complications Trial;[6] the results emphasized the importance of achieving the best possible glucose control in all persons with diabetes.
- Other risk factors for diabetic retinopathy include age, hypertension, hyperlipidemia, smoking, and genetic predisposition.
- Pregnancy and renal failure can potentiate retinopathy.

2 Diabetic retinopathy[3,4,7-9] occurs when the microvasculature that nourishes the retina is damaged, permitting leakage of blood components through the vessel walls. The retina is a layer of nerve tissue at the back of the eye that is responsible for focusing images and light, which then are relayed along the optic nerve to the brain (Figure 21.1). Retinopathy may vary from a mild asymptomatic form to a severe, rapidly devastating condition. Retinopathy is staged from its mildest to most advanced form using the terms nonproliferative, (mild, moderate, severe and very severe) and proliferative retinopathy. (Note: the terms background retinopathy and preproliferative retinopathy are no longer considered current).[10] (See Table 21.2).

FIGURE 21.1. NORMAL EYE

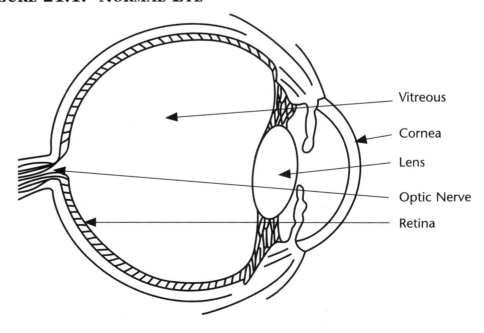

Vitreous

Cornea

Lens

Optic Nerve

Retina

Reprinted with permission: Noninsulin-Dependent Diabetes Mellitus: a curriculum for patients and health professionals, Michigan Diabetes Research and Training Center, The University of Michigan, 1988.

TABLE 21.2. STAGES OF DIABETIC RETINOPATHY

Early Stages *Mild NPDR*	• Retinal vascular microaneurysms and blot hemorrhages • Increased retinal vascular permeability • Cotton wool spots

Middle Stages
   Moderate NPDR
   Severe NPDR
   Very Severe NPDR
	• Venous caliber changes or beading
	• IRMA
	• Retinal capillary loss
	• Retinal ischemia
	• Extensive intraretinal hemorrhages and microaneurysms

Advanced Stages *PDR*	• NVD • NVI • Neovascularization of the iris • Neovascular glaucoma • Preretinal and vitreous hemorrhage • Fibrovascular proliferation • Retinal traction, retinal tears, retinal detachment

Reprinted with permission: Aiello LP, Gardner TW, King GL, Blankship G, et al.[10]

A Retinopathy before the development of retinal neovascularization is termed nonproliferative diabetic retinopathy (NPDR). Mild NPDR often causes no visual disturbance. It may remain asymptomatic for years, and the following specific features may be noted on ophthalmoscopic exam:

- *Microaneurysms* are seen as sacular outpouchings along weakened vascular walls.
- *Hard exudates*, the residue of fluid and lipid components that leak from the blood vessels, appear as round, yellow deposits on the retina.
- *Intraretinal hemorrhages* may appear as dots or flame shapes.
- *Cotton wool spots* or soft exudates represent infarcts of the nerve fiber layer of the retina.

B As the disease progresses, there is evidence of further vascular damage, capillary obstruction or closure, and retinal ischemia. Persons with very severe NPDR have a 45% risk of proliferative changes within one year but may not experience detectable vision impairment. More advanced nonproliferative retinopathy is characterized by:

- *Intraretinal hemorrhages* are more extensive in both size and number.

- *Venous beading* appears as changes in the appearance of the retinal veins as they become tortuous and swollen, loop back upon themselves, and take on the appearance of a string of sausages or beads.
- *Intraretinal microvascular abnormalities* (IRMA) appear as dilated capillaries that arise around ischemic areas where there is capillary closure.

C Once proliferation of new retinal vessels occurs it is referred to as *proliferative diabetic retinopathy* (PDR). PDR is thought to develop as a result of retinal ischemia and hypoxia following capillary closure. Proliferative changes, the process of *neovascularization* (NVE), is defined as the growth of new blood vessels along the surface of the retina; these vessels may extend into the vitreous chamber using the vitreous surface as a scaffold. The vessels are fragile and rupture easily, producing preretinal and vitreous hemorrhage. The resulting vision impairment may vary from mild blurring with cobweb-like wisps in the visual fields to severe obstruction of vision due to large, dense opacities.

- Neovascularization of the disc (NVD) refers to new vessel growth on or near the optic disc as opposed to neovascularization elsewhere (NVE) on the retina. Preretinal or vitreous hemorrhage in combination with or NVD that is greater than 25% of the surface area of the disc are considered high-risk features for major vision loss.
- Another potential threat to vision results as fibrous components of the neovasculature contract, leading to retinal traction, detachments, and tears.

D *Macular edema* is a serious consequence of leakage of fluid and exudate from the vessels in the macula, which is the specialized portion of the retina responsible for central vision.

- Macular edema may accompany nonproliferative or proliferative retinopathy.
- Vision loss may vary from mild blurring to an acuity of 20/200 or less (legal blindness).
- Ocular involvement, which is assessed by slit lamp biomicroscopy and fluorescein angiography, requires early treatment.

E Neovascular glaucoma (rubeosis iridis) is a relatively rare complication associated with proliferative retinopathy.

- New vessels proliferate from the surface of the iris, blocking aqueous outflow from the anterior chamber of the eye.
- The condition is painful, progresses rapidly, and is devastating to vision.

3 Treatment of retinopathy begins with preventive measures such as optimizing blood glucose and blood pressure, and smoking cessation. Routine annual screening and follow-up by an ophthalmologist are essential to assure that any intervention is appropriately timed.[4,7,9-12]

A Mild-to-moderate nonproliferative retinopathy requires only observation.

B Fundus photography and fluorescein angiography may be recommended to document progression of retinopathy and to evaluate macular edema and/or macular ischemia.

C Macular edema is treated with focal argon photocoagulation to seal leaking blood vessels. Multiple applications are often necessary. Early treatment reduces vision loss by 60%.[12]

D Proliferative retinopathy with high-risk characteristics should be treated with pan-retinal photocoagulation in which laser treatments are applied to the peripheral retina in a scatter pattern. Some patients with less than high-risk characteristics or with severe to very severe NPDR may also benefit from photocoagulation.

- Advise patients that multiple treatment sessions are often necessary and there may be mild eye discomfort. For patients with severe pain, a local anesthetic injection to the eye may be used, although most patients require only anesthetic eye drops.

- Side effects of therapy may include a small loss of visual acuity (about one line on the Snellen chart), as well as some decrement in peripheral vision, dark adaptation, and color discrimination. These effects are offset by preservation of the central vision.

- Treatment is performed on an outpatient basis. Patients can return to normal activities the next day.

E Surgical vitrectomy is considered for hemorrhages that do not resolve over 6 months or when there is a threatened or actual retinal detachment. An ultrasound may be used to detect detachments when there is dense vitreous hemorrhage.

- The vitreous contents, including hemorrhage and fibrous proliferation, are removed and replaced by a clear solution. Repair of the retina may be undertaken during the procedure.

- Surgical complications such as corneal edema, retinal tears, recurrent hemorrhage, and rubeosis, may be as high as 25%.[4] The risks and benefits should be carefully explored with the patient.

F Pan-retinal photocoagulation may be of benefit in neovascular glaucoma prior to attempting surgical filtration procedures.

G An important aspect of treatment is meeting the patient's needs in adapting to loss of vision.[13-15]

- Offer psychosocial counseling before there is actual deterioration of vision to help allay anxiety and depression.

- Low-vision evaluation is indicated as soon as vision loss impacts normal daily activities.

- Referral to rehabilitation services as early as possible will allow the patient to acquire adaptive skills and maintain participation and independence in work and recreational activities.

- Patients need information and instruction in adaptive diabetes self-care as soon as vision is compromised, preferably before adaptive equipment is actually required.

4 Other ocular complications are associated with diabetes.[2,7,8]

A Common senile cataracts occur more frequently, at younger ages, and progress more rapidly in persons with diabetes.

B The diabetic cataract is a rare type of cataract associated with osmotic irregularity that can mature in a few days and progress very rapidly.

C There is increased risk of primary open-angled glaucoma, the most common kind of glaucoma in the US.

D Ischemic optic neuropathy refers to irreversible optic nerve damage due to microvascular impairment. This ocular complication occurs more frequently in persons with diabetes and leads to permanent visual impairment.

E Ocular palsies result from ischemia to the third, fourth, and sixth cranial nerves. Impairment of extraocular muscle function leads to strabismus or diplopia. The condition is temporary and normal function usually returns within a few months.

F Blurring of vision due to instability of blood glucose is related to osmotic changes in the lens of the eye. This problem occurs commonly at the onset of diabetes and during periods of fluctuating control. Reassure the patient that this condition is transient. Instruct patients to delay testing for new refractive lenses until the blood glucose has been stabilized for 6 to 8 weeks.

G Temporary visual changes such as dimming of vision, bright flashing lights, or double vision may be experienced during periods of hypoglycemia.

5 All persons with diabetes should receive routine ophthalmologic screening and follow-up. Indirect ophthalmoscopy with slit-lamp examination and measurement of the intraocular pressure are essential.[9,17]

   A A dilated examination is recommended annually beginning 3 to 5 years after the diagnosis of diabetes for type 1 patients once the patient is age 10 or over and beginning at the time of diagnosis for type 2 patients.

   B Since pregnancy potentiates retinopathy, women should have an examination during preconception planning, the first trimester of pregnancy, and close follow-up as needed.

   C If retinopathy is identified, fundus photography or fluorescein angiography may be recommended, and more frequent eye examinations are needed (Table 21.3).

TABLE 21.3. SCHEDULE FOR OPHTHALMOLOGIC EXAMINATION

Stage of Retinopathy	Frequency of Examination
No retinopathy	Annually
Mild nonproliferative retinopathy	Annually
Moderate nonproliferative retinopathy/macular edema	6 to 12 months
Clinically significant macular edema or severe to very severe proliferative retinopathy	3 to 4 months
Proliferative retinopathy without high-risk characteristics	2 to 4 months
Proliferative retinopathy with high-risk characteristics	Individualized to patient needs

ASSESSING VISUAL FUNCTION AND ADAPTATION TO LOW VISION

1 The individual's functional ability is a reflection of the measurable visual acuity and field, as well as the capacity for adaptation to the vision loss.

   A Individuals with diabetic retinopathy can experience daily fluctuations in vision that may be influenced by postural changes, ambient lighting, and glucose levels. Measurements in the ophthalmologist's office may not reflect the true degree of vision impairment that the patient experiences in other environments.

B Persons who have had time to adapt to vision loss or who have had rehabilitation training may function better in activities of daily living than those who have had less severe vision impairment for a shorter interval. Some totally blind individuals will function more independently than other persons who have an acute milder loss of vision.

2 *Visual acuity*, or the sharpness of the central vision, is most often measured through the use of the Snellen chart. Acuity, as defined by the Snellen fraction, is the ratio of the distance at which an individual can read certain letters on the chart compared with the distance required for an individual with normal vision.

A A person with normal vision is said to have 20/20 vision, which means letters intended to be read at 20 feet can be seen at that range.

B An individual with 20/40 vision would need to stand at 20 feet to read letters that a normally sighted person could distinguish at 40 feet.[18]

3 The visual field is a measurement of peripheral vision. The normal visual field is 180 degrees. Loss of peripheral vision can cause significant dysfunction despite maintenance of good central visual acuity.[19]

A A decreased visual field may reflect narrowing of the total angle of vision.

B The visual field may also be reduced due to specific blind spots in the central or peripheral vision.

4 Definitions of vision impairment and blindness can vary according to the source.[19, 20]

A The American Foundation for the Blind suggests using the term *blind* only for persons who have no usable sight. The term *low vision* is used for persons with some usable vision.

B The term *visually impaired* may apply to persons with all levels of visual disability.

C *Legal blindness* was originally defined by the federal government to denote the level at which individuals are eligible to receive certain benefits. The standard for legal blindness is acuity of less than 20/200 in the better eye with corrective lenses and/or a visual field of less than 20 degrees.

D Standards for mild, moderate, severe and profound vision impairment are shown in Table 21.4.

5 In addition to assessment of visual acuity and field, the ability to use vision or adaptive alternatives in the practical settings of daily living also needs to be assessed. The following areas need to be addressed:

A Does the patient have adequate vision to perform necessary self-care tasks and use standard instruction materials?[21]

B Does the patient's vision fluctuate? If so, assess all of the following questions for times when the patient's vision is at its worst.

  • Can the patient read the lines on a syringe (if using insulin)?

  • Can the patient see the display on a blood glucose meter and the spot on which to apply a blood drop?

  • Can the patient read standard print or large print, either with or without magnification and appropriate lighting? If not, can the patient use audiotapes or Braille?

TABLE 21.4. CLASSIFICATION OF VISUAL LOSS[19]

| Classification | Acuity | | Level of Disability |
	ICD-9	WHO*	
Mild	20/30 to 20/60	<20/25	No special aids necessary
Moderate	20/70 to 20/160	<20/70 or 20/80	Special aids necessary for some tasks (magnification)
Severe	20/200 to 20/400	<20/160	Can read with special aids at reduced speed and endurance
Profound	20/500 to 20/1000	<20/400	Reading and mobility impaired, relies on other senses for some tasks
Near total blindness	—	—	Light perception, relies completely on other senses
Total blindness	—	—	No vision, relies on other senses

*WHO = World Health Organization

C If there is inadequate eyesight to perform vision-dependent diabetes self-care skills, is neuromuscular function adequate to acquire tactile skills? Different tactile devices require varying levels of sensory and motor ability.

D Does the patient currently need assistance in any of the following areas?[20]
  - Shopping and preparing food appropriate to the meal plan
  - Walking about the home
  - Transportation to medical appointments, social activities, and other activities important to the patient
  - Personal hygiene

E Has the patient had any blindness rehabilitation education in daily living skills? Has the patient had any mobility instruction?[21]

F Does the patient have adequate cognitive ability to learn new skills?[20]
  - Is the patient so anxious or disoriented by the vision loss that learning a new skill would be extremely difficult? If so, more time may need to be allowed for the learning, or teaching of diabetes skills.
  - Has the patient experienced short-term memory loss? If so, does the patient have adequate memory to learn new ways of performing diabetes self-care reliably?

6 Refer patients to appropriate agencies or personnel for a thorough investigation of rehabilitative, psychosocial, and financial needs related to the visual impairment. In the US, every state has an agency that provides rehabilitation services to blind people. In addition, many cities have private blindness rehabilitation services available from nonprofit agencies. Furthermore, the federal Department of Veterans Affairs provides comprehensive blindness rehabilitation services to veterans. A phone call to one's state information office will yield information about how to contact the state blindness rehabilitation agent, who will, in turn, have information about local private agencies and access to veteran's services. Another way to find information about local services for the blind is to call the American Foundation for the Blind (800-AFBLIND), which maintains a comprehensive referral list.[21] (See additional resources for vision impairment services at the end of this chapter).

Adaptive Diabetes Education for the Visually Impaired Person

1   Although the goals of diabetes education for persons with visual impairment are the same as for sighted individuals, the manner in which the content is presented and how the content is adapted to meet their needs is different.

   A   Observe the following rules of courtesy with the patient who is visually impaired:[22]

   • Immediately upon entering the room, address the patient by name and introduce yourself using your name and position.

   • Use a natural tone and speed in conversation. It is only necessary to speak loudly and slowly when the patient also has a hearing impairment.

   • It is acceptable to use words that refer to vision during the conversation: *look, see*, and *watch* are part of everyday conversation. *Blind* and *visually impaired* are not derogatory terms.

   • Indicate the end of a conversation and announce if you will be leaving the room. This will prevent any embarrassment to the patient who may continue talking after you have left the room.

   • If you need to touch the patient's hands during an equipment demonstration, ask for permission before doing so.

2   Many adaptive devices are available for the nonvisual measurement of insulin.[23-25]

   A   The following options are available for measuring insulin doses:

   • For those patients with reliable low vision, using better lighting, contrasting color backgrounds, and/or a magnifier may be all that is necessary. Some magnifiers are made specifically to fit onto the insulin syringe.

   • Preset dose gauges are designed to measure the space between the ends of the insulin syringe barrel and the plunger. Commercially prepared gauges are more reliable than those made at home. The patient will require multiple gauges for mixed insulin dosages or for multiple dosages that differ throughout the day.

   • A measuring device that holds the insulin vial and syringe can be preset for one or two doses. The syringe plunger is pulled back to the preset stop which measures a specific amount of insulin. A sighted individual must preset the doses.

- Variable-dose devices measure insulin for single and mixed doses in 1-, 2-, and 10-unit increments. Each increment of insulin is measured by clicks that may be felt or heard.
- Although not designed specifically for the visually impaired, a variety of pen-like devices is available to measure insulin in 1- or 2-unit increments. Each device uses insulin cartridges and a disposable needle. The insulin pens can be operated nonvisually by following specific, precise steps.
- At least one of the needleless injectors includes tactual and auditory cues for setting the amount of insulin to be delivered.
- Insulin pumps have been used successfully by patients with visual impairment. Some models come with auditory cues to assist in programming.

B Appropriate equipment is selected based on the treatment plan and motor skills of each patient:
- Only certain insulin-measuring devices are suitable for mixed- and/or variable-dose regimens.
- The size of the insulin dose influences the choice of equipment. Some devices do not measure large doses, and some do not measure 1-unit increments.
- A deficit in fine motor skills or sensory impairment due to neuropathy may prevent the use of certain devices.
- Allow the patient to choose among several suitable devices. Do not assume that one device will be easier to use than another. Provide sufficient time to work with all available equipment and let patients select the devices which best meet their needs.

C The procedure for using each dose-measuring device differs, although certain principles are universal to their use.
- The insulin vial should first be prepared using the standard method.
- Textured tape, a rubber band, or some other tactile marker on the vial can be used to identify each type of insulin.
- When measuring insulin, the insulin syringe and vial need to be held in a vertical position. To confirm this position tactually, hold the vial and insert the syringe against a vertical object such as a wall, or hold the vial and syringe perpendicular to a horizontal surface such as a table.
- To expel air bubbles from the syringe, pull insulin into the syringe and push it quickly back into the vial at least three times before filling the syringe to the desired dose. When mixing insulin, instruct

the patient to follow this procedure with the first insulin; with the second insulin, teach the patient to pull back on the plunger very slowly to prevent air bubbles from entering the syringe. Variable-dose devices may have modified instructions for eliminating air bubbles.

- There are several methods to ensure that there is sufficient insulin inside the vial at all times. One approach is to determine how many doses that a vial of insulin contains without using the last 50 units of insulin. For example, if the patient takes a total of 40 units each day from a 1,000-unit NPH vial, one vial of NPH would last 23 days (950 ÷ 40). The patient could set aside 23 syringes and start a new vial when those syringes are used.

- Observe accurate measurement of insulin using the selected adaptive device at least three times on two separate occasions before suggesting unsupervised insulin measurement.[26]

D Review adaptive principles of insulin administration.

- Visually impaired patients can be taught to inject themselves with insulin by using a conventional syringe, automatic needle injectors, pen injectors, or needle-free jet injectors.

- When using the conventional syringe without an assistive device, the visually impaired patient is taught to choose the site, pinch the skin, gently place the needle on the skin, and insert the needle into the skin. This method eliminates the usual dart-like motion so that the patient can control where the needle is inserted.

- The injection site is chosen by creating a map of the area to be injected. When creating the map of injection sites, a sighted person can alert the visually impaired person to areas to avoid, such as varicosities, scar tissue, or other areas (see Chapter 10, Pharmacologic Therapies, for injection sites).

- Some of the injection devices available for purchase are not specifically designed for use by persons with visual impairment. The needs of each patient will differ and need to be continually reassessed. Some visually impaired patients are able to inject themselves but are unable to fill the syringe because of multiple health problems. Guidelines for prefilling conventional syringes are found in Chapter 10, Pharmacologic Therapies.

3 Specialized adaptive equipment is available to assist the patient with visual impairment in blood glucose monitoring.[25,26]

A Evaluate individual needs to assure that the correct adaptive devices are chosen.

- For those with reliable low vision, monitors with large display screens and easy-to-use features may be appropriate. These monitors are made for the general population and are not marketed for individuals with vision impairment.
- Certain monitors can be adapted with an attachable voice module that verbalizes display messages. This type of monitor is convenient for the patient who is already familiar with the use of the system.
- Certain monitoring systems have been specifically designed for individuals with visual impairment and do not require additional adaptive components. The accuracy of these systems should be verified.[28]

B The techniques for obtaining a blood sample are universal. However, assuring an adequate blood sample and applying that sample to the reagent strip may require adaptive measures.

- The pad area and top surface of the strip need to be recognizable by using tactual methods without touching the target area. This task is accomplished by running a finger or fingernail along the edges of the strip to locate distinctive features.
- When checking for an adequate blood drop, patients who bleed easily can touch the puncture site with another finger to feel for wetness. The puncture site also may be touched lightly to the edge of the lip, which is another sensitive area for assessing wetness. Teach patients who find it difficult to obtain an adequate sample methods for increasing blood flow to the finger such as warming the hands before lancing, using a rubberband tourniquet around the finger, and using the wide tip of the lancet holder.
- Some meters have a feature that announces when an adequate blood drop has been applied.
- A few older monitoring systems require blood placement on the strip before it is inserted into the meter. A strip guide can be used to assist in the proper placement of the blood sample.
- Most newer systems allow blood sample placement on the strip after the strip is inserted into the meter. Commercially made blood drop guides can assist with this task. As a less expensive alternative to these devices, raised marks can be added to the monitor on either side of the target area.[21] The tactile marks can be used as a guide for placing the blood drop on the target area.

C Tactile labels such as rubberbands or textured tape are useful for identifying various control solutions.

D Because visually impaired patients cannot see when the meter needs to be cleaned, teach them to clean the meter routinely, especially if the blood is applied while the strip is in the meter. Certain meters with voice module attachments can "tell" the user that the monitor needs cleaning.

4 Proper foot care for the visually impaired patient with diabetes is imperative because of the increased potential for injury and the possible inability to recognize the early signs of infection. It is critical to the patient with visual impairment to be taught a nonvisual method of foot inspection.[29,30]

  A The visually impaired patient with diabetes can perform routine foot inspection using the senses of touch, smell, and temperature perception.

- If the sense of touch is reliable, the fingertips can be used to detect changes in the surface of the feet. Teach the patient to notice any breaks in the skin and new callouses, blisters, or objects imbedded in the skin. Teach the patient to inspect the feet on a daily basis, making note of any changes not present the day before.
- The back of the hand can be used to detect changes in temperature.
- When removing shoes and socks, ask the patient to make note of any changes in odor. The sense of smell can be used to detect infections, which can produce a foul odor.

  B Patients who are unable to reach their feet, who have neuropathic changes in their hands that affect their sense of touch, or those with an impaired sense of smell will require the assistance of a sighted person to visually inspect their feet.

- Even if the visually impaired patient can reliably perform nonvisual foot assessment, periodic visual assessment will still be necessary.
- Instruct patients with visual impairment and diabetes not to cut their toenails due to the increased risk of self-inflicted injury. Regular visits to a podiatrist or other foot care specialist are recommended.

5 Exercise recommendations and precautions vary depending upon the degree of vision loss. Visual impairment alone does not prevent a patient from participating in exercise if appropriate adaptations can be made.[31,32]

  A Patients with diabetes and proliferative retinopathy will need to take precautions to protect any usable remaining vision.

- There is concern that the increase in systolic blood pressure that occurs during exercise may aggravate underlying eye pathology.
- There is no clear evidence that intensive physical training programs accelerate the progression of diabetic retinopathy. However, certain types of exercises that increase systolic blood pressure with a concomitant increase in intraocular pressure are contraindicated (Table 21.5). See Chapter 9, Exercise, for information about diabetic retinopathy.

B Exercise routines for the visually impaired patient with diabetes includes a warm-up, aerobic activity, and cooldown.

- Muscle-stretching exercises such as toe touches can be performed while sitting in a chair and reaching for the extended leg to avoid bending at the waist, lowering head below the heart.
- For balance, stretching exercises can be done while standing near a wall or heavy chair.
- Walking is a safe and effective aerobic exercise. The patient with visual impairment and diabetes can walk with a sighted guide, on a treadmill, or with a guide rope installed around the yard or along the driveway. Those with adequate training can walk with a white cane or guide dog.
- Many other forms of exercise can be adapted and safely performed by visually impaired people, such as swimming, golfing, tandem bicycle riding, and horseback riding. A newly visually impaired patient who formerly enjoyed a particular form of exercise and wishes to continue it can consult a mobility instructor about possible adaptations.

TABLE 21.5. EXERCISE PRECAUTIONS FOR PATIENTS WITH ACTIVE DIABETIC RETINOPATHY[33]

Avoid activities that involve any of the following:
- Bending over so that the head is positioned lower than the waist
- Valsalva-type maneuvers that raise blood pressure
- Isometric and weight resistive activities
- Vigorous bouncing (eg, high-impact aerobics)
- Rapid head movements (eg, contact sports or jogging)
- Extreme changes in atmospheric pressure (eg, parachuting or scuba diving)

6 Adaptive devices are available to facilitate food preparation and assist with other diabetes-related activities.

    A Adaptive cooking devices include tactile and talking scales, timers, clocks, and kitchen utensils. Refer the patient to a blindness rehabilitation teacher for individualized instruction in this area.

    B To assist with diabetes related activities, patients can be provided with large-block color comparison charts for ketone testing, talking weight scales, talking sphygmomanometers, talking thermometers, and devices for organizing medications and facilitating the instillation of eye drops.

7 Some diabetes educators specialize in the care and education of visually impaired patients. Educators can refer to the Visually Impaired Specialty Practice Group of the American Association of Diabetes Educators.

PSYCHOSOCIAL ASPECTS OF DIABETES AND VISION LOSS

1 Visual impairment impacts all aspects of a person's life: family relations, social interactions, finances, employment, and recreation. Visual impairment coupled with diabetes creates added stress, anxiety, and depression. The patient must learn special skills not only to manage everyday activities but also to manage diabetes.[14-15,34]

    A Diabetes educators are in a key position to direct patients with vision impairment toward the resources they require.[26]

    B When vision is lost or severely diminished, routine tasks can cause the greatest frustration. Learning to pour a cup of coffee without it overflowing can provide a patient with the initial self-confidence needed to take on more complicated tasks.

        • Rehabilitation is essential for relearning activities of daily living such as safe mobility, household tasks, communication skills, vocational guidance, and education.

        • Rehabilitation counseling also can help the patient cope with the impact of visual loss on self-image and relationships.

    C Low-vision services have been designed to help a patient use remaining vision more efficiently.

        • Many visually impaired patients buy inexpensive magnifiers and are frustrated because the object or print may appear larger but not clearer. Inform patients that more effective options are available, such as audio and tactile devices as well a magnification devices prescribed by a low-vision specialist.

- Low-vision service begins with a comprehensive assessment of the patient's experience, attitude, and adjustment to vision loss. A detailed visual examination focuses on function. The exam is followed by the prescription of low-vision devices (eg, optical lenses) and visual aids (eg, lighting, reading stands, large print). The patient receives training in use of the aids and devices and is reevaluated when necessary.

D The diabetes educator can provide support to the patient with visual impairment and diabetes through active listening, recognizing effective and ineffective coping patterns, and referrals for counseling, rehabilitation, support groups, and education.

- Offer to refer the patient and family members for counseling to adjust to shifting roles and responsibilities within the family.

- The patient may grieve for the many losses associated with vision impairment such as loss of the visual aspects of communication, loss of the pleasure of visual sensory experience, loss of their own sense of personal competence, and loss of body image. If the patient becomes suicidal, or if the grieving is so intense or so prolonged as to interfere with necessary self-care activities, the diabetes educator should make an immediate referral to a mental health professional who is knowledgeable about adjustment to visual impairment.[21,35]

- Often, contact with other people who have adjusted successfully to living with visual impairment can be very helpful to patients with new vision loss. The diabetes educator can refer to peer counseling, support groups, or chapters of the national consumer advocacy organizations if available in the local area.[21]

- The person with visual impairment may need assistance in exploring all financial resources that are available.

KEY EDUCATIONAL CONSIDERATIONS

1 Diabetic retinopathy often occurs without symptoms until late in the disease process.

   A Treatment is most effective when instituted early.

   B Patients must understand the importance of having routine dilated eye exams by an eye care specialist.

2 Review the anatomy and function of the eye with the patient. Comparing the eye to a camera is one way to teach this information. The damaged retina can be compared to damaged film in a camera and a cataract to a camera lens with a scratch or crack. This analogy may help the patient understand why stronger refractive lenses may not correct the problem.

3 Instruct patients to immediately report any sudden loss of vision, sudden onset of floaters, the appearance of a shade or curtain coming across the visual field, eye pain, and photophobia to the ophthalmologist.

4 Conventional visual materials will not be useful when teaching patients with total or near-total visual impairment. Most patients may wish to receive audiotapes and a few may be able to use written instructions in Braille. Educators have the opportunity to be creative in developing tactile methods of teaching, such as plastic food models, raised T-shirt paint, and hands-on demonstrations.

5 Provide and encourage visually impaired patients to explore an adaptive aid with their hands before instruction. The device can then be named and its parts and their location can be described. Use the same name each time when referring to a specific part. Talk with the patient slowly through the entire procedure for using the device. If the process involves more than five steps, separate the steps into an easy-to-remember series of five or fewer steps.

6 Assist patients to select the syringe-filling device or glucose monitor that will be useful to them if fluctuation or deterioration of vision is anticipated

SELF-REVIEW QUESTIONS

1 List two risk factors for diabetic retinopathy.

2 Define the stages of diabetic retinopathy.

3 Describe the potential consequences of macular edema.

4 State the treatment modalities for each stage of diabetic retinopathy.

5 List three other ophthalmic complications associated with diabetes.

6 How is visual function determined?

7 Name three referral services that can be used by the visually impaired person with diabetes.

8 List three psychosocial issues that may impact the person with diabetes and visual impairment.

9 List three considerations in choosing the appropriate adaptive device for drawing up insulin.

10 List adaptations that will allow persons with diabetes and visual impairment to monitor their glucose level independently.

11 List two nonvisual methods of foot inspection.

12 List three adaptive devices to assist in diabetes-related activities of daily living.

13 Describe exercise restrictions that are appropriate for people who have diabetic retinopathy and at least some useful vision.

Case Study 1

BW, a 52-year-old woman, went to a neighborhood clinic complaining of blurred vision. She also noticed increased thirst and urination over the past few months. She has not been to a physician in the past few years. Her random blood glucose level was 294mg/dL (16 mmol/L). The physical examination revealed moderate obesity and a blood pressure of 168/96mmHg. The fundus was not sufficiently visible without pupillary dilation. The remainder of the exam was remarkable only for patchy loss of sensation in the lower extremities. Upon referral to an ophthalmologist, she was found to have cotton-wool spots, venous beading, hard exudates, IRMA, and a few small intraretinal (flame) hemorrhages. She was diagnosed as having severe nonproliferative diabetic retinopathy.

Questions for Discussion

1 What should be considered as likely causes of blurred vision in this patient?

2 What is the appropriate treatment for her condition?

3 What adaptations to standard diabetes teaching does this patient need right now?

Discussion

1 This patient has type 2 diabetes of unknown duration. Her blurred vision could be secondary to poor glucose control or serious underlying eye pathology. She needed immediate referral for ophthalmologic evaluation, which in this case revealed severe nonproliferative diabetic retinopathy.

2 In addition to ophthalmoscopy, she may need fluorescein angiography to evaluate the extent of involvement of the retina and macula.

3 Pan-retinal photocoagulation therapy may be performed for severe nonproliferative diabetic retinopathy, but is generally delayed until severe NPDR or proliferative retinopathy develops.

4 She will require focal photocoagulation to the macula if clinically significant macular edema is present.

5 In addition to immediate attention to her eye problems she needs to begin an appropriate treatment program for hyperglycemia and hypertension and receive diabetes self-management education. Adjustment to the diagnosis of diabetes and vision impairment needs to be assessed and referrals for counseling or other supportive services offered as needed.

6 This patient is likely to need to learn low-vision methods for blood glucose monitoring, foot inspection, and exercise. If insulin therapy is instituted, she will also need a low vision method for insulin measurement. If the patient has difficulty reading print, provide education materials in large print or audio format.

Case Study 2

RI, a 35-year-old man, is referred to you for diabetes self-management education. His home glucose record reveals erratic glycemic control with frequent hypoglycemic episodes. Although RI denies vision impairment, he is unable to accurately draw up his insulin dose when observed. Upon further questioning he reports occasional difficulty reading the newspaper. His physician referred him to an ophthalmologist, but RI has not yet made an appointment.

Questions for Discussion

1 What further assessment of this patient's functional status should be undertaken?

2 What can the diabetes educator do to assist this patient in managing his diabetes?

3 What other services could the diabetes educator recommend to this patient for further assistance?

Discussion

1 This patient appears to have fluctuating vision that is interfering with his diabetes self-care. He is reluctant to acknowledge the visual problem.

2 The patient should be strongly encouraged to undergo a complete ophthalmologic exam to determine if the problem is diabetes related and to ensure that appropriate treatment is initiated.

3 The diabetes educator should further assess RI's diabetes self-care skills, such as glucose monitoring, meal planning, foot care, etc. If he is unable to accurately fill his syringes using a magnifier, the need for an adaptive syringe-filling device is indicated.

4 Although he currently is able to use his glucose meter without difficulty, he can be reassured that there are adaptive devices available to assist with glucose monitoring should there be a change in his vision status.

5 If the assessment shows that RI is having difficulties in other areas due to his visual status, the diabetes educator can make referrals to appropriate rehabilitative or low-vision services. Since he is having difficulty acknowledging his vision problems, the diabetes educator should help explore his fears, provide reassurance, and make referrals for counseling if necessary.

REFERENCES

1   Javitt JC, Aiello LP. Cost effectiveness of detecting and treating diabetic retinopathy. Ann Intern Med 1996;124:164-69.

2   Klein R, Klein BEK. Vision disorders in diabetes. In: National Diabetes Data Group, eds. Diabetes in America. 2nd ed. National Institutes of Health, 1995:293-337.

3   Aiello LP, Cavallerano J, Bursell SE. Diabetic eye disease. Endocrinol Metab Clin North Am 1996;25:271-91.

4   Raskin P, Arauz-Pacheco C. The treatment of diabetic retinopathy: a view for the internist. Ann Intern Med 1992; 117:226-33.

5   Harris MI. Summary. In: National Diabetes Data Group, eds. Diabetes in America. 2nd ed. National Institutes of Health, 1995:1-13.

6   The Diabetes Control and Complications Trial Research Group. The effect of intensive treatment of diabetes on the development and progression of long-term complications in insulin-dependent diabetes mellitus. N Engl J Med 1993; 329:977-86.

7   Frank KJ, Dieckert JP. Diabetic eye disease: a primary care perspective. South Med J 1996;89:463-70.

8   Sanders R, Wilson M. Diabetes-related eye disorders. J Natl Med Assoc 1993; 85:104-8.

9   Ferris FL, III. Diabetic retinopathy. Diabetes Care 1993;16:322-25.

10 Aiello LP, Gardner TW, King GL, Blankship G, et al. Diabetic retinopathy: a technical review. Diabetes Care 1998;21:143-56.

11 The Diabetic Retinopathy Study Research Group. Preliminary report on effects of photocoagulation therapy. Am J Ophthalmol 1976;81:383-96.

12 Early Treatment Diabetic Retinopathy Study Research Group. Photocoagulation for diabetic macular edema. Early Treatment Diabetic Retinopathy Study report number 1. Arch Ophthalmol 1985;103:1796-1806.

13 Bernbaum M, Albert SG. Referring patients with diabetes and vision loss for rehabilitation—who is responsible? Diabetes Care 1996;19:175-77.

14 Bernbaum M, Albert SG, Duckro PN. Psychosocial profiles in patients with visual impairment due to diabetic retinopathy. Diabetes Care 1988; 11:551-57.

15 Jacobson AM. Current concepts: the psychological care of patients with insulin-dependent diabetes mellitus. N Engl J Med 1996;334:1249-53.

16 Wulsin LR, Jacobson AM, Rand LI. Psychosocial adjustment to advanced proliferative diabetic retinopathy. Diabetes Care 1993;16:1061-66.

17 American Academy of Ophthalmology Quality of Care Committee Retina Panel. Preferred practice pattern for diabetic retinopathy. San Francisco: American Academy of Ophthalmology, 1989.

18 Collins JF. Ophthalmic desk reference. New York: Raven Press, 1991:615.

19 Simons K. Visual acuity and the functional definition of blindness. In: Tasman W, Jaeger EA, eds. Duane's clinical ophthalmology. Philadelphia: Lippincott, 1991:1-21.

20 American Foundation for the Blind. Low vision questions and answers: definitions, devices, services. New York: American Foundation for the Blind, 1987.

21 Williams, AS, Teaching nonvisual diabetes self-care: choosing appropriate tools and techniques for visually impaired individuals. Diabetes Spectrum 1997;10:128-134.

22 American Foundation for the Blind. Sensitivity to blindness and visual impairment. New York: American Foundation for the Blind, 1991.

23 Petzinger RA. An eye on diabetes products. Diabetes Forecast 1995;48(5):48-53.

24 Petzinger RA. Adaptive medication measurement and administration. In: Cleary M, ed. Diabetes and visual impairment: an educators resource guide. Chicago: American Association of Diabetes Educators Education and Research Foundation, 1994:121-42.

25 Williams AS. Recommendations for desirable features of adaptive diabetes self-care equipment for visually impaired persons. Diabetes Care 1994;17:451-52.

26 ADEVIP Task Force. Guidelines for the practice of adaptive diabetes education for visually impaired persons (ADEVIP). Diabetes Educ 1994;20:111-112, 115-116, 118.

27 Petzinger RA. Adaptive self-monitoring strategies. In: Cleary M, ed. Diabetes and visual impairment: an educators resource guide. Chicago: American Association of Diabetes Educators Education and Research Foundation, 1994:143-57.

28 Bernbaum SM, Albert SG, Miller D, Hoffman JW, Mooradian AD. Reliability of the Diascan Partner glucose monitor for visually impaired people. Diabetes Spectrum 1995;8:322-24.

29 Plummer E, Albert SG. Foot care assessment in patients with diabetes: a screening algorithm for patient education and referral. Diabetes Educ 1995; 21:47-51.

30 Williams A. Foot care for the visually impaired. Diabetes Self Manage 1992; 9(6):41-43.

31 Albert SG, Bernbaum M. Exercise for patients with diabetic retinopathy. Diabetes Care 1995;18:130-32.

32 Bernbaum M. Adaptive exercise recommendations. In: Cleary M, ed. Diabetes and visual impairment: an educators resource guide. Chicago: American Association of Diabetes Educators Education and Research Foundation 1994:111-19.

33 Graham C, Lasko-McCarthey P. Exercise options for persons with diabetic complications. Diabetes Educ 1990;16: 212-20.

34 Bernbaum M, Albert SG, Duckro PN, Merkel W. Personal and family stress in individuals with diabetes and vision loss. J Clin Psychol 1993;49:670-77.

35 Carroll TJ: Blindness: what it is, what it does, and how to live with it. Boston: Little, Brown & Co, 1961.

Suggested Readings

Bernbaum M, Albert SG, Brusca SR, et al. A model clinical program for patients with diabetes and vision impairment. Diabetes Educ 1989;15:325-30.

Greenblatt S, ed. Meeting the needs of people with vision loss. Lexington, Mass: Resources for Rehabilitation, 1991.

Other Resources

Service Agencies
American Council for the Blind
1211 Connecticut Avenue, NW
Washington, DC 20036
800-424-8666

LIONS Club International
300 Twenty-Second Street
Oakbrook, IL 60570
708-415-2352

National Eye Institute
Information Officer
Building 31, Room 6A32
Bethesda, MD 20205
301-496-5248

National Federation of the Blind
1800 Johnson Street
Baltimore, MD 21230
410-659-9314

National Society to Prevent Blindness
79 Madison Avenue
New York, NY 10016
212-980-2020

**Sources for tapes or
reading material**
National Library Service for the Blind
and Physically Handicapped
Library of Congress
1291 Taylor Street, NW
Washington, DC 20542
202-287-5100

Braille Exchange Lists
Braille Institute
741 N. Vermont Avenue
Los Angeles, CA 90029
213-663-1111

American Printing House for the Blind
1839 Frankfort Avenue
Louisville, KY 40206
502-895-2405

Recording for the Blind and Dyslexic
20 Roszel
Princeton, NJ 08540
800-221-4792

Correspondence Course
Hadley School for the Blind
700 Elm Street
Winnetka, IL 60093
847-446-8111

COMPLICATIONS

Diabetic Neuropathy 22

Martha Mitchell Funnell, MS, RN, CDE
Michigan Diabetes Research and Training Center
University of Michigan Medical Center
Ann Arbor, Michigan

Douglas A. Greene, MD
Michigan Diabetes Research and Training Center
University of Michigan Medical School
Ann Arbor, Michigan

INTRODUCTION

1 While neuropathies can occur as a result of AIDS, leprosy, injury, systemic erythematosus lupus, and drugs, including alcohol and toxicity from heavy metals, the primary cause for peripheral neuropathy in the Western world is diabetes.[1] As the most common, symptomatic long-term complication of diabetes, peripheral neuropathy is responsible for a majority of limb amputations and causes a great deal of morbidity and suffering in patients who develop it.[2] Consequently, diabetic neuropathy represents an enormous and costly public health problem.

2 Diabetic neuropathy is thought to be the result of insulin deficiency and/or hyperglycemia.[1] It encompasses a group of clinical and subclinical syndromes with varying etiologies and manifestations, each of which is characterized by either diffuse or focal damage of the peripheral somatic or autonomic nerve fibers resulting from diabetes.[3] Treatment is directed toward prevention, early diagnosis, optimal glucose control, relief of symptoms, avoidance of secondary complications, and patient education for appropriate self-care.

3 Patients with neuropathy have often been told that the pain and other symptoms of neuropathy are just something they would have to live with. Because diabetic neuropathy has become the subject of intense research interest, however, there is new understanding of the causes and break-throughs in the treatment. The purpose of this chapter is to review the pathogenesis and approaches to the prevention and management of diabetic polyneuropathy as it affects the peripheral nervous system, and areas of current and future research.

OBJECTIVES

Upon completion of this chapter, the learner will be able to

1 Define diabetic neuropathy.
2 Explain the role of blood glucose control in the development and treatment of peripheral neuropathies.
3 List pharmacological and nonpharmacological treatments for peripheral neuropathy.
4 List the clinical manifestations of diffuse sensory neuropathy.
5 List the classifications and clinical manifestations of autonomic neuropathy.

6 State the primary symptom for each of the focal neuropathies.

7 Describe the key information about neuropathy that should be taught to all patients with diabetes.

KEY DEFINITIONS

1 *Axon.* The central core of nerve fiber that conducts impulses away from the nerve cell body.

2 *Inositol.* A crystalline substance resembling sugar found in nerve and other tissues, including the nerve.

3 *Myelin.* The fat-like substance forming a sheath around certain nerve fibers.

4 *Neuron.* The structural and functional unit of the nervous system.

5 *Plexus.* A network made up of nerve fibers.

6 *Radiculopathy.* Disease condition of the nerve roots in spinal nerves.

7 *Sorbitol.* A crystalline alcohol that is the intermediate product in the metabolism of glucose in the nerve and other tissues.

DEFINITION OF DIABETIC NEUROPATHY

1 *Diabetic neuropathy* is a descriptive term for a clinical or subclinical disorder that occurs in patients with diabetes without other causes for peripheral neuropathy.[4] Although this complication often is thought of in terms of the more common symptoms of pain and numbness, diabetic neuropathy actually comprises a large group of sensory and autonomic syndromes with a wide range of manifestations.[1]

2 Diabetic neuropathy can be defined as peripheral nerve dysfunction that occurs in people with diabetes, is of a type known to be more prevalent among people with diabetes, and cannot be attributed to any other disease.[4]

3 The diagnosis and staging of diabetic neuropathy are based on signs, symptoms, and objective measures. Objective evidence (eg, electrodiagnostic and sensory tests) is needed to detect subclinical neuropathy.

Clinical neuropathy is defined through symptoms, clinical signs, and objective measures, and subdivided into syndromes according to the distribution of peripheral nervous system involvement. The two subcategories of clinical neuropathy are diffuse polyneuropathy (multiple nerve involvement), which includes both sensory and autonomic impairment, and focal neuropathy (individual nerve involvement)[1] (see Table 22.1).

4 Each syndrome has a characteristic clinical presentation and course, although multiple syndromes may overlap and coexist.[5] The majority of patients experience diffuse neuropathies consisting of distal symmetric, primarily sensory, polyneuropathies that are often accompanied by diabetic autonomic neuropathy.[1]

5 The *diffuse neuropathies* are generally chronic, frequently progressive, and are associated with increased morbidity and mortality.[5] The focal neuropathies occur less often, are generally acute in onset, and are often self-limited.[6]

OCCURRENCE

1 Reliable prevalence estimates of diabetic neuropathy have been difficult to obtain because of the lack of standard diagnostic measures and consensus in diagnostic criteria.[7] Diabetic neuropathy occurs with similar frequency in patients with type 1 or type 2 diabetes, and also in patients with various forms of acquired diabetes.[8]

2 Estimates for the prevalence of neuropathy range from 5% to 60%, and up to 100% if patients with abnormalities of nerve conduction are included.[8-11] Pirat's[8] classic study reported 8% prevalence at the time of diagnosis (mostly in older type 2 patients) that increased in a linear manner to 50% after 25 years. A retrospective, population-based study[12] of subjects with type 1 and type 2 diabetes showed a cumulative incidence of distal symmetrical polyneuropathy of 4% after 5 years, 15% after 20 years, and a median time of 9 years after diagnosis to development of this neuropathy. In a large Italian study,[10] one third of type 1 and type 2 patients had neuropathy with increased severity related to both age and duration of diabetes.

TABLE 22.1. CLASSIFICATION AND STAGING OF DIABETIC NEUROPATHY

Class I: Subclinical Neuropathy*

1 Abnormal electrodiagnostic tests (EDX)

    A Decreased nerve conduction velocity

    B Decreased amplitude of evoked muscle or nerve action potential

2 Abnormal quantitative sensory testing (QST)

    A Vibratory/tactile

    B Thermal warming/cooling

    C Other

3 Abnormal autonomic function tests (AFT)

    A Diminished sinus arrhythmia (beat-to-beat heart-rate variation)

    B Diminished sudomotor function

    C Increased pupillary latency

Class II: Clinical Neuropathy

1 Diffuse neuropathy

    A Distal symmetric sensorimotor polyneuropathy

      • Primarily small-fiber neuropathy

      • Primarily large-fiber neuropathy

      • Mixed

    B Autonomic neuropathy

      • Genitourinary autonomic neuropathy

        — Bladder dysfunction

        — Sexual dysfunction

      • Gastrointestinal autonomic neuropathy

        — Gastric atony

        — Diabetic enteropathy

      • Cardiovascular autonomic neuropathy

      • Hypoglycemic unawareness

      • Sudomotor dysfunction

      • Abnormal pupillary function

2 Focal neuropathy

    A Mononeuropathy

    B Mononeuropathy multiplex

    C Plexopathy

    D Radiculopathy

    E Cranial neuropathy

---

* Neurological function tests are abnormal but no neurological symptoms or clinically detectable neurological deficits indicative of a diffuse or focal neuropathy are present. Class I, subclinical neuropathy, is further subdivided into class IA if an AFT or QST abnormality is present, class IB if EDX or AFT and QST abnormalities are present, and class IC if an EDX and either AFT or QST abnormalities or both are present.

Source: Adapted with permission from Greene et al[1]

3 Sensory symptoms (eg, pain) are reported by 30% of people with type 1 and 40% of people with type 2 diabetes in the United States. Those who have had diabetes 20 years or more have a twofold increase in symptoms.[13] As many as 20% to 30% of patients with long-standing diabetes have symptoms of gastroparesis.[14] Carpal tunnel syndrome occurs in 4% to 29% of people with both types of diabetes and also is related to duration.[9]

4 In type 1 diabetes, the prevalence of polyneuropathy appears to parallel the duration and severity of hyperglycemia. While this prevalence is probably also true in type 2 diabetes, undiagnosed patients may present initially with symptoms and signs of sensory and/or autonomic neuropathy and subsequently be diagnosed with diabetes.[8,9,15] The most likely explanation for this occurrence is the insidious nature of type 2 diabetes, which may be present but undiagnosed for years. Thus, the relationship of the duration of type 2 diabetes to neuropathy is difficult to determine.[2]

5 Diabetic neuropathy can be considered an extremely common problem that ultimately affects about half of all patients with diabetes.[8]

PATHOLOGY

1 The nervous system is divided into the central nervous system and the peripheral nervous system. The peripheral nervous system is made up of the autonomic nervous system (sympathetic and parasympathetic) and the sensorimotor nervous system. Autonomic nerves control involuntary functions, sensory nerves send information from the skin and internal organs about how things feel, and motor nerves send commands from the brain to the body about movement.

2 Most of the pathology of diabetic neuropathy occurs in the peripheral nervous system,[16] although there may be some central nervous system involvement. All types of neuropathies occur in the peripheral nervous system.

3 Diabetic neuropathy is believed to be a disease involving acute nerve fiber abnormalities, followed by more chronic nerve fiber injury, atrophy, and loss. The most common pathological lesion is demyelinization and atrophy of longer peripheral nerve axons.[16]

4 Neuropathies occur secondary to axonal degeneration that progresses from the distal to the proximal portions of the neurons[16]; the distal portions are eventually more seriously affected.[17] This process is further affected by microvascular dysfunction and blunted nerve fiber regeneration, and is linked with the effects of hyperglycemia on the cell constituents of peripheral nerve tissue and its supporting connective tissue and vascular elements.[18]

PATHOGENESIS

1 The association between diabetes and neuropathic symptoms in the legs and feet was first made by John Rollo over 200 years ago,[19] yet the pathogenesis of diabetic neuropathy is still unknown.[1] Evidence suggests that insulin deficiency and the related hyperglycemia contribute to the development of neuropathy.[8,13,20] Severity, however, does not always correlate with clinical findings or symptoms.[21] Cigarette smoking also has been implicated as a risk factor for neuropathy.[22]

2 Results from the Diabetes Control and Complications Trial (DCCT)[20] provided evidence that intensive therapy decreased the risk for neuropathy by 60% in a large sample of participants with type 1 diabetes. Although the results of the DCCT are generally believed to apply to persons with type 2 diabetes, there is less direct evidence of the influence of glucose control on the risk for neuropathy.[23,24] Poor glucose control, hypoinsulinemia, age, obesity, and duration of diabetes all have been linked with diabetic peripheral neuropathy in people with type 2 diabetes.[13,25-27] Overall, diabetic neuropathy is thought to result from the interaction between multiple metabolic, genetic, and environmental factors.[26,28] Prevention efforts are focused primarily on improved glucose control throughout the course of all types of diabetes.

3 There are several theories[29] about why neuropathy occurs: accumulation of sorbitol in the nerve cells, decrease in myoinositol, nerve glycosylation, and nerve hypoxia.

   A One theory is based on the conversion of glucose to sorbitol by the enzyme aldose reductase and secondary abnormalities in myoinositol, phosphoinositide, and Na, K-ATPase metabolism.[1]

- Unlike most other cells, insulin is not needed to move glucose into nerve cells. Therefore, high levels of blood glucose lead to high levels of glucose within the nerve cells.
- Once inside the cell, glucose is reduced to sorbitol by an enzyme called aldose reductase (the sorbitol pathway).
- Sorbitol is then oxidized to fructose by the enzyme sorbitol dehydrogenase (the polyol pathway).
- In diabetes, peripheral nerve glucose, sorbitol, and fructose levels are elevated, which alters normal intracellular metabolism and may be toxic to nerves. Specific aldose reductase inhibitors have been shown to improve nerve function by preventing the conversion of glucose to sorbitol.[16]

B The reasons why elevated sorbitol and glucose levels damage nerves are not known but may be related to decreased myoinositol levels.

- Myoinositol, the most common form of inositol, is found in most cells of the body, including nerve cells, and is needed for normal cellular function and metabolism.
- Activation of the polyol pathway may lead to a decrease in myoinositol levels. When myoinositol levels are decreased, nerve velocity is decreased.
- Myoinositol molecules are very much like glucose molecules in size and shape. In the presence of hyperglycemia, the large number of glucose molecules inhibits the transport of myoinositol into the peripheral nerves, causing a self-reinforcing cycle of metabolic disarrangement that results in peripheral nerve impairment.
- Agents that inhibit aldose reductase (aldose reductase inhibitors or ARIs) may improve nerve function by preventing the conversion of glucose to sorbitol; these agents are the subject of current research.[1,16]

C Additional theories are related to glycosylation of nerve myelin and microvascular disease. It has been hypothesized[5] that glycosylation of cellular proteins, which is similar to the processes resulting in glycosylation of nerve myelin, may lead to demyelination and a decrease in nerve conduction.

D The theory of hypoxia is based on the decreased blood flow and oxygen tension found in people with diabetes. The effects of decreased perfusion to peripheral nerve tissue are unclear, although the process may lead to microvascular disease and further hypoxia.[18] Large blood vessel occlusive disease alone does not produce peripheral neuropathy.[16]

4 The pathology of autonomic neuropathy is related to axonal degeneration and fiber loss in the sympathetic and parasympathetic systems. The intrinsic nerves of the gastrointestinal systems also are affected.[2] A metabolic basis for autonomic abnormalities similar to sensory polyneuropathy has been suggested, although autoimmunity also may play a role.[28] Focal neuropathies are thought to be caused by acute ischemic events and have a vascular basis for their occurrence.[2]

Diagnosis

1 Diagnosis is a process that involves excluding other potential causes of the signs and symptoms that are presented by a patient. Reported symptoms generally are of limited use in making a diagnosis of sensory neuropathy. However, monofilament testing for decreased tactile perception and clinical signs such as loss of ankle reflexes and decreased vibration sensation can be used as screening measures for sensory neuropathy.[29-31] Objective measures such as electrodiagnostic testing along with a clinical neurological exam are used to confirm and stage the diagnosis.[30]

2 Physical assessment of the person with diabetes needs to include evaluation of muscle strength, deep tendon reflexes, temperature, and position.

A Pain and light-touch sensations can be assessed using vibration and pinprick/monofilament testing. A safety pin can be touched lightly to the foot and the patient can be asked to describe the sensation as sharp or dull.[2]

B Temperature sensation can be assessed by touching a cool piece of metal (eg, a tuning fork) to the skin and asking the patient to describe the temperature.

C Position sense is assessed by flexing and extending the big toes and asking that the patient describe the position.

D Vibration sensation is assessed by applying a 128 Hz tuning fork to the distal first metatarsal head.

E The Valsalva-stimulated R-R response is sensitive to changes in autonomic function.[32]

F Routine assessment of blood pressures (lying, sitting, standing), cardiac status, and symptoms of autonomic neuropathic syndromes also need to be performed.

3 Annual risk categorization using monofilament testing for early detection of insensitive feet can have a substantial impact on preventing injury, sepsis, ulceration, and amputation.[31] See Chapter 16, Skin, Foot and Dental Care, for more information on monofilament testing.

TREATMENT

1 Treatment generally is palliative, supportive, and aimed at symptom relief, optimizing blood glucose control, addressing psychosocial distress or depression, protecting the feet, and providing patient self-management education.

2 Both pharmacological and nonpharmacological therapies may be useful for pain relief. Improved control of blood glucose levels may result in a decrease in symptoms for some patients. However, pain may initially worsen as a result of nerve regeneration.

3 Aldose reductase inhibitors (ARIs) prevent the breakdown of glucose into sorbitol in the nerve cells and may hold promise for future treatment of neuropathies.

OVERVIEW OF DIFFUSE SENSORY NEUROPATHIES

1 Distal symmetric sensorimotor polyneuropathy (sensory neuropathy) is the most widely known form of neuropathy, primarily involves the sensory nerves,[1] and affects 72% of patients with neuropathy.[12] Sensory deficits and symptoms begin in the distal portions of the lower extremities and progress to the upper extremities, spreading in a "stocking-glove" distribution. Lower extremities tend to be affected more seriously than upper extremities. The nerve fiber loss and atrophy is progressive, and the spread of symptoms is related to increasing duration and severity of the syndrome.[1] Manifestations in the early stages can include deterioration of nerve function and development of subtle sensory-motor deficits with minimal or absent symptoms. In the late stage, bands of sensory loss in the trunk area may occur.[16]

TABLE 22.2. SENSORY NEUROPATHY DEFICITS AND SYMPTOMS

Syndrome	Symptoms
Small-fiber damage	• Loss of ability to detect temperature • Pins-and-needles, tingling, or burning sensations • Pain, usually worse at night • Numbness or loss of feeling • Cold extremities • Swelling of feet • Pain on contact with clothing or bedsheets
Large-fiber damage	• Abnormal or unusual sensations • Loss of balance • Unable to sense position of toes and feet • Unable to feel feet when when walking
Motor nerve damage	• Loss of muscle tone in hands and feet
Foot deformities	• Callus formation • Charcot's joint • Misshapen or deformed toes and feet • Open sores or ulcers on feet

2   Sensory neuropathy can be viewed as a disease of progressive nerve fiber loss, atrophy, and injury. The signs and symptoms depend on the class and stage of nerve fiber loss (Table 22.2). Small fiber involvement impairs pain and temperature sensations, large fiber involvement produces diminished proprioception and light-touch sensation, and motor nerve damage results in loss of muscle tone. Most patients experience damage to more than one type of nerve.

DIFFUSE SENSORY NEUROPATHIES

1   Subclinical sensory neuropathy:

    A   The early stages of sensory neuropathy may be manifested as deterioration of nerve function and development of subtle sensory-motor deficits. Most patients have minimal symptoms at this stage.

    B   Some patients may present with neurological deficits that are found during a physical examination or with complications, such as undetected trauma to an insensate foot.[8]

C   Nerve fiber damage may be so mild that it is not apparent even with a careful physical examination but is evident only with nerve function testing or nerve biopsy.[18]

2   Small-fiber neuropathy:

A   Several types of spontaneous pain or discomfort may be associated with small-fiber neuropathy. Patients most often experience paresthesias (spontaneous uncomfortable sensations), dysesthesias (contact paresthesias), or pain. The pain is described as superficial and burning, shooting or stabbing, or bone-deep and aching or tearing, and is generally more severe at night. The pain can become disabling in and of itself, and depression may occur as a result of unremitting pain, sleep disturbance, or diminished quality of life.[2] In contrast, some patients have subjective symptoms of numbness or cold feet. Undetected trauma, particularly on the feet, is common.[2,16]

B   Sensory loss appears to correspond closely with the degree of nerve damage. However, pain corresponds more closely with independent processes such as fiber regeneration or structural deformities.[33]

C   In acute painful neuropathy, the pain develops and then remits in less than 6 months. Precipitous weight loss may occur.[2] In chronic painful neuropathy, symptoms appear and stabilize for more than 6 months, or disappear and are replaced by dense sensory deficits such as numb or cold feet.[1]

D   Diminished deep tendon reflexes of the Achilles tendon, and diminished temperature, pinprick, and monofilament sensations may be early signs of neuropathies, although these signs often are not striking.[2] Sensory impairment is clinically significant because it can predispose to ulceration.

E   Symptoms may occur in the absence of neurological deficits on physical examination.[2]

3   Large-fiber neuropathy:

A   Impaired balance and diminished proprioception and joint position sense are symptoms of large-fiber damage.[16] Pain is usually absent and sensory ataxia may occur in the most severe cases.

B   Clinical signs may include absent or reduced vibration sensation, impaired touch or pressure sensation, and diminished ankle reflexes.[2]

C Foot deformities are primarily the result of damage to the large fiber nerves in association with small fiber distal motor and autonomic abnormalities[2] (see Chapter 16, Skin, Foot, and Dental Care, for more information).

4 Motor neuropathy:
A Causes muscle weakness and atrophy of intrinsic foot muscles, leaving the pull of the long muscles unopposed.
B Ankle weakness and foot drop can then result.

TREATMENT OF DIFFUSE SENSORY NEUROPATHIES

1 Treatment is focused on glycemic control, pain management, relief from the depression that often accompanies chronic pain, and protecting deformed feet.

2 Improved glycemic control may decrease the pain and other symptoms for some patients, although the pain may initially worsen.[13,29]

3 Nonpharmacological therapies include walking to ease leg pains, gentle massage, stretching exercises, avoiding alcohol, relaxation exercises, biofeedback, hypnosis, acupuncture, use of transcutaneous nerve stimulation (TENS) units, body stockings or pantyhose to keep clothes away from hypersensitive skin, brief cold water foot soaks, and referral to a pain control clinic.

4 Pharmacological therapies include nonnarcotic analgesics such as ibuprofen and sulindac, phenytoin (Dilantin), carbamazepine (Tegretol), or gabapentin (Neurontin) in anticonvulsive doses, and amitriptyline (Elavil) or imipramine (Tofranil) in subclinical doses either alone or in combination with pheno-thiazine and mexiletine.[2,29,34] Narcotic agents are generally not recommended because of the chronic nature of neuropathy pain and the potential for addiction. Analgesics approved for other uses (eg, tramadol hydrochloride) have been found to be effective for pain relief. Topical capsaicin 0.075% (Zostrix HP) has been found to be effective for some patients[35] and is available without a prescription.

5 Lamb's wool padding, gentle filing of calloused areas, and specially made shoes and molded insoles or other orthotic devices can be used to protect deformed areas of the feet. Referral to a podiatrist or orthotic specialist is needed to identify abnormal weight-bearing and to prescribe mechanical measures to compensate.

6 One approach to treatment is to select a protocol based on the classification of the pain. Using this approach, capsaicin is recommended for people with superficial pain; imipramine and mexiletine for deep pain; and metaxalone, stretching exercises, and piroxicam for muscle pain.[36]

7 Aldose reductase inhibitors offer new hope for patients. ARIs have been found to be effective in halting or reversing the progression of nerve damage in patients with mild neuropathies.[37] Some of these agents are available in other countries and research efforts continue in this area.

COMPLICATIONS OF DIFFUSE SENSORY NEUROPATHIES

1 Neuropathic syndromes can culminate in the following severe tertiary complications of sensory and motor denervation that parallel severity and proximal extension of the sensory loss:[26] insensitivity to pain, limb deformity, ulceration, neuroarthropathy, infection, and amputation.

2 Neuropathic foot ulcers often occur in areas where the fat pad is decreased and callus formation subsequently occurs as a result of weight-bearing pressure. Autonomic neuropathy further leads to decreased perspiration and a tendency for dry, cracked skin and infection. Injuries may remain unnoticed due to diminished sensation until infection develops.

3 Neuropathic arthropathy (Charcot's Joint) can occur when motor function remains intact but sensation is impaired. The small joints of the foot (tarsals, metatarsals) are most commonly affected.[38] The foot is swollen, red, and painless in the early stages; multiple fractures, fragmentations, and disarticulations occur in the later stages. As the patient continues to walk on the injured, insensate foot, marked deformities occur such as a flattened arch and "bag of bones" appearance.[16]

4 Treatment for these complications is aimed at removing continued trauma, proper footwear, patient education concerning appropriate foot-care practices and aggressive follow-up and surveillance.

Overview of Autonomic Neuropathies

1 Diabetic autonomic neuropathies (DAN) can occur with all types of diabetes[39] and can affect any system in the body.[40]

   A The relationship of DAN to sensorimotor polyneuropathy varies, but these conditions generally coexist.

   B As many as 50% of patients with peripheral neuropathy may also have DAN.[40]

2 Because morbidity and mortality rates are closely linked to DAN, early diagnosis and treatment is of critical importance.[39,40]

3 The most common classifications of DAN, accompanying clinical manifestations, and interventions and self-management education for each syndrome are shown in Table 22.3.

Autonomic Neuropathies

1 Genitourinary impairment

   A Both bladder and sexual functioning may be affected.

   B Bladder dysfunction generally occurs in association with distal symmetric polyneuropathy and impotence among males.[2]

     • Afferent autonomic fibers transmit bladder fullness sensations (normally with 300 cc urine) and efferent parasympathetic fibers promote bladder contraction during micturition. Efferent sympathetic nerves maintain sphincter tone.[2] Damage can occur to all of these nerves; however, motor function usually remains intact.[40]

     • Symptoms of a neurogenic bladder are usually insidious and progressive. In the early stages, the sensation of the need to void may be blunted. This infrequent urination may be misinterpreted as decreased polyuria due to improved blood glucose control. In later stages, difficulty in emptying the bladder, dribbling, and overflow incontinence may occur.[39]

TABLE 22.3. DIABETIC AUTONOMIC NEUROPATHIES

Classification	Symptoms and Signs	Intervention/Patient Education
Genitourinary Neurogenic bladder	• Diminished urinary frequency • Incomplete or difficult bladder emptying • Frequent urinary tract infections • Bladder residual volume >150 mL	• Schedule urination every 2 hours • Prevention, signs, and symptoms of UTIs; seek treatment immediately • Credé maneuver, palpation for bladder distention, self-catheterization
Sexual dysfunction	*In males* • Retrograde ejaculation • Impotence *In females* • Diminished vaginal lubrication • Decreased frequency of orgasm	• Report symptoms to healthcare team; therapeutic options, uses, and potential side effects • Referral to impotence clinic; urologist/gynecologist
Gastrointestinal Gastroparesis	• Early satiety • Postprandial fullness • Postprandial hypoglycemia	Therapeutic options, uses and potential side effects; appropriate meal planning and frequent meals; importance of blood glucose control; frequent blood glucose monitoring; insulin adjustment; referral to a gastroenterologist
Intestinal	• Nocturnal diarrhea • Fecal incontinence	Adequate fiber and fluid intake and physical activity to prevent constipation; therapeutic options, uses, and potential side effects; importance of blood glucose control; judicious use of laxatives; bowel program, relaxation, or biofeedback
Cardiovascular Orthostatic hypotension	• Postural hypotension	Safety measures to prevent falls; rise slowly from a recumbent position; proper use of elastic body stockings; importance of blood glucose control; therapeutic options, uses, and potential side effects
Cardiac denervation	• Fixed heart rate • Painless MI, sudden death	• Avoid heavy exercise and straining • Prevent hypoglycemia
Abnormal cardiovascular response to exercise	• Hypotension with exercise	• Avoid aerobic exercise
Impaired Insulin Counterregulation	• Unawareness of hypoglycemia • "Brittle" diabetes	Frequent blood glucose monitoring, particularly before driving; prevention of hypoglycemia; wearing appropriate identification; treatment of hypo-glycemia, including glucagon; appropriate blood glucose goals
Sudomotor	• Areas of symmetrical anhydrosis • Gustatory sweating	• Check for fissures and lubricate feet daily; prevent heatstroke through avoidance of high heat and humidity • Avoid offending foods
Pupillary	• Decreased/absent responsiveness to light • Decreased pupil size	Caution regarding night driving; use of nightlights; safety measures to avoid falls such as turning on lights when entering a dark room

- Bladder insensitivity is diagnosed by a cystometrogram.[39] A postvoid urine residual volume of greater than 150 mL by ultrasound or postvoid catheterization confirms bladder dysfunction.

- Untreated neurogenic bladder often leads to urinary tract infections as a result of urinary stasis. These frequent infections may accelerate deterioration of renal function. More than two urinary tract infections per year among men and three among women are indicative of the need for further evaluation of bladder dysfunction.[39]

- Treatment involves frequent palpation for bladder fullness, scheduled urination every 2 to 4 hours during waking hours using manual suprapubic pressure (Credé method) to ensure that the bladder is empty, vigorous antibiotic therapy for infections, and parasympathomimetic drug treatment (eg, bethanechol) to improve nerve contraction.[40] Self-catheterization may be needed if the nerves to the bladder are severely damaged.

- Stress the need for frequent, complete urination, the signs and symptoms of urinary tract infections, and the importance of early treatment for infections. Patients can also be taught to palpate for bladder fullness with the Credé method.[40]

C Sexual dysfunction is common among people with diabetes. As many as 75% of men and 35% of women experience sexual problems due to diabetic neuropathy.

D Male sexual dysfunction involves impotence and retrograde ejaculation.

- Retrograde ejaculation is unusual and results in damage to the efferent sympathetic nerves that normally coordinate the simultaneous closure of the internal vesicle sphincter and relaxation of the external vesicle sphincter. Cloudy urine following intercourse and decreased volume of ejaculate are symptomatic of retrograde ejaculation. Retrograde ejaculation is diagnosed by the presence of oligospermia, azoospermia, and sperm in postcoital urine. Retrograde ejaculation may respond to the use of an antihistamine, desipramine, or phenylephrine.[2,40] Fertility may be possible by instructing patients to have intercourse with a full bladder or by harvesting sperm from the urine and artificially inseminating them into the prospective mother.

- Impotence is marked by impairment or loss of erectile ability sufficient for intercourse despite a normal libido.[40] Organic impotence is gradual in onset (from partial to complete in 2 years), is partner non-specific, and characterized by lack of erections during sleep.[2]

- Diagnosis of impotence involves ruling out other causes such as medications (eg, alcohol, antihypertensives), hormonal deficiencies, or psychological causes.[2] The assessment process can include penile blood flood and pressure measurements, blood hormone levels, nocturnal tumescence (eg, Snap Gauge®) testing, and referral to urologist for further evaluation. Diabetic autonomic neuropathy is specifically associated with diminished or absent testicular pain sensation to pressure and loss of perineal sensation. The sensations are lost because of parallel loss of somatic and autonomic sacral segments 2, 3, and 4.[40]

- Management for impotence often begins with referral to an impotence clinic or urologist for diagnosis and counseling for the patient and his partner. Treatment options include suction devices that produce an erection, rigid or semirigid penile prostheses (surgical implants), use of the alpha adrenergic agonist yohimbine, prostaglandin urethral suppositories (Muse®), injection of prostaglandins (Captoject®) directly into the corpus cavernosum to produce erection, or oral medications (sildenafil citrate [Viagra™]).

E Female sexual dysfunction involves difficulties in arousal, vaginal lubrication during stimulation, and anorgasmia despite a normal libido.[2]

- Symptoms such as dyspareunia, decreased lubrication, and delayed or absent orgasmic response should be assessed.

- Management includes application of estrogen or lubricant vaginal creams and referral to a gynecologist.

F Sexual difficulties not related to autonomic neuropathy include loss of libido related to depression as a result of diabetes and its complications, and the frequent occurrence of yeast and other vaginal infections in women with diabetes.[2]

G It is important for diabetes educators to address sexual concerns because these issues may be difficult for patients to discuss. Discuss sexual function, the potential for diabetes-related problems, and the need to bring problems to the attention of providers. Include both the patient and his or her partner in counseling for specific therapies.

2 Gastrointestinal impairment

   A Virtually all of the gastrointestinal system has autonomic innervation.[39] The parasympathetic nervous system stimulates intestinal and gastric peristalsis, dopaminergic innervation inhibits gastric peristalsis, and the sympathetic nervous system inhibits gastric emptying.[2]

   B In persons without diabetic autonomic neuropathy, the stomach empties liquids in about 30 minutes and solid foods in about 150 minutes.[14] If the nerves are affected by autonomic neuropathy, gastric emptying of both liquids and solids may be delayed. Most of the evidence supports the idea that vagal nerve dysfunction is responsible for the motility disturbances. Upper gastrointestinal dysfunction may involve the esophagus, stomach, and upper small intestine.

      • Symptoms of *gastroparesis* (delayed gastric emptying) can include heartburn, reflux, anorexia, early satiety, nausea, abdominal bloating, erratic blood glucose levels due to delayed absorption of food, and vomiting undigested food eaten several hours or days earlier.[2] Signs associated with gastroparesis include weight loss and gastrospasm, although delayed gastric emptying can also occur without symptoms.[40]

      • Visualization of the upper gastrointestinal tract with a barium series is useful to rule out obstruction and determine liquid-phase gastric emptying. While delayed liquid-phase emptying almost always indicates delayed solid-phase emptying, normal liquid-phase emptying does not rule out delayed solid-phase emptying. Therefore, a solid-phase gastric emptying phase study is the most specific way to diagnose delayed gastric emptying.[2]

      • Treatment includes referral to a dietitian for a low-fat/low-fiber diet; multiple small and mostly liquid meals eaten throughout the day; referral to a gastroenterologist; medications to decrease inhibition of gastric motility such as metoclopramide (Reglan), domperidone (Motilium), or octreotide taken one-half hour before all meals and snacks and at bedtime; or other medications that increase the motility of the stomach such as erythromycin, cisapride, or bethanechol. In the most severe stages jejunostomy tube feedings may be necessary.

      • Although normalizing blood glucose levels may improve gastric emptying, the presence of gastroparesis complicates balancing insulin doses with food absorption. Frequent monitoring of pre- and postprandial blood glucose levels is needed to detect hypo- and hyperglycemia and determine the insulin dose. Rapid-acting insulin (lispro) is probably not appropriate in gastroparesis.

C Lower intestinal tract dysfunction is the result of damage to the efferent autonomic nerves. This damage leads to hypotonia and poor contraction of the smooth muscles to the gut, which results in constipation.

- Constipation is fairly common and has been reported in up to 60% of all patients with diabetes.[2] Treatment involves increasing fiber in the diet; judicious use of laxatives; avoidance of excess fiber; adequate hydration; increased activity; stool softeners and bulk laxatives such as psyllium (Metamucil); and medications such as metoclopramide (Reglan), domperidone (Motilium), cisapride (Propulsid), or neostigmine (Prostigmin) to increase intestinal mobility.[41]

- Decreased small intestinal motility may lead to an overgrowth of the normal intestinal bacteria and diarrhea. Diarrhea can also occur as a result of hypermotility without bacterial overgrowth.[39]

- Although constipation is more common, diarrhea is usually more troublesome to patients. Diarrhea may be nocturnal, intermittent with constipation, associated with fecal incontinence, and occur without cramping or pain.[39] Treatment involves the use of antibiotics (eg, tetracycline) to decrease the bacterial overgrowth (if confirmed by a hydrogen breath test). Medications that may be useful for slowing intestinal motility are loperamide, codeine, diphenoxylate hydrochloride, or atropine sulfate. Fiber and psyllium may increase stool bulk and consistency. In addition, some patients may benefit from biofeedback, relaxation, and bowel training. Early treatment of diarrhea may help prevent the development of incontinence.[2]

- A discussion of these symptoms as they relate to diabetes and the importance of informing providers of symptoms to allow for early detection and treatment is an important part of patient education. Explanations of tests, test results, and therapies are also needed.

3 Cardiovascular impairment

A Cardiovascular dysfunction is associated with abnormalities in heart rate control and vascular dynamics. Parasympathetic nerves slow the heart rate, and sympathetic nerves increase the speed and force of heart contractions and stimulate the vascular tree to increase the blood pressure.[2] Cardiovascular impairment is present in up to 40%

of patients. The three major associated syndromes are orthostatic (postural) hypotension, cardiac denervation syndrome, and abnormal cardiovascular response to exercise.

B Blood pressure is normally maintained upon standing by a sympathetic reflex that increases the heart rate and by peripheral vascular resistance in association with an increase in norepinephrine levels. *Orthostatic (postural) hypotension* is defined as a drop in systolic blood pressure of more than 30 mmHg or a diastolic drop of more than 10mm Hg within 2 minutes of changing from a supine to standing position. This syndrome occurs late in diabetes and signals advanced autonomic impairment.[40]

- Orthostatic hypotension, which results from blood pooling in the feet, can occur without symptoms but often is accompanied by dizziness, lightheadedness, weakness, visual impairment, or syncope[2]; it also may lead to edema, which desensitizes the feet and places the patient at risk for injury from falls.

- Assessment of blood pressure and pulse rates in the lying, sitting, and standing positions is needed for all patients who have diabetes. Greater accuracy in the assessment can be achieved by having the patient rest in a supine position, then stand quietly while the blood pressure is measured at 1-minute intervals for 3 to 5 minutes.[42]

- Treatment of symptoms involves raising the head of the bed 30° at night; standing in stages; increasing venous pressure with supportive elastic body stockings that are applied while supine; wearing an antigravity suit; and correcting hypovolemia through glycemic control, increased salt intake, and/or fludrocortisone to expand the plasma volume.[40]

- Pharmacologic therapies can include fludrocortisone, yohimbine, metoclopramide, phenylephrine, ephedrine, neo-synephrine nasal spray, midodrine (Proamatine), beta blockers, clonidine, and somatostatin analog.[2]

- Patient education is focused on proper application and use of elastic body stockings and instructing patients to rise slowly from a recumbent position.

C *Cardiac denervation syndrome* is defined as a fixed heart rate that does not change in response to stress, exercise, breathing patterns, or sleep. This syndrome is the result of both parasympathetic and sympathetic system impairment. Initially, parasympathetic tone decreases, which causes a relative increase in sympathetic tone and an increase in heart rate. Progressive impairment of sympathetic tone causes a gradual slowing of the heart. Over time, both para-sympathetic and sympathetic tone become impaired, resulting in cardiac denervation syndrome.[2]

- Initially, a fixed heart rate of 100 to 120 beats per minute is common. In the later stages, the fixed heart rate will be in the range of 80 to 100 beats per minute.[2] The heart rate is unresponsive to stress, exercise, or tilting.[39]
- In the later stages, patients may suffer myocardial ischemia or myocardial infarction without experiencing pain. The resulting delay or failure to seek treatment contributes to increasing mortality rates. These patients are also at risk for cardiac arrhythmias and sudden death.[40]
- Cardiac denervation is assessed using the EKG to check the pulse or heart rate during deep breathing (6 breaths per minute) or before or after a valsalva maneuver or exercise. No variation in heart rate is indicative of cardiac nerve damage.[2]
- Teach patients with this syndrome to avoid heavy exercise, aerobic exercise, and straining. Stress testing is needed before initiating any type of exercise program. In addition, these patients need to be carefully evaluated prior to initiation of intensive insulin therapy because of the risk of hypoglycemia, which can cause a cardiac arrhythmia.[39]

D Some people with diabetic autonomic neuropathy may lose the normal increased cardiac output and vascular tone response to exercise and become hypotensive with aerobic activity.[26]

4 Impaired insulin counterregulation

A Maintaining blood glucose levels during times of food deprivation and increased insulin action depends on glucagon secretion and the adrenergic nervous system.[39] The acute counterregulatory response to low blood glucose levels is an increase in the secretion of glucagon, epinephrine, growth hormone, cortical, and glucose production by the liver.[2] Patients with autonomic neuropathy may have a defective adrenergic nervous system and defective glucagon secretion, both of which lead to impaired counterregulation and recovery from hypoglycemia. The decline in glucagon and epinephrine responses greatly diminishes the counterregulatory response and increases the risk for severe hypoglycemia.

- In people with type 1 diabetes, the normal glucagon response begins to deteriorate within 5 years of diagnosis. The epinephrine response declines with increasing duration of type 1 diabetes and may be lost after 15 to 30 years. Absent glucagon and epinephrine responses greatly increase the risk for severe hypoglycemia. The counterregulatory mechanism in type 2 diabetes is largely unknown.[26]

B People with diabetes of long duration may further experience hypoglycemia unawareness due to a lack of the classic adrenergic warning signs of hypoglycemia: anxiety, nervousness, sweating, and palpitations.[40] These patients may instead develop neuroglycopenia when hypoglycemic and become lethargic, irritable, dull, confused, and lose consciousness or have a seizure.[2]

  - A history of hypoglycemia warning symptoms and episodes of hypoglycemia coma should be elicited during patient visits.

  - The costs and benefits of more liberal glucose goals need to be discussed with patients who have hypoglycemia unawareness. Although improved metabolic control may reverse autonomic neuropathy, normoglycemia poses considerable risk for these patients. In general, normal glucose and glycosylated hemoglobin levels are not the therapeutic goal for these patients.[40] Long-acting insulins with only small boluses are generally recommended. These patients may benefit from using rapid-acting insulin (lispro) based on carbohydrate intake given just before or after a meal by injection or an insulin infusion pump.

  - Patient education includes avoidance of hypoglycemia, appropriate treatment, the value of frequent home blood glucose monitoring, caution while driving, and wearing appropriate diabetes identification. Teach family members the signs and treatment of hypoglycemia, including glucagon administration.[2] Blood glucose awareness training may improve functional capacity.[43]

5 Sudomotor dysfunction

  A This type of autonomic neuropathy is commonly manifested by anhidrosis in a stocking-glove pattern with compensatory hyperhidrosis of the face and trunk.[39] Bilateral symmetrical loss of the thermoregulatory response and gustatory sweating in response to foods (cheese, spicy foods) that normally induce salivation may also occur.[40]

   B Patients rarely think to report abnormal sweating. However, this symptom is important because of the potential for heat stroke and foot ulcers. A careful history should be taken and the feet should be examined for dryness and fissures at each visit.[2]

   C Propantheline hydrobromide or scopolamine patches may help to relieve severe gustatory sweating.[40] Dry feet need to be examined for fissures and should be lubricated daily.

   D Patient education includes appropriate foot inspection and care, avoidance of offending foods, and prevention of hyperthermia and heat stroke.

6 Abnormal pupillary response

   A The iris is innervated by both parasympathetic and sympathetic nerve fibers. Sympathetic nerve fibers cause the pupils to dilate and are generally more severely affected. Abnormal pupillary responses are related to duration of diabetes.[44]

   B Slow dilation of pupils in response to darkness may be observed during clinical examination. Patients may report slow adaptation when entering a dark room.

   C Stress using caution during night driving, the importance of turning on lights when entering a dark room, and using nightlights in darkened hallways and bathrooms to help prevent injuries when teaching patients with this syndrome.

OVERVIEW OF FOCAL NEUROPATHIES

1 The various focal neuropathies occur acutely and unpredictably. They are not specific to diabetes and are not thought to be related to duration of diabetes. There are no strategies to prevent these neuropathies or provide early detection, but this is offset by their self-limiting nature.[45]

2 The primary symptom of the focal neuropathies is acute local pain. Abnormal nerve conduction that corresponds to the distribution of a single nerve, multiple peripheral nerves, the brachial or lumbosacral plexus, or nerve roots will be noted. Focal neuropathies often occur in middle-aged patients or those with sensorimotor polyneuropathy.[2] There are four major focal neuropathies.

FOCAL NEUROPATHIES

1 Mononeuropathy and mononeuropathy complex

    A Isolated neuropathies of one or several nerves are more common among people with diabetes.[2] Examples of common mononeuropathies are compression or entrapment of the median nerve of the wrist (carpal tunnel syndrome), the ulnar nerve of the elbow leading to weakness and loss of sensation over the palmer aspect of the 4th and 5th fingers, the radial nerve of the upper arm leading to wrist drop, the lateral cutaneous nerve in the thigh, and the peroneal nerve at the head of the fibula leading to foot drop.[2] The most common mononeuropathy is carpal tunnel syndrome, which occurs three times more often in people with diabetes than in the general population.

    B Diagnosis is based on pain, wrist or foot drop, and abnormal electro-diagnostic studies.[2]

    C Treatment usually consists of surgical release of the nerve, physical therapy, or protection from further trauma using wrist splints, elbow pads, and ankle braces.

2 Plexopathy (femoral neuropathy)

    A The sacral plexus and femoral nerves are generally affected causing a pain that extends from the hip to the anterior and lateral surface of the thigh. Pain is generally worse at night and can cause weakness and wasting of thigh flexion and knee extension muscles.[15] Femoral neuropathy occurs most often among older adults.[2]

    B Nonnarcotic or simple analgesics may be used to relieve pain, which generally remits spontaneously but may recur periodically.[2]

3 Radiculopathy (intercostal neuropathy)

    A This focal neuropathy occurs as a result of damage to the nerve root, and is singular and unilateral with pain localized to the chest or abdominal wall. The patient generally presents with absent cutaneous sensation and pain or dysesthesia that is worse at night. Profound weight loss may also occur.

    B Nonnarcotic or simple analgesics may help control the pain, which generally remits spontaneously in 6 to 24 months.[2]

4 Cranial neuropathy (diabetic ophthalmoplegial)

    A The third cranial nerve is most often affected. The onset is generally abrupt with headache, eye pain, or dysesthesias of the upper lip that precede palsy by several days. Ptosis is marked and the affected person is unable to move the eye, although the pupil is generally spared.[2] Cranial neuropathy occurs most often in older adults.[15]

B Use of an eye patch for the affected eye may be helpful. Pain and oculomotor function will gradually improve after several weeks, with full recovery in 3 to 5 months.[2]

KEY EDUCATIONAL CONSIDERATIONS

1 The importance of foot inspection and care must be emphasized for patients with peripheral neuropathy (see Chapter 16, Skin, Foot and Dental Care, for detailed information).

2 Periodically assess patients with diabetes for the presence of modifiable risk factors for peripheral neuropathy, including hyperglycemia, alcohol abuse, smoking, and hypertension.

A Refer patients to counseling or organizations such as Alcoholics Anonymous if an alcohol abuse problem is identified.

B Discuss the added risk that smoking poses and ascertain the patient's thoughts about stopping. Provide information about local smoking cessation programs. Some patients may find that nicotine patches or gum will help in their attempts to stop smoking.

3 Because some manifestations of neuropathy (eg, sexual dysfunction, incontinence) may be embarrassing for the patient to discuss, tactfully assess these problems during each visit.

4 Inform patients about the symptoms of neuropathy and encourage them to report these symptoms to their provider. This topic can provide the basis for an effective group discussion. However, specific information about the neuropathic symptoms that a patient is experiencing, along with treatment options and approaches, is more effectively provided on an individual basis.

5 Because this content can be difficult to teach and learn, avoid detailed explanations of the complexity of the nervous system. Instead, present a simplified explanation such as, "Some nerves send information about how things feel, others tell the body to move, and others control automatic body functions." Focus teaching on what the patient needs to know (eg, symptoms and treatment) and discuss pathology only as needed. Visual aids can assist patient understanding.

A Reinforce the relationship between hyperglycemia and neuropathic pain, determine the patient's interest, and discuss specific individualized options for improving blood glucose levels.

B Open-ended questions will often yield information about the use of alternative therapies for pain.

C Offer patients options for both nonpharmacological and pharmacological treatment for pain.

D Because most therapies to relieve neuropathic pain take time to work, prepare patients for the delay and encourage them to give the therapies a fair trial.

E The depression that can accompany painful neuropathy may act as a barrier to learning and treatment. Therefore, treatment for depression is needed in conjunction with treatment for neuropathy. Focus teaching on what the patient can do to ease the discomfort and prevent other related problems; include significant others in education and offer options for support.

F Encourage patients with neuropathy to stay informed about new research studies and findings about the treatment of neuropathy.

G Provide education about complications with sensitivity and only after the patient's readiness to hear this information has been determined. Point out the value of early detection and the hope for future treatment of neuropathy.

SELF-REVIEW QUESTIONS

1 Define diabetic neuropathy.

2 List the classifications of peripheral neuropathy and the respective subcategories.

3 Describe the roles of aldose reductase, glucose, myoinositol, and ATPase in the pathology of diabetic neuropathy.

4 List therapies that are available for sensory neuropathies.

5 Describe the major symptoms, clinical manifestations, and treatments for the autonomic neuropathies.

6 What do all patients with diabetes need to know about neuropathy?

CASE STUDY 1

WJ is a 56-year-old African American male with a 10-year history of type 2 diabetes, which has been treated with glyburide 5.0 mg BID for the last 7 years. His HbA$_{1c}$ was 9.4 when measured today. He does not monitor his blood glucose levels at home because his insurance does not cover the cost of strips for non-insulin-requiring persons. He reports some blurred vision but denies any other symptoms of hyperglycemia. WJ is 5'8" (173 cm) tall and weighs 198 lb (90 kg). He was told by his doctor to follow a 1600-calorie ADA diet but states that he is hungry all of the time when he tries this diet; it also doesn't include the food that he likes to eat, particularly ethnic foods. His weight has been stable at about 200 lb (91 kg) since diagnosis. He is married, has three grown children, and works as a carpenter. WJ is a deacon in his church and describes church and family as important to him.

He presents today with burning and tingling sensations in his feet and occasional dizziness on standing. When asked about his greatest concern about his diabetes, he tells you it is that he has "lost his nature" for the past 3 months. His wife calls you aside and tells you that she is concerned because he appears to be depressed and is withdrawing from friends and family. She is also concerned because recently his cigarette smoking has increased to two packs per day. He reports some alcohol intake on social occasions.

On physical examination, WJ has diminished bilateral vibratory and monofilament responses, and dry feet. His sitting blood pressure is 148/84mmHg, supine is 136/82, and standing is 100/76. His fasting blood glucose is 196. When asked, he tells you he takes care of his feet by soaking them in vinegar once per week.

QUESTIONS FOR DISCUSSION

1 What information does WJ need to address his educational concerns?
2 What are strategies you can use to address his psychosocial concerns?

Discussion

1   Provide information about the potential costs and benefits of improved glycemic control. If he is interested, offer WJ options for achieving better blood glucose control through an individualized meal plan, addition of an insulin-sensitizing agent, or initiation of insulin therapy.

2   Offer WJ a referral for a new meal plan that better fits his lifestyle and preferred/cultural eating patterns, or to safely initiate insulin therapy. Because his wife does the shopping and cooking for the family, offering her the option of attending this session is likely be helpful to WJ.

3   Offer to provide self-management education about
    A   Neuropathy
    B   Foot care, emphasizing lubrication, appropriate footwear, and daily inspection. Point out that soaking and use of vinegar may cause dryness.
    C   Home blood glucose monitoring, including resources for strips.
    E   Safety issues related to carpentry work, particularly protecting feet and legs.

4   Determine whether WJ understands the impact of smoking on neuropathy and health in general. If he is interested, provide information about methods and support that are available for smoking cessation.

5   Offer a referral to a urologist, for further assessment of impotence.

6   Offer referral to a social worker for evaluation and nonpharmacological treatment of depression, and/or to a physician for pharmacological treatment of depression. Ask if his minister could be helpful with this issue and offer referral to a diabetes support group.

CASE STUDY 2

SH is as 36-year-old female who has had type 1 diabetes for 22 years. When she comes to the clinic, you notice that she has several fading bruises and is wearing a cervical collar. She tells you that she was recently in an automobile accident while on her way to pick up her children at school. She states that she had no warning signals of hypoglycemia and has no memory of the accident. Witnesses said that SH was driving erratically prior to the accident and was very confused when the ambulance arrived. Her blood glucose was 26 mg/dL in the emergency room, so she assumes that a low blood glucose level caused her collision.

Her husband is with her for this visit and is very concerned for her safety and that of their children because she frequently drives them to school and various activities. He is also concerned because her diabetes was not recognized initially by the paramedics who did not notice her medical identification bracelet. He tells you that he has had to tell her on several occasions that her blood glucose is low based on her behavior, but she had not noticed any symptoms. The most recent episode occurred last night, shortly after dinner. SH usually treats her hypoglycemia with a regular soft drink, but has noticed that her blood glucose level doesn't always respond as quickly as in the past.

While reviewing SH's blood glucose records you notice fairly wide variations in her glucose levels. She attributes these variations to the stress of her new part-time job. She denies nausea and vomiting but tells you that sometimes she has to force herself to eat all of the food in her meal plan because she feels full.

QUESTIONS FOR DISCUSSION

1　What information does SH need related to her safety?
2　What additional information is needed to better assess the potential causes of SH's hypoglycemia?

DISCUSSION

1 Provide information to SH and her husband about hypoglycemia unawareness, treatments other than beverages (glucose gel or tubes of cake icing), glucagon administration, training in recognition of subtle symptoms and the need for frequent blood glucose monitoring.

2 Discuss steps with SH that she can take to protect herself and others while driving, including testing her blood glucose prior to driving to be sure that it is over 100 mg/dL, testing frequently during extended driving times, carrying a form of treatment at all times, and having more visible diabetes identification.

3 Address SH's concerns and those of her husband about her safety when he is not available. Determine her comfort with providing co-workers and children with information about the signs of hypoglycemia and actions to take if they notice these signs.

4 Assess the cause of SH's erratic blood glucose levels through more comprehensive recordkeeping that includes the times and amounts of food eaten, timing, types and doses of insulin, and activity and stress levels. Review these records after 2 to 3 weeks, and consider gastric emptying studies if the erratic glucose levels do not appear to be related to these other factors.

REFERENCES

1 Greene DA, Sima AAF, Pfeifer MA, Albers JW. Diabetic neuropathy. Annu Rev Med 1990;41:303-17.

2 Herman WA, Greene DA. Microvascular complications of diabetes. In: Haire-Joshu D, ed. Management of diabetes mellitus. 2nd ed. St. Louis: CV Mosby, 1996:234-80.

3 Greene DA, Stevens MJ. Diabetic peripheral neuropathy: new approaches to treatment, classification and staging, introduction. Diabetes Spectrum 1993; 6:234-35.

4 American Diabetes Association. Consensus statement. Diabetic neuropathy. Diabetes Care 1996;19(suppl 1):S67-71.

5 Dyck PJ, Karnes J, O'Brien PC. Diagnosis, staging, and classification of diabetic neuropathy and associations with other complications. In: Dyck PJ, Thomas PK, Asbury AK, Winegrad AI, Porte D, eds. Diabetic neuropathy. Philadelphia: WB Saunders, 1987.

6 Asbury AK. Focal and multifocal neuropathies of diabetes. In: Dyck PJ, Thomas PK, Asbury AK, Winegrad AI, Porte D, eds. Diabetic neuropathy, Philadelphia: WB Saunders, 1987.

7 Melton LJ, Dyck PJ, Karnes J, O'Brien PC. Epidemiology. In: Dyck PJ, Thomas PK, Asbury AK, Winegrad AI, Porte D, eds. Diabetic neuropathy. Philadelphia: WB Saunders, 1987:27-35.

8 Pirart J. Diabetes mellitus and its degenerative complications: a prospective study of 4,400 patients observed between 1947 and 1973. Diabetes Care 1978;1:168-88, 252-63.

9 Dyck PJ, Kratz KM, Lehman JL, et al. The prevalence by staged severity of various types of diabetic neuropathy, retinopathy, and nephropathy in a population-based cohort: the Rochester Diabetic Neuropathy Study. Neurology 1993;43:817-24.

10 Fedele D, Comi G, Coscelli C, et al. A multicenter study on the prevalence of diabetic neuropathy in Italy. Diabetes Care 1997;20:836-43.

11 Harati Y. Frequently asked questions about diabetic peripheral neuropathies. Neurol Clin 1992;10:783-807.

12 Palumbo PJ, Elveback LR, Whisnant JP. Neurologic complications of diabetes mellitus: transient ischemic attack, stroke, and peripheral neuropathy. Adv Neurol 1978;19:593-601.

13 Harris M, Eastman R, Cowie C. Symptoms of sensory neuropathy in adults with NIDDM in the US population. Diabetes Care 1993;16:1446-52.

14 Clark DW, Nowak TV. Diabetic gastroparesis. Postgrad Med 1994; 95: 195-198,201-204.

15 McDaid EA, Monahan B, Parker AI, Hayes JR, Allen JA. Peripheral autonomic impairment in patients newly diagnosed with type II diabetes. Diabetes Care 1994;17:1422-27.

16 Broadstone VL, Cyrus J, Pfiefer MA, Greene DA. Diabetic peripheral neuropathy part I: sensorimotor neuropathies. Diabetes Educ 1987;13: 30-35.

17 Dolman CL. The morbid anatomy of diabetic neuropathy. Neurology 1963; 13:135-142.

18 Greene DA, Sima AAF, Stevens MJ, Feldman EL, Lattimer SA. Complications: neuropathy, pathogenic considerations. Diabetes Care 1992;15:1902-25.

19 Rollo J. Cases of diabetes mellitus. London: C. Dilly, 1798.

20 The Diabetes Control and Complications Trial Research Group. The effect of intensive treatment of diabetes on the development and progression of long-term complications in insulin-dependent diabetes mellitus. New Engl J Med 1993; 329:977-86.

21 Clements RS Jr. Diabetic neuropathy - new concepts of its etiology. Diabetes 1979;28:604-611.

22 Sands ML, Shetterly SM, Franklin GM, Hamman RF. Incidence of distal symmetric (sensory) neuropathy in NIDDM. Diabetes Care 1997; 20:322-29.

23 American Diabetes Association. Position statement. Implications of the diabetes control and complications trial. Diabetes Care 1998;21(suppl 1):S88-90.

24 Nathan DM. Inferences and implications: do the results from the Diabetes Control and Complications Trial apply in NIDDM? Diabetes Care 1995; 18:251-57.

25 Franklin GM, Shetterly SM, Cohen JA, Baxter J, Hamman RF. Risk factors for distal symmetric neuropathy in NIDDM. Diabetes Care 1994; 17:1172-77.

26 Greene DA, Sima AAF, Albers JW, Pfiefer MA. Diabetic neuropathy. In: Ellenberg and Rifkin's diabetes mellitus: theory and practice. 4th ed. New York: Elsevier Publishing Co, 1990.

27 Partanen J, Niskanen L, Lehtinen J, Mervaala E, Siitonen O, Uusitupa M. Natural history of peripheral neuropathy in patients with non-insulin-dependent diabetes mellitus. N Engl J Med 1995; 333:89-94.

28 Vinik AI, Milicevic Z, Pittenger GL. Beyond glycemia. Diabetes Care 1995; 18:1037-41.

29 Calissi P, Jaber L. Peripheral diabetic neuropathy: current concepts in treatment. Ann Pharmacother 1995; 29:769-77.

30 Feldman EL, Stevens MJ, Thomas PK, Brown MB, Canal N, Greene DA. A practical two-step quantitative clinical and electrophysiological assessment for the diagnosis and staging of diabetic neuropathy. Diabetes Care 1994; 17:1281-89.

31 Rith-Najarian SJ, Stolusky T, Gohdes DM. Identifying diabetic patients at high risk for lower-extremity amputation in a primary health care setting. Diabetes Care 1992;15:1386-89.

32 Levitt NS, Stansberry KB, Wynchank S, Vinik AI. The natural progression of autonomic neuropathy and autonomic function tests in a cohort of people with IDDM. Diabetes Care 1996;19:751-54.

33 Britland ST, Young RJ, Sharma AK, Clarke BF. Association of painful and painless diabetic polyneuropathy with different patterns of nerve fiber degeneration and regeneration. Diabetes 1990;39:898-908.

34 McQuay HJ, Tramer M, Nye BA, Carroll D, Wiffen PJ, Moore RA. A systematic review of antidepressants in neuropathic pain. Pain 1996; 68(2-3):217-27.

35 Capsaicin Study Group. Effect of treatment with capsaicin on daily activities of patients with painful diabetic neuropathy. Diabetes Care 1992; 15:159-65.

36 Pfeifer MA, Ross DR, Schrage JP, et al. A highly successful and novel model for treatment of chronic painful diabetic neuropathy. Diabetes Care 1993; 16:1103-15.

37 Giugliano D, Acampora R, Marfella F, et al. Tolrestat in the primary prevention of diabetic neuropathy. Diabetes Care 1995;18:536-41.

38 Sinha S, Munichoodapa CS, Kozak GP. Neuro-arthropathy (Charcot's joint) in diabetes mellitus: clinical study of 101 cases. Medicine (Baltimore) 1972; 51:191-210.

39 Cyrus J, Broadstone VL, Pfeifer MA, Greene DA. Diabetic peripheral neuropathy part II: autonomic neuropathies. Diabetes Educ 1987;13:111-15.

40 Vinik AI, Holland MT, LeBeau JM, Liuzzi FJ, Stansberry KB, Colen LB. Diabetic neuropathies. Diabetes Care 1992; 15:1926-75.

41 Haines ST. Treating constipation in the patient with diabetes. Diabetes Educ 1995;21:223-32.

42 Gilden JL. Orthostatic hypotension in the patient with diabetes. Practical Diabetol 1996;15(3):28-31, 34.

43 Cox, DJ Gonder-Frederick, Julian DM, Clark, W. Long-term follow up evaluation of blood glucose awareness training. Diabetes Care 1994;17:1-5.

44 Straub RH, Zietz B, Palitzsch K-D, Scholmerich J. Impact of disease duration on cardiovascular and pupillary autonomic nervous function in IDDM and NIDDM patients. Diabetes Care 1996;19:960-67.

45 Stevens MJ, Feldman EL, Funnell MM, Sima AAF, Greene DA. Optimal methods for detecting early neuropathy and its progression. In: Morgenstern CE, Standl E, eds. Concepts for the ideal diabetes clinic. Vol IV. Berlin: deGruyter Publications, 1993:315-32.

SUGGESTED READINGS

Albert L. Restraining pain. Diabetes Forecast 1988;41(1):39-41.

Barnett JL. Will the nausea ever end? Diabetes Forecast 1997;50(7):31-35.

Barnett JL. Taking care of constipation. Diabetes Forecast 1992; 45(5):25-27.

Bernstein G. Gastroparesis: dealing with a sluggish stomach. Diabetes Self-Manage 1997;14(2):62-65.

Campbell RK, Baker DE. New drug update: capsaicin. Diabetes Educ 1990; 16:313-14, 316.

Cohen SN. Treating impotence. Diabetes Forecast 1991; 44(12):54-57.

Cowley EP, Haines ST. Return to a regular life. Diabetes Forecast 1996; 49(12):42-48.

Cronin B. Nutritional concerns in gastrointestinal neuropathy. Diabetes Educ 1992;18:531-35.

Fogel CI. Sexuality and diabetes: an issue for both sexes. Diabetes Spectrum 1991;4:13-40.

Funnell MM, McNitt PM. Autonomic neuropathy. Am J Nurs 1986;86: 266-70.

Graham C. Neuropathy made you stop? Diabetes Forecast 1992; 45(12):47-49.

Greene DA, Stevens MJ. Diabetic peripheral neuropathy: new approaches to treatment, classification and staging. Diabetes Spectrum 1993;6:234-57.

Haire-Joshu D. Smoking cessation and the diabetes health care team. Diabetes Educ 1991;17:54-64.

Ivy J. Exercise and complications. Diabetes Forecast 1990;43(2):46-49.

Lagana DJ. Female sexuality: separating fact from fiction. Diabetes Self-Management 1992;9(4):40-42.

Leese DL. Diabetic cranial mononeuropathies: a patient's perspective. Diabetes Educ 1988;14:527-31.

Lorber DL. Complications of diabetes: neuropathy. Practical Diabetol 1994; 13(3):15-22.

Lyrenas EB, Olsson EHK, Arvidsson UC, Orn TJ, Spjuth JH. Prevalence and determinants of solid and liquid gastric emptying in unstable type I diabetes. Diabetes Care 1997;20:413-18.

Maser RE, Becker DJ et al. Pittsburgh epidemiology of diabetes complications study. Diabetes Care 1992;15:525-27.

Merio R, Festa A, Bergmann H, et al. Slow gastric emptying in type I diabetes: relation to autonomic and peripheral neuropathy, blood glucose, and glycemic control. Diabetes Care 1997; 20:419-23.

O'Dorisio TM, Cataland S. Gastrointestinal autonomic neuropathy. Diabetes Spectrum 1992;5:147-72.

Sands ML, Shetterly SM, Franklin GM, Hamman RF. Incidence of distal symmetric (sensory) neuropathy in NIDDM. Diabetes Care 1997;20:322-29.

Schover LR. Women, sexuality and diabetes. Diabetes Forecast 1992; 45(8):59-61.

Wakelee-Lynch J. Relieving pain with peppers. Diabetes Forecast 1992; 45(6):35-37.

Wyeth-Ayerst Consensus Conference. Proceedings of a consensus development conference on standardized measures in diabetic neuropathy. Diabetes Care 1992;15:1079-1107.

Yeap BB, Russo A, Faser RJ, Wittert GA, Horowitz M. Hyperglycemia affects cardiovascular autonomic nerve function in normal subjects. Diabetes Care 1996;19:880-82.

COMPLICATIONS

Nephropathy 23

Kristina L. Ernst, BSN, RN, CDE
Grady Health System Diabetes Clinic
Atlanta, Georgia

INTRODUCTION

1 The fight against diabetic complications requires a long-term or even life-long strategy. Diabetic nephropathy, the kidney disease associated with diabetes mellitus, is characterized clinically by albuminuria, hypertension, and progressive renal insufficiency.[1] In individuals with type 1 diabetes diabetic nephropathy is the leading cause of death and a major risk factor for cardiovascular disease.

2 Diabetes has become the most common single cause of end-stage renal disease (ESRD) in the United States and Europe. ESRD is a debilitating condition that requires renal replacement (ie, dialysis), or a kidney transplant. In the US, diabetic nephropathy accounts for approximately one-third of all cases of ESRD, and the cost for treatment of diabetic patients with ESRD is in excess of $2 billion annually.[2]

3 The number of new ESRD patients has increased dramatically at an average rate of 7.8% annually.[3]

   A The growth in the number of ESRD patients has been particularly dramatic in the elderly. Individuals over age 60 years represent 55% of all incident cases.

   B Racial differences also exist; incidence rates for African Americans, Hispanics (especially Mexican Americans), and Native Americans are three to six times higher than rates among non-Hispanic Caucasians.[4]

4 Caring for patients with diabetic nephropathy is challenging and requires expertise and services from the following disciplines: medicine, nutrition, nursing, mental health, social services, surgery, pharmacy, podiatry, and rehabilitation.

   A Studies[5] have demonstrated that the onset and course of diabetic nephropathy can be ameliorated to a very significant degree by attaining and maintaining glycemic and blood pressure control, but these interventions have their greatest impact if instituted very early in the course of this complication.

   B Striving to inform and involve patients and families is critical to health promotion and treatment during all phases of kidney disease and interventions.

5 The following interventions are aimed at optimizing health and quality of life for the patient with diabetes who has renal disease:

    A Controlling blood pressure and blood glucose levels

    B Preventing insults to the kidney

    C Using an angiotension-converting enzyme (ACE) Inhibitor

    D Decreasing dietary protein intake

    E Treating the symptomatic anemia of kidney disease with erythropoietin

6 When renal replacement therapy is required, careful consideration of individual needs must be incorporated into the decision-making process. Current options in uremia therapy include

    A No therapy (resulting in death)

    B Hemodialysis

    C Peritoneal dialysis

    D Kidney transplant

    E Simultaneous kidney-pancreas transplant for people with type 1 diabetes

7 Self-management education and medical and nutritional management are incorporated into both intervention and renal replacement modalities. Regardless of the stage of renal disease or type of renal replacement therapy, both the patient and the healthcare team must recognize that the patient's diabetes still requires daily attention, and that education, medical care, and meal planning will be integral components of that management.

8 Detection of microalbuminuria before diabetic nephropathy is clinically evident allows for early interventions that prevent the onset or slow the progression of microvascular disease.[6]

OBJECTIVES

Upon completion of this chapter, the learner will be able to

1 Discuss the epidemiology of diabetic nephropathy and end-stage renal disease.

2 Describe the basic functions of the kidney.

3 Describe the major stages in the natural progression of diabetic nephropathy.

4 List diagnostic tests used to assess and monitor renal function.

5 Review treatment modalities for diabetic nephropathy.

6 List treatment options for renal replacement therapy.

KEY DEFINITIONS

1 *Blood urea nitrogen (BUN)* The blood level of urea which is the end product of protein metabolism and is formed in the liver. After synthesis, urea travels through the blood and is excreted in the urine. The normal plasma value of urea is 8 to 20 mg/dL (2.9 to 7.1 mmol/L), varying with the quantity and quality of protein intake, state of hydration, and kidney function. The blood level rises as kidney function deteriorates.

2 *Creatinine (Cr).* A nitrogen compound formed mainly from the metabolism of muscle. The daily production rate of creatinine is relatively constant in an individual. The normal plasma value is 0.5 to 1.4 mg/dL (44 to 124 µmol/L), varying with body size and gender; males have higher levels than females. Serum creatinine rises as kidney function deteriorates.

3 *Creatinine clearance (CrCl).* The rate at which creatinine is removed from the blood by the kidney and is used as an estimate of glomerular filtration rate (GFR) and an approximate measure of kidney function. Creatinine clearance is used clinically (rather than GFR) because it is more easily determined. To calculate CrCl, a timed urine specimen and a serum or plasma sample are required. Since the clearance depends on protein intake, CrCl is a reflection of the individual's diet in the absence of renal disease. The CrCl of a typical Western diet in an adult male is 100 to 120 mL/minute. The clearance is slightly lower in females probably because they have less muscle mass, which is where creatinine is formed.

4 *Microalbuminuria* An abnormal excretion of slightly increased quantities of urinary albumin. An albumin excretion rate (AER) of up to 30 mg/24 hours is considered normal. Persistent microalbuminuria (30 to 300 mg/day or 20 to 200 µ/minute measured on three different occasions) is often the first laboratory evidence of kidney damage.

5 *Glomerulus.* The filtering component of the nephron. It is a tuft of capillaries in which filtration of blood takes place. A kidney biopsy will show structural changes in the glomerulus in a patient with diabetic nephropathy.

6 *Glomerular basement membrane.* A selectively permeable structure located between the glomerular capillaries and Bowman's capsule that serves as a dialyzing membrane to regulate the passage of water and solutes.

7 *Glomerular filtration.* A process that initiates the production of urine with the formation of an ultrafiltrate as blood passes through the glomerular capillaries.

8 *Glomerular filtration rate (GFR).* The rate at which the kidney produces glomerular filtrate. GFR represents the amount of fluid that passes from the blood into the capsular space over a given period of time. Normal GFR is ~100 to 125 mL/minute. This rate is determined using a precise technique that measures the renal clearance of a marker substance; GFR values are used primarily in research. GFR decreases with aging, the presence of kidney or vascular diseases, sodium and water depletion, hemorrhage, and vigorous exercise. The rate increases with dietary protein intake, hyperglycemia, and pregnancy. Repeated measurements of GFR over time provide more useful information than a single value.

9 *Mesangium* The central core tissue in the glomerulus, bounded by the capillary endothelium and the glomerular basement membrane. The mesangium may play a role in regulating glomerular blood flow.

10 *Nephrons.* The functional unit of the kidneys that serves to clear the blood of waste materials and form urine. Each kidney contains about 1 million nephrons. Each nephron consists of a glomerulus leading to a long tubule in which the filtrate is concentrated and modified before it is eliminated as urine.

11 *Proteinuria.* A urinary albumin excretion (UAE) rate of ≥300 mg/24 hours or 500 mg/24 hours of total protein in the urine. Persistent proteinuria indicates progression to clinical or overt nephropathy.

12 *Nephrotic syndrome.* A state characterized by urinary protein excretion >3.5 g/24 hours, edema, hypercholesterolemia, and hypoalbuminemia Typically the rate of protein excretion can increase from 4 to 30 g protein/ 24 hours, resulting in low blood proteins and massive fluid retention. Weight gain and peripheral edema are common clinical manifestations of nephrotic syndrome. Although many people with diabetes manifest nephrotic range proteinuria, true nephrotic syndrome occurs in only 10 to 20% of patients.

13 *Uremia.* A syndrome characteristic of ESRD that develops as renal function declines, causing an accumulation of urea, creatinine, and other metabolic waste products in the blood. This extra amount of urea results in anemia, osteodystrophy, neuropathy, and acidosis. Nausea, hypertension, susceptibility to infection, and generalized organ dysfunction frequently accompany this syndrome.

14 *End-stage renal disease (ESRD).* The term used to describe advanced kidney failure. Renal replacement therapy (eg, dialysis or transplantation) must be implemented for life to continue.

RENAL PHYSIOLOGY

1 Normally, people have two kidneys located posterior to the abdominal cavity. Each kidney is the size and shape of an Idaho potato, weighs approximately 5 oz (150g), and contains about 1.25 million nephrons.

2 Urine formation begins in the glomerulus. Blood from the systemic circulation enters each glomerulus through its afferent arteriole and exits through its efferent arteriole. The kidneys help to maintain the internal environment of the body by regulating the quality of plasma.

3 Blood flow to the kidneys is approximately 1300 mL/minute and accounts for 25% of the cardiac output.

4 The kidney, which is an excretory organ, performs several important metabolic and endocrine functions:[7]
  A Removal of water, urea, creatinine and other metabolic wastes and toxins from the body (ie, formation of urine)
  B Maintenance of blood volume
  C Preservation of acid-base and electrolyte (sodium, potassium) balance
  D Regulation of blood pressure
  E Synthesis of erythropoietin, a hormone that stimulates and regulates the production of red blood cells
  F Formation of 1,25 vitamin D

Incidence and Prevalence of Diabetic Nephropathy

1 The United States Renal Data Systems (USRDS) collects information about ESRD in the United States.[4,6]

  A Diabetes is the most common cause of ESRD in the US.

  B There are currently over 80 500 prevalent cases of ESRD caused by diabetes, accounting for almost 37% of all new cases of ESRD.[4]

  C Over 15 000 new patients are enrolled in the ESRD program annually.

2 The incidence rate of ESRD among patients with diabetes has been increasing at a striking rate.[4]

3 The incidence of ESRD among persons with diabetes increased twelve-fold in the group over age 45 years. This increase likely reflects the prevalence of type 2 diabetes as a frequent cause of ESRD in this age group.

  A African Americans with diabetes are four to five times more likely to develop ESRD than Caucasians with diabetes.[4,8]

  B Hispanics and Native Americans have an incidence of diabetic ESRD that is 6.3 times higher than Caucasians with diabetes.[3,4]

4 Renal failure occurs in about 30% to 40% of persons with type 1 diabetes within a mean time of approximately 30 years after diagnosis (Figure 23.1). Individuals who do not develop microalbuminuria or other clinical signs of nephropathy after 25 to 30 years of diabetes are unlikely to develop nephropathy.

5 Renal failure occurs in 20% to 30% of patients with type 2 diabetes and accounts for 60% of the prevalent cases of diabetes-related ESRD.[9]

  A The natural history of nephropathy in type 2 diabetes is less well defined than in type 1 diabetes. Uncertain duration of diabetes and coexisting conditions, including hypertension, make it more difficult to isolate the role of diabetes in ESRD in type 2 diabetes.

  B In some individuals, microalbuminuria or proteinuria is present at the time of diagnosis of type 2 diabetes, perhaps reflecting a long period of unrecognized hyperglycemia.

  C The morphological changes in type 2 diabetic nephropathy are also similar to those of type 1 and include renal hypertrophy, glomerular basement membrane thickening, mesangial expansion, and diffuse intercapillary glomerulosclerosis.

FIGURE 23.1. NATURAL HISTORY OF NEPHROPATHY IN TYPE 1 DIABETES

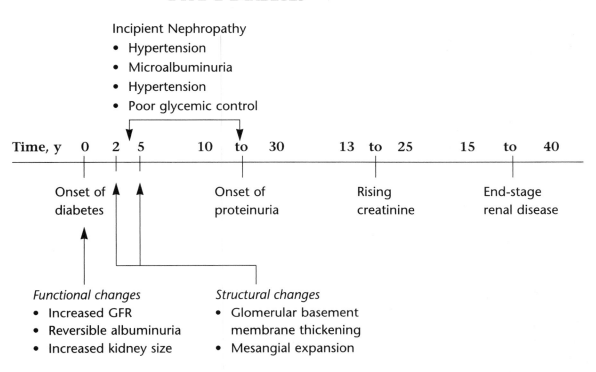

Source: Adapted from Selby JV et al[10] and Breyer JA.[11]

STAGES IN THE DEVELOPMENT OF RENAL CHANGES

1 Mogensen et al[12] proposed five distinct stages of renal changes in the course of diabetic nephropathy in type 1 diabetes (Tables 23.1 and 23.2).

   A Stage 1 is characterized by hyperfiltration and renal hypertrophy.

   • These changes frequently are seen at the time of diagnosis of diabetes.

   • Near normal glycemic control at this stage has been shown to restore alterations in kidney function and size.

   B Stage 2 involves structural changes, including glomerular basement membrane thickening and mesangial expansion.

   • Renal hyperfunction and hypertrophy are detectable on biopsy and progress silently over several years.[12]

   • These structural changes appear to initiate the decline in renal function. GFR is elevated and may be related to suboptimal glycemic control.

Table 23.1. Stages of Renal Disease in Patients with Type 1 Diabetes

Stage	Characteristics	Onset	% Progressing to Next Stage (without treatment)
1	*Functional changes* • Early hypertrophy and hyperfiltration	Onset of diabetes	100%
2	*Structural changes* • Renal lesions	2 to 3 years	35% to 40%
3	*Incipient nephropathy*	7 to 15 years	80% to 100%
4	*Overt nephropathy* • Proteinuria	10 to 30 years	50% to 75%
5	End-stage renal disease	20 to 40 years	75% to 100%

Source: Adapted from Selby JV, et al[10] and Mogensen CE, et al.[12]

C Stage 3, incipient diabetic nephropathy, develops after 7 to 15 years of diabetes duration when microalbuminuria first appears.

- Functional and structural renal alterations lead to abnormal filtration of microscopic amounts of protein into the urine. Once albumin excretion rate exceeds 70 μg/minute, GFR begins to fall.
- Blood pressure during this stage may be normal or slightly elevated; patients are generally asymptomatic.
- The presence of microalbuminuria in type 1 diabetes appears to be a strong predictor of clinical or overt diabetic nephropathy.

D Stage 4 is overt (clinical) diabetic nephropathy.

- Abnormal filtration of protein increases progressively and becomes persistent in this stage.
- Without intervention, GFR declines at the rate of 1 mL/min/month.
- Nephrotic syndrome and hypertension are usually present. Suboptimal blood pressure and glucose control are positively correlated with the rate of GFR decline.

E Stage 5, end-stage renal disease, develops in 75% to 100% of patients with overt nephropathy within 20 years.[6]

- GFR is less than 15 mL/minute and uremia is present.
- Usually, patients with a serum creatinine level greater than 5 mg/dL (>442 μmol/L) are unable to resume their normal activities because of signs and symptoms of uremia (Table 23.3).

TABLE 23.2. PROGRESSION OF RENAL DISEASE IN TYPE 1 DIABETES

	At Diagnosis	Early Renal Changes	Incipient Nephropathy	Clinical Nephropathy	ESRD
GFR	↑HF	HF, ↑GFR	Still HF initially, ↓GFR	Fall rate: 2 mL per year, HF likely	Close to zero
UAER	High* or normal	HF (total normal, but slightly ↑ <30 mg/day)	↑microalbuminuria	↑proteinuria	↑proteinuria
BP or hypertension	BP usually normal	↑BP (in ~5% to 10% of individuals)	BP increasing 3% per year	BP ↑7% per year	High BP
	Metabolic and hemodynamic change, plus hyperphagia	Metabolic changes ↑glycemia ↑ARI ↑hormones	Metabolic changes ↑glycemia ↑ARI ↑hormones	Metabolic changes ↑glycemia ↑ARI ↑hormones	Nephron closure
		Hemodynamic changes Normal BP, intrarenal HT likely	Hemodynamic changes Systemic, intrarenal HT	Hemodynamic changes Systemic, intrarenal HT	
Other concomitant abnormalities	↑HBA1c, many metabolic changes	Possibly hyperperfusion	Retinopathy, neuropathy, lipid and vascular disease in general	As in incipient nephropathy with increasing severity	Uremia
Main structural counterparts	Hypertrophy of nephrons	Hypertrophy of nephron, Basement membrane thickening after ~2 years, mesangial expansion after ~5 years	Microalbuminuria associated with more advanced ultrastructural lesions	Advancing structural lesion, especially mesangial expansion, glomerular closure	Nephron closure

ESRD = end-stage renal disease, GFR = glomerular filtration rate, UAER = urinary albumin excretion rate, BP = blood pressure, HF = hyperfiltration, HT = hypertension, ARI = aldose reductase activity, BM = basement membrane
*Reversible
Source: Adapted with permission from Mogensen CE et al.[12]

- Patients with diabetes are clinically sicker at equivalent levels of kidney dysfunction than patients without diabetes.

Other Considerations in the Progression of Renal Disease

1 One-fourth to one-third of injected insulin is catabolized by the kidney. As kidney function declines, exogenous insulin acts longer and in an unpredictable manner, characterized by recurrent or severe hypoglycemia in some patients. The use of multiple daily insulin injections and hypoglycemia awareness training may reduce the frequency and severity of hypoglycemic episodes.

2 Management and rehabilitation of these patients are further complicated by the fact that more than 95% of patients with diabetic nephropathy have some degree of retinopathy, with 50% being blind or having lost significant vision (renal-retinal syndrome).

4 The prognostic significance of microalbuminuria and proteinuria in patients with type 2 diabetes indicates increased cardiovascular mortality.

5 70% to 80% of patients with diabetes do not develop ESRD and may live without significant renal complications throughout their lives.[4,6]

Table 23.3. Signs and Symptoms of Uremia

- Anorexia
- Nausea
- Vomiting
- Anemia
- Acidosis
- Pruritus
- Dyspnea
- Lethargy
- Hypertension
- Fluctuating blood glucose levels

Pathogenesis of Diabetic Nephropathy

1 Hyperglycemia plays a role in the pathogenesis of diabetic nephropathy (Table 23.4).

  A Alteration in tubuloglomerular feedback occurs, resulting in renal vasodilation, increased renal blood flow, and hyperfiltration.

B Abnormalities in polyol (eg, sorbitol) metabolism occur.

   • Because the kidney does not require insulin for glucose uptake, excess glucose in renal tissue is metabolized by aldose reductase through the polyol pathway to sorbitol. This action initiates a chain of biochemical alterations that lead to depletion of tissue myoinositol concentrations in the glomerulus.

C Accelerated formation of nonenzymatic advanced glycosylation endproducts (AGEs) in tissues is directly correlated with hyperglycemia.

   • An increase in circulating AGE peptides parallels the severity of renal dysfunction in diabetic nephropathy.

   • Glycosylation of proteins in the capillary basement membrane may stimulate mesangial growth leading to mesangial expansion.

   • Glycation of albumin can also contribute to its loss across the glomerular basement membrane.

2 Other hormonal imbalances, aside from insufficient insulin, have been implicated in the pathogenesis of diabetic nephropathy (Table 23.4).

   A Growth hormone and glucagon, which are both elevated in poorly controlled diabetes, have been shown to produce glomerular hyperfiltration.

   B Increased levels of atrial natriuretic factor (ANF) may also contribute to glomerular hyperfiltration, perhaps as a result of chronic plasma volume expansion.

   C Changes in circulating levels of angiotensin II, catecholamines, and prostaglandins, or altered responsiveness to these vasoactive hormones may also result in hyperfiltration. It is theorized[13] that angiotensin II may promote cellular and glomerular hypertrophy, as well as mesangial expansion.

3 Renal hemodynamic changes play a role in the pathogenesis of diabetic nephropathy (Table 23.4). Defects in glomerular cellular metabolism lead to hemodynamic changes in the kidney.[14]

   A Glomerular hypertension contributes to increased pressure and flow across the glomerular membrane, resulting in hyperfiltration.

   B Glomerular hypertension and the associated renal vasodilation and hyperfiltration increase transglomerular protein filtration, leading to proteinuria and mesangial deposition of circulating proteins.

   C Mesangial expansion and glomerulosclerosis result in destruction of nephrons. Unaffected nephrons must then work harder.

D In response to the destruction of nephrons, a positive feedback stimulus for compensatory hyperfiltration is initiated, with further increasing GFR and progressive renal injury.

E Self-destruction of the surviving glomeruli occurs. Glomerular hypertension mediates the progressive destruction of nephrons.[15]

TABLE 23.4. THEORIES OF THE PATHOGENESIS OF DIABETIC NEPHROPATHY

Hyperglycemia	• Alterations in tubuloglomerular feedback • Abnormalities in polyol (eg, sorbitol) metabolism • Advanced glycosylation end-products (AGEs)
Hormonal Imbalances	• Decreased insulin • Increased growth hormone and glucagon • Altered concentrations of or responsiveness to vasoactive hormones – Angiotensin II – Catecholamines – Prostaglandins
Renal Hemodynamic Changes	• Glomerular hypertension • Glomerular hyperfiltration

RISK FACTORS FOR DIABETIC NEPHROPATHY

1 Multiple factors have been identified that place individuals at increased risk of diabetic nephropathy, including hypertension, genetic predisposition, smoking, increased dietary protein intake, and poor glycemic control. No single risk factor is consistently associated with all cases; a combination of risk factors are likely to be responsible for increasing the risk for diabetic nephropathy.

A Hypertension is twice as prevalent among individuals with type 1 and type 2 diabetes than in the nondiabetic population.

• Diabetic nephropathy increases the risk of hypertension, and hypertension exacerbates the progression of diabetic nephropathy.[16]

• Clinical hypertension is uncommon at the time of diagnosis of type 1 diabetes, whereas blood pressure is frequently elevated at the time of diagnosis in type 2 diabetes.

- Adequate systemic blood pressure control[17] and use of ACE inhibitors have been shown to independently reduce the rate of progression of early diabetic renal disease in randomized, controlled trials of persons with type 2 diabetes.[18,19]

B Hyperglycemia is one of the most important risk factors for persistent proteinuria; the level of fasting hyperglycemia at the time of diagnosis is associated with subsequent chronic renal failure in type 2 diabetes. The rate of progression of diabetic nephropathy in type 1 diabetes can be significantly reduced by optimizing glycemic control, as evidenced in the Diabetes Control and Complications Trial (DCCT)[20] and the Stockholm Diabetes Intervention Study.[21]

C Genetic predisposition to hypertension, including a positive family history of hypertension and renal disease, as well as susceptibility to nephropathy in patients with type 1 diabetes has been identified by Krolewski et al.[22]

D Diabetic nephropathy is more common among African American, Hispanic and Native American persons with type 2 diabetes than among Caucasians. This is reflected in an overall incidence of ESRD in type 2 diabetes that is significantly higher in the US than in Europe.

E A high-protein diet has been shown to increase both renal size and GFR.
- Increases in GFR, or hyperfiltration, occur early in diabetic nephropathy.
- Hyperfiltration increases intrarenal pressure within the glomerulus and is believed to be instrumental in the destruction of the kidneys.

F Non-modifiable risk factors:
- Duration of diabetes
- Age at diagnosis
- Male gender
- Family history of nephropathy

DIAGNOSIS AND RENAL FUNCTIONS TESTS

1 Individuals are asymptomatic throughout the early stages of diabetic nephropathy.

2 Diagnostic tests focus on early detection of microalbuminuria.

A Annual screening for microalbuminuria in type 1 diabetes should begin with puberty and after a 5-year disease duration. Among people with type 2 diabetes, screening for microalbuminuria should begin at the time of diagnosis (Figure 23.2). Screening for microalbuminuria can be performed by three methods[6]:

- Measurement of the albumin-to-creatinine ratio in a random spot urine collection.
- 24-hour urine collection with creatinine, allowing simultaneous measurement of creatinine clearance.
- Timed (eg, 4-hour or overnight) collection.

B Creatinine clearance (CrCl) is the most widely used direct method of estimating GFR. This value is measured based on results of a carefully timed urine collection, usually over 24 hours.

C Serum creatinine (SCr) is an indirect measurement of GFR. Subtle changes in serum creatinine (eg, 0.8 mg/dL to 1.3 mg/dL) may in fact indicate major functional loss and should command attention.

- It is well accepted that changes in SCr between 1.4 mg/dL and 6.0 to 7.0 mg/dL parallel changes in GFR as measured by inulin clearance.[23]

D Blood urea nitrogen (BUN) is an indirect measurement of GFR.

- BUN is a less sensitive marker of renal function in early diabetic nephropathy, but is frequently used along with SCr to evaluate patients on a day-to-day basis due to the ease of measurement.
- BUN is affected by a variety of conditions other than renal disease; despite these limitations, however, the BUN and SCr values remain useful, valid, and inexpensive measures of GFR.

CLINICAL MANIFESTATIONS

1 Clinical manifestations of diabetic nephropathy (Table 23.5) are evident when GFR is 20% to 35% of normal and patients become nephrotic with a urinary protein excretion greater than 4 g per day. The clinical management of diabetes with nephrotic syndrome presents a great challenge. Management of glucose control becomes more difficult as loss of renal function diminishes renal catabolism of insulin, resulting in an increased half-life.

A Proteinuria is generally 4 to 8 g per day, but urinary protein loss can reach 20 to 30 g per day.

B Fluid retention is often massive, resulting in weight gain, peripheral edema, congestive heart failure and pulmonary edema as uremia progresses.

FIGURE 23.2. SCREENING FOR MICROALBUMINURIA

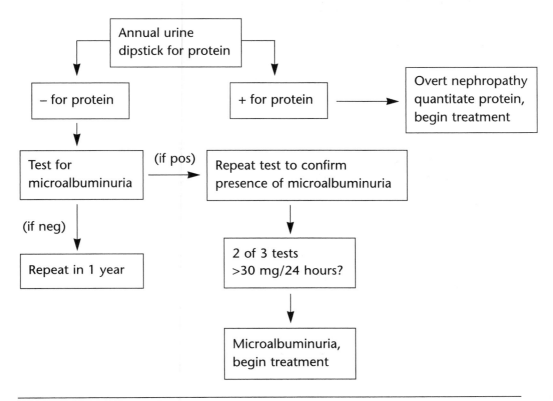

Source: Adapted from Vijan S, et al.[27]

- Fatigue and shortness of breath result in a reduction of daily activities.
- Hypertension may become uncontrolled secondary to fluid volume overload.

C Uremia becomes evident due to the accumulation of metabolic wastes and toxins.

- Anorexia, hiccups, nausea, and vomiting are gastrointestinal manifestations of uremia.
- Neuromuscular disturbances range in severity from early subtle changes in concentration, behavior, and level of consciousness to stupor, seizures, and coma.
- Anemia and its ensuing fatigue reflect the loss of renal synthesis of erythropoietin resulting in decreased red blood cell production. Other hematologic and immunologic abnormalities increase the risk of bleeding and infection.

TABLE 23.5. CLINICAL MANIFESTATIONS OF RENAL FAILURE

Gastrointestinal	• Anorexia • Hiccups • Nausea, vomiting
Fluid and Electrolyte	• Fluid retention, weight gain • Electrolyte imbalance (ie, hyperkalemia)
Neuromuscular	• Fatigue • Muscle cramps • Changes in concentration, consciousness, behavior • Seizures • Coma • Asterixis
Cardiovascular and Pulmonary	• Congestive heart failure • Accelerated atherosclerosis • Pleural effusion
Hematologic and Immunologic	• Anemia ⬇ white blood cell count ⬆ risk of bleeding ⬆ risk of infection
Endocrine and Metabolic	• Increased risk for skeletal fractures • Osteomalacia • Altered calcium, phosphate metabolism

- Renal osteodystrophy occurs due to impaired vitamin D metabolism and associated hypocalcemia resulting in secondary hyperparathyroidism.

2 Individuals with diabetic nephropathy appear to be more ill at equivalent levels of renal insufficiency than nondiabetic individuals. Underlying diabetes-induced neurologic abnormalities such as gastroparesis can exacerbate uremia-induced nausea and vomiting.

INTERVENTIONS FOR PATIENTS WITH DIABETES AT RISK OF RENAL DISEASE

1 Interventions are aimed at different stages of disease progression and include optimizing glycemic control, controlling blood pressure, and limiting dietary protein intake to 10% to 20% of total calories.[24]

A Primary prevention strategies such as optimizing glycemic control, prevent the development of diabetic nephropathy.

B Secondary prevention strategies prevent or delay the progression from microalbuminuria to overt proteinuria.
- Aggressive control of blood pressure
- ACE inhibitor therapy

C Tertiary prevention strategies prevent or delay the progression of overt diabetic nephropathy and improve clinical outcomes. Tertiary care reduces morbidity and mortality by delaying time to dialysis or transplant.

2 The Diabetes Control and Complications Trial (DCCT)[20] and the Kumamoto Study[25] demonstrated that maintaining strict glycemic control with intensive insulin and dietary therapy delays the onset and slows the progression of early microvascular complications in patients with type 1 and type 2 diabetes.

3 Treatment for hypertension must be preceded by careful patient assessment.

A Assessment includes using the following questions to evaluate specific areas for intervention including weight, usual sodium, potassium, alcohol intake, tobacco use, and activity pattern.
- At what weight are you most comfortable?
- What would have to happen in order for you to attain that weight?
- Have you noticed any swelling in your hands or your feet and legs?
- Does the swelling cause you any distress?
- Do you add salt to your food?
- Can you identify foods that you eat that are especially high in sodium?
- What are some ways that you can reduce your sodium intake?
- Do you use tobacco in any form? Have you ever considered quitting? What has to happen in order for you to reduce your tobacco consumption, and eventually quit?
- We've talked about a lot of changes you'd like to make. On what are you most interested in working?

B Is the patient taking any drug (prescribed or over-the-counter) known to raise the blood pressure or glucose levels?

C Does the patient have a surgically correctable form of hypertension (renovascular disease or Cushing's syndrome)?[26]

4 Antihypertensive drug therapy may slow the decline in renal function. However, all antihypertensives do not exert the same effect on the kidney in the presence of diabetes. ACE inhibitor therapy is considered as first line therapy for all patients with diabetic nephropathy unless contraindications are present or side effects are intolerable.[27] Given the multisystem nature of diabetes, drug effects on renal function, metabolic control, and the cardiovascular and peripheral vascular systems must be considered (Table 23.6).

TABLE 23.6. CHARACTERISTICS OF THE IDEAL ANTIHYPERTENSIVE DRUG FOR PATIENTS WITH DIABETES

- Neutral metabolic effects
- Does not cause or mask symptoms of hypoglycemia
- Does not increase lipid levels
- Does not promote orthostatic hypotension
- Does not cause impotence
- Does not aggravate coronary or peripheral vascular disease
- Preserves renal function

A A single elevated blood pressure reading does not constitute a diagnosis of hypertension but indicates that additional observation is necessary.

B A blood pressure greater than 130/85 mmHg is abnormal in patients with diabetic nephropathy or with evidence of microvascular or macrovascular disease.[28]

C Supine hypertension and orthostatic hypotension sometimes occur in patients with autonomic neuropathy. In this situation, it is recommended that blood pressure be determined supine, immediately on standing, and after 1 minute in the upright position.

D To help prevent extreme orthostatic reduction in blood pressure, the blood pressure in the standing position must be considered the therapeutic end point when evaluating treatment with hypertensive agents.

E To establish timing and proper dosage of antihypertensive drugs, 24-hour ambulatory blood pressure recordings or home measurements can be obtained.

- Self-monitoring of blood pressure enhances educational efforts and allows the patient and the healthcare team to work together for detection, treatment, and evaluation.

- Reviewing patients' technique and checking blood-pressure monitoring devices regularly can help ensure accurate readings,

F The initial pharmacological agent chosen is often an angiotensin-converting enzyme (ACE) inhibitor. Studies have demonstrated that ACE inhibitors given alone or with another antihypertensive agent produce a reduction in urinary albumin excretion rate.[18,19]

G Certain calcium antagonists have also demonstrated the ability to reduce microalbuminuria and proteinuria, and therefore, theoretically, will reduce the progression of diabetic nephropathy.

- Some members of the dihydropyridine class of calcium channel blockers may increase urinary albumin excretion and should be avoided in patients with microalbuminuria and overt proteinuria.[29]
- Recent evidence suggests that the use of calcium channel blockers may increase the risk of sudden death from acute myocardial infarction in patients with diabetes.[30]

H Loop diuretics, alpha-1 receptor blockers, thiazide diuretics in low dosages, and β-blockers are all effective antihypertensive agents.

I Side effects can occur when using antihypertensive agents.

- Worsening of lipid levels and glycemic control from diuretics or β-blockers.
- Altered symptoms of hypoglycemia from β-adrenergic blockers.
- Fluid retention from sympathetic inhibitors, calcium channel blockers, and vasodilators.
- Hyperkalemia and worsening azotemia when using an ACE inhibitor in patients with kidney disease.

J Sodium restriction is also a central component of antihypertensive therapy.

5 The amount of protein in the diet affects renal size, structure, and function. Prospective studies[31] have shown that in patients with type 1 diabetes with nephropathy, even moderate protein restriction resulted in a stabilization of renal function. Studies also indicate vegetable protein may have less of an effect on hyperfiltration before nephropathy is diagnosed. The role of a diet containing <0.8 g protein/kg body weight remains controversial.

A The Recommended Dietary Allowance (RDA) for adults is an intake of 0.8 g protein/kg of ideal body weight (IBW).

B The usual dietary intake of protein in US diets is 1.2 to 1.4 g/kg of body weight per day.

C Studies[31,32] have demonstrated that meal plans containing a protein restriction of ≤0.8 g/kg body weight per day can be achieved without compromising nutritional status and without danger to metabolic control. Low-protein meal plans may have positive effects on lipid profiles.

D Low-protein meal plans, such as 0.6 g/kg of IBW per day, have been shown to decrease blood pressure, reduce the rate of decline in GFR, and decrease albumin excretion in some patients.

E The feasibility of long-term patient use of such a restricted meal plan must be initially and continuously assessed by the dietitian and health-care team.

F Reduction of daily dietary protein intake to between 0.6 and 0.8 g/kg of IBW by patients with early nephropathy has been recommended by some, but further research is needed to define appropriate medical nutrition therapy at different levels of kidney function (Table 23.7).

G Low protein (0.6 g/kg body weight) meal plans should be used cautiously because of the difficulties maintaining such a restricted diet and because of the risk for malnutrition and associated muscle weakness.[24]

H Use of protein restricted meal plans can be assessed by measurement of urinary urea nitrogen (UUN). Patients using a protein restricted meal plan must be continuously monitored for signs of malnutrition.
- Weight loss
- Muscle weakness
- Hypoalbuminemia

6 Preventive measures to reduce the risk of insult to the kidneys are recommended for patients with diabetes who are at risk for renal disease. Early identification and aggressive treatment of urinary tract infections are imperative to prevent further insult to the kidneys.

A Guidelines for prevention and early treatment of urinary tract infections are listed in Table 23.8.

B Avoid nephrotoxic drugs.
- If such agents (eg, aminoglycosides such as gentamicin) must be used, monitor blood levels and reduce the dosage of the drug administered to patients with impaired renal function.
- Teach patients to use acetaminophen rather than nonsteroidal anti-inflammatory drugs because of the latter's effect of reducing prostaglandins.

C Avoid contrast dyes. If contrast media agents are necessary for tests, adequate hydration must be maintained before and after the study.

TABLE 23.7. NUTRITIONAL RECOMMENDATIONS AT VARIOUS STAGES OF DIABETIC NEPHROPATHY

	Prevention of Nephropathy	Predialysis	Hemodialysis	CAPD	Post Transplant
Protein	10% to 20% of total calories	0.8 g/kg (50% high biological value protein)	1 to 1.4 g/kg (50% high biological value protein)	1.2 to 1.5 g/kg (50% high biological value protein)	1.3 to 2. g/kg initially then 0.8 to 1. g/kg
Fat	30% of total calories	35%*	30%	30%	25% to 30%
Carbohydrate	50% of total calories	Remainder of non-protein kcal	Remainder of non-protein kcal	Remainder of non-protein kcal	Based on assessment. ≤50% of kcal with CHO intolerance
Calories	Adequate for desired body weight	35 kcal/kg DBW	35 kcal/kg DBW	35 kcal/kg DBW	Assess basal and activity needs; for weight gain add 300 to 500 kcal/day
Calcium	RDA	1200 to 1600 mg/day	1400 to 1600 mg/day	1000 to 1500 mg/day	1500 mg/day
Phosphorus	RDA	10 mg/kg	17 mg/kg	17 mg/kg	No restriction
Sodium	3000 mg/day 2400 mg/day if hypertensive	1000 to 2000 mg	2000 mg	No restriction	No restriction unless hypertensive
Potassium	No restriction	No restriction unless hyperkalemia	2000 mg	No restriction unless hyperkalemia	No restriction
Fluid	No restriction	1500 to 3000 mL restrict if hypo-natremia develops	700 to 1000 mL plus urine output in 24 hours	2000 to 3000 mL	Adequate fluid to prevent dehydration

CAPD = Continuous ambulatory peritoneal dialysis; DBW = desired body weight.
* With restricted protein, fat is >30% to meet caloric needs.

Table 23.8. Urinary Tract Infections

Patient Education	Guidelines for Health Professionals
• Teach patients about the signs and and symptoms of a urinary tract infection	• Obtain cultures to detect specific organisms
• Teach patients to seek treatment right away if urgency, dysuria or other signs of cystitis or a urinary tract infection occur	• Repeat urine cultures after treatment with antibiotics
• Teach female patients about emptying the bladder following sexual intercourse	• Determine whether bladder dysfunction is contributory
• Recommend consumption of cranberry juice, which acidifies the urine and has shown to reduce the incidence of urinary tract infections in elderly women	• Avoid placing an indwelling Foley catheter

D Contrast media should not be administered to any person with diabetes whose serum creatinine level is greater than 2 mg/dL (>265 μmol/L) unless the information sought is not available by any other means.

Choosing a Treatment Option for End-Stage Renal Disease

1 Treatments for ESRD are aimed at replacing the work of diseased kidneys. People with diabetes who receive transplants or dialysis experience higher morbidity and mortality than patients without diabetes because of coexisting complications such as coronary artery disease, retinopathy, and neuropathy. Providing education and information on each treatment option allows the patient and family to make an informed choice and enhances the chances for a positive outcome.

    A Benefits and risks of each treatment option should be reviewed with patients and family members for a comparison of options in uremia therapy (Table 23.9).

    B Direct contact with other patients who are receiving different forms of therapy for ESRD may be valuable for education, emotional support, and instilling hope.

TABLE 23.9. COMPARISON OF UREMIA TREATMENT OPTIONS FOR PATIENTS WITH DIABETES AND END-STAGE RENAL DISEASE

	Renal Transplantation	CAPD	Home Hemodialysis
Advantages	• Permits long intervals away from treatment facility • Best rehabilitation • Reverses uremic state completely • Patient survival often >10 y	• Avoids major surgery • Minimizes cardiovascular stress (volume shifts) • Facilitates glucose control (when insulin added to dialysate) • Can be readily taught for home dialysis • No need for vascular access	• Avoids major surgery • Type 2 patients have survived >10 yr • rHuEPO* may improve rehabilitation
Disadvantages	• Steroids exacerbate poor metabolic control • Cyclosporine exacerbates hypertension • Risk of infection • Inability to predict risk of diabetes in familial donors • May not be appropriate in severe cardiovascular disease, chronically infected patients • Risk of recurrent diabetic nephropathy • Retinopathy progresses in 30% of patients	• High technique failure rate, mortality • Risk of peritonitis • Retinopathy progresses • Risk of patient burnout from daily repetitive nature of technique	• Requires committed partner • "Failure-to-thrive" in about one third of patients • Mortality similar to cadaveric kidney recipients • Retinopathy progresses • Requires vascular access

*rHuEPO = recombinant human erythropoietin.
Source: Adapted with permission from Markell MS, Friedman EA. Care of the diabetic patient with end-stage renal disease. Semin Nephrol 1990;10:274-86.

C   Common medications used when treating ESRD:[33]

- Multivitamins or vitamins B and C are taken to replace those vitamins lost in dialysis.
- Calcium carbonate is used to prevent renal bone disease or renal osteodystrophy. Calcium is usually taken with meals to bind the phosphorous, but it can also be taken without regard to meals to raise the calcium level in the body.
- Calcitriol (1,25 – dihydroxycholecalciferol) may be prescribed to help improve absorption of calcium. It is the most potent form of vitamin D available.
- Ferrous sulfate is taken to restore iron stores depleted by anemia or administration of erythropoietin therapy. Iron supplements should be taken separately from calcium carbonate (phosphorous binders) to improve absorption.
- Epoetin alpha (EPO) is given to correct anemia associated with ESRD. It is given subcutaneously or intravenously to increase the hematocrit.

2   Planning for treatment should begin early, usually when the serum creatinine level reaches 3 mg/dL (265 µmol/L).

A   Planning includes tissue typing of family members for possible kidney transplant donation, being placed on a cadaveric waiting list, and/or creating vascular access for dialysis.

B   Circumstances may exist that limit the patient's choice of treatment. For example, those with cardiovascular disease or vascular access problems might be less suitable candidates for hemodialysis, or those unable to tolerate fluid in the peritoneal cavity would not be appropriate candidates for peritoneal dialysis.

TREATMENT OPTIONS FOR END-STAGE RENAL DISEASE

1   No treatment

A   If no treatment is administered, death will result usually within 7 months. This option is an elective decision for some patients.

B   The patient and family should consider the no treatment option after the patient is dialyzed and nonuremic because of uremia's effect on mental status.

C   Encourage the patient and family to discuss this decision with clergy, a psychologist, a social worker, the healthcare team and other family members.

D Planning supportive care (eg, home care, hospice care) is necessary for the patient who wishes to forego treatment.

2 *Hemodialysis* is a process of cleansing or filtering the blood of nitrogenous wastes. The patient's blood is circulated and cleansed outside of the body. With effective dialysis treatments, uremia can be treated and the patient can return to an improved level of health and well-being, including a vigorous appetite. The following hemodialysis process and factors should be considered.

    A The filter used for hemodialysis is a semipermeable membrane. This membrane is a thin material with holes that permits the passage of small particles but retains larger particles.

    B During dialysis, the patient's blood passes on one side of the membrane, while dialysate (prepared dialysis solution) passes on the other side of the membrane. The solution removes fluid and particles (waste products) from the blood by diffusive clearance.

    C Blood is withdrawn through a needle inserted in a specially prepared blood vessel, usually a synthetic graft or an arteriovenous fistula (using the patient's own blood vessels) located in the patient's forearm. The needle is attached by plastic tubing to a hemodialysis machine. A pump keeps blood moving through the dialyzer as wastes and fluid are filtered out. The cleansed blood returns to the patient through another needle in the same or an adjacent blood vessel.

    D Hemodialysis can be performed in an ambulatory setting or in the patient's home. Treatments are usually given 3 times per week and take 3 to 6 hours to complete.

    E Because the blood is not being cleansed 24 hours a day, the patient must still use an individualized renal meal plan with fluid restriction.

    F Treatment of the associated anemia has a significant effect on rehabilitation in this population, improving quality-of-life indicators and employment status.[34]

    G Patients with diabetes receiving dialytic therapy might be oliguric and therefore not experience the osmotic diuresis that typically accompanies hyperglycemia in a patient with diabetes not undergoing dialysis. Satisfying the thirst that accompanies hyperglycemia might be an additional challenge for the patient while on a fluid restricted diet.[22] Chewing gum, hard candy or sucking on lemon wedges may help.

H Factors that can alter glucose levels for the patient receiving hemo-dialysis treatment include the glucose concentration in the dialysate bath, appetite alteration on dialysis days and "off" days, decreased activity on dialysis days, and emotional stress.

I The following questions can be used to help elicit information regarding causes of blood glucose variability in patients with diabetes who are receiving hemodialysis treatments.

- What is your glucose pattern on days you are having dialysis?
- What is your pattern on other days?
- When (and how much) do you eat on days you are having dialysis?
- What about other days?
- What is your activity pattern like on days you are having dialysis?
- What is your activity pattern on other days?
- What is your hematocrit?
- What is the acceptable hematocrit range for the meter you are using?
- On a scale or 1 to 10, with 1 being very low and 10 being very high, how would you rate your level of stress on dialysis days? How does this compare to other days?

J Sometimes a change in the type of glucose meter used may be warranted to avoid measuring erroneous blood glucose values. Meter manufacturers provide specifications of hematocrit ranges for their meters (see Chapter 11, Monitoring, for more information).

3 Peritoneal dialysis takes place inside the body by employing the body's own capillary and serosal membranes.

A Blood is filtered through the peritoneal membrane that lines the abdominal cavity.

- Surgery is required to place a catheter through an opening in the wall of the abdominal cavity. This opening is needed so that the dialysis solution can be instilled into the peritoneal cavity and waste products can pass from the bloodstream into the dialysis solution.
- The used solution is drained and replaced with a new solution on a regular basis.

B Currently, three types of peritoneal dialysis are being used.

- Continuous ambulatory peritoneal dialysis (CAPD) is a manual method of performing peritoneal dialysis. The patient exchanges new fluid (dialysate) every 4 to 6 hours during a 24-hour period each day. The dialysate passes from a plastic bag through the catheter and stays in the patient's abdomen with the catheter sealed. The dialysate is drained after several hours, then the process begins again with fresh dialysate solution.

- Continuous cyclic peritoneal dialysis (CCPD) is like CAPD except a machine that is connected to the catheter automatically fills and drains the dialysate solution from the patient's abdomen. This type of dialysis can be performed at night while the patient is sleeping. Assistance from a family member, friend or health professional is needed to perform CCPD.

- Intermittent peritoneal dialysis (IPD) uses the same type of machine as CCPD to fill and drain the dialysate solution from the patient's abdomen. IPD treatments take longer than CCPD, and assistance is needed from a family member, friend, or health professional.

C Patients requiring insulin can administer regular insulin directly into the dialysate before the dialysate is instilled into the peritoneal cavity. Intraperitoneal insulin regimen has the following advantages:

- Provides a continuous insulin infusion.
- Eliminates the need for injections.
- May provide a more physiologic route of absorption, since the exogenous insulin is absorbed into the portal vein which mimics the action of pancreatic insulin.

D Intraperitoneal insulin has the following disadvantages:

- Provides an additional source of bacterial contamination for the dialysate during injection of insulin into the bags.
- Results in higher total insulin doses due to loss of spent dialysate.

E Regular insulin works to metabolize the dietary glucose that is consumed as well as the highly concentrated dextrose in the dialysate solution. Table 23.10 outlines insulin adjustments for dialysis.

F Visually impaired and blind patients have been successful in performing peritoneal dialysis.

G Factors that can affect glucose regulation for patients on peritoneal dialysis include the concentration of the dialysate solution, method(s) of insulin delivery (eg, intraperitoneal, subcutaneous, or both), and infection (peritonitis).

H The following questions can be used to help assess factors that may contribute to variability in blood glucose levels.

- What is the dextrose concentration of the solution you are using for your peritoneal dialysis: 1.5%, 2.5%, or 4.25%?

- What type(s) of insulin are you using?
- When are you taking your insulin?
- Where on your body are you injecting the insulin?
- Are there any signs of infection (catheter-related or peritonitis)?

TABLE 23.10. INSULIN ADJUSTMENTS FOR PATIENTS ON CAPD OR CCPD

Concentration of glucose in dialysate (g/dL)	Additional insulin in units/liter of dialysate solution
0.005	0
1.5	1
2.5	2
4.25	3

Fasting blood glucose	1 hour post-prandial glucose	Change in baseline insulin in units per 2 liters of dialysate solution
	<40 mg/dL	-6 units
<40 mg/dL	40 mg/dL	-4 units
40 mg/dL	80 mg/dL	-2 units
80 to 140 mg/dL	120 to 180 mg/dL	No change
180 mg/dL	240 mg/dL	+2 units
240 mg/dL	>240 mg/dL	+4 units
>40 mg/dL		+6 units or more May need additional subq

Reprinted with permission: Tzamaloukas, AH. Diabetes. In: Handbook of Dialysis, 2nd ed. Daugirdas JT, Ing TS, eds. Little & Brown, Boston, 1994:422-32

4 Kidney transplantation can be performed using a kidney from a living related donor, a living unrelated donor, or a suitable cadaveric donor.

   A Once transplantation has occurred, immunosuppressive medications are required throughout the patient's life to prevent the body from rejecting the transplanted organ.

B Patients with diabetes must take additional insulin following transplantation because the newly functioning kidney catabolizes insulin once again, posttransplant steroid therapy has a hyperglycemic effect, and the patient experiences a notable increase in appetite which can lead to weight gain.

C Following transplantation, blood glucose control may be altered by the following factors:

- Degree of function of the transplanted kidney
- Treatment for transplant rejection
- Changes in steroid dose
- Patient's increased appetite and ability to consume a more liberal diet with subsequent weight gain
- Diuretic therapy
- Presence of infection (transplant patients are more susceptible to infection because of immunosuppression)

D The following questions can be used to help detect the cause of variability in blood glucose levels:

- What is your current immunosuppression regimen?
- Does that regimen represent an increase or decrease from your usual dose of immunosuppressive medication?
- How much weight have you gained since your transplant?
- Are you being treated for any infection?
- What antihypertensive/diuretic agents are you currently taking?
- What is your current exercise/activity schedule?

5 Patients with type 1 diabetes may be considered for a simultaneous kidney-pancreas transplantation.

A A kidney-pancreas transplantation restores both glucose metabolism and kidney function.

B Criteria for patient selection vary at each transplant center but typically include the following:

- Diagnosis of type 1 diabetes
- Evidence of secondary complications such as renal insufficiency or preproliferative retinopathy
- Metabolic instability
- Adequate financial resources/insurance coverage (insurance carriers review eligibility for payment on a case-by-case basis)

C Contraindications for kidney-pancreas transplantation include

- Presence of HIV

- Malignancy
- Psychosis
- Any active infection
- Severe neuropathies
- Inoperable cardiovascular disease

D Complications of kidney-pancreas transplantation include
- Cardiac incompetence
- Arterial or venous thrombosis
- Anastomotic leaks, bleeding
- Side effects of immunosuppression (Table 23.11)
- Pancreatitis
- Metabolic acidosis related to exocrine pancreatic function

E Transplantation can be justified if the complications of diabetes are more dangerous than the side effects of immunosuppression.

F Renal transplant function is easier to measure than pancreas function.
- A rise in serum creatinine is a primary indicator of kidney rejection.
- A decrease in urinary amylase production can signal a pancreas in jeopardy.
- Hyperglycemia occurs late in pancreas rejection.
- Signs of rejection can be detected earlier in the kidney and treatment can be initiated, thus providing some protection for the pancreas.
- Living related donors must be screened carefully because of their risk for developing diabetes. Brain-dead cadavers are a more common donor source.[35,36]

Psychosocial Issues in End-Stage Renal Disease

1 Rates of depression, anxiety, and stress may be higher among dialysis patients than among the general population. These psychological reactions may occur in response to the losses associated with diabetes and renal disease (eg, loss of physical capacities and loss of control from the complications associated with diabetes).

2 Patients respond in a variety of ways to receiving a diagnosis of renal disease. Some typical responses include:

A "No one ever told me this could happen."

B "My life is over."

C "It's all my fault, if only I had taken better care of myself."

TABLE 23.11. SIDE EFFECTS OF IMMUNOSUPPRESSION

Prednisone	• Sodium, water retention	• Increased stomach acid
	• Increased appetite	• Night sweats
	• Increased fat deposits	• Increased hair
	• Hyperkalemia	• Acne
	• Muscle wasting	• Blurred vision
	• Increased serum cholesterol	• Slowed healing
	• Calcium loss	• Muscle weakness
	• Sun sensitivity	• Susceptibility to infection
	• Mood swings	
Cyclosporine	• Flushing	
	• Hair growth	
	• Fine tremor	
	• Gingival hyperplasia	
	• Paresthesias	
	• Hypertension	
	• Gastrointestinal distress	
	• Nephrotoxicity	
Sulfa drugs	• Liver toxicity	
	• Decreased leukocytes	
	• Allergy	
	• Sun sensitivity	
	• Gastrointestinal symptoms	
	• Renal toxicity	
Azathioprine	• Decreased leukocytes	
	• Liver toxicity	
	• Hair loss	
	• Allergy	
Antacid drugs	• Diarrhea or constipation	
	• Low phosphorous	
	• High magnesium	
Antilymphocyte globin	• Allergy	
	• Decreased leukocytes	
	• Decreased platelets	

Source: Adapted with permission from the American Association of Diabetes Educators.[35]

D "It's all my doctor's fault."
E "I feel like my body is falling apart, piece by piece."

3 It is imperative to assess and comprehend how each patient and family respond to the patient's illness.

   A A variety of healthcare professionals, including mental health professionals, need to be involved in helping patients and families adjust to their losses and to a new, often complex treatment regimen.[37]

   B Some patients blame themselves when they develop complications of diabetes.

   C Scare tactics (eg, "If you don't control your blood glucose, you will go into kidney failure.") are not an effective behavior change strategy.

   D Avoid giving "pat" answers or responses which can sound patronizing. By asking, "would it help to know that complications such as diabetic nephropathy can develop in patients who have done their best to maintain optimal glucose control" the healthcare team can communicate this possibility to the patient and family and perhaps help lessen the feelings of guilt and blame that can occur with a diagnosis of end-stage renal disease.

4 An effective intervention for some patients with ESRD is to invite them to join a support group or to pair new patients with patients who have had success using one of the various renal replacement therapies.

   A Patients can learn new information, coping skills and behaviors, and positive attitudes from these role models.

   B Patients, their families, and the healthcare team can benefit from having members from a support group available in the clinic setting to meet with new patients who face a diagnosis of renal disease.

Self-Review Questions

1 What is the annual cost of treatment for ESRD in the US in patients with diabetes?

2 Define creatinine clearance, BUN, and nephrotic syndrome.

3 State four of the seven functions of the kidney.

4 What percentage of people with type 1 diabetes develop renal failure?

5 What percentage of people with type 2 diabetes develop renal failure?

6 Describe the progression of renal disease in patients with type 1 diabetes.

7 Identify four risk factors for diabetic nephropathy.

8 Identify the laboratory tests used most frequently to diagnose diabetic nephropathy and monitor renal function.

9 Name the first clinical sign indicative of kidney damage for a person with diabetes and how often an assessment should be conducted.

10 List the clinical manifestations of diabetic kidney disease.

11 Describe interventions used to prevent or slow the progression of diabetic nephropathy.

12 Summarize the characteristics of the ideal antihypertensive agent for patients with diabetes.

13 Describe potential dietary modifications that may be needed at different stages of diabetic nephropathy.

14 Name other factors that can harm the kidneys, and describe how these factors can be minimized.

15 Describe treatment options for ESRD and their impact on diabetes management.

16 Contrast microalbuminuria with proteinuria.

CASE STUDY 1

MB is a 53-year-old engineer who is married and is the mother of 3 grown children. She has been referred because of an elevated hemoglobin HbA_{1c} despite taking a combination of glyburide 20 mg and metformin 1500 mg daily. The only other medication she takes is hydrochlorothiazide 25 mg daily. She is familiar with SMBG but stopped testing because her glucose was always high. She denies a previous history of known complications from diabetes. MB is of normal weight, her blood pressure is 130/98 with no postural change, and both fundi show moderate background retinopathy. She has trace pedal edema, and mild stocking-glove sensory deficit in both lower extremities. Laboratory results show a BUN of 32, creatinine of 2.4, potassium of 4.3, 24-hour urine protein excretion of 945 mg, and creatinine clearance of 38 mL/minute. Her HbA_{1c} is 9.8% (normal = 3.4% to 6.2%). After reviewing the answers to MB's diabetes knowledge and self-care questionnaire, you determine she demonstrates a lack of knowledge about both diabetes management and kidney disease.

QUESTIONS FOR DISCUSSION

1 What teaching plan would you develop with MB and how would you begin?

2 What interventions could the healthcare team employ immediately?

3 What are potential psychosocial issues for this patient?

Discussion

1 A priority at this first visit is to begin to establish rapport and a relationship between MB and the other key members of the healthcare team.

    A Team members should meet with MB over the next few weeks in order to individually assess her needs, and desired level of involvement in her care. This time is an opportunity for MB to identify specific goals toward which she would like to work. These visits give the educator the opportunity to provide information to MB and allow for discussion regarding the importance of her role in her care.

    B Initiate regular visits and telephone contact to answer questions and reinforce MB's desired behavior change.

    C Review MB's SMBG technique. Her feelings and concerns regarding SMBG also need to be explored.

    D Ask what would make SMBG relevant for her and discuss how often she believes she needs to test to reach her blood glucose goals.

    E Assist MB in learning how to use the information she obtains through SMBG.

    F Let MB know that this can be her opportunity to take charge of her diabetes which may help to slow the progression of kidney damage.

    G Offer MB and her family introductory information on kidney disease, including function, preventive measures, terminology, and what tests are used to track kidney function and how often they are needed.

    H Preventive measures related to eye and foot care must be reviewed and reinforced. The educator can use the time during MB's foot exam to stress the importance of daily self-inspection of shoes and feet.

2 Interventions that could be employed include

    A Metformin should be discontinued immediately; this medication is contraindicated in patients with an elevated serum creatinine due to increased risk of lactic acidosis.

    B If MB expresses a desire to improve her glucose control, review options for optimizing glycemic control.

    C If MB is agreeable, insulin therapy can be initiated.

    D Blood pressure control must be achieved. The addition of an ACE inhibitor to her current diuretic therapy is warranted. This medication may not only reduce her blood pressure, but the level of proteinuria may also be decreased.

- Discuss the benefits of a lower BP on her kidney function and the value of frequent BP measurement. MB may be interested in monitoring the effects of her sodium intake and the addition of the ACE inhibitor on her daily blood pressure.
- Options for frequent BP measurements include obtaining a blood pressure monitor for home use.

E Because MB is at risk for hyperkalemia with the addition of the ACE inhibitor, she will need a review of the usual sources of potassium-rich foods in her diet.

F Decreasing sodium may eliminate her pedal edema.

G Provide a referral to the ophthalmologist for a baseline retinal examination and develop a treatment plan to further evaluate for MB's moderate background retinopathy.

3 Potential psychosocial issues for MB include
  A The emotional impact of the diagnosis of kidney damage.
  - MB and her family will need support from the healthcare team with time allotted to discuss fears and concerns related to the diagnosis.
  - A referral to a social worker or psychologist may help MB explore her feelings and coping ability concerning the diagnosis of kidney disease and identify sources of emotional and financial support.

  B Given changes in diabetes and hypertension management, new medications, and the amount of education needed, the educator can work with MB to prioritize her teaching, according to MB's stated goals.

  C The educator should be available to MB by telephone, and schedule a series of return visits to answer questions and provide further information, support, or referral.

  D Although renal replacement therapy is not currently indicated, when MB displays readiness and asks about the treatment for ESRD, a discussion regarding her options for renal replacement therapy should be initiated.

References

1 Herman W, Hawthorne V, Hamman R, Keen, H, et al. Consensus statement. Am J Kidney Dis 1989;13(1):2-6.

2 Brennan DT, ed. Diabetic nephropathy: monograph for diabetes educators and nephrology nurses. Chicago: American Association of Diabetes Educators, 1995.

3 Cowie CC, Port FK, Wolfe RA. Disparities in incidence of diabetic and end-stage renal disease according to race and type of diabetes. N Engl J Med 1989;321:1074-79.

4 National Institute of Diabetes and Digestive and Kidney Diseases. United States Renal Data Systems (USRDS) 1996 Annual Report. Bethesda, Md: National Institute of Diabetes and Digestive and Kidney Diseases, April 1996.

5 Bennett PH, Haffner S, Kasiske BL, et al. Screening and management of microalbuminuria in patients with diabetes mellitus. Am J Kidney Dis 1995;25:107-12.

6 American Diabetes Association. Position statement. Diabetic nephropathy. Diabetes Care 1998;21(suppl 1)S50-3.

7 Guyton AC. Formation of urine by the kidney. Renal blood flow, glomerular filtration, and their control. In: Textbook of medical physiology. 8th ed. Philadelphia: WB Saunders, 1991:286-97.

8 Brancati, FL, Whittle JC, Whelton PK, Seidler AJ, Kiag, MJ. The excess incidence of diabetic end-stage renal disease among blacks: a population-based study of potential explanatory factors. JAMA 1992;268:3079-84.

9 Nathan DM. Long-term complications of diabetes mellitus. N Engl J Med 1993; 328:1676-85.

10 Selby JV, FitzSimmons SC, Newman JM, et al. The natural history and epidemiology of diabetic nephropathy. Implications for prevention and control. JAMA 1990;263:1954-60.

11 Breyer JA. Diabetic nephropathy in insulin-dependent patients. Am J Kidney Dis 1992;20:533-47.

12 Mogensen CE, Christensen CK, Vittinghus E. The stages in diabetic renal disease with emphasis on the stage of incipient diabetic nephropathy. Diabetes 1983;32(suppl 2):64-78.

13 Lewis EJ, Hunsicker LG, Bain RP, Rhode RD. The effect of angiotensin-converting-enzyme inhibition on diabetic nephropathy. N Engl J Med 1993; 329:1456-62.

14 Tuttle KR, DeFronzo RA, Stein JH. Treatment of diabetic nephropathy: a rational approach based on its pathophysiology. Semin Nephrol 1991; 11:220-35.

15 Castellino P, Shohat J, DeFronzo RA. Hyperfiltration and diabetic nephropathy: is it the beginning? Or is it the end? Semin Nephrol 1990;10:228-41.

16 Marcus AO. Diabetes mellitus: nephropathy and hypertension. Clin Diabetes 1996;14:91-94.

17 Savage S, Nagel NJ, Estacio RO, Lukken N, Schrier RW. Clinical factors associated with urinary albumin excretion in type 2 diabetes. Am J Kidney Dis 1995;25: 836-44.

18 Ravid M, Lang R, Rachmani R, Lishner M. Long-term renoprotective effect of angiotensin-converting enzyme inhibition in non-insulin-dependent diabetes mellitus: a 7-year follow-up study. Arch Intern Med 1996;156:286-9

19 Ravid M, Savin H, Jutrin I, Bental T, Katz B, Lishner M. Long-term stabilizing effect of angiotensin-converting enzyme inhibition on plasma creatinine and on proteinuria in normotensive type 2 diabetic patients. Ann Intern Med 1993; 118:577-81.

20   The Diabetes Control and Complications Trial Research Group. The effect of intensive treatment of diabetes on the development and progression of long-term complications in insulin-dependent diabetes. N Engl J Med 1993;329:977-86.

21   Reichard P, Nilsson BY, Rosenqvist U. The effect of long-term intensified insulin treatment on the development of microvascular complications of diabetes mellitus. N Engl J Med 1993;329:304-9.

22   Krolewski AS, Canessa M, Warram JH, et al. Predisposition to hypertension and susceptibility to renal disease in insulin-dependent diabetes mellitus. N Engl J Med 1988;318:140-45.

23   Carlson JA, Harrington JT. Laboratory evaluation of renal function. In: Schrier RW, Gottschalk CW, eds. Diseases of the kidney. 5th ed. Boston: Little & Brown, 1993:361-405.

24   American Diabetes Association. Position statement. Nutrition recommendations and principles for people with diabetes mellitus. Diabetes Care 1997;20:(suppl 1)S14-17.

25   Ohkubo Y, Kishikawa H, Araki E, Miyata T, et al. Intensive insulin therapy prevents the progression of diabetic microvascular complications in Japanese patients with non-insulin dependent diabetes mellitus: a randomized prospective 6-year study. Diabetes Research and Clinical Practice 1995;28:103-17.

26   National High Blood Pressure Education Program Working Group report on hypertension and chronic renal failure. Arch Intern Med 1991;151:1280-87.

27   Vijan S, Stevens DL, Herman WH, Funnell MM, Standiford CJ. Screening, prevention, counseling, and treatment for the complications of type 2 diabetes mellitus. J Gen Intern Med 1997;12:567-80.

28   American Diabetes Association. Consensus statement. Diagnosis and management of nephropathy in patients with diabetes mellitus. Diabetes Care 1996; 19:(suppl 1) S103-6.

29   Abbott K, Smith A, Bakris G. Effects of dihydropyridine calcium antagonists on albuminuria in patients with diabetes. J Clin Pharmacol 1996;36:274-9.

30   Estacio R, Jeffers, B, Hiatt, W, et al. The effect of nisoldipine as compared with enalapril on cardiovascular outcomes inpatients with non-insulin-dependent diabetes and hypertension. N Engl J Med 1998;338:645-52.

31   Zeller K, Whittaker E, Sullivan L, Raskin P, Jacobson HR. Effect of restricting dietary protein on the progression of renal failure in patients with insulin-dependent diabetes mellitus. N Engl J Med 1991; 324:78-84.

32   Scopelite JA. Dietary modifications: impact on diabetic nephropathy. ANNA J 1992;19:447-52.

33   Kleinbeck C. Challenges of diabetes and dialysis. Diabetes Spectrum 1997; 10:135-41

34   Delano BG. Improvements in quality of life following treatment with rHuEPO in anemic hemodialysis patients. Am J Kidney Dis 1989;14(suppl 1):14-18.

35   Nettles AT. Pancreas transplantation: a University of Minnesota perspective. Diabetes Educ 1992;18:232-38.

36   Trusler LA. Simultaneous kidney-pancreas transplantation. ANNA J 1991; 18:487-91.

37   Kopp J. Psychosocial correlates of diabetes and renal dysfunction. ANNA J 1992;19:432-37.

SUGGESTED READINGS

Alzaid AA. Microalbuminuria in patients with NIDDM: an overview. Diabetes Care 1996;19:79-89.

Barbosa J, Steffes NW, Sutherland DE, Connett JE, et al. Effect of glycemic control on early diabetic renal lesions. JAMA 1994;727:600-06.

Bloomgarden ZT. Nephropathy. Diabetes Care 1995;18:1402-05.

Bojestig M, Arnqvist HJ, Hermansson G, Karlberg BE, Ludvigsson J. Declining incidence of nephropathy in insulin-dependent diabetes mellitus. N Engl J Med 1994;330:15-18.

Brennan DR. CAPD in IDDM: initial treatment strategies. Diabetes Spectrum 1994;7:327-28.

Coonrod BA, Ellis D, Becker DJ, et al. Predictors of microalbuminuria in individuals with IDDM. Pittsburgh epidemiology of diabetes complications study. Diabetes Care 1993;16:1376-83.

Freidman EA. Treatment options for diabetic nephropathy. Diabetes Spectrum 1992;5:6-16.

Henry RR. Protein content of the diabetic diet. Diabetes Care 1994;17:1502-13.

Hoops S. Renal and retinal complications in insulin-dependent diabetes mellitus: the art of changing the outcome. Diabetes Educ 1990;16:221-33.

Irvin B. Maximizing nutrition therapy at every stage of diabetic nephropathy Diabetes Spectrum 1997;10:304-8.

Kelly M. Chronic renal failure. Am J Nurs 1996;96(1):36-37.

Klahr S, Levey AS, Beck GJ, Caggiula AW, et al. The effects of dietary protein restriction and blood-pressure control on the progression of chronic renal disease. N Engl J Med 1994;330:877-84.

Kleinbeck C. Challenges of diabetes and dialysis. Diabetes Spectrum 1997; 10:135-41.

Kopple JD. Nutrition management of non-dialyzed patients with chronic renal failure. In Nutrition Management of Renal Disease. Kopple JD, Shaul GM eds. Baltimore: Williams and Wilkins, 1997:479-531.

Markell MS, Friedman EA. Diabetic nephropathy: management of the end-stage patient. Diabetes Care 1992;15:1226-38.

Molitch ME. ACE inhibitors and diabetic nephropathy. Diabetes Care 1994; 17:756-60.

Raal FJ, Kalk WJ, Lawson M, Esser JD, et al. Effect of moderate dietary protein restriction of the progression of overt diabetic nephropathy: a 6-month prospective study. Amer J Clinl Nutrit 1994;60:579-85.

Rodby RA. Fabulous filters. Diabetes Forecast 1997;50(3):32-36.

Smulders YM, Rakic M, Stehouwer CDA, Weijers RNM, Slaats EH, Silberbusch J. Determinants of progression of microalbuminuria in patients with NIDDM. Diabetes Care 1997;20:999-1005.

Striker G. Report on a workshop to develop management recommendations for the prevention of progression in chronic renal disease. J Am S Neph 1995;5:1537-40.

Thom S. Protein: the last macronutrient frontier. Diabetes Spectrum 1993; 6:332-33.

Tzamaloukas AH. Diabetes. In: Handbook of Dialysis, 2nd ed. Daugirdas JT, Ing TS eds. Boston: Little & Brown, 1994;422-32.

Wang S-L, Head J, Stevens L, Fuller JH. WHO Multinational Study Group. Excess mortality and its relation to hypertension and proteinuria in diabetic patients. Diabetes Care 1996;19:305-12.

COMPLICATIONS

Macrovascular Disease   **24**

Frank Vinicor, MD, MPH
Centers for Disease Control and Prevention
Division of Diabetes Translation
Atlanta, Georgia

INTRODUCTION

1 *Arteriosclerosis* is a general term that describes the condition in which the walls of blood vessels (both arteries and veins) are thick, hard, and nonelastic.

2 *Atherosclerosis* is a specific term that refers to the process of deposition of materials along blood vessel walls (especially arterial).

3 *Macrovascular disease* is a term that refers to both arteriosclerotic and atherosclerotic changes in moderate- to large-sized arteries and veins. Coronary, cerebral, and peripheral macrovascular diseases are particularly significant because of the associated morbidity and mortality.[1,2]

4 Atherosclerosis, which is common in diabetes, is literally a "soft" hardening in which mounds of lipid material mixed with smooth muscle cells and calcium accumulate in the inner walls of blood vessels. These mounds, called *plaques,* enlarge over time.

   A Eventually the plaque completely blocks blood flow or causes the formation of a blood clot.

   B Plaque may also initiate vascular spasm, which further reduces blood flow.

   C Plaque formations occur by several different mechanisms.

     • Smooth muscle cells, which normally lie behind the inner wall, or intima, of a blood vessel, may migrate into this intima, spread across its surface, and form the base of plaque. What starts this process of migration is not known for certain. Injury to the intima may initiate this smooth muscle migration, the injury itself reflecting mechanical insult, oxygen deficiency, or lipid deposition. As the plaque forms, cholesterol becomes a major component.

     • Calcium deposits may also cause further hardening of plaque.

     • All plaques are not the same, and recent investigations[3] have identified vulnerable, thinly-capped plaques, which are common in diabetes mellitus, as being associated with greater morbidity and mortality than stable plaques with a thick fibrous cap over the fatty compartment.

OBJECTIVES

Upon completion of this chapter, the learner will be able to

1   Identify the types of macrovascular disease that occur among patients with diabetes mellitus.

2   Explain the contribution of macrovascular disease to the overall disease and economic burden associated with diabetes mellitus.

3   Describe risk factors that may contribute to the prevalence, morbidity, and mortality of macrovascular disease in diabetes.

4   Describe assessment and intervention strategies that may prevent and/or minimize macrovascular disease in diabetes mellitus.

TYPES OF MACROVASCULAR DISEASE THAT AFFECT PATIENTS WITH DIABETES

1   The three major types of macrovascular disease are coronary artery, cerebral vascular, and peripheral vascular disease.[1]

   A   In persons with diabetes, atherosclerotic vascular disease of the coronary vessels develops at an earlier age than in the nondiabetic population and involves coronary vessels more extensively and diffusely.

   •   The incidence of early-onset or midlife *atherosclerotic coronary artery disease* (CAD), which is much lower among the nondiabetic female population than the nondiabetic male population, is relatively comparable in men and women with diabetes. Women with diabetes lose their gender protection from atherosclerosis.

   •   The adverse consequences of an acute coronary event, (eg, death, congestive heart failure) and the likelihood of a recurrent myocardial infarction are greater in persons with diabetes.

   B   Persons with diabetes appear to be prone to *cerebral vascular disease* developing at an earlier age than nondiabetic individuals. (The data are not quite as strong or extensive for cerebral vascular disease when compared with coronary artery disease.) Persons with diabetes also seem to be at risk for both transient ischemic attacks and thrombotic cerebral vascular accidents.

   C   *Peripheral vascular disease* (PVD) is very common in persons with diabetes; it is clinically characterized by intermittent claudication, lower leg and foot ulcers, and the need for amputations. Smoking, dyslipidemia, and other conditions may contribute to the progression or clinical expression of peripheral vascular disease.

2 Complications associated with macrovascular disease contribute significantly to the morbidity, disability, mortality, and costs associated with diabetes, particularly in those persons with long-standing diabetes.[4,5]

   A Most clinical and epidemiological studies[6,7] indicate that coronary artery disease accounts for 50% to 60% of all deaths in patients with diabetes.

- Persons with type 2 diabetes are particularly at risk for coronary-associated mortality.[6,7] Coronary artery disease is also the greatest cause of mortality in persons with type 1 diabetes.[6]

- In general, mortality ratios for coronary artery disease in patients with diabetes are two- and fourfold greater in men and women with diabetes, respectively, than in a comparable nondiabetic population.[8,9]

   B Most persons with diabetes who experience acute coronary insufficiency display the usual symptoms (eg, angina, diaphoresis, anxiety). However, an important element of coronary artery disease in patients with diabetes is the so-called silent or atypical myocardial infarction in which patients do not manifest the typical symptoms of acute coronary ischemia.

- Silent myocardial infarctions also occur in the general population, but are about two to three times more common in persons with diabetes, especially if the diabetes is of long-standing duration.

- Because of autonomic neuropathy, classic symptoms such as chest pain may not occur. Instead other symptoms (eg, nausea, shortness of breath, sweating, and vomiting) may be present.

- When considering patient symptoms in activities such as exercise programs, silent coronary artery disease and possible atypical manifestations of coronary artery disease should be considered.

   C There is little relationship between the duration of type 2 diabetes and the presence of coronary events (see discussion in this chapter about impaired glucose tolerance, Syndrome X, and improper intrauterine nutrition for possible explanations). For persons with type 1 diabetes, however, the longer the duration of diabetes, the more likely it is that the person will experience a coronary event.

   D Studies of cerebral vascular disease in patients with diabetes are limited but suggest that mortality ratios are from three to five times greater than for the nondiabetic population.

- There is a relationship between the level of glycemic control at admission for a stroke in persons with diabetes and subsequent mortality.[10]

- The increased likelihood of cerebral vascular death applies to both males and females.

D Peripheral vascular disease infrequently leads to fatal complications during the first few years after clinical expression. Thus, most epidemiologic investigations are based on nonfatal complications, symptoms, or clinical findings associated with peripheral vascular disease (see Chapter 16, Skin, Foot, and Dental Care, for more information about lower-extremity complications).

- About 50% of all nontraumatic lower-extremity amputations performed on patients with diabetes are due to peripheral neuropathy and/or vascular disease. People with diabetes have a 15 times higher age-related risk for amputation than nondiabetic individuals.[11,12]
- Absent peripheral pulses due to occlusive peripheral arterial disease are seen considerably more often in patients with type 2 diabetes than in patients with type 1 diabetes.
- The incidence of occlusive peripheral arterial disease is approximately four to six times higher in men and women with diabetes, respectively, than in those without diabetes.[13] Thus, the need for preventive education about foot care is particularly important in persons with diabetes. Recent health services research studies[13] of the diabetic foot support this need for foot care education.

MAGNITUDE OF THE PROBLEM

1 Determining how common, serious, and costly a diabetes complication is assists in characterizing and describing the dimension of the disease problem.

A Of the approximately 190 000 deaths in 1995 to which diabetes was listed as an underlying or contributing factor, almost 125 000 were due to CAD.[14]

B The greatest cause of mortality among persons with either type 1 or type 2 diabetes is cardiovascular disease (CVD), with 61% of life lost prematurely due to a combination of CVD and cerebral vascular disease.[5]

2 Regarding health resource utilization (eg, hospitalizations, clinic visits), PVD and CVD accounted for approximately 26% of all days in the hospital and hospital discharges among those with diabetes in 1997.[5] Furthermore, 15% of the almost 70 million nursing home days for persons with diabetes were due to the sequelae of cerebral and cardiovascular disease, and 6% of the over 30 million physician visits for persons with diabetes in 1997 were primarily for assessment of cerebral vascular and cardiovascular disease.[5]

3 In terms of costs, almost 20% of the $44 billion healthcare expenditures in 1997 directly attributable to diabetes were for cardiovascular and peripheral vascular disease. Furthermore, 58% of mortality costs attributable to diabetes in 1997 reflect premature death in persons with diabetes due to either cerebral vascular or cardiovascular disease.[5]

4 CVD is the most lethal, devastating, and costly complication of diabetes. Even small risk reductions in diabetes-associated cardiovascular disease would have a substantial impact on the overall diabetes burden.

RISK FACTORS

1 A remarkable number of risk factors may contribute to the accelerated atherosclerotic vascular disease in patients with diabetes, including lipid abnormalities, hypertension, smoking, obesity, physical inactivity, nutrition, hyperinsulinemia, insulin resistance, blood flow dynamics and coagulation factors, albuminuria, hyperglycemia per se, and perhaps even the treatment of diabetes itself.[15]

A Elevated plasma triglyceride and lowered high-density lipoprotein (HDL) levels are often found in patients with insulin resistence and type 2 diabetes. Total cholesterol and LDL-cholesterol are generally comparable between persons with type 2 diabetes and matched nondiabetic individuals. In persons with well-controlled type 1 diabetes, lipoprotein levels are similar to control subjects. Qualitative abnormalities in lipid components have been identified in persons with diabetes, including very dense lipoproteins and increased amounts of lipoprotein [Lp(a)].[16,17]

- There is controversy regarding whether elevated triglycerides are an independent risk factor for coronary artery disease, both in the general population as well as in persons with diabetes.[18,19] Evidence is accumulating that controlling triglycerides is important for those with diabetes.[20] Postprandial elevations of triglycerides in the form of chylomicrons may be particularly serious.[21]

- Plasma triglyceride levels correlate positively with blood glucose and glycosylated hemoglobin levels. In both type 1 and type 2 patients, improved metabolic control results in lowered triglyceride levels and some degree of reciprocal increase in high-density lipoprotein (HDL) levels.

- The impact of plasma cholesterol levels on the subsequent development of cardiovascular disease is probably similar in individuals with and without diabetes. Thus, if an elevated cholesterol level doubles the chance of a myocardial infarction in a nondiabetic individual, a similar cholesterol level will likely have a comparable effect in a patient with diabetes.[15]

- Persons with diabetes seem to start from a higher baseline regarding mortality in the absence of any other risk factor (eg, cholesterol), probably as a direct result of diabetes. The deleterious interaction of the several risk factors for macrovascular disease also continues for several years.[22] The qualitative nature of lipid structures (eg, glycosylation and/or oxidation of lipoproteins) may be as important as the absolute levels.

B Elevated plasma fibrinogen levels and other indicators of defective clotting dynamics exist in diabetes and appear to be strongly associated with diabetic macrovascular disease.[9,15] In recent epidemiologic studies in the general population, an elevated plasma fibrinogen level was identified as a potent risk factor for future cardiovascular morbidity and mortality. Fibrinogen levels are raised by both cigarette smoking and hyperglycemia, thus underscoring the importance of smoking cessation and glycemic control in the possible prevention of coronary disease.

- In both type 1 and type 2 diabetes, the correlation between hyperglycemia and HDL levels is poor, suggesting a complex interrelationship (ie, achieving glycemic control, by itself, will not necessarily increase HDL levels).

- Effective and safe ways to increase HDL levels need to be identified, because low HDL levels are a powerful and independent predictor of subsequent vascular events.[15]

C Hypertension is approximately twice as common in patients with diabetes than in nondiabetic individuals. Hypertension is an independent risk factor for cardiovascular disease in the general population as well as in patients with diabetes.

- In type 1 diabetes there is a correlation between duration of diabetes, the presence of renal dysfunction, and the development of hypertension.
- In persons with type 2 diabetes, the pathogenesis of hypertension may be associated with Syndrome X. In this syndrome, at least four elements commonly seen together in clinical practice—hyperglycemia, hyperlipidemia, hypertension, and central obesity—are apparent.[23,24] A central role of insulin resistance and subsequent hyperinsulinemia and hypertension, even prior to the onset of hyperglycemia, is proposed. An atherosclerotic environment may thus exist for years before the onset of hyperglycemia, including during a time of impaired glucose tolerance.[6] This scenario would explain the lack of a time relationship between the onset of hyperglycemia and hypertension in persons with type 2 diabetes.[25,26]
- Recent studies[27,28] have indicated that an impaired intrauterine nutritional environment associated with a smaller fetus and newborn, also is associated with a high likelihood of developing Syndrome X, coronary artery disease, and type 2 diabetes many decades later. This exciting concept may both explain the common association between the "deadly quartet", and offer opportunities for preventive interventions during pregnancy.

D Persons with diabetes smoke tobacco, on average, with the same frequency as the general population. Unfortunately, younger people with diabetes smoke more often than their nondiabetic peers.[29] In any case, smoking appears to have an independent additive impact on the risk of subsequent cardiovascular disease developing for patients with diabetes.

- It is unclear whether the mechanisms for the effects of smoking on vascular function in persons with diabetes are due to cigarette toxins, or are mediated through lowered HDL or elevated fibrinogen levels.
- More recent studies[30] suggest that, like diabetes itself, smoking is associated with an increase in protein glycosylation, including advanced glycosylated end products (AGEs).
- The combination of having diabetes and smoking cigarettes could result in a substantial increase in permanent protein glycosylation and subsequent microvascular dysfunction.

E Obesity is a problem for the majority of patients with either impaired glucose tolerance[6] or type 2 diabetes. The independent contribution of obesity to atherosclerotic vascular disease in these patients has not yet been established, perhaps because these same individuals also often have dyslipidemia and/or hypertension.

F Little direct information is presently available on the relationship between physical activity and the risk of atherosclerotic vascular disease among patients with diabetes. However, a well-planned cardiovascular exercise program, with careful cardiovascular assessment prior to exercise, is a prudent adjunct to therapy for hyperglycemia.[15,31] Lifestyle and behavioral interventions, including physical activity, are presently being studied to determine whether a reduction in the progression of impaired glucose tolerance to type 2 diabetes will occur.[32]

G The influence of a diet high in saturated fat and cholesterol on lipids and CAD is well known (see Chapter 8, Nutrition, for more information).

H Because blood coagulation factors are important in the formation and dissolution of arterial thrombi, they may contribute to both acute and chronic atherosclerotic lesions. A number of platelet and clotting-factor abnormalities have been reported in patients with diabetes. Importantly, platelet behavior tends to improve with better metabolic control.[4,15]

I Both microalbuminuria and macroalbuminuria appear to be highly associated with the incidence and mortality of macrovascular disease. Whether albuminuria is a risk marker for macrovascular disease (ie, not causative) or a true risk factor is not clear.[33,34]

J In the past, attention has been directed to a possible role of therapeutic agents used to treat diabetes and associated conditions in the pathogenesis of macrovascular disease.
  - While results from the University Group Diabetes Program (UGDP) suggested an increased risk of cardiovascular complications in patients with diabetes treated with an oral antidiabetes drug, subsequent overall experience with sulfonylureas as well as newer oral agents does not support this association.
  - In nondiabetic subjects, hyperinsulinemia is associated with increased risk of coronary artery disease. Some clinical studies of patients with type 2 diabetes suggest that high plasma insulin levels may also be associated with atherosclerotic vascular disease. Considerable controversy exists regarding the relationships among

insulin resistance, hyperinsulinemia, and macrovascular disease in diabetes, but at present no evidence that exogenous insulin causes atherosclerosis exists.[35,36]

- In the treatment of hypertension, concern has been expressed that side effects from certain antihypertensive agents (eg, diuretics, β-blockers, calcium channel blockers) may attenuate, if not reverse, the benefits of blood-pressure-lowering medications perhaps in part by increasing insulin resistance.[37] Although blood pressure medication must be selected carefully for persons with diabetes, it is very important to establish normal blood pressure in persons with diabetes.

K Because hyperglycemia is the hallmark of diabetes, the possible contribution of chronically elevated levels of blood glucose to the development of atherosclerotic vascular disease must be considered.

- With hyperglycemia, sorbitol accumulates in the intima and causes this layer to enlarge, possibly contributing to atherosclerotic plaque formation.

- In an environment of hyperglycemia, protein glycosylation within the artery wall may contribute to atherosclerotic vascular disease by altering the normal protein function within the intima.

- Red blood cell deformability and oxygen release are reduced when diabetes is poorly controlled, interfering with tissue oxygen delivery and affecting blood flow.

- Problems with the oxidative state in association with hyperglycemia may also contribute to tissue damage.

- At present, several observational studies have demonstrated a direct relationship between glycemia and atherosclerosis. However, this relationship was not firmly established in the Diabetes Control and Complications Trial[38] although observed in a prospective study among Japanese insulin-requiring type 2 patients.[39] Results from the pilot Veterans Administration study[40] suggest a potential deleterious effect of improved glucose control on atherosclerotic events. The atherogenic process may have begun well before the hyperglycemia began (eg, during insulin resistance or impaired glucose tolerance),[23-26] so that glucose control is a very late intervention for atherosclerosis.

2 A number of risk factors may account for excessive macrovascular disease in diabetes, however, their exact individual role is unclear. It is likely that each risk factor for macrovascular disease contributes to the overall prevalence of coronary artery, cerebral vascular, and peripheral vascular disease.

A The strength of the relationship between the three major risk factors—elevated plasma cholesterol level, high blood pressure, and smoking—and the development of atherosclerotic vascular disease is probably the same in patients with diabetes and comparable individuals without diabetes.[15]

B Studies indicate, however, that only a modest proportion of the excess atherosclerotic vascular disease seen in diabetes can be explained by the levels of the general risk factors for vascular disease. Excess atherosclerotic vascular disease in patients with diabetes is probably due to the effects of hyperglycemia through the substantial number of mechanisms.

- Other factors only recently being investigated such as homocysteine, an amino acid that recent studies indicate may affect vascular disease.[41]

C Some of these problems can be improved by achieving and maintaining better glycemic control.

D Interventional strategies directed at stopping smoking and treating dyslipidemia and hypertension may further reduce the tendency for macrovascular disease.

ASSESSMENT OF ATHEROSCLEROTIC VASCULAR DISEASE

1 The medical history should focus on coronary symptoms (eg, angina, dyspnea, etc), cerebral symptoms (eg, dizziness, transient weakness, etc), and peripheral symptoms (claudication, foot ulcers, etc). The presence of risk factors such as smoking, family history of atherosclerotic vascular disease, personal history of elevated cholesterol levels or blood pressure readings, etc. should also be noted.

2 The physical assessment includes blood pressure measurement (at least two measurements either lying or sitting), evaluation for the presence of vascular bruits, and determination of the status of the feet, including the presence of peripheral pulses and evaluation of orthostatic hypotension.

3 Laboratory assessment includes glycemic control measures and a lipid profile (HDL, cholesterol, low-density lipoprotein [LDL], triglycerides).

4 The educational and psychosocial assessments focus on dietary and exercise/activity habits, coping skills, smoking, and relevant knowledge, beliefs, attitudes.

INTERVENTION STRATEGIES

1 Because macrovascular disease accounts for such significant morbidity, mortality, and costs among patients with diabetes, therapeutic measures to reduce atherosclerotic risk are imperative. In general, efforts can be classified as

   A Primary: trying to decrease the incidence or onset of cardiovascular disease and/or symptoms

   B Secondary: preventive strategies after the onset of clinical cardiovascular disease

   C Tertiary: interventions in association with an acute event (eg, myocardial infarction)

2 Primary and secondary interventions for patients with diabetes are very similar and include aggressive treatment of hypertension, cessation of cigarette smoking, reduction in possible coagulation tendencies, treatment of hyperlipidemia, and optimal control of hyperglycemia.

   A All of these strategies are designed to slow the development and/or progression of atherosclerotic disease.

   B Underlying each of these are self-management education, medical nutrition therapy, and physical activity.[42] Meal planning for weight loss, reduction of cholesterol and saturated fat intake, and increasing consumption of soluble fibers are some of the important strategies that can be presented to patients as therapeutic options (see Chapter 8, Nutrition, Chapter 9, Exercise, and Chapter 13, Hyperglycemia, for more information about these topics).

3 There are several generally accepted principles regarding the treatment of hypertension in persons with diabetes.

   A Pharmacologic treatment is likely to be initiated in persons with diabetes who have only modest elevations of blood pressure compared with the general population.

   B The selection of initial antihypertensive agents for persons with diabetes will differ from the selection for nondiabetic individuals because of the presence of diabetes.

- Angiotensin-converting enzyme (ACE) inhibitors or calcium-channel blockers are often selected as initial therapy, in part because of apparent beneficial effects on kidney function.
- If thiazide diuretics or β-blockers are selected, they should be used very cautiously and at the lowest possible dose. Thiazide diuretics potentially promote hyperglycemia and β-blockers potentially interrupt symptoms of hypoglycemia.

C Serious efforts should be made to achieve normalization of blood pressure, with frequent reassessment and change in medication if acceptable blood pressures are not being achieved.[15,37]

D Self-management education includes the benefits of blood pressure monitoring and control, target levels, and therapeutic options.

4 Smoking status must be routinely assessed in all patients. Self-management education includes the additional risk of smoking for the person with diabetes, use of alternative nicotine delivery systems, written or video materials and other resources, including availability of smoking cessation programs. Generally, if members of the healthcare team demonstrate concern about smoking and its seriousness and display persistence in efforts to help the individual with diabetes to stop smoking, patients are more likely to succeed in this important goal.

5 In approaching persons with diabetes and dyslipidemia, the following sequence of interventions should be considered:

A Self-management education emphasizing medical nutrition therapy, the benefits of physical activity, limitations in total saturated fat, cholesterol reduction, and meal planning for glycemic control and weight loss is essential for patients with lipid abnormalities. See Chapter 8, Nutrition and Chapter 9, Exercise, for more information.

B Optimal glycemic control is sought in concordance with any pharmacologic therapy for dyslipidemia.

C Pharmacologic treatment includes several classes of lipid-lowering agents for treatment of dyslipidemia. Several of these agents have been carefully studied regarding their metabolic effects as well as prevention of adverse macrovascular outcomes. In the past, however, persons with diabetes have either been excluded from these studies or participated in inadequate numbers to make firm judgments about specific agents for this patient population. Fortunately, additional studies[16,17] have been completed and more explicit recommendations now exist.

- Bile acid binding resins (eg, cholestyramine) are effective but difficult to use over long periods and may increase triglyceride levels.
- Fibric acid derivatives (eg, gemfibrozil) do not alter diabetes control and seem effective in controlling dyslipidemia. Their full effect may not be achieved for 3 to 6 months, however.
- Nicotinic acid is inexpensive and effective but is associated with side effects such as flushing and worsening of glycemic control in type 2 diabetes.
- Antioxidant agents that may prevent LDL oxidation are still being evaluated in ongoing coronary prevention trials.
- Estrogen replacement for women with diabetes is quite logical given the loss of gender protection from atherosclerosis. However, there is still some concern about the effect of estrogens on triglyceride levels.
- Subanalyses of recent primary and secondary lipid reduction trials[43] on cardiovascular disease have for the first time allowed some scientific judgment about the benefits of ß-hydroxy-ß-methylglutaryl-coenzyme A (HMG-CoA) reductase inhibitors. It is clear that persons with diabetes experience even a greater benefit from lipid reduction with the "statins" than persons without diabetes. Thus, even before glycemic control has been achieved, or if it has not been possible to substantially improve glucose regulation, specific antilipid medication should be initiated, probably with the "statins."[17]

D Clearly there are a number of therapeutic pharmacologic agents; selection of the most appropriate medication must be based on individual patient characteristics.

E Interest in aspirin therapy in the prevention of CVD in persons with diabetes has increased. At present, it is reasonable and appropriate to prescribe aspirin to persons with diabetes who are at risk for the progression of CAD.[44]

6 For the person with diabetes who experiences an acute myocardial infarction, many treatment options are now available that were not routinely considered a decade ago. Given the reality that persons with diabetes are not only more likely than persons without diabetes to have a myocardial infarct, die from the infarct, have complications from the heart attack (congestive heart failure), and experience a subsequent myocardial infarct, aggressive interventions at the time it occurs seem warranted (ie, tertiary prevention).

A The rapid application of thrombolytic therapy is appropriate, with no evidence of greater adverse consequences.[45] Recent studies[46] have also indicated the benefit of an insulin/glucose/potassium solution. Other agents that should be strongly considered are anticoagulation,[47] ACE inhibitors,[48] and β-blockers.[47]

B Regarding interventions such as angioplasty, bypass grafting, etc, recent studies[49] have indicated that coronary artery bypass grafting is preferable in persons with diabetes because of a high 5-year mortality rate among those receiving angioplasty. In persons with diabetes, the diffuse nature of the coronary atherosclerotic lesions as well as the tendency for re-stenosis may well be so substantial that percutaneous coronary angioplasty is not as effective.

KEY EDUCATION CONSIDERATIONS

1 Explain the significant problem of macrovascular disease in diabetes—the increased susceptibility of patients with diabetes, the synergistic effect of risk factors, which risks are modifiable, and the manifestations of macrovascular disease in diabetes.

2 Inform the patient and family of the importance of monitoring the status of lipid and blood pressure control in addition to blood glucose levels. Antilipid and aspirin therapy also may be used. Familiarize the patient with normal and elevated levels of lipids and blood pressure and strategies to lower.

3 Present the benefits of a meal plan that is low in fat, with special emphasis on consuming low amounts of saturated fat and high amounts of soluble fiber, at the onset of diabetes.

4 Resources (programs and materials) related to coping skills and modifying cardiovascular risk factors should be explored and made available to patients as appropriate.

5 Nutritional, physical activity, and/or pharmacologic therapy for hyperlipidemia or hypertension brings an additional element of complexity to an already challenging treatment program. Thus, health professionals need to recognize patient efforts and make available needed referrals and resources. Priorities need to be clear to all team members, especially the patient and family. Blood glucose, blood pressure, and lipid goals need to be established by the patient and healthcare team.

SELF-REVIEW QUESTIONS

1 Define macrovascular disease and distinguish it from microvascular complications of diabetes.

2 State how macrovascular complications contribute to morbidity and mortality in patients with diabetes.

3 List factors that may contribute to accelerated macrovascular disease in patients with diabetes.

4 Describe ways you would assess for the presence of these risk factors in your patients with diabetes.

5 Describe interventional programs that should be initiated to minimize the chance of macrovascular disease developing in patients with diabetes.

CASE STUDY

TM, a 46-year-old African American woman and mother of three teenagers, with a 13-year history of type 2 diabetes, is being seen in your clinic for the first time. She has been treated with insulin (24 units NPH insulin in the morning, 8 units NPH insulin before dinner), but has used no particular meal plan or exercise program. She tests her blood glucose level periodically, usually when she feels bad. She has come to the clinic to be evaluated for shortness of breath and headaches. Both symptoms have been present for about 2 months but have been increasing in severity over the past 2 weeks. TM has not been routinely followed in any health facility over the past 4 years; she occasionally visits an emergency room for care.

Initial questioning reveals that TM doesn't adjust her insulin but does take her shots each day. She had a random blood glucose reading of 283 mg/dL (15.7 mmol/L) last week. She urinates frequently and has never had a low blood sugar reaction (she does know what this means). She had been told during a past emergency room visit that she had some high blood pressure, but she wasn't prescribed any medication and has not had her blood pressure checked in about 2 years. TM has smoked cigarettes for 18 years. She is unaware of any cholesterol, heart, or kidney problems.

Physical assessment reveals that her blood pressure is 195/108 mm Hg, and she has background diabetic retinopathy, bilateral rales, a heart gallop, 2+ edema, left ventricular hypertrophy by ECG, proteinuria and glucosuria, and a random capillary glucose level of 268 mg/dL (14.9 mmol/L).

QUESTIONS FOR DISCUSSION

1   What general approaches can be used with complex patients such as TM?
2   What would you do first?
3   What would you include in an educational assessment with TM?
4   What are the approaches that the healthcare team can use that demonstrate cultural appropriateness and sensitivity?

DISCUSSION

1   The fact that TM has not been receiving regular evaluation and care is disturbing. However, because she has now come to the clinic when this has not been her pattern over the past 4 years, the healthcare team needs to be particularly sensitive to her presenting concerns.

2   Because of the complexity of the case and the fact that TM is new to your clinic, you need to obtain a lot of information during this first visit. This information is essential for appropriate treatment. In addition, depending on the way this information is collected, the process of interacting with her in a sensitive and appropriate way can help establish rapport so that the chances of her returning are enhanced.

3   The concerns of the healthcare team for TM are
    A   Her diabetes has not been regularly evaluated and her glucose control is inadequate.
    B   She has microvascular (eye) and likely macrovascular (heart) problems, the latter associated with hypertension and tobacco use.
    C   She also may have lipid problems, although this information is not yet known.

4 Some initial attention to her glycemic and blood pressure status is essential. While it might seem reasonable to admit TM to the hospital to initiate treatment, she indicates that she must return home to care for her family; she also notes that she has only very basic health insurance. The following tasks can be completed at this initial visit:

   A Offer referral to a registered dietitian for meal planning and alter her insulin program to begin to improve her blood glucose control.

   B Start an ACE inhibitor for her hypertension.

   C Establish some mechanisms for follow-up at home (ie, call from nurse) before her scheduled return visit.

5 The educator should be concerned with establishing rapport, addressing TM's concerns, and not overwhelming her with too much information at this first visit. Plans for ongoing care and education need to be established with TM.

   A Assess her diabetes knowledge, skills, self-management activities, and attitudes, as well as her socioeconomic situation and the status of cardiovascular risk factors. Asking about her concerns and why she came to the clinic today will provide information about areas to address during this first visit.

   B Because attention to her blood pressure and blood glucose control is indicated, assessment of her monitoring technique and ability (including financial) and willingness to do more frequent blood glucose monitoring is needed. Ask about her interest in smoking cessation to assess her readiness to quit.

   C If she is able to test her blood glucose levels reliably and more frequently, a plan can be developed to determine when to test and how to use the results to improve her glycemic control. A plan for telephone follow-up may be useful.

6 Part of the reason that TM may not have sought health care may be related to negative experiences in the healthcare system. It is therefore important to address TM by her last name, treat her with respect, and avoid making judgments about her self-care behaviors and lack of past medical care. It is also important to assess her cultural and religious beliefs and practices that may influence the way she cares for her diabetes. Incorporate ethnic foods into her meal plan as appropriate, and ask about her use of alternative therapies.

REFERENCES

1   Haffner S. The prediabetic problem: development of non-insulin-dependent diabetes mellitus and related abnormalities. J Diabetes Complications 1997; 11:69-76.

2   Nattrass M. Managing diabetes after myocardial infarction. Br Med J 1997; 314:1497.

3   Libby, P. Molecular bases of the acute coronary syndromes. Circulation 1995; 91:2844-50.

4   Vinicor F. Features of macrovascular disease of diabetes. In: Haire-Joshu D, ed. Management of diabetes mellitus: perspectives of care across the life span. 2nd ed. St. Louis: Mosby-Year Book Inc, 1996:281-308.

5   American Diabetes Association. Economic consequences of diabetes mellitus in the US In 1997. Diabetes Care 1998;21:296-309.

6   The Expert Committee on the Diagnosis and Classification of Diabetes Mellitus. Report of the Expert Committee on the Diagnosis and Classification of Diabetes Mellitus. Diabetes Care 1997;20: 1183-97.

7   Eastman RC, Vinicor F. Science: moving us in the right direction. Diabetes Care 1997;20:1057-58.

8   Kannel WB. Coronary heart disease risk factors: Framingham study update. Hosp Pract 1990;25:119-27.

9   Kannel WB, D'Agostino RB, Wilson PW, Belanger AJ, Gagnon DR. Diabetes, fibrinogen and risk of cardiovascular disease: the Framingham experience. Am Heart J 1990;120:672-76.

10 Mankovsky B, Metzger B, Molitch M, Biller J. Cerebrovascular disorders in patients with diabetes mellitus. J Diabetes Complications 1996;10:228-42.

11 Pecoraro R, Reiber GE, Burgess EM. Pathways to diabetic limb amputation: basis for prevention. Diabetes Care 1990;13:513-21.

12 Reiber G, Pecoraro RE, Koepsell TD. Risk factors for amputation in patients with diabetes mellitus: a case-control study. Ann Intern Med 1992;117:97-105.

13 Levin ME. Preventing amputation in the patient with diabetes. Diabetes Care 1995;18:1383-94.

14 Centers for Disease Control and Prevention. National diabetes fact sheet. Atlanta: US Department of Health and Human Services, Centers for Disease Control and Prevention, Division of Diabetes Translation, 1997.

15 American Diabetes Association. Role of cardiovascular risk factors in the prevention and treatment of macrovascular disease in diabetes. Diabetes Care 1989;12:573-79.

16 Haffner SM. Management of dyslipidemia in adults with diabetes: a technical review. Diabetes Care 1998;21: 160-78.

17 American Diabetes Association. Management of dyslipidemia in adults with diabetes. Diabetes Care 1998;21:179-82.

18 Criqui MH, Heiss G, Cohn R, et al. Plasma triglyceride level and mortality from coronary heart disease. N Engl J Med 1993;328:1220-25.

19 Stewart MW, Laker MF. Triglycerides in diabetes: time for action? Diabetic Med 1994;11:725-27.

20 Manninen, V, Tenkanen L, Koskinen P, et al. Joint effects of serum triglyceride and LDL cholesterol and HDL cholesterol concentrations on coronary heart disease risk in the Helsinki Heart Study. Implications for treatment. Circulation 1992;85:37-45.

21 Nakamura H, Ikewaki K, Nishiwaki M, Shige H. Postprandial hyperlipidemia and coronary artery disease. Ann N Y Acad Sci 1995;748:441-46.

22 Yusuf H, Giles W, Croft J, Anda R, Casper M. Impact of multiple risk factor profiles on determining cardiovascular disease risk. Prev Med 1998;27:1-9.

23 Reaven GM. Role of insulin resistance in human disease. Diabetes 1988;37:1595-607.

24 Kaplan NM. The deadly quartet. Upper-body obesity, glucose intolerance, hypertriglyceridemia, and hypertension. Arch Intern Med 1989;149:1514-20.

25 Haffner SM, Stern MP, Hazuda HP, Mitchell BD, Patterson JK. Cardiovascular risk factors in confirmed pre-diabetic individuals. Does the clock for coronary heart disease start ticking before the onset of clinical diabetes? JAMA 1990; 263:2893-98.

26 Saudek CD. When does diabetes start? JAMA 1990;263:2934.

27 Barker DJ. Fetal nutrition and cardiovascular disease in later life. Br Med Bull 1997;53:96-108.

28 Hales CN, Desai M, Ozanne SE. The Thrifty Phenotype hypothesis: how does it look after 5 years? Diabetic Med 1997; 14:189-95.

29 Ford ES, Newman J. Smoking and diabetes mellitus. Findings from 1988 Behavioral Risk Factor Surveillance System. Diabetes Care 1991;14:871-74.

30 Vlassara H. Advanced glycation endproducts and atherosclerosis. Ann Med 1996;28:419-26.

31 Helmrich S, Ragland DR, Leung RW, Paffenbarger RS Jr. Physical activity and reduced occurrence of non-insulin-dependent diabetes mellitus. N Engl J Med 1991;325:147-52.

32 National Institutes of Health. Non-insulin dependent diabetes primary prevention trial. NIH guide grants Contracts 1993; 22:1-20.

33 Dinneen SF, Gerstein HC. The association of microalbuminuria and mortality in non-insulin-dependent diabetes mellitus. A systematic overview of the literature. Arch Intern Med 1997;157:1413-18.

34 Rossing P, Hougaard P, Borch-Johnsen K, Parving HH. Predictors of mortality in insulin dependent diabetes: 10 year observational follow-up study. Br Med J 1996;313:779-84.

35 Stout RW. Insulin and atheroma. 20-year perspective. Diabetes Care 1990;13: 631-54.

36 Home PD. Insulin resistance is not central to the burden of diabetes. Diabetes Metab Rev 1997;13:87-92.

37 Joint National Committee on Prevention, Detection, Evaluation and Treatment of High Blood Pressure. The sixth report of the Joint National Committee on prevention and treatment of high blood pressure. Arch Intern Med 1997;157:2413-46.

38 The Diabetes Control and Complications Trial Research Group. The effect of intensive treatment of diabetes on the development and progression of long-term complications of insulin-dependent diabetes. N Engl J Med 1993;329:977-86.

39 Ohkubo Y, Kishikawa H, Araki E, Miyata T, Isami S, Motoyoski S, et al. Intensive insulin therapy prevents the progression of diabetic microvasular complications in Japanese patients with non-insulin dependent diabetes mellitus: a randomized prospective 6-year study. Diabetes Res Clin Practice 1995;18:103-17.

40 Abraira C, Colwell J, Nuttall F, et al. Cardiovascular events and correlates in the Veterns Affairs Diabetes Feasibility Trail: Veterans Affairs Cooperative Study on glycemic control and complications in type 2 diabetes. Arch Int Med 1997;157:181-88.

41 Colwell JA. Elevated plasma homocysteine and diabetic vascular disease. Diabetes Care 1997;20:1805-6.

42 US Department of Health and Human Services. Physical activity and Health: a report of the Surgeon General. Atlanta, Ga: US Department of Health and Human Services, Centers for Disease Control and Prevention, National Center for Chronic Disease Prevention and Health Promotion, 1996.

43 Gotto AM Jr. Cholesterol management in theory and practice. Circulation 1997; 96:4424-30.

44 Colwell JA. Aspirin therapy in diabetes: a technical review. Diabetes Care 1997; 20:1767-71.

45 Granger CB, Califf RM, Young S, et al. Outcome of patients with diabetes mellitus and acute myocardial infarction treated with thrombolytic agents. The Thrombolysis and Angioplasty in Myocardial Infarction (TAMI) Study Group. J Am Coll Cardiol 1993;21: 920-25.

46 Malmberg K, Ryden L, Hamsten A, Herlitz J, Waldenstrom A, Wedel H. Mortality prediction in diabetic patients with myocardial infarction: experiences from the DIGAMI study. Cardiovasc Res 1997;34:248-53.

47 Aronson D, Rayfield EJ, Chesebro JH. Mechanisms determining course and outcomes of diabetic patients who have had acute myocardial infarction. Ann Intern Med 1997;126:296-306.

48 Nesto R, Zarich S. Acute myocardial infarction in diabetes mellitus: lessons learned from ACE inhibition. Circulation 1998;97:12-15.

49 The Bypass Angioplasty Revascularization Investigation (BARI) Investigators. Comparison of coronary bypass surgery with angioplasty in patients with multivessel disease. N Engl J Med 1996;335: 217-25.

SUGGESTED READINGS

Atherosclerosis and diabetes. Diabetes Reviews;1997,5(4).

American Diabetes Association. Role of cardiovascular risk factors in prevention and treatment of macrovascular disease in diabetes. Diabetes Care 1989;12:573-79.

Colwell J, Lopes-Virella M. A review of the development of large vessel disease in diabetes mellitus: the genesis of atherosclerosis in diabetes mellitus. Am J Med 1988;85:113-18.

Jarrett RJ. Cardiovascular disease and hypertension in diabetes mellitus. Diabetes Metab Rev 1989;5:547-58.

Jarrett RJ. Type II (non-insulin-dependent) diabetes mellitus and coronary heart disease - chicken, egg, or neither? Diabetologia 1984;26:99-102.

Pyorala K, Laasko M, Uusitupa M. Diabetes and atherosclerosis: an epidemiologic view. Diabetes Metab Rev 1987;3:463-524.

Diabetes and Arteriosclerosis. International Diabetes Federation Bulletin 1997(Nov); V 42.

RESEARCH

The Importance of Research and Outcomes **25**

James A. Fain, PhD, RN, FAAN
University of Massachusetts Medical Center
Graduate School of Nursing
Boston, Massachusetts

Introduction

1 Whether diabetes educators practice in an acute-care facility, community agency, or outpatient setting, quality care and education is expected to reflect the translation of strong scientific evidence and professional consensus into practice.

2 Diabetes educators have a responsibility for assuming an active role in this process by:

   A Having knowledge of the research process to improve the ability to determine what constitutes good research.

   B Developing the skills of reading and evaluating research reports to determine the accuracy and applicability of the findings of a study.

   C Participating in research opportunities.

3 Diabetes educators must examine how research opportunities can best be incorporated into their everyday practice.

4 This chapter provides an overview of the value of research and the application of the scientific method; the research process with several types of research methods; and, the role of research consumer and outcome measures.

Objectives

Upon completion of this chapter, the learner will be able to

1 Explain the importance of research for diabetes educators.

2 Describe how the scientific method is applied in research.

3 Distinguish between a quantitative and qualitative approach to research.

4 List the five general phases of the research process.

5 Identify the basic elements of a research report.

6 Distinguish between experimental and nonexperimental research.

7 Explain strategies for participating in research opportunities.

The Importance of Research

1 The challenges confronting the healthcare system today have made it necessary for all health practitioners to document the effectiveness of their clinical decisions and educational efforts. Diabetes educators must validate their practice by applying the knowledge and skills gained through ongoing scientific investigations.

2 New information that is discovered through research helps explain, describe, and predict relationships about individuals and their health care experiences, expected outcomes associated with new therapies, and helps with the evaluation of clinical care and education programs. This discovery is essential for gaining new knowledge and skills that can contribute to the continued growth of the profession. Diabetes educators who base their clinical decisions and educational strategies on scientifically documented information are acting in the most professional and accountable manner.

   A The development of a discipline such as diabetes education is marked by the growth of knowledge that is useful in solving problems that are encountered in practice. By actually conducting research studies or understanding the research results of other investigators, diabetes educators contribute to the knowledge base that serves as a reference for the practice of diabetes care and education.

   B Diabetes educators must focus on improving their understanding of the research process, developing skills to evaluate published research reports, and incorporating relevant findings into their practices.

Definition of Research

1 *Research* is defined as a systematic process in which the scientific method is employed to answer questions.[1] The goal of research is to explain, predict, and/or control phenomena.

2 Research often is considered synonymous with problem-solving. This notion is incorrect because the focus of research is discovering or generating new knowledge, whereas problem-solving involves using current knowledge.

3 The scientific method is a rigorous process for generating new knowledge.

   A Two characteristics that are unique to the scientific method are objectivity and the use of empirical data.[2]

B The following research tasks are part of the scientific method:
- Selecting and defining a problem
- Formulating research questions and/or hypotheses
- Collecting data
- Analyzing data
- Reporting results

4 The two major types of scientific inquiry are quantitative research and qualitative research.

    A Quantitative vs. qualitative research

- *Quantitative research* is defined as a systematic, formal process that involves the use of quantitative methods such as questionnaires, surveys, and experiments, such as controlled clinical trials to describe variables, examine relationships among variables, and determine cause-and-effect interactions between variables. Data are collected, quantified, and translated into numbers to be statistically analyzed.
- The quantitative research approach is viewed by some researchers as a "hard" science that reflects the rigor of the scientific method.
- Quantitative methods have long been used for research in the basic sciences of physics, chemistry, and medicine. More recently, quantitative methods have been used in applied sciences such as nursing, nutrition, and pharmacology.
- A description of a quantitative approach to research[3] is shown in Figure 25.1. The aim of this study was to evaluate the effectiveness of several diabetes education programs that provided a range of self-care instructions to patients with type 2 diabetes who had not previously undergone diabetes education. Note how several types of data were collected and analyzed across time (eg, glycosylated hemoglobin levels, height, weight, blood pressure, cholesterol levels, and knowledge of diabetes).

    B *Qualitative research* is defined as a systematic, subjective approach that involves the use of methods of inquiry that emphasize subjectivity and the meaning of the experience for the individual.

- Qualitative methods incorporate the subject's own words and narrative summaries of observable behavior to express data, rather than using numbers. Questions that lend themselves to qualitative inquiry are generally broad and seek to understand why particular phenomena occur.

TABLE 25.1. TYPES OF QUANTITATIVE AND QUALITATIVE RESEARCH

1   Quantitative Approach
    A   Experimental research
        • Experimental designs
        • Quasi-experimental designs
    B   Nonexperimental research
        • Descriptive designs
        • Correlational designs
        • Longitudinal designs
        • Time-Series designs
2   Qualitative Approach
    A   Grounded theory research
    B   Phenomenological research
    C   Ethnographic research

FIGURE 25.1. EXAMPLE OF A QUANTITATIVE RESEARCH APPROACH

In this randomized trial, patients with NIDDM [type 2 diabetes] were assigned to one of four programs: a minimal instruction program (n=59), an education program of individual visits (n=57), an education program incorporating a group education course (n=66), and a behavioral program (n=59). The four programs involved different amounts of patient contact time, delivery format, and instructional strategies. The following outcome measures were assessed at baseline and at 3, 6, and 12 months: glycosylated hemoglobin (HbA_{1c}); Body Mass Index (BMI)—height and weight were measured to allow this calculation; blood lipids (fasting total cholesterol, HDL); blood pressure (systolic and diastolic); and knowledge of diabetes—diabetes knowledge scale (DKNA).

Source: Excerpted from Campbell et al.[3]

• Qualitative research is typically used for investigation of human behavior in the fields of psychology, sociology, and education.
• A description of a qualitative approach to research[4] is shown in Figure 25.2. The purpose of this qualitative approach (grounded theory) was to investigate the experience of living with type 1 diabetes. Data were collected from interviews with four participants and from analyzing their diabetes papers and personal journals.

Figure 25.2. Example of a Qualitative Research Approach

In grounded theory, data collection and data analysis occur simultaneously. In this study, transcriptions of interviews, diabetes papers, and journals were examined and coded line-by-line to identify the underlying processes. Coded data that seemed related were grouped into categories. Throughout the coding, data collected through interviews, diabetes papers, and journals were constantly compared for similarities and differences. As data collection and analysis continued, categories were collapsed into more general categories until the underlying theory of "becoming diabetic" emerged; a theory of integration. Throughout the process, memos were written containing ideas and questions that has been sparked by the interview and coding activities. These memos helped to delineate the emerging theory. Recruitment into the study was terminated after the fourth participant because of the wealth of data that had been collected with all four participants corroborated the three-phase process of integration.

Source: Excerpted from Hernandez.[4]

5   Regardless of the research methods used, researchers have the responsibility of conducting a study with rigor and skill. *Rigor* is defined as the striving for excellence in research using discipline, scrupulous adherence to detail, and strict accuracy.[5]

   A   The use of both quantitative and qualitative methods to collect data is referred to as *triangulation*.[5]

   B   Several different types of quantitative and qualitative research approaches are shown in Table 25.1.

The Research Process

1   The research process is a decision-making process that involves considering various alternatives and deciding what methods will provide answers for particular research question(s) or for testing hypotheses.

2   The research process is flexible. There are no correct answers but rather multiple possibilities from which researchers must choose, each with its own strengths and weaknesses.

3 The research process is circular. When conducting a study, researchers may need to rethink and reconceptualize a problem several times. For example, researchers continually review the literature to keep up with the most current information and refer to previous research reports to get ideas for sampling, operational definitions, and research designs. In addition, research is circular in that research leads to further research and the process starts over again.

4 The intent of the research process is to describe the general thinking of researchers who plan the study rather than to present a set of rules. Although many different research models exist, the research process consists of standard elements; the order may vary and the steps may overlap in different research situations. The five general phases of the research process[6] are presented in Figure 25.3.

HOW TO READ A RESEARCH REPORT

1 As consumers of research, diabetes educators need to develop the ability to understand and apply research findings to their practices. Becoming familiar with research terminology assists the diabetes educator in reading published research reports.

2 Research reports are divided into sections with headings and subheadings that follow a standardized format. The following elements are used in this sequence: abstract, introduction, research questions and/or hypotheses, methods, results, and discussion of conclusions.[7]

A The abstract is located at the beginning of a research report and provides a brief, concise summary of the study. Many journals use a structured abstract form, limiting the number of words to approximately 100.

   • The following information about the study is included in the abstract: purpose, objectives, or hypotheses; brief explanation of data collection and analysis procedures; and summary of important findings.

   • The abstract presented in Figure 25.4 summarizes the purpose, number, and type of subjects; type of analysis; and summary of results.[8] The abstract is written in a brief, concise manner to help readers determine whether the research is appropriate for their needs and if the complete article is something they may want to read.

FIGURE 25.3. PHASES OF THE RESEARCH PROCESS

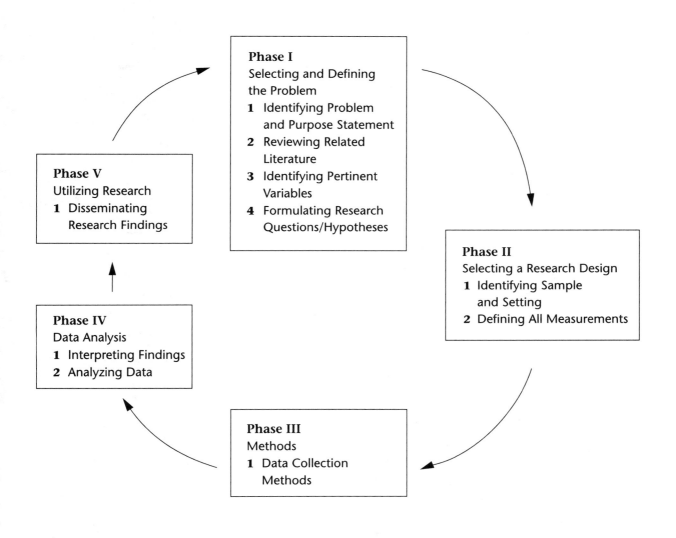

Figure 25.4. Example of a Typical Abstract

The purpose of this research study was to explore personal illness models of preadolescents and adolescents regarding diabetes mellitus. Personal illness models were defined as the adolescents' cognitive representations of their disease. Sixty children ages 10-17 years with a diagnosis of IDDM [type 1 diabetes] were interviewed using a semi-structured questionnaire. Data were content analyzed for common themes. Although most participants expressed an understanding that their disease would last a lifetime, they were hopeful for a cure. Participants wanted healthcare professionals to provide strategies for controlling blood glucose to prevent future complications. Family and friends who followed the same diet as the adolescent with diabetes were viewed as supportive. The majority of adolescents were responsible for much of their own disease management. Their greatest fears concerned insulin reactions and long-term complications such as amputation of limbs.

Source: Excerpted from Standiford DA et al.[8]

B The introduction of a research article contains three parts: a problem statement, a review of related literature, and a purpose statement.

- The problem statement provides direction for the research study and is typically stated at the beginning of a research article. The problem statement provides a justification for the study by citing background information about the problem to support the need for conducting the proposed study.[1,2,7] The discussion of previous research can be as brief as one or two sentences or as long as several pages.

- Literature reviews involve identifying and analyzing relevant publications that contain information related to the proposed research problem. Literature reviews are conducted to uncover what is already known about the topic and problem, to determine consistencies and gaps in knowledge about the problem, to describe strengths and weaknesses of designs and methods of inquiry, and to generate useful research questions and/or hypotheses.[1,2,7] A review of literature can be as brief as three or four sentences or as long as two or three pages. Comprehensive reviews of the literature are usually not found in most research reports due to space limitations, but may be published separately as a literature or technical review study.

FIGURE 25.5. EXAMPLE OF A PROBLEM STATEMENT WITH A PURPOSE STATEMENT

Problem Statement:

Approximately 14 million Americans have diabetes. People with diabetes are at risk for chronic complications of the disease affecting the heart, kidneys, eyes, nervous system, and lower extremities. Diabetes-related foot complications result in amputation of the lower extremities and millions of dollars in medical cost. African Americans have a higher rate of lower-extremity amputation than the general population. The US Public Health Service has stated as one of its goals the reduction of lower-extremity amputations in African Americans. The goal is to reduce the 1987 rate of 10.2 per 1000 to 6.1 per 1000 by the year 2000.

Studies have shown that proper foot care can reduce the number and severity of diabetic foot problems. Proper foot care requires daily care and maintenance and can be effectively implemented with the necessary knowledge, attitudes, and self-care skills. Educating people with diabetes to care for their feet is recognized as a key to the prevention and early detection of podiatric problems. To date, few diabetes education programs for foot self-care have been systematically developed and evaluated or targeted for a special population.

Purpose Statement:

The purpose of this project was to develop, formatively evaluate, and pilot test a self-care, take-home program for the prevention of foot problems in African Americans with diabetes.

Source: Excerpted from Ledda et al.[9]

- The problem statement presented in Figure 25.5 provides the reader with a clear understanding of the problem being studied and why it is important.[9] The literature review is concise (two paragraphs) and reflects the relevant background that is necessary to support the rationale for the study. The literature review ends with a purpose statement that delineates the variables to be studied and identifies the study population.
- The purpose statement is a single statement that identifies why the problem is being studied, specifies the overall goal and intent of the research, and clarifies the knowledge to be gained.[1,2,7] The purpose statement is usually shown after the problem statement and some-

times under the subheading of introduction, literature review, or background.[7]

C Hypotheses and/or research questions are formulated after the literature review has been completed. Before stating hypotheses and/or research questions, the researcher need to identify variables that are pertinent to the study.

- A *hypothesis* is defined as a statement that explains or predicts the relationship or differences between two or more variables in terms of expected results or outcomes of a study.[1,2,7] Hypotheses provide direction for the research design, and the collection, analysis, and interpretation of data. Hypotheses are not needed for research that is descriptive (describing rather than explaining). When the purpose of a study is to explain the nature and strength of relationships among variables, hypotheses are used.

- Researchers do not set out to prove a hypothesis but rather to collect data that either support or refute the hypothesis.

- The variables that are identified in hypotheses are operationally defined. An operational definition specifies how the variables will be measured in terms of the instruments and/or scales to be used.[1,2,7]

- The following statement is an example of a hypothesis: Individuals with type 2 diabetes who receive service from a home health agency that provides a multidisciplinary approach to diabetes care will have a shorter length of service (LOS) than those individuals who receive services from an agency that does not provide a multidisciplinary approach to diabetes care.

- Research studies do not always contain hypotheses but may instead be organized around research questions. A *research question* is defined as a concise, interrogative statement that is written in the present tense and includes one or more variables.[1,2,7] Research questions focus on describing the variable(s), examining relationships among variables, and determining differences between two or more groups regarding the selected variable(s).

- The type of research question that focuses on determining differences between groups is described in Figure 25.6.[10] In this study, 61 parents of children with type 1 diabetes completed a modified version of the Hypoglycemic Fear Survey (HFS). Parents also indicated their child's history of hypoglycemic-related seizures (SLC), or loss of consciousness events. In the first research question, parents of children with type 1 diabetes *with* a history of SLC were compared with parents of children with type 1 diabetes *without* a history of SLC. In the second research question, adolescents *with* a history of SLC were compared with adolescents *without* a history of SLC.[10]

- The dependent variable, or outcome, represents the area of interest under study and reflects the effect of or the response to the independent variable. Dependent variables are sometimes thought of as the results of conducting a study, or the outcome measure. The dependent variable for both research questions in Figure 25.6 was fear of hypoglycemia as measured by the HFS.

FIGURE 25.6. EXAMPLE OF RESEARCH QUESTIONS

The present study was designed to address the dearth of knowledge in this subject area. The following research questions were posed:

1 Do parents of IDDM [type 1 diabetes] children with a history of hypoglycemic SLC events have a greater fear of hypoglycemia compared with parents of IDDM children without a SLC history?

2 Do adolescents with IDDM [type 1 diabetes] who have a SLC history have a greater fear of hypoglycemia than those without a SLC history?

Source: Excerpted from Marrero et al.[10]

- The independent variable is perceived as contributing to or preceding a particular outcome. It is sometimes referred to as the variable that is manipulated by the researcher, and its effect on the dependent variable is observed. Depending on the research approach, the independent variable may be classified as an experimental, treatment, intervention, or predictor variable. History of SLC versus no history of SLC was the independent variable for both research questions in Figure 25.6 that affects the fear of hypoglycemia, or the dependent variable.

D The methods section of a research report contains information about how a study is conducted. This section is the most important part of the research report and needs to be written clearly and concisely. The first part of the methods section, the overall study design that will be employed to test the hypotheses or answer the research question(s), is identified.

- The *research design* is defined as a set of guidelines by which a researcher obtains answers to the research question(s). The research design provides a methodological direction and specifies procedures such as site selection, sampling techniques, selection of instruments, and data analysis.

- A wide variety of study designs are used in research. Most research designs are classified as experimental or nonexperimental.

- Experimental designs refer to studies in which the researcher manipulates and controls one or more variables and observes the effect(s) on another variable.[1,2,7] Several types of research designs (eg, experimental and quasi-experimental) are used in experimental research.[1,2,7]

- Experimental designs are referred to as intervention studies whereby a particular method or treatment is expected to influence one or more outcomes. Such studies enable researchers to assess the effectiveness of various teaching methods, curriculum models, and other variables at influencing the characteristics of individuals or groups.

- Quasi-experimental designs refer to a modified experimental approach. Researchers may use a quasi-experimental design and still be able to manipulate the independent variable (experimental condition) and exercise some control over the study. However, random assignment of subjects to control or experimental groups is not feasible using quasi-experimental designs.

- Nonexperimental designs refer to studies in which the researcher examines variables in natural environments and does not include researcher-imposed treatments.[1,2,7] Nonexperimental research is classified as descriptive and/or correlational.

- Descriptive research provides information about the characteristics of a particular individual, event, or group for the purpose of discovering new information, describing what exists, and determining the frequency with which something occurs.[1,2,7]

- Correlational research provides a description of the relationship between two or more variables and the nature of that relationship (eg, positive or negative).[1,2,7] Descriptive correlational research, which is very common, attempts to describe what exists and identify several interrelationships. Variables are not manipulated and the setting is not controlled. Analysis of data often leads to forming hypotheses that can be tested experimentally.

- An example of a descriptive correlational study[11] is provided in Figure 25.7. The authors have described the differences between African American and Caucasian patients with respect to their self-reported dietary adherence as stated in the first research question.

FIGURE 25.7. EXAMPLE OF A DESCRIPTIVE CORRELATIONAL STUDY

Nutrition therapy is a cornerstone of diabetes care and often the primary form of treatment for persons with NIDDM [type 2 diabetes]. Because of the impact of food choices on diabetes management and because of the significant difficulty many patients have in following dietary recommendations, it is important to identify beliefs, attitudes, and behaviors that influence the ability of patients to successfully implement dietary recommendations.

Health beliefs and health behaviors are influenced by ethnic, cultural, and socioeconomic factors. The impact of diabetes-related dietary recommendations is likely to vary among different ethnic and cultural groups. Meal plans recommended by health professionals may not accommodate existing dietary habits, thus making self-care more difficult for patients.

The following research questions were proposed: (1) Do African American and Caucasian patients with NIDDM differ in self-reported dietary adherence? and (2) Does adherence to dietary recommendations have the same relationship with other psychosocial factors for African Americans and Caucasians with NIDDM?

Source: Excerpted from Fitzgerald et al.[11]

The second research question focuses on the relationships between dietary adherence and psychosocial factors.

- *Longitudinal designs* collect data over time, usually for the purpose of describing developmental changes in a particular group.
- *Time series designs* assess changes over time, prior to and following administration of a treatment.
- *Grounded theory* is a qualitative research method, a form of field research. It is the discovery of theory from data that have been systematically obtained through research.
- *Phenomenological research* is a qualitative research approach. Researchers use a phenomenological approach to describe experiences as they are lived. In the phenomenological terms this is referred to as the "lived experience."
- *Ethnographic research* is a qualitative approach that can provide the opportunity for researchers to conduct studies regarding the need for intimacy among members of the culture. The researcher becomes

intimately involved in the data collection process and seeks to understand fully how life unfolds for the individual or group under study.

E Details of the methods section are presented in the following subsections: subjects/setting, data collection procedures, data collection instruments, and specific statistical procedures for analyzing data.

- Discussion of the subjects (study sample) includes the criteria for selecting the subjects, sample size, sample characteristics, and setting. Research reports also include a statement documenting that subjects have read and signed an informed consent form and that the study was approved by an institutional review board (IRB) for the protection of human subjects' rights.

- The example in Figure 25.8 illustrates criteria for study eligibility along with a rationale for why only women participated in the study. A statement about approval from an Office of Regulatory Compliance is mentioned along with how subjects were invited to participate in the study. Data collection procedures are described so that the reader can follow the procedural flow of the study. These procedures include a detailed explanation of what subjects were asked to do, who collected the data, and how often measurements were taken. Data collection instruments (surveys, scales) identify the variables that are measured.

F The results section of a research report provides a description of the findings from the study based on statistical analysis of the data. The results of a study are organized according to the research purpose or objectives and the hypotheses and/or research questions.

G The discussion section of a research report combines and gives meaning to information from the other sections and includes major findings, limitations of the study, conclusions drawn from the findings, and implications/recommendations for further research.

3 The first step in reading a research report is to skim the article to gain a broad overview of the content.[7] Read the title, author's name, abstract, major headings, and one or two sentences under each heading. Skimming allows you to make a preliminary judgment about the value of the source.

4 Read the entire study carefully to comprehend the findings that are presented.

FIGURE 25.8. EXAMPLE OF A METHODS SECTION WITH INCLUSION CRITERION AND DATA COLLECTION

Women between the age of 40 and 60 years and diagnosed with NIDDM [type 2 diabetes] at least 12 months prior to the initiation of the study were recruited from a rural community. Age was restricted to 40 to 60 years because NIDDM is usually diagnosed after the age of 40 years and the label reading habits of older women (>65 years) differ from those of younger women. Women were the focus of this study because they were frequent label readers as well as primary food shoppers. A uniform group of women in terms of diagnosis and use of nutrition labels was desired.

Participants were recruited through advertisements in newspapers and public service announcements on television. The study was described as a general consumer research study rather than a nutrition study to minimize social desirability effects. All methods were approved by the Office for Regulatory Compliance at a major university.

Three procedures were followed for data collection: (1) a telephone screening interview to determine subject eligibility; (2) written questionnaire about location and frequency of grocery shopping, diabetes education, and demographic characteristics mailed to participants to be completed at home; and (3) participation in either a focus group or an in-depth interview. Both the data collection and data analysis of the focus groups and in-depth interviews are further described.

Source: Excerpted from Miller et al.[12]

A Focus on understanding the major concepts and the logical flow of ideas within the study.

B Use the glossary of key terms at the end of most research textbooks to to review the definition of words that are unfamiliar.

C Highlight the parts of the research report that are difficult to read and understand to be reviewed again later.

5 Identify the steps of the research process in the margins of the research report to easily locate the problem, purpose, major variables, study design, sample size, data collection and analysis techniques, and findings.

6 Divide the content of the report into sections to examine for accuracy, completeness, and organization. Determine whether the steps of the research process flow logically or whether steps are missing or incomplete.

The Use of Outcomes as Performance Measures

1 *Outcome measures* are defined as data that describe a patient's health status.[13]

2 Patient health outcomes (eg, morbidity/mortality, surgical infection rates, quality of life, patient satisfaction) have been measured for years. The use of patient health outcomes has been increasing steadily as more researchers perceive these outcomes as the gold standard for measuring the performance of providing health care.[13]

3 Improved patient health outcomes are the ultimate goal of all healthcare services.

4 The need to examine outcomes is evidenced by mandates by the Health Care Financing Administration (HCFA), the Agency for Health Care Policy and Research (AHCPR), and accrediting bodies such as the Joint Commission on Accreditation of Health Care Organizations (JCAHO).

5 Diabetes-specific health outcomes measures can be divided into three categories: quality of life (QoL), clinical outcomes, and essential processes.

   A Diabetes affects general health status in addition to causing complications and functional problems related to the disease. Several instruments exist for assessing QoL, including the SF-36 used in the Medical Outcomes Study[14] for individuals with type 2 diabetes. Other diabetes-specific QoL measures have been used.[15-17] It is important for the researcher to conceptualize and define QoL as it relates to the research problem being studied so that appropriate instrumentation can be used.

   B Several clinical outcomes that should be measured in individuals with diabetes include glycosylated hemoglobin (HbA$_{1c}$), quantitative urinary protein, lipids (total cholesterol, HDL, LDL, triglycerides), blood pressure (systolic and diastolic), frequency of self-monitoring of blood glucose (SMBG), frequency of hypoglycemic reactions, and frequency of diabetic ketoacidosis.

   C Several important measures or essential processes for individuals with diabetes include an annual retinal exam, foot exam for new ulcers/ infections, and yearly chart review for reports of amputation.

6 Patient satisfaction outcomes are likewise important. Satisfaction may be evaluated in a variety of areas, including amenities of care (eg, waiting time, comfort, privacy), the art of care (whether healthcare providers are perceived as courteous, thorough, and respectful), and the results of care (patients' perception of improved health and well-being). Raising the level of perceived quality can improve an organization's level of effectiveness and ability to achieve better outcomes.[18]

7 Evaluation of diabetes education programs is critical when educators/clinicians need to document the effectiveness of their clinical decisions and educational efforts. When measuring the effects of diabetes patient education, there are several important steps to take:

    A Use an unbiased selection process when choosing the sample. The sample need to be representative of all patients who participate in the program.[19]

    B Obtain an adequate sample to make sure the number of patients studied is sufficient to conduct statistical analysis.[19]

    C Use standardized measures with proven validity and reliability. Evaluation measures themselves are sometimes invalid and do not provide accurate information about program effectiveness.[19]

    D Collect data that are longitudinal or prospective in nature (eg, data gathered at the beginning of the program, at the end of the program, and again at one or more follow-ups after the program). Retrospective measurements (eg, only asking patients at some point after the program whether they have learned anything or whether their behavior has changed) should be avoided. This type of measurement represents retrospective bias.[19]

    E Obtain follow-up measures two or three times. The first time is immediately after the educational program, with another 2 to 3 months later. The purpose of these follow-ups is to see whether patients are making an effort to implement the goals and intentions they formulated at the end of the program. The next follow-up should be 3 to 6 month after the initial program was completed. In conducting follow-ups, a representative number of those individuals who participated in the program should be sampled. If there was a large percentage of dropouts, the results of follow-up data may be questioned.[19]

8 Outcome measures associated with diabetes education programs include medical, behavioral, and psychosocial factors.[19]

A Medical factors are identified in the patient's medical history (eg, present health status, health resource utilization, risk factors).

B Behavioral factors focus on goals and intentions that mediate the program effect on self-care (eg, blood glucose, monitoring, medications, diet, exercise, prevention/management of complications, knowledge). The most common technique for measuring self-care is patient self-report or, in the case of young children, parent reports, and in the case of the elderly, caregiver reports.

C Psychosocial factors evaluate social support systems (eg, family, peer, health professional), and health beliefs and attitudes. In addition, barriers to learning and socioeconomic factors are addressed.

9 The outcomes of many individuals are pooled to provide aggregate outcome data, which are more useful for attributing patterns of outcomes to the performance of a particular program organization or provider than single-patient data.

10 Limitations in the use of outcomes measures concern data reliability and validity. Choosing instruments that are valid and reliable provides confidence in the results.

A *Reliability* is defined as to the consistency with which an instrument, scale, or test examines a particular measure.

B *Validity* is defined as the degree to which an instrument, scale, or test measures what it is supposed to measure.[20] "Choosing instruments that are valid and reliable provides confidence in the results."

RESEARCH AND THE DIABETES EDUCATOR

1 The role of the researcher is defined on a continuum by the degree of active or passive participation in the research process. At one end of the continuum are those diabetes educators who are consumers of research.

2 The role of the research consumer includes the ability to read and evaluate research reports. Diabetes educators are increasingly expected to maintain, at minimum, this level of involvement in research. Developing skills to critically read and understand research takes time, knowledge of the research process, and repeated practice.

3 At the other end of the continuum are those diabetes educators who are Principal Investigators (PI) and conduct research and actively participate in designing and implementing a study. Diabetes educators who are members of a research team collaborate on the development of an idea and actually participate in the design and production of a study.

4 Participation in research activities is shared by diabetes educators at all levels. Several research-related activities in which diabetes educators may participate are listed in Table 25.2

TABLE 25.2. RESEARCH-RELATED ACTIVITIES

1 Participating in a journal club that involves regular meetings among educators to discuss research articles

2 Attending research presentations at professional meetings and conferences

3 Evaluating published research for possible use in the practice setting

4 Assisting in collecting research information (eg, distributing questionnaires to patients/clients or observing/recording behaviors)

5 Collaborating in the development of an idea for a research project

6 Joining an institutional review board where ethical aspects of a proposed study are examined

7 Serving on committees or task forces of professional organizations

8 Developing clinical guidelines

9 Publishing review papers

10 Serving as principal investigator (PI) or co-principal investigator of a study

---

KEY EDUCATIONAL CONSIDERATIONS

1 Diabetes educators are responsible for assuming an active role in developing a body of knowledge that serves as a reference for the science and art of diabetes education and care. As research consumers, diabetes educators need to develop the skills of reading and critiquing published research reports.

2 Quantitative and qualitative approaches to research refer to an organizing framework that contains a set of assumptions or values that relates to the purpose of the study.

3 The five general phases of the research process are
   A Selecting and defining the problem
   B Selecting a research design
   C Collecting data
   D Analyzing data
   E Using research findings

4 Published research reports are divided into several sections and may include the following:
   A Abstract
   B Introduction
   C Research question/hypotheses
   D Methods
   E Results
   F Discussion of conclusions

5 The problem statement (usually located within the introduction) presents the topic to be studied along with a description of the background and rationale for its significance.

6 A literature review involves identifying, obtaining, and analyzing literature that is related to the research problem.

7 The purpose statement is expressed as a single statement or research question that specifies the overall goal of the study.

8 Hypotheses provide direction to the study and determine research methodologies and type of data to be collected. Hypotheses state clearly and concisely the expected relationship between two or more variables.

9 Research questions are cited in published research reports when prior knowledge about a particular phenomenon is limited and the researcher seeks to identify and/or describe that phenomenon (exploratory or description studies).

10 Independent variables are used to explain or predict a result or outcome, and sometimes are referred to as experimental or treatment variables.

11 Dependent variables reflect the effects of or responses to the independent variables and sometimes are referred to as outcome variables.

12 Research designs are classified as experimental versus nonexperimental.

13 Several organizations have come together to evaluate the quality of care delivered to individuals with diabetes. Diabetes-specific health outcomes can be classified into three categories:

    A Quality of life measures

    B Clinical outcomes

    C Essential processes related to individuals with diabetes (eg, eye and foot examinations)

14 Evaluation of diabetes education programs include

    A Assessment of medical factors (health status, health resources)

    B Behavioral factors (diabetes knowledge and skills, health behaviors and goals)

    C Psychosocial factors (social support systems, health beliefs and attitudes)

SELF-REVIEW QUESTIONS

1 Describe the value of research for diabetes educators.

2 Identify several research-related activities in which diabetes educators can participate.

3 Define the difference between a quantitative and qualitative approach to research.

4 Describe the type of information usually found in an abstract associated with a published research report.

5 Define the difference between a problem statement and purpose statement.

6 Describe why is it important for a researcher to review literature pertinent to the research topic before planning a study.

7 State the purpose of a hypothesis.

8 Define an independent variable, a dependent variable.

9 Describe differences between true experiments and quasi-experiments. In what ways are true experiments better than quasi-experiments? In what ways are quasi-experiments better than true experiments?

10 As consumers of research, diabetes educators must be able to read, understand, and analyze research to apply the findings to practice. What are strategies you can use as you go about reading research reports?

Case Study

Read the following excerpt from the literature about gender orientation and healthcare attitudes and behaviors to respond to the Questions for Discussion.

Research indicates that men and women have different attitudes and behaviors related to health care. Verbrugge[21] suggested that men and women have different illness orientations. Women are more sensitive to illnesses, more able and likely to rest during an illness, and more willing to seek medical advice, while men pay less attention to these matters and are less likely to seek medical advise. In another study,[22] women were found to have a greater interest and concern for health and were more likely to perceive symptoms. Women make greater use of health services and have a larger network of people with whom to discuss medical problems. In general, women appear to be more knowledgeable about and sensitive to the symptoms of illnesses and seek care more frequently than men.

Differences between men and women with regard to their attitudes and behaviors associated with chronic disease have not received as much attention in the literature. Verbrugge[21] found that women reported illness more frequently than men but the illnesses usually were less serious. Verbrugge also suggested that the differences between men and women were most pronounced for prolonged and mild (nonfatal) conditions. Furthermore, psychosocial factors were important in these chronic and less severe diseases. A study[23] of patients with heart disease revealed that women report more symptoms than men and the symptoms reported are of greater intensity. However, gender-related adherence to heart disease management recommendations differed only in exercise behavior; men adhered more than women.

Diabetes is a chronic disease for which self-care is crucial for disease management. The impact of diabetes on a patient's lifestyle can be dramatic, and self-care recommendations often require substantial time and effort from the patient. Not surprisingly, low adherence to the different components of a diabetes regimen (eg, self-monitoring of blood glucose, foot inspection, and diet) has been reported. Demographic variables such as gender have been thought to have little impact on diabetes self-management. However, it is reasonable to assume that men and women have different perceptions of diabetes and adherence to diabetes self-care given their different societal roles and the behavior modification required for effective management of diabetes.

The purpose of this case study was to determine whether men and women with diabetes differ in their attitudes and self-reported adherence to self-care recommendations. An additional question for consideration was whether health professionals provide different recommendations to men and women that might account for differences in their attitudes and behaviors.

The three key questions of this study were

1 Are there gender differences in the attitudes toward diabetes for men and women with diabetes?

2 Are there gender differences in the recommendations given by health professionals for self-treatment of diabetes?

3 Are there gender differences in self-reported adherence to diabetes self-care recommendations?

QUESTIONS FOR DISCUSSION

1 What is the pertinent background information leading to the proposed study?

2 What is the significance/importance of the proposed problem in relation to diabetes education?

3 Based on the information provided within the problem statement/review of literature, what level of knowledge exists about the proposed problem?

4 What are the information gaps that will be addressed in this case study.

5 What was the purpose(s) of this case study?

DISCUSSION

1 Research findings have suggested that men and women have different attitudes and behaviors related to health care. In particular, women report more illness than men, they are more knowledgeable about and sensitive to the symptoms of illness, and seek care more frequently when compared with men. At present, there is a lack of studies regarding gender differences in attitudes and behaviors associated with chronic disease.

2 Diabetes is a chronic disease that requires self-management. Healthcare professionals need to understand how men's and women's attitudes and behaviors are different. If men and women have different attitudes and behaviors related to diabetes, their different educational needs must be addressed when developing educational programs. Diabetes educators

are in an ideal position to assess and discover these differences, so that appropriate strategies can be designed to address these individual needs.

3   Existing knowledge is limited on attitudes and behaviors related to diabetes and gender. Only information related to adherence and self-management has been reported. To date, no studies have examined differences between men and women in terms of attitudes toward diabetes or aspects of the diabetes regimen.

4   The following information will be gathered in this case study: whether men and women with diabetes differ in their attitudes and self-reported adherence to care recommendations, and whether healthcare professionals provide different recommendations to men and women that might account for gender differences in attitudes and behavior.

5   The purposes of this case study were to:
    A   Determine if there are gender differences in the attitudes toward diabetes between men and women with diabetes.
    B   Determine if there are differences in recommendations given by healthcare professionals to men and women for the self-treatment of diabetes.
    C   Determine if there are gender differences between men and women in self-reported adherence to diabetes self-management recommendations.

REFERENCES

1   Polit DF, Hungler BP. Nursing research: principles and methods. 5th ed. Philadelphia: JB Lippincott Co, 1995.

2   Wilson HAS. Introducing research in nursing. 2nd ed. New York: Addison-Wesley, 1993.

3   Campbell EM, Redman S, Moffitt PS, Sanson-Fisher RW. The relative effectiveness of educational and behavioral instruction programs for patients with NIDDM: a randomized trial. Diabetes Educ 1996;22:379-86.

4   Hernandez CA. The experience of living with IDDM: lessons for the diabetes educator. Diabetes Educ 1995;21:33-37.

5   Burns N, Groves SK. The practice of nursing research: conduct, critique, and utilization. 2nd ed. Philadelphia: WB Saunders, 1993.

6   Fain JA. Reading, understanding, and analyzing nursing research. Philadelphia: FA Davis Publishing Company, In press, 1998

7   Huck SW, Cormier WH. Reading statistics and research, 2nd ed. New York: Harper Collins Publishers, 1996.

8   Standiford DA, Turner AM, Allen SR, Drozda DJ, McCain GC. Personal illness models of diabetes: preadolescents and adolescents. Diabetes Educ 1997;23: 147-51.

9   Ledda MA, Walker EA, Basch CE. Development and formative evaluation of a foot self-care program for African Americans with diabetes. Diabetes Educ 1997;23:48-51.

10 Marrero DG, Guare JC, Vandagriff JL, Fineberg NS. Fear of hypoglycemia in the parents of children and adolescents with diabetes: maladaptive or healthy response? Diabetes Educ 1997;23: 281-86.

11 Fitzgerald JT, Anderson RM, Funnell MM, et al. Differences in the impact of dietary restrictions on African Americans and Caucasians with NIDDM. Diabetes Educ 1997;23:41-47.

12 Miller CK, Probart CK, Achterberg CL. Knowledge and misconceptions about the food label among women with non-insulin-dependent diabetes. Diabetes Educ 1997;23:425-32.

13 Schoenbaum SC. Using clinical practice guidelines to evaluate quality of care. Vol 1 (issues), and Vol 2 (methods). Washington, DC: US Department of Health and Human Services, Agency for Health Care Policy and Research, 1995; NIH publication no. 95-0045.

14 Ware JE Jr, Sherbourne CD. The MOS 36-item short-form health survey (SF-36). I. Conceptual framework and item changes. Med Care 1992;30:473-83.

15 Anderson RM, Fitzgerald JT, Wisdom K, Davis WK, Hiss RG. A comparison of global versus disease-specific quality of life measures in patients with diabetes. Diabetes Care 1997;20:299-305.

16 Hammond GS, Aoki TT. Measurement of health status in diabetic patients. Diabetes impact measurement scales. Diabetes Care 1992;15:469-77.

17 Nerenz DR, Repasky DP, Whitehouse FW, Kahkenan DM. Ongoing assessment of health status in patients with diabetes mellitus. Med Care 1992;30(suppl 5): S112-24.

18 Glasgow RE. A practical model of diabetes management and education. Diabetes Care 1995;18:117-26.

19 Peyrot M. Evaluation of patient education programs: how to do it and how to use it. Diabetes Spectrum 1996; 9:86-93.

20 Fink A. Evaluation fundamentals: guiding health programs, research, and policy. Newbury Park, Calif: Sage Publications, 1993.

21 Verbrugge LM. Sex differentials in health. Public Health Rep 1982;97:417-37.

22 Hibbard JH, Pope CR. Gender roles, illness orientation and use of medical services. Soc Sci Med 1983;17:(2)129-37.

23 Sharpe PA, Clark NM, Janz NK. Differences in the impact and management of heart disease between older women and men. Wom Health 1991;17(2):25-43.

SUGGESTED READINGS

Beauchamp TC, Childress JF. Principles of biomedical ethics. 4th ed. New York: Oxford University Press, 1994.

Denzin N, Lincoln Y. Handbook of qualitative designs. Thousand Oaks, Calif: Sage Publications, 1994.

Funk SG, Champagne MT, Wiese RA, Tornquist EM. Barriers to using research findings in practice. The clinician's perspective. Appl Nurs Res 1991;4:90-95.

Funk SG, Tornquist EM, Champagne MT. A model for improving the dissemination of nursing research. West J Nurs Res 1986;11:361-72.

Lekander BJ, Tracy MF, Lindquist R. Overcoming the obstacles to research-based clinical practice. AACN Clin Issues 1994;5:115.

Lincoln Y, Guba E. Naturalistic inquiry. Beverly Hills, Calif: Sage Publications, 1985.

Locke LF, Spirdusco WW, Silverman SJ. Proposals that work. 3rd ed. Newbury Park, Calif: Sage Publications, 1995.

Titler MG, Kleiber C, Steelman V, et al. Infusing research into practice to promote quality care. Nurs Res 1994;43:307-13.

Wylie-Rosett J, Wheeler M, Krueger K, Halford B. Opportunities for research-oriented dietitians. J Am Diet Assoc 1990;90:1531-34.

CONTINUING EDUCATION POST-TEST QUESTIONS

Continuing education is available for nurses, dietitians and pharmacists through use of post-test questions which are included on the following pages. A complete set of answer sheets can be purchased through the AADE Order Department. CE credits are granted on successful completion of each test and payment of appropriate processing fee. For more information and to order test answer sheets contact the AADE at 800-338-3633, ext. 812.

A project of this nature involves many hours of "behind the scenes" work. A very dedicated group of volunteer members wrote post-test questions and reviewed questions written by others. An equally dedicated group participated in the pilot testing of the questions for each chapter. We appreciate their willingness to share their expertise and their insightful comments. We applaud their contribution and wish to recognize them for this effort.

Anne H. Skelly, PhD, RN, ANP
Chair, AADE Psychometric Committee

American Association of Diabetes Educators
100 West Monroe, 4th Floor
Chicago, Illinois 60603

Post-Test Writers

Robert L. Beamer, RPh, PhD
University of South Carolina
College of Pharmacy
Columbia, South Carolina

Mary Kinney Bielamowicz, PhD, RD,
LD, CFCS
Texas Agricultural Extension Svcs
College Station, Texas

Patricia M. Butler, PhD, RN, CDE
The University of Michigan
Educational Services for
Nursing Dept.
Ann Arbor, Michigan

Patrice M. Carmichael, PharmD
Midwestern University Chicago
College of Pharmacy
Downers Grove, Illinois

Dee A. Deakins, RN, MS, CDE
Veteran Affairs Medical Center
Lexington, Kentucky

James A. Fain, RN, PhD, FAAN
University of Massachusetts/Med Ctr.
Graduate School of Nursing
Worcester, Massachusetts

Karen Forbes, RN, PhD, CDE
College of New Rochelle
School of Nursing
New Rochelle, New York

Shirley A Le Clair, RN, PhD, CDE
Rochester Psychiatric Center
Dept. Education and Training
Rochester, New York

Anne H. Skelly, PhD, RN, ANP
Univ of NC-Chapel Hill School
of Nursing
Community Mental Health
Chapel Hill, North Carolina

Alice L. Tobias, EdD, RD, CDE
Lehman College CUNY
Bronx, New York

Post-Test Volunteers

Angela Bacque, MPA, RPh, CDE
Rahway Hospital
Rahway, New Jersey

Rosemary Baldys, RPh, CDE
Osco Pharmacy
Brookfield, Illinois

Jean C. Baltz, RD, MMSc, CDE
Mission St. Josephs Hospital
Health System
Asheville, North Carolina

Jo-Ann D. Barrett, RN, BSN, CDE
St. Elizabeth
Medical Center
Boston, Massachusetts

Lori D. Berard, RN, DRTC
Winnipeg, Canada

James V. Berger, BS
Marsh Drugs
Indianapolis, Indiana

Sharon Berger, RPh
NCS Healthcare
Indianapolis, Indiana

Rosemary L. Briars, RN, CDE
Larabida Childrens Hospital
Chicago, Illinois

Vanessa J. Briscoe, RN, CDE
Tennessee State University
Nashville, Tennessee

Brenda A. Broussard, RD, MPH,
MBA, CDE
Healthcare Consultant
Albuquerque, New Mexico

Laurie S. Caday, RPh, CDE
Rite Aid
Corvallis, Oregon

Susanne M. Chapman, RN, CDE
St. Joseph Hospital
Elgin, Illinois

Stephanie M. Cosentino, RD
North Kansas City, Missouri

Sharon Dinse, BSN, BSEd, MA
St. Luke's Healthcare Assoc.
Saginaw, Michigan

Wendy Drew, RN, BSN, CDE
St. Joseph Health Center
Kansas City, Missouri

Mary Beth Fisher, RN, MSN, CDE
North Kansas City Hospital
North Kansas City, Missouri

Jo-Ann Franczek
Riverside Diabetes Center
Kankakee, Illinois

Sharon R. Gladden, RN, BS, CDE
Naval Hospital
Dept. of Health Education
Jacksonville, Florida

Dean E. Goldberg, RPh, CDE
Abbott Northwestern Hospital
Minneapolis, Minnesota

Karen R. Halderson, RD, MPH, CDE
Alaska Native Medical Center
Diabetes Program
Anchorage, Alaska

Jean R. Halford, RD, CDE
Western Colorado
Physicians Group
Grand Junction, Colorado

Annissia N. Neal Janifer, PharmD
Pfizer Pharmaceuticals
New York, New York

Carita Dale Johnson, RPh
Osco Drug Pharmacy
Chicago, Illinois

Jean M. Kerver, MS, RD
University of Chicago
DRTC
Chicago, Illinois

Connie Kleinbeck, RN, CDE
St Luke's Hospital
Diabetes Center
Kansas City, Missouri

John F. McAloon, RPh, CDE
Our Lady of Resurrection
Medical Center
Chicago, Illinois

Barbara M. McCloskey,
PharmD, BCPS, CDE
Baylor Medical Center of Irving
Irving, Texas

Randy Patrick McDonough, MS, RPh
University of Iowa
Iowa City, Iowa

Melissa B. McGuire, RD, CDE
Shawnee Mission Medical Center
Shawnee Mission, Kansas

Jacquelyn S. McKernan,
MSN, CCRN, CDE
Edwards Hospital
Naperville, Illinois

Darryl M. Nomura, RPh, CDE
LifeScan Inc.
Milpitas, California

Lora Page, RN, CDE
Rocky Mountain HMO
Grand Junction, Colorado

Carole Post, RD, LDN, CDE
Baton Rouge General Medical Center
Baton Rouge, Louisiana

Anthony A. Provenzano, PharmD, CDE
American Drug Stores
Franklin Park, Illinois

Karen M. Rezabek, RD, MMSC, CDE
Rush Presbyterian-St. Lukes
Chicago, Illinois

Jane W. Schultz, RN, MSN, CDE
Mary Washington Hospital
Fredericksburg, Virginia

Robert Scurr, RPh
Mill Street Clinic Pharmacy
Naperville, Illinois

Elizabeth T. Silvers, RD, CDE
Diabetes Management Services
Belmont, North Carolina

Marla C. Solomon, RD, CDE
Illinois Masonic Medical Center
Diabetes Care Center
Chicago, Illinois

Maria M. Spaeth, RD, LD, CDE
Elmhurst Memorial Hospital
Elmhurst, Illinois

Kim M. Sterk, MSN, RN, CDE
Lehigh Valley Hospital
Center for Health Promotion &
Disease Prevention
Allentown, Pennsylvania

Joan R. Thompson, PhD, MPH, RD
La Clinica De La Raza
Oakland, California

Donna M. Tomky, MS, APRN, CDE
Diabetes Health Center
Salt Lake City, Utah

Marianne Vasquez, RN, CDE
Maui Memorial Hospital
Wailuku, Hawaii

Patricia Wegner, PharmD
Edward Hospital/Owen Healthcare
Naperville, Illinois

CONTINUING EDUCATION POST-TEST QUESTIONS

Education Principles and Strategies   1

1 The best instructional approach to use in planning a class on self-monitoring of blood glucose for adults with type 2 diabetes would be:
- **A** Content oriented, primarily didactic in approach
- **B** Task centered or problem oriented
- **C** Interactive group discussion
- **D** Computer simulations

2 The factor that makes the most significant difference when deciding whether to use a lecture method or a group discussion approach to learning is:
- **A** Relevance of the material to the learner
- **B** Educator facilitation skills
- **C** Opportunities to reinforce learning
- **D** Availability of audiovisual resources

3 DR is planning a diabetes self-management class for the adults at the health maintenance center and trying to decide how much time she should take to present the key concepts for the class. As a diabetes educator, you advise her to allow:
- **A** 10 minutes and focus on a single topic
- **B** 15 - 20 minutes with time to ask questions
- **C** 30 minutes lecture, 30 minutes discussion
- **D** 50 - 60 minutes to adequately cover the subject material

4 JB, a diabetes educator, frequently communicates to the patient the idea that he or she has the ability to perform the skill being taught and provides feedback to that effect to build confidence. This strategy facilitates learning in that it encourages:
- **A** Self-efficacy
- **B** Values clarification
- **C** Knowledge acquisition
- **D** Problem solving skills

5 A 65 year-old widower with type 2 diabetes is referred for education regarding weight reduction. Which of the following strategies would be best to try with this person?
- **A** Develop a calorie-exchange meal plan and explain to the patient
- **B** Discuss his dietary habits, food choices and meal preparation skills
- **C** Teach him how to use carbohydrate-counting approach
- **D** Have him attend lecture on dietary goals for type 2 diabetes

6 What would be the best learning strategy for a college athlete who is starting insulin therapy?
- **A** Have the person demonstrate how to draw up and administer insulin
- **B** Discuss insulin administration procedure using printed material
- **C** Have him or her watch a videotape on insulin administration
- **D** Enroll him or her in a class on insulin therapy

7 When is the use of role-playing most effective?
- **A** To help people with diabetes develop rapport with the educator
- **B** When a high level of trust exists
- **C** When learners are still in denial
- **D** When time is limited

8 What level of diabetes education is most appropriate for a person taking insulin who wants to learn how to make medication adjustments?
- **A** Survival skills
- **B** Self-management education
- **C** Behavior change therapy
- **D** Lifestyle education

9 Which of the following persons with diabetes is most likely to exhibit an increased readiness to learn?

    A An acutely ill patient

    B A patient who thinks he has "a touch of diabetes"

    C A person who exhibits low-to-moderate anxiety about his condition

    D A person dealing with multiple stressors

10 An effective educational program for persons with diabetes

    A Uses statements of measurable and observable behaviors to achieve goals

    B Presents specific, single-topic sessions on an as-needed basis

    C Emphasizes disease type and needs over cultural background of patient

    D Incorporates the empowerment approach as the only standard for its patient population

CONTINUING EDUCATION POST-TEST QUESTIONS

Teaching Patients with Low Literacy Skills 2

1 Which instrument can be used by the diabetes educator to assess the health literacy of an adult in less than 5 minutes?
  A The Test of Functional Health Literacy in Adults (TOFHLA)
  B The Rapid Estimate of Adult Literacy in Medicine (REALM)
  C The Medical Achievement Reading Test (MART)
  D Slossen Oral Reading Test (SORT_R)

2 Which literacy assessment test is available in Spanish?
  A The Test of Functional Health Literacy in Adults (TOFHLA)
  B The Rapid Estimate of Adult Literacy in Medicine (REALM)
  C The Medical Achievement Reading Test (MART)
  D Slossen Oral Reading Test (SORT_R)

3 The most effective way to determine the literacy level of a person with diabetes who is referred to you for counseling is to:
  A Ask the patient how well he or she reads.
  B Obtain information about the patient's background since the reading level will be the equivalent to the reported final educational level.
  C Gauge the patient's reading level from the newspapers and magazines that he or she likes to read.
  D Ask the patient to read an educational pamphlet on diabetes and explain the meaning of what was read.

4 Literacy was defined in the 1991 National Literacy Act as "an individual's ability to read, write and speak in English and to compute and/or solve problems." Which of the following approaches would be best to use with a patient who has an elementary school functional level?
  A Give repeated demonstrations on the use of a glucose meter.
  B Have patient read a simple brochure and follow up with one-on-one counseling to ensure the material is adequately understood.
  C Have patient complete a glucose monitoring log.
  D Provide written materials explaining the connection between food intake, exercise and insulin on blood glucose levels.

5 REALM and MART are designed to gauge a patient's:
  A Intelligence and learning ability
  B Ability to understand and perform quantitative operations
  C Reading ability and comprehension
  D Ability to comply with written instructions

6 FG, a 50 year-old obese man with type 2 diabetes has low literacy skills. What is likely to be the most effective way of teaching him about weight control in diabetes management?
  A Use videos to explain the effects of overweight and excessive body fat on blood sugar levels.
  B Give him written information in which key terms are underlined and explained in simple language.
  C Provide a low caloric diet and ask him to comply with the suggested food pattern.
  D Have him maintain a glucose log and a food diary so you can show how food intake influences blood sugar levels.

7 You are working with BT, a 60 year-old patient with newly-diagnosed diabetes and low literacy skills. Which strategy would be appropriate in the planning, implementation and evaluation of instruction?

 A Use only short term learning objectives and limit the number

 B Use audiovisual teaching aids to cover all major conceptual points

 C Repeat major points during the instruction process

 D Use written test to evaluate learning

8 Strategies for diabetes education should include all of the following except:

 A Limit the number of learning objectives to what is essential for meeting patient's needs

 B Limit the amount of material taught in a particular session

 C Emphasize the philosophic rationale and general concepts around which the program is designed

 D Emphasize actions and behaviors over theories and concepts

9 A diabetes educator who assesses functional literacy needs to know that:

 A Grade-level equivalents are the best predictor of a person's level of literacy.

 B Literacy skills are closely correlated with intelligence and motivation.

 C The patient's ability to function in everyday life affects literacy skills.

 D Appearance, race and speech patterns are often useful indicators of literacy level.

10 When developing patient education materials for a low literacy population, it is important to:

 A Employ a passive writing style and use few definitions

 B Use all-capital letters in the layout to emphasize key concepts

 C Incorporate commercially-produced audio/visual materials

 D Introduce definitions in one section to establish a working vocabulary

CONTINUING EDUCATION POST-TEST QUESTIONS

Cultural Appropriateness in Diabetes Education and Care   3

1   A goal of culturally appropriate diabetes care is to:
   A Acknowledge and accommodate the patient's beliefs about health and illness
   B Change the patient's beliefs about health and illness
   C Reinforce the need to abandon "folk remedies" that may be doing harm
   D Help the patient with the acculturation process and self-care management

2   Cultural competence or intercultural sensitivity
   A Is innate to all human beings
   B Requires active awareness and practice
   C Is not achievable by most people
   D Has a great deal of historic precedent

3   A set of beliefs or behaviors that are learned and shared by members of a group is known as:
   A An ethnicity
   B Cultural relativism
   C A culture
   D A worldview

4   The belief that one's culture is superior to others is known as:
   A Ethnicity
   B Cultural relativism
   C Enculturation
   D Ethnocentrism

5   ZW has recently moved to the US from Thailand. He seeks your advice as he begins to adapt his diet to what is available in his local markets. This process is known as:
   A Enculturation
   B Acculturation
   C Cultural adjustment
   D Ethnocentrism

6   DD is a diabetes educator serving a large multicultural population. She seeks to become more sensitive to the needs of her patients and provide culturally appropriate care. To do so, she can include all of the following except:
   A Learn about the patient's health beliefs by asking him or her
   B Negotiate mutually acceptable treatment plans
   C Stress the importance of adjusting to new ways of doing things
   D Incorporate patient's concerns and perspectives

7   An example of how DD might demonstrate her understanding and respect for different cultural beliefs and preferences is by:
   A Demonstrating to patients and families how they might adapt their favorite ethnic dishes to the diabetes meal plan.
   B Organizing screening programs in high-risk communities.
   C Pointing out to patients and families the areas that need improvement in their diet.
   D Asking local community agencies to distribute diabetes literature.

8   Healthcare professionals in the US who seek to increase their cultural competence recognize that:
   A Barriers such as language and vocabulary can be more easily overcome when English is the common language
   B Their own ethnocentric worldview is based on a biomedical model of health and illness and can be a barrier to improved care
   C Positive patient outcomes are an appropriate indicator that cultural barriers have been addressed
   D The patient's own cultural beliefs are a more important reference than their own

9 Which of the following is the most accurate statement about the prevalence of diabetes among high-risk populations:

A Puerto Ricans have a higher incidence of diabetes in the US than Mexican Americans.

B Among ethnic Asian groups, Chinese have the highest incidence of diabetes.

C Among African Americans, the prevalence of type 2 diabetes is greater for males than females.

D With the exception of the Pima Indians, the prevalence of diabetes among Native Americans is slightly higher than that of Caucasians.

10 African Americans with type 2 diabetes:

A Have the highest rates of diabetes in the US

B Have a higher incidence of diabetes and greater disability from complications

C Are three times more likely to have diabetes than Caucasians

D Are at less risk statistically for the development of complications of diabetes

11 DD has been working with AR, a Hispanic woman with type 2 diabetes, on issues related to her meal plan. In developing a culturally-appropriate intervention, DD would need to consider all of the following factors except:

A Culturally-defined roles within the family

B Cultural constraints on behaviors related to food preparation

C Cultural norms of the Caucasian population in the US

D Cultural differences in the expectations of the patient and healthcare provider

12 DD feels that as a diabetes educator it is her responsibility to learn more about the culture of her patients. One of the most important techniques she can utilize to do this is to:

A Avoid sensitive areas of religious and political beliefs

B Ask her patients questions about their specific health beliefs and values

C Categorize behaviors and beliefs by culture

D Share with them what she considers to be the main problems with their healthcare practices.

13 In this chapter, the author presents a set of four tenets for conducting successful diabetes community outreach programs for African Americans. A good example of these tenets is:

A Involve community members only at the beginning of a health education program

B Base education efforts more on ethnicity and less on social and economic class

C Increase research to study culturally diverse populations

D Involve community members in determining which services to offer

14 DD, in her interactions with AR, a Hispanic woman with type 2 diabetes, has encouraged AR to bring in some of her favorite family recipes so that they can review and adapt them to fit her meal plan. This approach is an example of all of the following except:

A Cultural sensitivity

B Cultural relativism

C Patient empowerment

D Ethnocentrism

15 DD is concerned about AR's use of traditional remedies to help her diabetes. One approach she might use is to:

A Ask AR to bring in her home remedies and send them to the lab for analysis.

B Ask AR to tell her more about these remedies and how she uses them.

C Explain to AR the potential side effects of many of the natural remedies.

D Impress on AR the importance of adhering to the medical treatment plan.

CONTINUING EDUCATION POST-TEST QUESTIONS

Psychosocial Assessment   4

1 Which of the following contextual factors need to be assessed to determine a person's ability to effectively manage diabetes:
   A Self-care ease, financial stability, and educator's concerns
   B Cultural influences, socioeconomic factors, & learning barriers
   C Organizational factors, regimen simplicity, and ego strength
   D Learning style, regimen complexity, and cultural biases

2 Based on the Locus-of-Control Theory, ML exhibits a "powerful others" orientation. Which of the following behaviors would be consistent with this orientation?
   A He blames his poor glucose control on his wife's pasta meals.
   B He claims he knows more about what's good for his health than the doctors do.
   C He states that diabetes runs in the family and that he knows from being with his mother and brother who have diabetes that managing this condition is out of his hands.
   D He compares his outcomes with others in the doctor's waiting room.

3 Issues of psychosocial adjustment are critical regarding diabetes management because they:
   A Assess emotional well being and mental illness presentation
   B Point out specific problems posed in self-management skills
   C Are essential to successful efforts in improving self-care
   D Allow the diabetes educator to not teach mentally unstable people

4 A diagnosis of clinical depression is made when:
   A A patient reports feeling depressed
   B A patient exhibits two specific symptoms on a consistent basis for at least 4 weeks
   C Laboratory data confirm the diagnosis of depression
   D Patient exhibits five or more specific symptoms over a minimum 2 week period

5 In relationship to Health Beliefs, there are four perceptions which influence a person's behavior in diabetes self-care. These include:
   A Self-care benefits, social supports, susceptibility, and cost
   B Susceptibility, severity, self-care activity benefits and cost
   C Severity, self-care cost and limitations, and susceptibility
   D Social supports, severity, susceptibility, and limitations

6 JP is considered to have an internal locus-of-control. Which of the following responses related to an elevated blood glucose value is more reflective of this type of orientation?
   A "I overate at my last meal without taking an adequate amount of insulin to cover the carbohydrates."
   B "My mother gave me a piece of regular cake with icing and ice cream because it was my sister's birthday."
   C "My primary care practitioner did not raise my insulin dosage so I couldn't take extra, it's not my fault."
   D "I guess that my blood sugar is high because it is winter now. That's the way it's supposed to be."

7 Diabetes self-care skills may be best assessed by:

   A Observing the person performing specific diabetes psychomotor activities

   B Asking what he/she things about a given diabetes regimen

   C Allowing someone to learn self-care tasks through trial and error

   D Giving someone a written examination of diabetes management questions

8 A stated intention to psychological behavior mode by a person who has diabetes is:

   A A poor predictor of behaviors

   B More likely to occur if it involves self-management behaviors

   C More likely to result in positive outcomes if achieved within 6 to 12 weeks

Please answer the remaining 2 questions based upon the following case scenario.

LJ was recently diagnosed with type 2 diabetes mellitus after her opthamologist found advanced retinopathy in both her eyes. In addition to her problem with vision, she is grieving the death of her husband of 40 years. Since his death 4 months ago, she has become exceptionally concerned and frustrated dealing with the losses in her life: Living alone, being unable to drive at night due to poor vision, generally poor appetite and having to structure meals around medication and blood testing.

---

9 At this time, which psychological presentation is LJ most at risk for?

   A Anxiety disorder

   B Eating disorder

   C Depressive disorder

   D Personality disorder

10 Which approach is best for the educator to use with LJ?

   A Uncaring and politically correct

   B Caring and actively listening

   C Distant and matter of fact

   D Structured and firm

CONTINUING EDUCATION POST-TEST QUESTIONS

Behavior Change   5

1   How have diabetes self-care behaviors
    been affected by technological
    advances?
    A Offers better health but involves
       greater self-care
    B Has little or no effect on
       self-care demands
    C Reduces self-care demands on
       persons with diabetes who are not
       using with insulin
    D Requires less active decision-making
       skills of patients

2   What is one effective way for diabetes
    educators to facilitate
    self-management skills?
    A Encourage rigid adherence to a
       treatment program to maintain
       better blood glucose control.
    B Teach using a didactic approach to
       enhance patient-knowledge of
       diabetes-related concepts.
    C Work with the patient to set realistic
       self-care goals.
    D Use experiences of other patients to
       teach coping and self-care skills.

3   The main difference between a
    compliance model and empowerment
    approach to behavior change is the:
    A Clinical outcomes
    B Financial cost
    C Individual's role in self-management
    D Degree of behavior change

4   A diabetes education program that
    encourages patients to become active
    learners focuses on:
    A Skills orientation, practice and
       direct feedback
    B Oral instructions supported with
       written educational materials
    C Checklists, monitoring logs and
       self-administered questionnaires
    D Sporadically scheduled practice
       review sessions, and a coping skills
       assessment

5   The empowerment approach
    A Focuses exclusively on the strengths
       of the person with diabetes
    B Offers solutions to problems for the
       patient to choose
    C Provides education to help patients
       make informed choices
    D Enables the healthcare team to
       formulate a intervention plan early
       in the treatment process and have
       everyone follow it

6   If a patient makes negative comments
    about the burden of self-care, admits to
    feeling overwhelmed, and states he is a
    failure, the diabetes educator should:
    A Listen and help the individual to
       focus on specific problem areas
    B Offer solutions
    C Agree with the patient to help him
       move beyond the negative thoughts
    D Give examples of other patients who
       have overcome difficulties

7   Which of the following may be an
    expectation of diabetes educators as a
    result of using the empowerment
    approach?
    A They experience feelings of guilt
       when patients do not
       follow suggestions.
    B They accept that patients
       may choose to ignore
       their recommendations.
    C They hold themselves accountable
       for patient decisions.
    D They expect to invest significant time
       and energy to motivate patients.

8   Which of the following statements is the
    most accurate?
    A Self-management training is about
       self-awareness.
    B Coping skills training is about
       providing information and
       treatment options.
    C Empowerment concerns a person's
       self-management and coping skills
       and the pace at which they proceed.
    D Treatment plans need structure and
       repetition to be effective.

9 The organization and structure of an educational and treatment program can affect a patient's ability to make change. All of the following are components of a program except:
  A Interdisciplinary staff
  B Patient protocols
  C Group support
  D On-call availability and follow-up contact

10 Taking into account a patient's readiness to change, which of the following is an appropriate action for a diabetes educator?
  A Recommend a support group for patients in the precontemplation stage
  B Encourage patients in the contemplation stage to set specific goals
  C Refer patients in the preparation stage to a self-management program
  D Help patients problem-solve and anticipate difficult situations when they're in the maintenance stage

11 Which of the following actions facilitates patient empowerment?
  A Start with the patient's agenda
  B Focus on outcomes rather than behavior
  C Use a standardized set of questions to elicit information
  D Address general issues with a problem-solving approach

CONTINUING EDUCATION POST-TEST QUESTIONS

Psychological Disorders 6

1 Research indicates that depression may be more severe in persons with diabetes due to:
   A Higher rates of substance abuse
   B Neuroendocrine effects caused by both diabetes and depression
   C Reluctance to seek mental health services
   D Lack of family support with diabetes care

2 Which of the following contributes to the underdiagnosis of depression in persons with diabetes:
   A The lack of reliable, valid tools for diagnosing depression in diabetes
   B The fact that depression manifests itself differently in persons with diabetes
   C The perception that depression is secondary to the medical condition itself
   D The lack of recognized primary-care based interventions for depression

3 Interpersonal therapy (IPT) seeks to help depressed individuals:
   A Sublimate feelings of anxiety and hostility
   B Cognitively reframe and restructure negative thoughts and actions
   C Avoid stressful and conflicted relationships
   D Improve skills in communication and social interaction

4 Which of the following actions taken by the diabetes educator exemplifies application of Cognitive Behavioral Therapy (CBT)?
   A Work with patients to build skills for more effective coping.
   B Refer patients with depressive symptoms for treatment with antidepressants.
   C Stress the relationship of glycemic control to moods.
   D Educate the patient to the prevalence of depression in persons with diabetes.

5 The advantages of the selective serotonin reuptake inhibitors (SSRIs) include:
   A Less gastrointestinal side effects
   B Less sedation
   C Less agitation
   D Less sexual dysfunction

6 One of the major barriers to effective treatment with antidepressants is:
   A The lack of sufficient choices among effective agents
   B Patient reluctance to accept medication therapy
   C The length of time between initiation of treatment and improvement in symptoms
   D The high degree of drug interactions with other medications

7 Anxiety disorders are characterized by:
   A Compulsive, repetitious rituals
   B Auditory hallucinations
   C Disjointed thought patterns
   D Exaggerated emotional responses to normal fears

8 SS, a 44 year-old school teacher with type 2 diabetes, has just started an antianxiety agent for her symptoms. During your assessment, what potential adverse clinical concern would you have related to the medication?
   A Skin rash
   B Oversedation
   C Palpitations, tremors
   D Loss of glycemic control

9 Often individuals with eating disorders are reluctant to acknowledge the problem. It is important for the diabetes educator to recognize that to an individual with an eating disorder:
   A Exerting control over eating is extremely important
   B Control of blood sugar is of crucial importance
   C Weight gain is desirable
   D Purging is a means of self punishment

10 An early indicator that a person with diabetes may be suffering from a psychological/ psychiatric disorder is:
  A Recurrent diabetic ketoacidosis
  B Family report
  C Exhibition of obvious clinical symptomatology
  D Referral by other health professional

11 The incidence of psychological disorders in the population of persons with diabetes:
  A Is likely to be detected earlier because of their more frequent inter-actions with health professionals
  B Has the same incidence as in the general population
  C Has a higher incidence than in the general population
  D Is well understood and effectively treated by healthcare providers

12 Symptoms of depression and anxiety are dramatically elevated in persons with diabetes who:
  A Have two or more diabetes related complications.
  B Have elevated blood glucose levels.
  C Have less access to medical care.
  D Have had diabetes for longer than 10 years.

13 The use of psychopharmacological agents in the treatment of persons with diabetes who experience anxiety
  A Has limited effectiveness in select patients
  B Is the most promising area of treat-ment and intervention modalities
  C Is supported by a number of studies in persons with diabetes
  D Has the potential to improve metabolic control

CONTINUING EDUCATION POST-TEST QUESTIONS

Pathophysiology of the Diabetes Disease State   7

1   Gluconeogenesis is the:
   A Mechanism of breaking down complex carbohydrate for storage
   B Process of glucose production in the liver from precursors
   C Attachment of insulin with glucose at cell receptor sites
   D Transport of glucose across cell membrane for cell usage

2   Glycogenolysis is the metabolic conversion of:
   A Glycogen into glucose
   B Glucagon into glucose
   C Glucose into glycogen
   D Glucose into glucagon

3   A characteristic of the normal Phase II postabsorbtive state is:
   A Plasma insulin levels are high and glucagon levels are low
   B Triglyceride and free fatty acids are stored in the adipocyte
   C Carbohydrate and lipid stores are mobilized
   D Renal gluconeogenesis contributes to high blood glucose levels

4   Which of the following individuals would be diagnosed with diabetes mellitus using the present criteria on a subsequent day:
   A A 44 year-old woman with unexplained weight loss, fatigue, and casual plasma glucose concentrations of 180 mg/dL and 170 mg/dL
   B A 50 year-old male with a fasting plasma glucose of 138 mg/dL and 146 mg/dL
   C A 28 year-old male with a 2-hour plasma glucose (OGTT) of 160 mg/dL and 140 mg/dL
   D A 60 year-old female with casual plasma glucose concentrations of 145 mg/ dL and 130 mg/dL

5   Which statement best describes the differences in the characteristics between type 1 and type 2 diabetes:
   A Persons with type 2 diabetes usually require lower doses of insulin because of the presence of some functioning ß-cells.
   B Persons with type 1 diabetes may be asymptomatic at the time of diagnosis but rapidly develop complications.
   C Persons with type 1 diabetes require endogenous insulin, and persons with type 2 diabetes utilize exogenous insulin to regulate blood glucose levels.
   D Autoimmune factors are more likely to be a cause or contributing factor for type 1 diabetes than for type 2 diabetes.

6   JJ, a 16 year-old male, is frequently leaving class, going to the bathroom to urinate and stopping by the water fountain for a drink. Despite the fact that he eats a lot in school and at home, he is losing weight. John is exhibiting symptoms of:
   A Hyperglycemia
   B Hypoglycemia
   C Ketoacidosis
   D Hyperosmolarity

7   People who do not have diabetes can have impaired fasting blood glucose values. One example of this is:
   A A school aged child with FBSs of 86 and 89 mg/dL
   B An active teenager with FBSs of 101 and 103 mg/dL
   C An employed adult with FBSs of 122 and 125 mg/dL
   D An elderly adult with FBSs of 140 and 142 mg/dL

8 The pathophysiological states in the stages of development of type 1 diabetes include all of the following, except:

A Ongoing ß-cell function

B An environmental trigger

C A genetic predisposition

D Overt diabetes mellitus

9 ß-cell function in persons with type 2 diabetes is best characterized by:

A Hypertrophy and hyperfunction caused by hyperglycemia

B 10% to 20% reduction in cell mass leading to diminished response to hyperglycemia

C Altered or impaired insular receptor function

D Abnormal insulin secretion in response to impaired recognition of glucose

10 DP only eats once a day. After 16 to 24 hours her circulating blood glucose levels are maintained through the breakdown of all of the following substances, except:

A Lactate

B Amino acids

C Fatty acids

D Glycogen

11 Which of the following individuals is at greatest risk for developing type 1 diabetes?

A A person who is shown to have a genetic predisposition for type 1 diabetes

B An identical twin in whom type 1 diabetes has developed in the other twin

C Individuals with high levels of glutamic acid decarboxylase antibodies

D Persons exposed to an environmental trigger independent of autoimmune factors

CONTINUING EDUCATION POST-TEST QUESTIONS

Nutrition   8

1   Which of the following persons with type 2 diabetes would most benefit from medical nutrition therapy (MNT)?
    A 42 year-old female with a cholesterol of 205
    B 51 year-old male with low density lipoproteins (LDL) of 179
    C 36 year-old female with triglycerides of 150
    D 60 year-old male with high density lipoproteins (HDL) of 50

2   An effective strategy for achieving blood glucose goals in a person with type 1 diabetes is:
    A Moderate caloric restriction
    B Eat meals and snacks at specific times
    C Increase NPH insulin if carbohydrate intake exceeds usual consumption
    D Adjust insulin based on blood glucose patterns

3   The macronutrient that exerts the greatest influence on postprandial blood glucose levels is:
    A Protein
    B Carbohydrate
    C Fat
    D Fiber

4   Insulin affects the use and storage of nutrients in each of the following ways except:
    A Facilitates cellular transport
    B Promotes lipolysis by inactivating lipoprotein lipase
    C Stimulates glycogen synthesis
    D Accelerates gluconeogenesis (glucose production by the liver)

5   Which of the following intakes of the sugar substitute aspartame on a daily basis exceeds the acceptable daily intake (ADI) for a female who weighs 130 pounds?
    A 14 cans of diet soft drinks
    B 20 cartons of fruited yogurt
    C 75 packets of a tabletop sweetener
    D 30 servings of a frozen dessert

6   ML is a 39 year-old person with type 1 diabetes who weighs 121 lb. (55 kg) and has overt nephropathy. Her protein requirement is:
    A 35 g
    B 44 g
    C 50 g
    D 55 g

7   If ML eats a meal which includes 1 serving from the starch group, 1 serving of meat (1 oz), 1 serving of fruit (1/2 c) and 1 serving of milk (8 oz), what will be her intake of protein?
    A 10 g
    B 14 g
    C 18 g
    D 20 g

8   Which of the following MNT strategies is consistent with the goal of attaining optimal lipid levels?
    A Limit fat consumption to 20% of total calories in a person with normal lipid levels
    B Restrict saturated fat intake to 20% total calories if triglycerides are elevated
    C Limit dietary cholesterol to less than 200 mg/day if LDL-cholesterol is the primary concern
    D Increase polyunsaturated fat to 15% of total fat calories if VLDL levels are a primary concern

9   Assuming that blood glucose goals are being met, the guidelines for the use of alcohol in persons with diabetes include all of the following except:
    A Teach patients with type 1 diabetes to limit consumption to 2 drinks with their regular meal plan
    B Eliminate one or more food items for each alcoholic beverage consumed
    C Count the calories from the alcoholic beverage as part of the meal plan if alcohol is consumed daily
    D Avoid consumption of alcoholic beverages if triglycerides are elevated.

10 Persons with type 2 diabetes who are sodium sensitive and taking medications for hypertension should:

A Limit their intake of sodium to 3000 mg daily

B Use no more than 2 tsps (5g) of table salt as part of their total daily intake

C Be encouraged to consume entrees with 800 mg sodium or less

D Limit their intake to low sodium foods having 140 mg of sodium or less

11 Guidelines for the role of carbohydrate in meal planning include:

A The amount of carbohydrate to be included in the meal plan is determined before the protein and fat.

B The amount of carbohydrate included will depend on the individual's current eating patterns and nutrition goals.

C It is more important to count the carbohydrate from simple sugars that the total daily intake of carbohydrate.

D The amount of fiber in the diet can be ignored since it is not digested (available to the body).

12 Which of the following statements accurately describes the carbohydrate counting approach to meal planning?

A An individual is ready to learn pattern management once they learn carbohydrate-to-insulin ratios.

B Use of the basic diet planning guidelines is integral to a carbohydrate counting approach.

C Individuals who have used the exchange system for meal planning may more easily grasp the carbohydrate counting approach.

D Addresses the relationship of food, activity and medication at level one as a basis for meal planning.

13 PS is a marketing director with type 1 diabetes who learned about carbohydrate-to-insulin ratios a month ago and has managed to reach her glucose goals since she implemented this approach. She now wants to adjust her insulin for a corporate dinner she will be attending and asks your assistance. Her usual CHO-to-insulin unit ratio is 2 and she usually takes 8 units of regular with her evening meal. She anticipates that she will select 6 carbohydrate choices at this affair which is more than her usual. How many additional units of insulin will she need to take?

A 1

B 2

C 4

D 6

14 With her new flexibility in meal planning, she has also started to work out and has lost 5 pounds. You advise her that:

A Her carbohydrate-to-insulin ratio will probably not change

B She'll need to recheck her carbohydrate-to-insulin ratios if the exercise program continues to go well

C The protein content of her meals or snacks will not be as important as the carbohydrate content

D She should eat higher calorie snacks with sufficient fat content to adjust for the increase in flexibility in carbohydrate intake and to cover for exercise

15 GH is an assembly line worker with type 2 diabetes and the equivalent of a fifth grade education. She was referred to you by her employer for nutrition counseling because she has had to take more than the usual number of bathroom breaks while working. Which approach to meal planning is more likely to be appropriate for her?

A Carbohydrate counting

B Exchange system

C Diabetes nutrition guidelines

D Booklets featuring monthly menus

CONTINUING EDUCATION POST-TEST QUESTIONS

Exercise   9

1 Which of the following are benefits of exercise?
  - **A** Reduced plasma cholesterol and triglycerides, and enhanced fibrinolysis
  - **B** Reduced body fat, muscle mass and weight
  - **C** Improved glucose tolerance and hypercoagulability
  - **D** Increased insulin sensitivity and decreased high-density lipoproteins

2 In persons without diabetes, during the first 5 to 10 minutes of exercise, the major fuel for energy is:
  - **A** Free fatty acids from adipose tissue
  - **B** Intramuscular glucose from glycogen
  - **C** Hepatic glucose from glycogenolysis
  - **D** Hepatic glucose from gluconeogenesis

3 In persons without diabetes, during the post-exercise recovery period, there is:
  - **A** Replenishment of glycogen stores for 12 hours
  - **B** Lessened insulin sensitivity
  - **C** Increased uptake of glucose by muscle
  - **D** Suppression of glucogenesis by the liver

4 After exercise, which factor contributes to hypoglycemia in type 1 diabetes?
  - **A** Mobilization of free fatty acids
  - **B** Depletion of muscle glycogen stores
  - **C** Normal counterregulatory hormonal response
  - **D** Accelerated absorption of insulin

5 BD has type 1 diabetes and is on the high school track team. He runs the 4th leg of the 200-meter relay which is a short, very intense workout. Ten minutes after the race, BD's blood glucose is 350 mg/dL. He should:
  - **A** Inject himself with some regular insulin to cover the high blood sugar.
  - **B** Test his urine for ketones.
  - **C** Eat a snack of 1 bread exchange and 1 meat exchange.
  - **D** Run for about 40 more minutes to decrease his blood glucose.

6 CN is age 55 years and has had type 2 diabetes for 10 years. He is 6'1" and weighs 300 lbs His fasting blood glucose is 145 mg/dL and he is on metformin. He wants to start an exercise program. Which of the following would be the least important to teach him?
  - **A** See his provider and have a stress test before beginning to exercise
  - **B** Wear properly fitting exercise shoes
  - **C** Carry glucose tablets for hypoglycemia
  - **D** Have an eye examination prior to his exercise program

7 What frequency of exercise is optimal for weight loss for CN?
  - **A** 2 to 3 days/week
  - **B** 3 to 4 days/week
  - **C** 4 to 5 days/week
  - **D** 5 to 7 days/week

8 What maximum age-adjusted heart rate would provide an optimum aerobic workout for CN?
  - **A** 50% to 70%
  - **B** 55% to 75%
  - **C** 60% to 85%
  - **D** 65% to 90%

9 Which exercise routine is most appropriate for an elderly patient with a degenerative joint disease?
  - **A** No exercise at all
  - **B** Aerobic exercise only
  - **C** Anaerobic exercise only
  - **D** Alternating aerobic and anaerobic exercise

10 A patient with moderate non-proliferative retinopathy should:
  - **A** Avoid all strenuous activity.
  - **B** Avoid exercise that dramatically increases their blood pressure.
  - **C** Limit exercise to two days a week.
  - **D** Gradually incorporate resistance training into their normal exercise routine.

CONTINUING EDUCATION POST-TEST QUESTIONS

Pharmacologic Therapies   10

1 Insulin exerts all of the following effects on the body tissues except:
  A Stimulate entry of glucose into muscle cells for utilization as an energy source
  B Enhance fat storage
  C Promote breakdown of liver glycogen to maintain blood glucose levels
  D Stimulate entry of amino acids into cells enhancing protein biosynthesis

2 When the pancreas is stimulated by an elevated blood glucose level, insulin enters the blood stream:
  A In equimolar quantities with proinsulin
  B In equimolar quantities with C-peptide
  C In equimolar quantities with glucagon
  D With a small amount of C-peptide

3 Lispro insulin analog is a:
  A Rapid-acting insulin which has an onset of action in 15 to 30 minutes, reaches a peak in 1 to 2 hours, and has a therapeutic duration of 3 to 4 hours.
  B Long-acting insulin which has an onset of action in 4 to 6 hours, reaches a peak in 18 hours, and has a therapeutic duration of 24 to 36 hours.
  C Intermediate-acting insulin which has an onset of 1 to 4 hours, reaches a peak in 8 hours, and has a therapeutic duration of 10 to 16 hours.
  D Rapid-acting insulin which has an onset of 30 minutes to 1 hour, reaches a peak in 2 to 4 hours, and has a therapeutic duration of 6 to 8 hours.

4 MJ is planning a trip to Europe for 21 days. She asks how her insulin should be stored while traveling. Which of the following is the best advice for MJ?
  A "Carry ice packs to keep your insulin at 36° to 46° F."
  B "Store your open insulin at room temperature for 7 days, after which time it must be discarded."
  C "Insulin may be stored at 59° to 86° F for the entire trip provided it is used within 1 month."
  D "People with diabetes in all foreign countries use U100 insulin, so there should be no difficulty obtaining insulin when traveling in Europe."

5 A patient asks you if she can reuse her syringes and needles. Which of the following is the best answer?
  A "Needles and syringes should never be reused because of increased risk of infection."
  B "Needles and syringes may be used indefinitely since the new needles are thin and never become dull."
  C "Needles and syringes may be reused provided they are kept refrigerated."
  D "Syringes and needles can be reused. The needle should be safely recapped and the syringe should be stored at room temperature."

6 The action of troglitazone is to:
  A Enhance insulin action without affecting insulin secretion
  B Stimulate the ß-cells of the islets of Langerhans to produce more insulin
  C Inhibit α-glucosidase
  D Enhance insulin-stimulated glucose transport into skeletal muscle

7 The most dangerous complication of sulfonylurea therapy is:
  A Weight gain
  B Skin rashes
  C Gastrointestinal disturbance
  D Hypoglycemia

8 What laboratory test is needed before a person starts taking metformin?
  A Creatinine clearance test
  B Alkaline phosphatase, and CBC with differential
  C Cardiac enzymes
  D Blood chemistry panel

9 GW, a 70 year-old patient with type 2 diabetes, has a blood creatinine level of 3.0 mg/dL. Which of the following drugs is contraindicated for GW?
  A Troglitazone
  B Glipizide
  C Glyburide
  D Metformin

10 A contraindication for troglitazone is:
  A Hepatic dysfunction
  B Renal dysfunction
  C Hypoglycemia
  D Dyslipidemia

11 An oral agent for diabetes that may be especially useful in patients who have type 2 disease with elevated triglycerides and LDL cholesterol is:
  A Glyburide
  B Glimepiride
  C Metformin
  D Troglitazone

12 The role of exogenous glucagon is to:
  A Stimulate hepatic glucose release
  B Counteract hyperglycemia
  C Delay gastric emptying
  D Increase the postprandial glucose levels

13 At what point can combination therapy be recommended for a person with type 2 diabetes?
  A Upon initial diagnosis
  B Only after a person develops two or more complications
  C When sulfonylurea dose approaches half of the maximum dose
  D When sulfonylurea dose is at the maximum dose

CONTINUING EDUCATION POST-TEST QUESTIONS

Monitoring
11

1   The most important benefit to patients of SMBG is:
A It facilitates problem-solving and decision-making skills
B It decreases the number of medical visits they make
C It enables them to make medication adjustments based on a single reading
D It may reveal psychosocial issues

2   What is a decision concerning diabetes control that can be made from a single blood glucose reading?
A Adjustment of a patient's split insulin regimen
B Treatment of a blood glucose reading less than 70 mg/dL
C Understanding the impact of a daily walking program
D Adjustment of meal plan

3   The most common SMBG user error is:
A Failure to get an adequate blood sample
B Improper storage of meter and equipment
C Failure to calibrate the meter
D Inadequate reporting of high and low BG values

4   Which of the following is not a factor that can affect the accuracy of SMBG systems?
A Altitude
B Temperature and humidity
C Blood cholesterol concentrations
D Hypoxia and hypotension

5   Glycosolated hemoglobin:
A Represents an average blood glucose concentration within a defined period of time
B Is a weighted mean over a relative period of time
C Should be measured at the onset of symptoms and during each routine medical check-up
D Is easily measured by a single method with a known range using a defined component

6   JG brings in her blood glucose monitor to a diabetes education session. She states that it has not worked properly since she purchased it through a mail-order discount device company. What would be the educator's first assessment step to determine the problem?
A Demonstrate proper technique of the meter and give the patient a videotape of instructions.
B Use the glucose control solution to determine the meter's accuracy.
C Ask the patient to demonstrate SMBG using her meter.
D Get a venipuncture to determine the patient's random blood glucose level.

7   The expiration date on JG's reagent strip-container indicate that her strips are current. Could they still be a source of error in SMBG determinations?
A No, reagent strips are extremely durable and rarely are a source of SMBG error.
B No, even expired reagent strips are commonly used by patients with diabetes.
C Yes, the date could be printed wrong by the manufacturer.
D Yes, environmental changes in temperature and atmosphere could degrade strips.

8   An effective approach for teaching patients how to use a blood glucose meter is:
A Show how to calibrate the meter before demonstrating its use
B Change your gloves every hour
C Evaluate the patient's technique whenever hyperglycemia occurs
D Wait for the patient to master BG monitoring technique before teaching meter cleaning and monitoring records

9 Urine testing of ketones is primarily determined by the detection of which of the following free fatty acids?

  A Acetone

  B Acetoacetate

  C ß-hydroxybutyrate

  D Nitroprusside

10 Which of the following is a feature of available blood glucose meters?

  A Blood glucose strips can be automatically calibrated

  B Control solutions adjust for differences in hematocrit levels

  C Sensor-type meters rely on enzymatic reactions to determine blood glucose concentrations

  D Noninvasive monitoring of blood glucose does not require a blood sample from a fingerstick

CONTINUING EDUCATION POST-TEST QUESTIONS

Pattern Management   12

1   Components of an intensive diabetes management program can include:
    A Generalized glycemic goals that follow a pre-established pattern
    B Interaction with the healthcare team 2 to 3 times a year
    C Self-monitoring of blood glucose levels when symptoms occur
    D Self-management education and reliable support systems

2   The main reason to use an algorithmic approach to insulin therapy is to:
    A Increase insulin dosages by 10% to 20% to avoid hyperglycemia
    B Provide flexibility in usual insulin dosages to maintain euglycemia
    C Decrease insulin dosages by 10% to 20% to avoid hypoglycemia
    D Avoid using a meal plan and offset eating as desired

3   An adult with previously controlled diabetes, has been experiencing hyperglycemia with blood glucose values over 225 mg/dL 2 hours after every meal for the past 2 weeks. Which would be the best initial action for the diabetes educator to take?
    A Evaluate food consumption of the person, especially protein intakes
    B Encourage more vigorous aerobic exercise be done by the individual
    C Assess all areas of diabetes self-management
    D Check the appearance and expiration date of the individual's insulin

4   Effectiveness of lispro insulin is best determined by measuring:
    A Pre-meal glucoses
    B Fasting glucoses
    C 2 hour postprandial glucoses
    D 3 AM glucoses

5   Pattern management of blood glucose levels involves reviewing:
    A Several days of glucose records and making changes in the diabetes management program when a problem persists
    B Sporadic glucose records and making corrections in the diabetes management program after problems have occurred
    C Glycosolated hemoglobin values and making adjustments in diabetes management before the onset of long-term complications
    D Fasting serum glucose values and making modifications in diabetes management before a problem surfaces

6   One reason sliding scale insulin administration is less desirable as a pattern management approach is:
    A It is based on patient's current weight
    B It varies according to patient's food intake
    C It may contribute to rapid shifts in glucose levels
    D It may confuse patients trying to remember amount of insulin to administer

7   Pattern management for a pregnant woman is likely to be:
    A Fasting blood glucoses of 100 mg/dL
    B Postprandial blood glucoses less than 120 mg/dL
    C Testing glucose levels 2 to 4 times/day
    D Sliding scale plan to cover blood glucose shifts

8 Which of the following statements about combination therapy is most accurate?

   A Addition of troglitazone to existing therapy produces a therapeutic response within a week

   B Combination therapy improves glycemic control in persons with type 1 diabetes

   C When oral agents are combined, the medications should be taken 1 hour before meals

   D Individuals starting combination therapy will need to monitor post-prandial blood glucose levels

9 Examples of SMBG data that can be useful for managing blood glucose levels and making changes to the treatment plan include all of the following except:

   A Using pre-meal testing to determine regular insulin dose for multiple injections

   B Testing at 3 AM at least once a week when fasting glucose levels are elevated.

   C Testing daily for people who have asymptomatic hypoglycemia

   D Using pre-meal testing before administering a supplemental insulin bolus during acute illness

CONTINUING EDUCATION POST-TEST QUESTIONS

Hyperglycemia   13

1   Prolonged hyperglycemia from
    uncontrolled diabetes mellitus can
    lead to one of two metabolic crises.
    They are:
    A Ketoacidosis and hyperglycemic
        hyperosmolar nonketotic syndrome
    B Diabetic neuritis and hyperosmolar
        hypertension
    C Cerebral vascular accident and severe
        dehydration
    D Diabetic nephrosis and acute
        dehydration

2   Which of the following is not likely to
    be a precipitating factor in the
    development of diabetic ketoacidosis?
    A Illness or infection
    B Insufficient insulin
    C Hypertension
    D Emotional stress

3   HHNS is a life-threatening emergency
    with high mortality rate. It is often seen
    in which type of patients?
    A Middle-aged type 1
    B Youthful type 2
    C Teenage Gestational
    D Elderly type 2

4   A prominent respiratory symptom
    present in diabetic ketoacidosis is:
    A Shallow breathing
    B Hyperpnea
    C Wheezing
    D Hypoventilation

5   During HHNS and DKA, mental
    function is most directly affected by:
    A Plasma sodium level
    B Serum osmolality
    C Degree of acidosis
    D Hyperglycemia

6   The reason the outcome of diabetic
    ketoacidosis is frequently less severe
    than that of HHNS is that:
    A A person experiencing DKA
        frequently receives medical help
        when symptoms first appear
    B DKA generally occurs among older
        adults who are more likely to take
        better care of themselves.
    C A person has some insulin reserves
        that tend to blunt symptoms
    D A person is not likely to lose
        consciousness during a DKA episode

7   During acidosis, the serum-bicarbonate
    concentration, blood pH, and carbon
    dioxide pressure will be:
    A Elevated
    B Lower
    C Unchanged
    D Variable

8   Patients with HHNS may have focal
    neurological signs that mimic:
    A Myocardial infarction
    B Diabetic ketoacidosis
    C Multiple sclerosis
    D Cerebral vascular accident

9   Which of the following features is not
    present in HHNS?
    A Severe hyperglycemia
    B Neurologic manifestations
    C Presence of ketosis
    D Profound dehydration

10 The immediate treatment goal for
    diabetic ketoacidosis is to:
    A Assess and correct fluid and
        electrolyte imbalance
    B Provide education and follow-up
        with the family
    C Diminish insulin administration
        and acidosis
    D Prevent long-term degenerative
        complications

11 A person has been admitted to the emergency room with the following symptoms: severe hyperglycemia (>800 mg/dL), absence of ketoacidosis, profound dehydration, and neurologic signs ranging from depressed nerve sensation to coma. What life threatening emergency may be occurring?

A Diabetic ketoacidosis

B Hyperglycemic hyperomolar non-ketotic syndrome

C Cerebral vascular accident

D Chronic obstructive pulmonary disease

12 Kussmaul's respirations are the physiologic response to:

A Metabolic alkalosis

B Dehydration

C Metabolic acidosis

D Hypotension

13 Which is the most accurate statement regarding the impact of dehydration?

A If the deficit of sodium is greater than that of water, the sodium level will be high

B If the deficit of sodium is greater than that of water, the sodium level will be low

C If the deficit of sodium is greater than that of water, the two deficiencies will be roughly equal

D The sodium level does not correspond to the H_2O level

CONTINUING EDUCATION POST-TEST QUESTIONS

Hypoglycemia   14

1   When a patient with type 1 diabetes of 10 years suddenly begins trembling, shaking and experiencing other symptoms indicating a hypoglycemic reaction, the body responds by releasing:
    A   Acetylcholine
    B   Epinephrine
    C   Hydrocortisone
    D   Glucagon

2   Neuroglycopenic symptoms now have been shown to:
    A   Occur before autonomic symptoms
    B   Occur later than autonomic symptoms
    C   Be cholinergic in origin
    D   Occur at about the same time as autonomic symptoms

3   Which of the following is not a symptom of neuroglycopenia?
    A   Extremely high energy and excitation
    B   Slurred or rambling speech
    C   Mental confusion and disorientation
    D   Irrational or unusual behavior

4   When neuroglycopenic symptoms first occur, patients should:
    A   Wait for help from a health care professional
    B   Not treat themselves because of the possibility of an accident
    C   Treat themselves quickly
    D   Wait before any treatment because their symptoms may eventually disappear

5   Consumption of coffee may:
    A   Be a first aid treatment for hypoglycemia
    B   Increase autonomic symptoms
    C   Enhance neuroglycopenia
    D   Interfere with gluconeogenesis

6   Hypoglycemia can be defined as any blood glucose level of:
    A   85 mg/dL or lower
    B   80 mg/dL of lower
    C   75 mg/dL or lower
    D   70 mg/dL or lower

7   Physical activity by the person with diabetes:
    A   May require an increase in carbohydrate consumption and/or insulin reduction
    B   May be beneficial to prevent hypoglycemia
    C   Has no effect on hypoglycemia
    D   May require an increase in the insulin dose

8   Over the course of type 1 diabetes, defective hormonal counterregulation can cause:
    A   Neuroglycopenic symptoms to diminish
    B   Decreased epinephrine secretion leading to a diminished or delayed onset of symptoms
    C   Decreased glucagon secretion leading to a diminished or delayed onset of symptoms
    D   Fewer or delayed symptoms because of diminished cortisol secretion

9   Patients with type 1 diabetes and their families/significant others:
    A   Should not be given information concerning hypoglycemia on diagnosis because it increases their anxiety level
    B   Should be given written materials on hypoglycemia and instruction on administering glucagon
    C   Should be given written material, but no instruction on glucagon administration, because it is dangerous for a nonprofessional to administer
    D   Should be given instructions in glucagon administration but not on hypoglycemia to avoid information overload

10 Patients with type 2 diabetes who are taking sulfonylureas and meglitinides:
   A Do not require instruction in hypoglycemia because they are less at risk due to a maintenance of integrity of hormonal counterregulation
   B Have an increased risk of hypoglycemia because of a lack of hormonal counterregulation
   C Need to be taught about hypoglycemia, although they appear to be at less risk for severe hypoglycemia due to a maintenance of the integrity of hormonal counterregulation
   D May experience occasional hypoglycemic attacks, but these are mild and never require corrective measures

11 Problems with hypoglycemia
   A Are minimal for persons with type 2 diabetes receiving combination therapy
   B Are more significant because of current treatment approaches and blood glucose goals
   C Are less problematic as a result of the more intensive insulin therapies
   D Only occur with patients using insulin therapy

12 Symptoms associated with hypoglycemia
   A May vary for a person from one hypoglycemic episode to the next
   B Are well-documented and occur consistently in patients with diabetes
   C Are less likely to be affected by physiological or psychological factors
   D Are only slightly affected by food, alcohol or medications

13 Most hypoglycemic episodes
   A Occur within two hours after taking intermediate-acting insulin
   B Are likely to occur during the night
   C Occur despite a consistent carbohydrate consumption and regularly-scheduled meals
   D Are unrelated or unaffected by physical activity

14 Physical activity can have immediate and prolonged effects on blood glucose levels. One of these effects is
   A Increased glucose utilization combined with decreased glucose production
   B Decreased glucose utilization by muscle tissue
   C Delayed insulin absorption
   D Accelerated glycogenolysis by the liver during exercise

CONTINUING EDUCATION POST-TEST QUESTIONS

Illness and Surgery 15

1 Postsurgical stress involving an increased release of cortisol may be expected to cause:
   A Hypoglycemia from increased glucose uptake by muscles
   B Hyperglycemia from increased glycogenolysis by the liver
   C Hyperglycemia from increased gluconeogenesis from amino acids by the liver
   D Hypoglycemia from increased glycogen synthesis by the liver

2 Increased ketone levels in a post-surgical patient are most likely to be caused by:
   A Insufficient insulin and/or food intake
   B Decreased lipolysis and/or food intake
   C Decreased protein catabolism and/or food intake
   D Increased protein anabolism and/or food intake

3 In addition to completing an admission history, reviewing laboratory data and performing a physical exam, what additional information would be most useful in a preoperative assessment of a 42 year-old patient with type 2 diabetes and no cardiovascular risk factors?
   A Medical records from previous hospital admission
   B Cardiovascular enzyme activity laboratory data
   C Information about the patient's cognitive and affective needs
   D Postoperative glucose and insulin protocol of hospital

4 Cardiac problems can be serious, even fatal, in a person with diabetes and should be assessed prior to surgery. During surgery, which of the following could occur?
   A Anesthesia agents could stimulate heart muscle function
   B Hyperglycemia could cause excessive bleeding
   C Patients risk hypotension, hypovolemia and rhythm disturbances
   D Metabolic stresses cause carotid bruits to develop

5 A particular postoperative concern for a type 2 patient whose blood glucose level is higher than 200 mg/dL is:
   A Fluid restrictions
   B Discontinuation of oral hypoglycemic agents
   C Peripheral vascular disease
   D Impaired wound healing

6 To maintain adequate hydration, caffeine-free, calorie-free liquids should be used. The reason such liquids should be caffeine-free when given to a patient with diabetes during 'sick days' is because:
   A Caffeine is a stimulant and causes insomnia
   B Caffeine is a diuretic
   C Caffeine will raise blood glucose levels
   D Caffeine will decrease blood glucose levels

7 Surgical patients with type 2 diabetes who are taking antidiabetes agents:
   A Will not need insulin before surgery
   B Will need to take insulin after surgery as a permanent replacement of their previous treatment
   C Should be informed that they may need insulin before, during, and immediately after their surgery
   D Should not be told that their insulin may be adjusted during surgery because they may become fearful of giving others decision-making responsibility for insulin adjustment

8 On discharge from a hospital, patients with diabetes need:

A Oral instructions on sick-day management of their disease sufficient to avoid medical emergencies

B To be told to contact healthcare providers only at certain times of the day so that proper attention can be given to their condition

C Not be given any instructions on discharge since they will be too overwhelmed by all the procedures to grasp the meaning

D Survival skills that include written instructions on sick-day management

9 When patients with diabetes are too sick to eat or tolerate large volumes of fluids, they are advised to consume something that contains 15 g of carbohydrate every 1 to 2 hours. An example of this would be:

A Milk shake (1/3 cup lowfat milk and 1/4 cup vanilla ice cream)

B 1 can diet Coca Cola®

C ½ cup of sugar-free Jell-O®

D 2 double-stick Popsicles®

10 Elevation of epinephrine secretion in a patient with diabetes who is under stress causes:

A Hyperglycemia from increased biosynthesis of glucose by the liver from non-carbohydrates such as alanine

B Hypoglycemia because of increased uptake of glucose by the muscles

C Hyperglycemia from increased glycogenolysis by the liver

D Hyperglycemia from increased glycogenolysis by the muscles

CONTINUING EDUCATION POST-TEST QUESTIONS

Skin, Foot and Dental Care 16

1 Which of the following factors is the most important in maintaining skin integrity in a person with diabetes?
   A Avoid exposure to sun
   B Maintain blood glucose levels within target ranges
   C Wear only white socks with closed toed shoes
   D Use oil-based creams to prevent dry, flaky skin

2 In addition to elevated blood glucose levels, a reason that people with diabetes may be at increased risk for infection is:
   A Impaired circulation
   B Excessive perspiration
   C Anhidrosis
   D Overuse of oil-based lotions

3 Common pathogens causing skin infections in people with diabetes include all except:
   A Beta-hemolytic streptococci
   B Fungus
   C Haemophilus influenzae type b
   D Staphylococci

4 A characteristic of foot ulceration is that it:
   A Causes irreversible damage to the foot
   B Usually involves joint spaces and bone
   C Is usually caused by minor, repetitive pressure
   D May not be preventable in persons with long standing diabetes

5 The best indicator of peripheral sensory neuropathy is:
   A Intermittent claudication
   B Inability to perceive the 5.07 monofilament
   C Callus over the metatarsal heads
   D Maceration between the toes

6 A sign of peripheral vascular disease is:
   A Cracked, reddened, flaky skin
   B Venous filling time greater than 20 seconds
   C Palpable pedal pulses
   D Prominent metatarsal heads

7 All of the following should be included in every diabetic foot risk screening examination except:
   A History of foot ulceration or amputation
   B History of vascular disease
   C Frequency of hypoglycemia
   D Changes in foot shape

Please answer the remaining questions based upon the following case scenario.

BG was diagnosed with type 2 diabetes 15 years ago. At the time of diagnosis he was told he had "a little sugar and not to worry about it". He has recently retired and seeks your assistance after noting a painless, non-healing sore on his right heel.

8 BG's right heel demonstrates significant erythema, edema, warmth, fluctuance and moderate foul drainage. Initial treatment should include all except:
   A Optimal blood glucose control
   B Duplex doppler studies
   C Deep tissue culture
   D Oral antibiotics

9 Venous filling time as a measure of vascular disease is normal if:
   A ≤ 40 seconds
   B ≥ 40 seconds
   C ≤ 20 seconds
   D ≥ 20 seconds

10 The most effective treatment for peripheral vascular disease resulting from arteriosclerosis is:
    A A low-fat diet
    B Angioplasty
    C Cessation of smoking
    D Diuretics to reduce edema

11 Instruct patients with dry, cracked skin
on their feet to:

   A Smooth skin with a pumice stone

   B Soak feet in warm water daily for
10-15 minutes

   C Apply powder or cornstarch after
bathing

   D Apply an emollient between the toes
after washing the feet

CONTINUING EDUCATION POST-TEST QUESTIONS

Childhood and Adolescence   17

1 A 14 year-old boy with type 1 diabetes plays soccer 2 days a week after school. Which of the following actions could he take to avoid possible delayed hypoglycemia?
   A Reduce his AM NPH insulin by 2 units
   B Reduce his PM NPH insulin by 2 units
   C Eat additional carbohydrates at lunch
   D Eat additional food at his bedtime snack

2 A 3 year-old with type 1 diabetes will not eat his evening meal. Which of the following would be the most appropriate action to take?
   A Save the food and re-offer it in 30 minutes
   B Substitute milk or juice for CHO foods
   C Check blood glucose; give simple CHO only if blood glucose is below 90 mg/dL
   D Reward the child with sweets if he eats well

3 Which of the following is appropriate when treating hypoglycemia in an infant with diabetes?
   A 4 oz undiluted baby fruit juice
   B 1 large tube of glucose gel
   C 5 tsp Karo syrup
   D ½ can regular soda

4 A 4 year-old with diabetes is resisting his insulin injections. Which of the following strategies would be the most appropriate in this situation?
   A Have the child learn to give his own insulin injections under parental supervision
   B Reward the child if he cooperates at injection times
   C Utilize play therapy to act out his injection fears
   D Have the child select his injection sites

5 Which of the following is the most appropriate expectation of an 8 year-old child involving her diabetes care?
   A Have the child perform all glucose testing and insulin injections
   B Share diabetes tasks between parents and the child
   C Have parent only administer insulin without involving the child in site selection
   D Have the child observe the tasks while parents do them

6 Which of the following metabolic changes that occurs during puberty can lead to deterioration of diabetes control?
   A Increased insulin resistance
   B Decreased insulin resistance
   C Decreased epinephrine responses
   D Elevated ketone production

7 A child's ability to manage self-care tasks is best determined by
   A Age and performance in school
   B Availability of self-management education programs
   C Parental approval of self-care tasks
   D Learning readiness and maturity

8 The best indicator that diabetes management in a child is appropriate is:
   A Normal growth and sexual maturation patterns
   B Parental satisfaction with treatment
   C Child's ability to verbalize self-care abilities
   D Child's ability to implement the self-management program

9 Which of the following is consistent with recommended caloric intake for children with diabetes?

   A 20% of the total calories from protein to meet growth requirements

   B 40% of the total calories from carbohydrate to decrease the need for insulin

   C 55% to 60% of total calories from carbohydrate to cover growth and activity needs

   D 15% of total calories from fat to reduce the risk of future cardiovascular complications

10 Emotional and physical stress in an adolescent with diabetes can impact self-care issues. If an adolescent experiences several episodes of DKA, the diabetes educator should suspect:

   A Increased physical activity

   B Manipulation of insulin doses

   C Increased sexual activity

   D Changes in physical maturation or an accelerated growth spurt

CONTINUING EDUCATION POST-TEST QUESTIONS

Pregnancy: Preconception to Postpartum   18

1 Which of the following is not true regarding diabetes and pregnancy?
   A Insulin may be necessary to achieve euglycemia during pregnancy in type 1, 2, and gestational diabetes.
   B Women who develop gestational diabetes during pregnancy need screening for vascular complications.
   C Pregnant women with type 1 or type 2 diabetes are at risk for having a baby with congenital anomalies if they are not in good glycemic control prior to pregnancy.
   D Gestational diabetes is usually diagnosed during the latter part of pregnancy.

2 Which of the following statements is true about preconception care?
   A Spontaneous abortion rates have been found to correlate with glycosylated hemoglobin values during the first trimester.
   B Good preconception glucose control can eliminate the risks for congenital anomalies and spontaneous abortion.
   C Most women in the US with type 1 or type 2 diabetes achieve optimal glycemic control prior to pregnancy.
   D Major malformations occur after the eighth week of gestation.

3 The following metabolic changes are seen during the latter part of pregnancy except:
   A Accelerated starvation characterized by higher concentration of ketones during the fasting state
   B Prolonged postprandial blood glucose that promote fetal growth
   C Transplacental delivery of insulin to the fetus promotes fetal growth
   D Insulin resistance is related to human placental lactogen, prolactin, and cortisol levels

4 Vaginal delivery is contraindicated in the patient who has:
   A A macrosomic infant
   B Gastroparesis
   C Neuropathy
   D Untreated proliferative retinopathy

5 Neonatal complications due to diabetes may occur in both preexisting and gestational diabetics. Which of the following complications is not associated with gestational diabetes?
   A Macrosomia and hyperbilirubinemia
   B Birth defects and small for gestational age
   C Hypoglycemia and hyperbilirubinemia
   D Macrosomia and hypoglycemia

6 Which of the following has been identified as a predictor of poor perinatal outcome?
   A Age of onset of maternal diabetes
   B Duration of maternal diabetes
   C Presence of vascular complications of diabetes
   D Mild nonproliferative retinopathy

7 TS has type 2 diabetes and has been taking metformin for one year. Her glycosylated hemoglobin is within normal range. She is using her meal plan but is still 25 pounds overweight. During preconception care, which of the following is the most likely recommendation?
   A Do not attempt conception until she has lost 25 pounds
   B Discontinue metformin and start patient on insulin
   C Start on prenatal vitamins
   D Discontinue metformin and start patient on glyburide

8 Women with diabetes should seek preconception counseling 3-6 months prior to conception. The main goal of preconception counseling is:

   A To normalize glycosylated hemoglobin levels

   B To start calcium supplementation

   C To add an oral agent to the existing medication regimen

   D To achieve desirable body weight

9 According to the American Diabetes Association, which of the following are desirable blood glucose goals for pregnancy?

   A Fasting 60-105 mg/dL, 1 hour post prandial 100-140 mg/dL

   B Fasting 60-90 mg/dL, 1 hour post prandial 100 - 140 mg/dL

   C Fasting 60-90 mg/dL, 1 hour post prandial 100-120 mg/dL

   D Fasting 70-100 mg/dL, 1 hour post prandial 100-120 mg/dL

10 Which of the following is not true when working with women who have type 1 diabetes and who are breastfeeding?

   A They are at risk for hypoglycemia

   B Their infants are at risk for hyperglycemia

   C Their insulin dosage will need to be adjusted

   D The meal plan during lactation is similar to that of the 3rd trimester

11 According to the recommendations by the Expert Committee on Diagnosis and Classification of Diabetes Mellitus, universal screening for gestational diabetes is still recommended at 24 to 28 weeks gestation for women who meet all of the following high risk criteria:

   A Glycosuria, obese, >25 years of age, first degree relative with diabetes

   B Obese, >25 years of age, member of high risk ethnic group, first degree relative with diabetes

   C Obese, >35 years of age, member of high risk ethnic group, first degree relative with diabetes

   D Glycosuria, >25 years of age, member of high risk ethnic group, first degree relative with diabetes

CONTINUING EDUCATION POST-TEST QUESTIONS

Diabetes and The Life Cycle: Diabetes in the Elderly   19

1   The physiological changes of aging include all of the following except:
    A   Increased GFR
    B   Slower reaction time
    C   Decreased muscle mass and strength
    D   Increased vascular resistance

2   When counseling a 65 year-old man with type 2 diabetes who has never exercised in the past, it would be important to first:
    A   Assess his functional capacity and existing comorbidities
    B   Caution him against participating in strenuous activity
    C   Advise him to join an aerobic class
    D   Advise him to swim for 45 minutes every other day

3   *Failure to thrive* in older people:
    A   Occurs in patients who have one or more changes in functional ability
    B   Occurs in patients who experience recent weight loss
    C   Usually results from a combination of changes in physical and cognitive function
    D   Is seldom related to rates of depression

4   When considering blood glucose monitoring for an older adult, it is important to take into account all of the following except:
    A   Finances
    B   Manual dexterity
    C   Blood glucose goals
    D   Age of patient

5   When providing education to the elderly an appropriate strategy is to:
    A   Be technical and complete
    B   Direct your message only to the individual with diabetes
    C   Be meaningful and practical
    D   Be directed by agency policies and protocols

6   In your teaching with an elderly patient you note markedly poor short term memory. You should do all of the following except:
    A   Reassess mental status after glycemic control is achieved
    B   Provide supplemental sources of information
    C   Limit time for practice
    D   Slow the pace of teaching

7   Hypoglycemia is more problematic in the elderly due to:
    A   Greater sensitivity to glucagon
    B   Resultant fatal cardiovascular events
    C   Greater total body fat
    D   Subsequent rebound hyperglycemia

8   Which of the following statements about the elderly is true?
    A   Depression is uncommon in persons with diabetes
    B   Depression may be masked in the elderly by physical symptoms
    C   Assessment of signs and symptoms of depression should only be done by mental health professionals
    D   Aside from feeling sad, depression has no serious effects

9   All of the following actions are appropriate in reducing the risk of hypoglycemia in the elderly except:
    A   A regular review of signs and symptoms of hypoglycemia
    B   The use of appropriate bedtime snacks to avoid nocturnal hypo-glycemia
    C   Use of blood glucose monitoring
    D   Lowering target blood glucose goals to avoid risk of complications of hypoglycemia

10 One of the most serious complications of type 2 diabetes in the elderly is:
    A   Hyperglycemic Hyperosmolar Nonketotic Syndrome (HHNS)
    B   Diabetic Ketoacidosis (DKA)
    C   Nocturnal hyperglycemia
    D   Cataracts

CONTINUING EDUCATION POST-TEST QUESTIONS

Chronic Complications of Diabetes: An Overview 20

1 Risk factors: (Choose one)
   A Are unique to persons with diabetes and are a significant predictor of the progression of the disease.
   B Can be attributed to a single etiology and are important to the development of diabetic complications.
   C May vary for each complication contributing to a highly variable, individual and complex pattern of disease progression.
   D Affect individuals with diabetes similarly at approximately similar ages and stages of diabetes patho-genesis.

2 Which of the following statements best describes the role of hyperglycemia in the development of complications of diabetes?
   A There is strong evidence that control of hyperglycemia will result in a decrease in cardiovascular events.
   B Improved glycemic control has a marginal impact, if any, on the total cholesterol levels, platelet adherence factors and LDL cholesterol.
   C Elevated blood glucose levels can interfere with nerve membrane func-tioning and nerve transport.
   D Hyperglycemia leads to suppression of the polyol pathway and the for-mation of advanced glycation end products (AGE).

3 When compared to Caucasians with diabetes, African Americans with dia-betes have a lower overall prevalence rate for:
   A Myocardial infarction.
   B Hypertension.
   C Neuropathy.
   D Nephropathy.

4 Patients with elevated homocysteine levels may lower their levels by use of:
   A "Statin" drugs
   B Sulfonylureas
   C Metformin
   D Vitamin B12

5 In addition to the non-modifiable risk factors of duration of diabetes, race, genetics and age, for which of the following complications of diabetes is height and autoimmunity a factor?
   A Cardiovascular complications
   B Neuropathies
   C Nephropathies
   D Retinopathies

6 Adiposity or obesity is a modifiable risk factor for which of the following complications of diabetes?
   A Cardiovascular complications
   B Neuropathies
   C Nephropathies
   D Retinopathies

7 Hyperglycemia can damage the glomerulus by:
   A Causing glycosylation of the proteins of the glomerular tuft.
   B Deactivating the polyol pathway.
   C Increasing protein in urine.
   D Increasing lipid levels in the glomerulus.

8 Studies with hypertensive diabetic patients have demonstrated that:
   A Hypertension is not linked to diabetic neuropathy.
   B Diastolic hypertension is linked more to the development of diabetic neuropathy than systolic hypertension.
   C Systolic hypertension is linked more to the development of diabetic neuropathy than is diastolic hypertension.
   D Treatment with ACE inhibitors is unlikely to change nerve conduction in patients with neuropathies.

9 Diabetic neuropathy may be affected by:
   A The type of medication used in diabetes treatments
   B The type of diabetes
   C Specific diets
   D Alcohol intake

10 Platelet adherence:
   A Is not decreased by improved glucose control.
   B May contribute to plaque formation.
   C Is a non-modifiable risk factor.
   D Principally causes circulatory problems in larger arteries.

CONTINUING EDUCATION POST-TEST QUESTIONS

Eye Disease and Adaptive Diabetes Education for Visually Impaired Persons

21

1   Hard exudates and microaneurysms in the vascular walls are characteristics at what stage of retinopathy?
   A   Mild nonproliferative diabetic retinopathy
   B   Moderate to severe nonproliferative retinopathy
   C   Proliferative retinopathy
   D   Neovascular retinopathy

2   For a person with visual impairment to be categorized as legally blind, he or she would have to have:
   A   A visual acuity that is < 20/80 in the better eye with corrective lenses and/or a visual field of < 40 degrees.
   B   A visual acuity that is < 20/160 in the better eye with corrective lenses and/or a visual field of < 30 degrees.
   C   A visual acuity that is < 20/200 in the better eye with corrective lenses and/or a visual field < 20 degrees.
   D   The level of disability in which the individual has no light perception.

3   Which type of activity should not be recommended to a patient with active diabetic retinopathy?
   A   Jogging
   B   Warm ups
   C   Walking
   D   Modified Stretching

4   MB, a newly diagnosed patient with type 2 diabetes, needs referral for a routine ophthalmologic screening and follow-up:
   A   Annually, beginning at the time diabetes is diagnosed
   B   Semiannually, beginning 2 years after the time that diabetes was diagnosed
   C   Every 4 to 6 months, beginning 5 years after the time that diabetes was diagnosed
   D   Wait until visual changes occur and then begin to schedule semi-annually

5   The most common form of glaucoma seen in people with diabetes is:
   A   Angle-closure glaucoma
   B   Lenticular glaucoma
   C   Open-angled glaucoma
   D   Neo-vascular glaucoma

6   Treatment of mild-to-moderate retinopathy includes all of the following except:
   A   Normalizing blood glucose levels
   B   Monitoring blood pressure
   C   Smoking cessation
   D   In-office laser treatments

7   TC, a 52 year-old blind woman with diabetes is being taught to calculate and plan for the number of days a vial of insulin will last. TC uses a total of 35 units of NPH insulin each day. How many syringes should she use before starting a new vial and setting aside a new batch of syringes?
   A   25
   B   27
   C   29
   D   31

8   Which method of insulin administration does not assist the patient with visual impairment to control the insertion of the needle into the skin?
   A   Pinch the skin at the selected spot and then place the needle on the skin and insert
   B   Select the site and then use a dart like motion to inject the needle into the skin
   C   Use of an automatic needle injector
   D   Use of a pen injector

9 A diabetes educator is teaching a blind patient to monitor his/her own blood glucose levels. Which is not an appropriate method for determining if there is adequate blood to apply to the reagent strip?

    A Use a meter with a feature that checks that an adequate blood drop has been applied.

    B Teach patients to touch the puncture site with another finger to feel for wetness.

    C Teach patients to touch the reagent strip with the edge of the needle tip.

    D Teach patients to lightly touch the side of their lips to check for wetness.

10 Temporary visual changes such as bright flashing lights or double vision may be symptomatic of:

    A Hyperglycemia

    B Ketosis

    C Hypoglycemia

    D Macular edema

CONTINUING EDUCATION POST-TEST QUESTIONS

Neuropathy   22

1   Diabetic neuropathy is described as
    a condition:
    A Which affects the peripheral and
       central nervous systems
       almost equally
    B With a narrowly defined range of
       manifestations
    C Which results from the interaction
       of multiple metabolic, genetic,
       environmental factors
    D That is not generally painful but is
       self-limiting in nature

2   The most common pathological lesion
    in diabetic neuropathy is:
    A Excitation of postsynaptic
       membranes
    B Demyelinization and atrophy of
       peripheral nerve axons
    C Loss of active transport mechanisms
       of neurotransmitters
    D Loss of white matter within the
       central nervous system

3   The prevalence of subclinical signs and
    clinical symptoms of neuropathy in
    diabetes appear to be strongly
    correlated with:
    A The degree of pain and numbness
       experienced by patient
    B Number of episodes of symptomatic
       hypoglycemia
    C Duration of the disease
    D Type of medication used to achieve
       glycemic control

4   A characteristic that distinguishes the
    focal neuropathies from the diffuse
    polyneuropathies is
    A Focal neuropathies are associated
       with higher rates of morbidity and
       mortality
    B Diffuse polyneuropathies
       are asymmetrical
    C Focal neuropathies are acute in onset
       and self-limiting in nature
    D Diffuse polyneuropathies are limited
       to autonomic impairment only

5   Teach patients with peripheral
    neuropathy that improved glycemic
    control may:
    A Improve long term prognosis
       but cause increased discomfort
       temporarily
    B Have no long term effect but
       temporarily increase discomfort
    C Improve long term prognosis and
       result in rapid relief of symptoms
    D Have no long term effect but result
       in rapid relief of symptoms

6   The most common mononeuropathy is
    involvement of the:
    A Medial nerve leading to carpal
       tunnel syndrome
    B Peroneal nerve leading to foot drop
    C Radial nerve leading to wrist drop
    D Ulnar nerve leading to weakness and
       paresthesia of the lateral fingers

7   Treatment for orthostatic hypotension
    related to diabetic autonomic
    neuropathy with cardiovascular
    involvement includes all of the
    following except:
    A Increased salt intake
    B Use of supportive elastic
       body stockings
    C Improved glycemic control
    D Raise head of bed to a 60% angle

8   MH is a 45 year-old female who has
    had type 1 diabetes for 25 years. She
    takes her insulin regularly but does not
    do SMBG. Concerned about several
    recent episodes of hypoglycemia, her
    provider recently reevaluated her med-
    ication and self-care and found them to
    be adequate. Lab tests were
    unremarkable. What would be the
    most likely cause of her hypoglycemia?
    A Autoimmune response to the insulin
    B Development of gastroparesis with
       delayed gastric emptying
    C Inappropriate glucagon response
    D Changes in renal clearance of insulin

9 Diabetic neuropathy includes all of the following except:

    A Acute nerve fiber abnormalities

    B Chronic nerve fiber injury or loss

    C Atrophy of longer peripheral nerve axons

    D Central nervous system impairment due to macrovascular dysfunction

10 LM is a 55 year-old female with type 2 diabetes who was recently diagnosed with a neurogenic bladder. Which of the following interventions would be most helpful to her at this stage:

    A Teach her the Crede method

    B Encourage an aerobic exercise program to promote circulation

    C Instruct her on the signs and symptoms of urinary tract infections

    D Teach her self-catheterization

11 LM is least likely to experience dysfunction or disruption of:

    A Efferent autonomic fibers signaling bladder fullness

    B Efferent sympathetic fibers responsible for maintaining sphincter tone

    C Efferent parasympathetic fibers promoting bladder contraction

    D Motor function signaling release of urine

12 JH complains of altered sensations and impaired feeling. Which test would you expect to be ordered to determine nerve conduction velocity?

    A Electrodiagnostic test (EDX)

    B Quantitative sensory testing (QST)

    C Autonomic function test (AFT)

    D Transcutaneous nerve stimulation (TENS)

13 The most accurate statement about gastroparesis associated with autonomic neuropathy and gastrointestinal dysfunction is that it:

    A Involvement is to the stomach.

    B Is easily detected because of occurrence of overt signs and symptoms.

    C Is treated with a high-protein/high-fiber diet to stimulate motility.

    D Requires frequent monitoring of pre- and postprandial blood glucose levels.

CONTINUING EDUCATION POST-TEST QUESTIONS

Nephropathy 23

1 Which of the following statements is most accurate about diabetic nephropathy?

A Both persons with type 1 and type 2 diabetes can expect to experience some symptoms and complications of nephropathy.

B Persons with microalbuminuria and proteinuria usually have some retinopathy.

C Persons with diabetes experience the same frequency of kidney dysfunction as individuals who do not have diabetes.

D Symptoms of nephropathy usually occur 2 to 3 years after diagnosis is first made.

2 The functions of the kidney include:

A The removal of water, urea, iron and protein from the body

B The maintenance of blood volume and formation of 1,25 vitamin D

C The conservation of potassium and excretion of sodium

D The inhibition of erythropoietin production

3 Structural changes characteristic of nephropathy include:

A Basement membrane thickening which precedes mesangial expansion

B The presence of microalbuminuria, indicating that the nephrons have closed

C Hypertrophy of the nephrons, which usually occurs in the second decade after diagnosis

D Elevated blood pressure in 70% of individuals at the time of diagnosis

4 Which of the following is not true?

A Diabetes accounts for more than 35% of new cases of ESRD.

B In the person with diabetes over 45, the incidence of ESRD has increased twelve-fold.

C The incidence of ESRD in Hispanics and Native Americans is six times higher than Caucasians with diabetes.

D The development of ESRD in African-Americans with diabetes is approximately equal to that occurring in Caucasians with diabetes.

5 The stage of renal disease at which microalbuminuria first appears is:

A Functional changes

B Structural change

C Incipient nephropathy

D Overt nephropathy

6 At which stage of kidney involvement has improved glycemic control been shown to restore alterations in function?

A Functional changes

B Structural changes

C Incipient nephropathy

D Overt nephropathy

7 What effect does declining renal function have on insulin catabolism?

A Increased insulin catabolism prolongs insulin availability resulting in hypoglycemia.

B Increased insulin catabolism decreases availability of insulin resulting in hyperglycemia.

C Decreased insulin catabolism prolongs insulin availability resulting in hypoglycemia.

D Decreased insulin catabolism decreases insulin availability resulting in hyperglycemia.

8 Risk factors for diabetic nephropathy include all of the following except:

A Hypertension

B Hyperglycemia

C Low-protein diet

D Genetic predisposition

9 SW is having a creatinine clearance test. You explain to her that this is a test that involves:

    A The collection of all urine for 24 hours

    B A urine specimen treated with dye and its clearance timed

    C A blood specimen used to measure her creatinine.

    D Urine collected for a 4-hour period

10 Which strategy would be best to consider when evaluating treatment options for ESRD?

    A Begin to plan treatment when serum creatinine reaches 1.8 mg/dL.

    B Discuss only the treatment option the healthcare team believes is best for the person.

    C Suggest patient meet others who are experiencing the treatment modalities being considered.

    D Recommend that patients with cardiovascular disease not consider renal transplantation.

11 GA is a 75 year-old man who has had diabetes for 25 years. He has glaucoma, is blind in the left eye, and has limited mobility. He has requested no renal replacement for his ESRD. In your discussion with him, which of the following would you not include?

    A No renal replacement for ESRD is an option but it will result in death

    B This decision must be made when he is in a non-uremic state

    C His wife, children and grandchildren should be his reason to live and choose treatments that keep him alive

    D Resources are available to him and his family if he decides on no renal replacement

12 Which of the following are not manifestations of renal failure in diabetes?

    A Weight gain, pedal edema, shortness of breath

    B Hiccups, nausea and vomiting

    C Skeletal fractures, changes in concentration, muscle cramping

    D Diaphoresis, shaking, blurred vision

13 JC is being taught about the prevention renal damage. Important information for her to know would be:

    A Kidney infections should be treated with aminoglycoside drugs.

    B Contrast dyes can be used for diagnostic tests if necessary.

    C If she has symptoms of a urinary tract infection, she should push fluids and call her provider after 2 to 3 days if symptoms persist.

    D She should empty her bladder after sexual intercourse.

14 The laboratory test indicating first evidence of kidney damage is:

    A Serum creatine levels over 2mg/dL on two occasions

    B Blood urea nitrogen over 20 mg/dL on more than one occasion

    C Protein excretion ≥ 3.6 g/ 24 hours

    D Albumin excretion rate of 30 to 300 mg/day on three different occasions

15 A limitation of renal transplant surgery as a treatment option for nephropathy is:

    A The new kidney will function effectively for a limited time only

    B The patient must use immunosuppressive drugs for the remainder of his/her life

    C Patient will still need to follow a restricted diet to avoid damaging the new kidney

    D Blood glucose levels are not likely to change or will improve only slightly following surgery

16 An effective approach for the diabetes educator in dealing with the psychosocial issues associated with end-stage renal disease is:

    A Reassure the patient it is not his or her fault

    B Assess on an on-going basis the patient's ability to cope with loss and handle complex treatments

    C Use scare tactics only when other attempts to get patient's attention fail

    D Recommend support groups only when patient seems motivated to succeed

CONTINUING EDUCATION POST-TEST QUESTIONS

Macrovascular Disease   24

1   Fifty to sixty percent of all deaths in persons with diabetes can be attributed to:
    A Microvascular disease
    B Coronary artery disease
    C Peripheral vascular disease
    D Cerebral vascular disease

2   What impact does diabetes have on the development of coronary artery disease for women compared to men?
    A Women have a higher risk than men
    B Men have a higher risk than women
    C The risk is minimal in both sexes
    D The risk is the same for both sexes

3   Which of the following is not a usual symptom of acute coronary insufficiency?
    A Angina
    B Sweating
    C Diaphoresis
    D Anxiety

4   Improved glycemic control does which of the following:
    A Decreases triglycerides and increases HDL
    B Increases plasma fibrinogen levels
    C Increases HDL levels independent of changes in lipid levels
    D Has little effect on platelet behavior

5   The presence of hypertension in persons with type 1 diabetes is correlated with:
    A Weight and insulin resistance
    B Duration of diabetes and renal function
    C Low HDL levels and physical inactivity
    D Presence of AGEs and elevated glucose levels

6   Which of the following medications should be used with caution when treating hypertension in persons with diabetes?
    A Beta blockers
    B Angiotensin-converting enzyme inhibitors
    C Statins
    D Aspirin therapy

7   Which of the following statements is the least accurate about peripheral vascular disease (PVD)?
    A Absent peripheral pulses occur with approximately the same frequency in persons with type 1 and type 2 diabetes.
    B Patient education efforts should emphasize foot care.
    C People with diabetes have a 15 times higher age-related risk for amputation.
    D PVD is clinically characterized by intermittent claudication and foot ulcers.

8   The elements that commonly characterize Syndrome X are:
    A Hyperglycemia, central obesity, neuropathy, and microalbuminuria
    B Hyperglycemia, hyperlipidemia, hypertension, and central obesity
    C Hyperlipidemia, hypertension, and family history of cardiovascular disease
    D Hypoglycemia, neuropathy, hyperinsulinemia, and pregnancy

9   In the development of cardiovascular disease, smoking is associated with:
    A Elevated HDL levels
    B Decreased fibrinogen levels
    C Development of advanced glycosylated end products (AGEs)
    D Formation of stable plaques with a thick fibrous cap

10 JS is a 45 year-old female patient with type 2 diabetes. Her blood pressure is 170/95. She has an elevated LDL cholesterol and an elevated total cholesterol. Her fasting blood sugar is 130mg/dL. What additional information would be most helpful to complete your assessment and develop an intervention strategy for her cardiovascular complications?
    A Food habits
    B Age at time diabetes was first diagnosed
    C Ethnicity and family history of cardiovascular disease
    D Use of anti-hypertensive agents

CONTINUING EDUCATION POST-TEST QUESTIONS

Importance of Research and Outcomes   **25**

1   The scientific method incorporates the procedures used by researchers in the pursuit of new knowledge. The first step of the scientific method is:
   - **A** Developing a theoretical framework
   - **B** Reviewing the related literature
   - **C** Formulating a research problem and purpose
   - **D** Formulating research objectives, questions, and hypotheses

2   A research approach to acquire knowledge that describes life experiences is classified as:
   - **A** Quantitative
   - **B** Qualitative
   - **C** Experimental
   - **D** Quasi-experimental

3   Triangulation refers to the process of:
   - **A** Reaching agreement among members of a research team
   - **B** Collecting data using more than one research approach
   - **C** Abstracting themes into theoretical constructs
   - **D** Examining problems to gain knowledge about improving healthcare

4   Research uses a systematic approach to explain or predict phenomena. The research process itself may best be characterized as a:
   - **A** Random manner of assigning people to various groups to prove a hypothesis
   - **B** Set of steps carried out in prescribed order as part of the research design
   - **C** Set of regulations which must always be followed in the implementation phase
   - **D** Flexible and circular planning and decision-making process

5   A problem statement includes all of the following except:
   - **A** Justification for the study
   - **B** Population
   - **C** Statement of need
   - **D** Design

6   Abstracts of research reports include information about all of the following except:
   - **A** Purpose and importance of study
   - **B** Description of methods
   - **C** Overall project costs
   - **D** Highlights of data analysis

Consider the following hypothesis:

"Patients with type 2 diabetes who receive instruction on an individual basis will be more compliant than those who receive instruction in a group setting."

7   What is the dependent variable in the hypothesis above?
   - **A** Type 2 diabetes mellitus
   - **B** Individual vs. group setting
   - **C** Type of instruction undergone
   - **D** Patient compliance

8   What is the independent variable?
   - **A** Type 2 diabetes mellitus
   - **B** Individual vs. group setting
   - **C** Content of instruction undergone
   - **D** Patient compliance

9   Where in the research report would you expect to find the following statement, "The study was conducted within the Grady Health Systems, a public health-care facility serving two urban counties in Atlanta."
   - **A** Introduction
   - **B** Methods
   - **C** Results
   - **D** Conclusions

10   Where in the research report would you expect to find the following statement, "The purpose of this study was to examine the relationship between caregiving burden and social support in spouses of individuals with type 1 diabetes."
   - **A** Introduction
   - **B** Methods
   - **C** Results
   - **D** Conclusions

11 In choosing a quasi-experimental design over a true experimental design, the researcher realizes that the study would involve less:
   A Bias
   B Control
   C Rigor
   D Significance

12 A correlational study identifies:
   A Relationships among variables
   B Causal link between an independent variable and an outcome
   C Difference between an independent and dependent variable
   D The effect of one variable on another

13 In order to execute research responsibilities, the diabetes educator will need to use
   A Patient health outcomes as performance measures
   B Staff satisfaction with methods employed
   C Patient reports of satisfaction with treatment
   D Records showing the patient's commitment to continuing the tested treatment

14 Choosing a validated instrument as an outcome measure provides:
   A Confidence in the results
   B Reliable results regardless of when the instrument is administered
   C A biased sampling of the target population
   D Qualitative research data

15 The purpose of an operational definition is to:
   A Assign numerical values to investigational variables
   B Specify how variables will be explained and measured
   C Stipulate expected relationship between the variables
   D Designate the overall plan which drives the research

INDEX

THIRD EDITION ERRATA

Corrections are shown in italics.

PAGE 191

TABLE 8.1. RECOMMENDED LIPID VALUES FOR ADULTS[3,7]

	Cholesterol Levels Levels	LDL-Cholesterol Levels	HDL-Cholesterol Levels
Acceptable	≤200 mg/dL (5.17 mmol/L)	<100 mg/dL (2.59 mmol/L)	≥45 mg/dL (1.17 mmol/L)
Borderline	200-239 mg/dL (5.17-6.18 mmol/L)	100-129 mg/dL (2.59-3.34 mmol/L)	35-45 mg/dL (0.9-1.17 mmol/L)
High	≥240 mg/dL (6.20 mmol/L)	≥130 mg/dL (3.36 mmol/L)	<35 mg/dL (0.9 mmol/L)
Adults with preexisting cardiovascular disease (CVD)		*≤100 mg/dL (2.59 mmol/L)*	

PAGE 305

6 Velosulin® Human BR insulin is usually recommended for insulin pump use because it contains phosphate buffers that may minimize crystallization or aggregation of insulin in the infusion tubing. *The chemical and pharmacokinetic properties of lispro insulin suggest that it would be an efficacious choice for insulin pump use; however, product labeling does not currently reflect this indication.*

PAGE 373 (first bullet)

• Patents with type 1 diabetes who are restricting calories to lose weight require decreased dosages of insulin to prevent hypoglycemia. Too much of a reduction of insulin will result in *hyperglycemia*, ketonuria and, if not corrected, metabolic decompensation to ketoacidosis.

PAGE 429

FIGURE 13.3. SAMPLE APPROACH FOR LOW-DOSE INSULIN INFUSION FOR DKA

7 Subcutaneous insulin may be started when the patient is able to eat. Administer four to *10 units* short-acting insulin before stopping the insulin infusion to maintain blood glucose in a safe range.

PAGE 488

1A These patients may respond metabolically like type 1 patients so the treatment *approach* is the same.

PAGE 489

2 Patients whose diabetes is well controlled with medical nutrition therapy (MNT) or MNT-plus-oral antidiabetes agents do not require specific therapy. Patients with fasting blood glucose levels lower than 140 mg/dL (7.8 mmol/L) treated with an oral agent can be given their medication and started on a glucose infusion the morning of surgery; however, it is sometimes suggested to stop the oral agent the evening before surgery. Discontinue the longer-acting chlorpropamide 48 to 72 hours prior to the surgical procedure.

PAGE 591, MISSING TABLE

TABLE 18.7. ADA RECOMMENDED CALORIC INTAKE DURING PREGNANCY FOR WOMEN WITH DIABETES

Current Body Weight	Caloric Intake, Kcal/kgBW/d
<90% desirable weight	36-40
At desirable weight	30
120% to 150% desirable weight	24
>150% desirable weight	18

PAGE 754 (D, second bullet)

• Without intervention, GFR declines at the rate of *25-30 mL/min/month*.

POST-TEST QUESTIONS

CHAPTER 2—TEACHING PATIENTS WITH LOW LITERACY SKILLS

7 You are working with BT, a 60 year-old patient with newly-diagnosed diabetes and low literacy skills. Which strategy would be *not be* appropriate in the planning, implementation and evaluation of instruction?

A Use only short term learning objectives and limit the number

B Use audiovisual teaching aids to cover all major conceptual points

C Repeat major points during the instruction process

D Use written test to evaluate learning

CHAPTER 4—PSYCHOSOCIAL ASSESSMENT

8 A stated intention to *change* behavior *made* by a person who has diabetes is:

A A poor predictor of behaviors

B More likely to occur if it involves self-management behaviors

C More likely to result in positive outcomes if achieved within 6 to 12 weeks

D *More likely to occur if it involves lifestyle changes*

CHAPTER 8—NUTRITION

4 Insulin affects the use and storage of nutrients in each of the following ways except:

A Facilitates cellular transport

B Promotes lipolysis by inactivating lipoprotein lipase

C Stimulates glycogen synthesis

D *Suppresses* gluconeogenesis (glucose production by the liver)

CHAPTER 9—EXERCISE

9 Which exercise routine is most appropriate for an elderly patient with a degenerative joint disease?

A No exercise at all

B Aerobic exercise only

C Anaerobic exercise only

D Alternating aerobic and *strength training* exercise

CHAPTER 10—PHARMACOLOGIC THERAPIES

7 The most *acutely* dangerous complication of sulfonylurea therapy is:

A Weight gain

B Skin rashes

C Gastrointestinal disturbance

D Hypoglycemia

CHAPTER 16—SKIN, FOOT, AND DENTAL CARE

11 Instruct patients with dry, cracked skin on their feet to:

A Smooth skin with a pumice stone

B Soak feet in warm water daily for 10-15 minutes

C Apply powder or cornstarch after bathing

D Apply an emollient, *except* between the toes after washing the feet

CHAPTER 22—NEUROPATHY

5 Teach patients with peripheral neuropathy that improved glycemic control may:

A Improve long term *effects* but cause increased discomfort temporarily

B Have no long term effect but temporarily increase discomfort

C Improve long term prognosis and result in rapid relief of symptoms

D Have no long term effect but result in rapid relief of symptoms

6 The most common mononeuropathy is involvement of the:

A *Median* nerve leading to carpal tunnel syndrome

B Peroneal nerve leading to foot drop

C Radial nerve leading to wrist drop

D Ulnar nerve leading to weakness and paresthesia of the lateral fingers

13 The most accurate statement about gastroparesis associated with autonomic neuropathy and gastrointestinal dysfunction is that:

A Involvement is *limited* to the stomach.

B Is easily detected because of occurrence of overt signs and symptoms.

C Is treated with a high-protein/high-fiber diet to stimulate motility.

D It requires frequent monitoring of pre- and postprandial blood glucose levels.